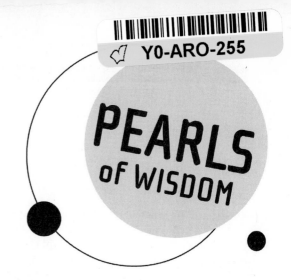

PEARLS of WISDOM

Plastic and Reconstructive Surgery
BOARD REVIEW

Samuel J. Lin, M.D.
John B. Hijjawi, M.D.

McGraw-Hill
Medical Publishing Division

New York Chicago San Francisco Lisbon London
Madrid Mexico City Milan New Delhi
San Juan Seoul Singapore
Sydney Toronto

Plastic and Reconstructive Surgery Board Review

1 2 3 4 5 6 7 8 9 0   CUS/CUS   0 9 8 7 6 5

ISBN 0-07-146447-6

Notice

Medicine is an ever-changing science. As new research and clinical experience broaden our knowledge, changes in treatment and drug therapy are required. The authors and the publisher of this work have checked with sources believed to be reliable in their efforts to provide information that is complete and generally in accord with the standards accepted at the time of publication. However, in view of the possibility of human error or changes in medical sciences, neither the authors nor the publisher nor any other party who has been involved in the preparation or publication of this work warrants that the information contained herein is in every respect accurate or complete, and they disclaim all responsibility for any errors or omissions or for the results obtained from use of the information contained in this work. Readers are encouraged to confirm the information contained herein with other sources. For example and in particular, readers are advised to check the product information sheet included in the package of each drug they plan to administer to be certain that the information contained in this work is accurate and that changes have not been made in the recommended dose or in the contraindications for administration. This recommendation is of particular importance in connection with new or infrequently used drugs.

The editors were Catherine A. Johnson and Marsha Loeb.
The production supervisor was Phil Galea.
The cover designer was Handel Low.
Von Hoffmann Graphics was printer and binder.

This book is printed on acid-free paper.

Cataloging-in-Publication data for this title is on file at the Library of Congress.

DEDICATION

To my parents, S.C. and Anne, and my wife Valerie
For all the love and support you have given me.

Sam

To my mother Amal,
For giving me big dreams to dream and the constant
love to reach them.

To my wife Sarha,
For your love, support and confidence.

John

ACKNOWLEDGMENTS

Special thanks to Vanessa Ho, M.D. for help with editing and production of the book

and

Many thanks to Scott H. Plantz, M.D. and Terri Lair for this wonderful opportunity

EDITORS IN CHIEF:

Samuel J. Lin, M.D.
Chief Resident
Division of Plastic and Reconstructive Surgery, Department of Surgery
Northwestern University Feinberg
School of Medicine
Chicago, IL

John B. Hijjawi, M.D.
Assistant Professor of Surgery
Department of Plastic Surgery
Medical College of Wisconsin
Milwaukee, WI

CONTRIBUTING AUTHORS:

Cori Agarwal, M.D.
Private Practice
Plastic Surgery
Merrillville, IN

Jayant Agarwal, M.D.
Resident Physician
Division of Plastic Surgery
Department of Surgery
University of Chicago
Chicago, IL

Ali Al-Attar, M.D.
Resident Physician
Department of Plastic Surgery
Georgetown University Medical Center
Washington, D.C.

Alexander Anzarut, M.D., MSc
Division of Plastic and Reconstructive Surgery
University of Alberta
Edmonton, Alberta, Canada

Jugpal S. Arneja, M.D.
Fellow, Pediatric Plastic Surgery
Department of Plastic Surgery
Medical College of Wisconsin
Milwaukee, WI

George Athwal, M.D., FRCSC
Assistant Professor of Surgery
Hand and Upper Limb Centre
University of Western Ontario
London, Ontario, Canada

Cesar Bravo, M.D.
Special Fellow, Hand and Microsurgery
Division of Hand Surgery
Department of Orthopedic Surgery
Mayo Clinic and Foundation
Rochester, MN

Reuben A. Bueno, Jr., M.D.
Staff Plastic Surgeon
Children's Mercy Hospital
Kansas City, MO

Gregory M. Buncke M.D.
Attending Plastic Surgeon
The Buncke Clinic
San Francisco, CA

Rudolf F. Buntic M.D.
Attending Plastic Surgeon
The Buncke Clinic
San Francisco, CA

Laurie Casas, M.D.
Attending Plastic Surgeon
Northwestern University Feinberg
School of Medicine
Chicago, IL

Rakesh K. Chandra, M.D.
Assistant Professor
Department of Otolaryngology-Head &
Neck Surgery
University of Tennessee Health Science Center
Memphis, TN

Ming-Huei Cheng, M.D.
Assistant Professor
Department of Plastic Surgery
Chang-Gung Memorial Hospital
Taipei, Taiwan

Mark A. Codner, M.D., FACS
Assistant Professor of Surgery
Emory University School of Medicine
PACES Plastic Surgery
Atlanta, GA

Alvin Cohn, M.D.
Resident Physician
Division of Plastic Surgery
Department of Surgery
University of Chicago

Stephen H. Colbert, M.D.
Chief Resident
Division of Plastic and Reconstructive Surgery
University of Missouri at Columbia
Columbia, MO

Matthew J. Concannon, M.D., FACS
Associate Professor, Director, Hand and
Microsurgery
Division of Plastic and Reconstructive Surgery
University of Missouri at Columbia
Columbia, MO

Julia Corcoran, M.D.
Attending Physician
Division of Pediatric Plastic Surgery
Children's Memorial Hospital
Chicago, IL

Dimitrios Danikas, M.D.
Division of Plastic Surgery
New York Presbyterian Hospital/Weill Medical
College of Cornell University
New York, NY

Wellington Davis III, M.D.
Fellow
Division of Plastic and Reconstructive Surgery
Loyola University Stritch School of Medicine
Chicago, IL

Mary Talley Dorn, M.D.
Department of Otolaryngology
University of Texas Medical Branch
Galveston, TX

Benjamin Eskra, M.D.
Private Practice, Plastic Surgery
Wyomissing, PA

Jules A. Feledy, M.D.
Clinical Specialist
Department of Plastic and
Reconstructive Surgery
MD Anderson Cancer Center
Houston, TX

Julius W. Few, M.D.
Assistant Professor of Surgery
Division of Plastic Surgery
Northwestern University Feinberg
School of Medicine
Chicago, IL

Robert E. H. Ferguson, Jr., M.D.
Resident Physician
Division of Plastic and Reconstructive Surgery
University of Kentucky
Lexington, KY

Christine Fisher
Division of Plastic Surgery
University of Texas Medical Branch-Galveston
Galveston, TX

Christopher Forrest, M.D., MSc, FRCS(C), FACS
Head, Division of Plastic Surgery
Hospital for Sick Children
Assistant Professor, Division of Plastic Surgery,
Department of Surgery
University of Toronto
Toronto, Canada

Jeffrey B. Friedrich, M.D.
Division of Plastic and Reconstructive Surgery
University of Washington
Seattle, WA

Viki Fripp, M.D.
Fellow
Plastic and Reconstructive Surgery
New York Presbyterian Hospital
New York, NY

Alberto S. Gallerani, M.D.
Chief of Plastic and Reconstructive Surgery, Chief of
Tissue Engineering
Medici Institute For Plastic Surgery
Miami, FL

Lloyd B. Gayle, M.D.
Division of Plastic Surgery
New York Presbyterian Hospital/Weill Medical
College of Cornell University
New York, NY

Brian S. Glatt, M.D.
Fellow, Plastic and Reconstructive Surgery
Memorial Sloan-Kettering Cancer Center
New York, NY

Arun K. Gosain, M.D.
Attending Plastic Surgeon
Department of Plastic Surgery
Medical College of Wisconsin
Milwaukee, WI

Karol Gutowski, M.D.
Attending Plastic Surgeon
Division of Plastic and Reconstructive Surgery
University of Wisconsin
Madison, WI

Matthew M. Hanasono, M.D.
Assistant Professor of Surgery
Department of Plastic Surgery
M.D. Anderson Cancer Center
Houston, TX

Scott Hansen, M.D.
Assistant Professor of Surgery
Plastic and Reconstructive Surgery
University of California at San Francisco
San Francisco, CA

Steven L. Henry, M.D.
Resident Physician
Division of Plastic Surgery
University of Missouri Hospital and Clinics
Columbia, MO

Daron C. Hitt, M.D.
Assistant Professor
Division of Plastic and Reconstructive Surgery
East Carolina University Brody School of Medicine
Greenville, North Carolina

Karen Horton, M.D., MSc, BScH
Senior Clinical Microsurgery Fellow
The Buncke Clinic
San Francisco, CA

Lawrence Iteld, M.D.
Assistant Professor of Surgery
University of Miami
Miami, FL

Abdulaziz Jarman, MB.BS, FRCSC
Division of Plastic and Reconstructive Surgery
University of Alberta
Edmonton, Alberta, Canada

Craig Johnson, M.D.
Chairman
Division of Plastic and Reconstructive Surgery
Surgery, Department of Surgery
Mayo Clinic and Foundation
Rochester, MN

Ajaipal S. Kang, M.D.
Attending Physician
Department of Plastic Surgery
Division of Surgery
Hamot Medical Center
Erie, PA

Mark W. Kiehn, M.D.
Assistant Professor of Surgery
Division of Plastic Surgery
University of Wisconsin
Madison, WI

Thomas A. Knipe, M.D.
Resident Physician
Department of Otolaryngology-Head & Neck
Surgery
University of Tennessee Health Science Center
Memphis, TN

Anthony Labruna, M.D.
Division of Plastic Surgery
Weill Medical College of Cornell University
New York, NY

Charles K. Lee, M.D.
Attending Plastic Surgeon
The Buncke Clinic
San Francisco, CA

Clinton McCord, M.D.
Assistant Professor of Surgery
Emory University School of Medicine
PACES Plastic Surgery
Atlanta, GA

Cay Mierisch, M.D.
Special Fellow, Hand and Microsurgery
Division of Hand Surgery
Department of Orthopedic Surgery
Mayo Clinic and Foundation
Rochester, MN

Michael Morhart, MSc, M.D., FRCSC
Division of Plastic and
Reconstructive Surgery
University of Alberta
Edmonton, Alberta, Canada

Arian Mowlavi, M.D.
Cosmetic Surgery Clinics
Laguna Beach, CA

Ananth S. Murthy, M.D.
Fellow, Pediatric Plastic Surgery
Boston Children's Hospital
Harvard Medical School
Boston, MA

Nicole Nemeth, M.D.
Resident Physician
Division of Plastic Surgery
University of Texas Medical Branch-Galveston
Galveston, TX

Robert I. Oliver, Jr., M.D.
Private Practice, Plastic Surgery
Birmingham, AL

Lee Q. Pu, M.D., Ph.D.
Assistant Professor of Surgery
Division of Plastic and Reconstructive Surgery
University of Kentucky
Lexington, KY

C. Lin Puckett, M.D., FACS
Chief, Division of Plastic and Reconstructive Surgery
University of Missouri Health Care
Columbia, MO

Russell Reid, M.D., Ph.D.
Fellow, Pediatric Plastic Surgery
University of Pennsylvania
Philadelphia, PA

Gary Ross, MBChB, MRCS, M.D.
Division of Plastic Surgery
Wythenshawe Hospital
Manchester, United Kingdom

Michel Saint-Cyr, M.D.
Assistant Professor of Surgery
Department of Plastic Surgery
UT Southwestern Medical Center
Dallas, TX

Douglas M. Sammer, M.D.
Resident Physician
Division of Plastic Surgery
University of Michigan Medical School
Ann Arbor, MI

Clark Schierle, M.D., Ph.D.
Resident Physician
Division of Plastic and Reconstructive Surgery
Northwestern University Feinberg
School of Medicine
Chicago, IL

Christiaan Schrag, BSc, M.D., FRCSC
Department of Plastic and Reconstructive Surgery
Chang Gung Memorial Hospital
Taipei, Taiwan

Hisham Seify, M.D.
Oculoplastic Fellow
Division of Plastic Surgery
Emory University School of Medicine
Atlanta, GA

Alex Senchenkov, M.D.
Resident Physician
Division of Plastic and Reconstructive Surgery
Department of Surgery
Mayo Clinic and Foundation
Rochester, MN

Ned Snyder, M.D.
Division of Plastic Surgery
University of Texas Medical Branch-Galveston
Galveston, TX

Mia Talmor, M.D.
Attending Plastic Surgeon
New York Presbyterian Hospital/Weill Medical
College of Cornell University
New York, NY

Hanif Ukani, M.D., FRCSC
Clinical Specialist
Department of Plastic and
Reconstructive Surgery
MD Anderson Cancer Center
Houston, TX

Betul Gozel Ulusal, M.D.
Department of Plastic and
Reconstructive Surgery
Chang Gung Memorial Hospital
Taipei, Taiwan

Fu Chan Wei, M.D.
Chairman
Department of Plastic and
Reconstructive Surgery
Chang Gung Memorial Hospital
Taipei, Taiwan

W. Stites Whatley, M.D.
Chief Resident
Department of Otolaryngology-Head and
Neck Surgery
University of Tennessee Health Science Center
Memphis, TN

Thomas Wiedrich, M.D.
Attending Plastic and Hand Surgeon
Bell Stromberg Chicago Hand Surgery
Division of Plastic and Reconstructive Surgery
Northwestern University
Feinberg School of Medicine
Chicago, IL

INTRODUCTION

Plastic and Reconstructive Surgery Board Review: Pearls of Wisdom is designed to help you prepare for the ABPS Board Examination and the In-service Examination in Plastic and Reconstructive Surgery. This book is one in a series of *Pearls of Wisdom* texts.

We aimed to produce a text that would serve as a study aid for Plastic Surgery residents, fellows, and first year attendings. The book is structured in question and short answer format in order to move through a large body of information. This format will hopefully facilitate reviewing for the standardized examinations and quickly assess strengths and weaknesses in various topics. The question/short answer format will also hopefully allow for fast review before morning rounds, in between cases, and during any other time during the day.

Plastic and Reconstructive Surgery Board Review should be used as a learning tool in conjunction with subject-specific textbooks. Incorporating these facts into a structure of knowledge requires further reading on surrounding concepts.

There may be concepts that are repeated in separate chapters – redundancy is key for recall, and the more variations of a concept that are presented the better in depth the learning.

Plastic and Reconstructive Surgery Board Review does have limitations. We have made great efforts in reviewing, editing, and cross-referencing factual information. However, discrepancies and inaccuracies sometimes occur. Many times this is due to variance between original sources. Keep in mind that some answers may not be the answers you have learned.

Furthermore, new research and practice occasionally deviates from that which likely represents the correct answer for test purposes. Remember, this book is designed to maximize your score on a test. Refer to your most current sources of information and mentors for direction in practice.

Each question is preceded by a hollow bullet. This permits you to check off areas of interest, weakness or simply note that it has been read. This also allows for re-reading without having uncertainty about what was reviewed earlier.

We welcome your comments, suggestions and criticism. Please make us aware of any errors you find. We hope to make continuous improvements and would greatly appreciate any input with regard to format, organization, content, presentation, or about specific questions. We look forward to hearing from you!

Best of luck on the In-Service and the Boards!

S.J.L. and J.B.H.

TABLE OF CONTENTS

HEAD AND NECK REGION

INTEGUMENT

PEDIATRICS

RECONSTRUCTION

STRATEGIES FOR STUDYING

Julia Corcoran, MD, FACS

Outline

Strategies for Studying

1. Take an inventory
2. Plan your attack
3. Set achievable goals
4. Set aside time to study
5. Make your study effective

Study Techniques

1. How do you study
2. How do you learn?
   a. Audio
   b. Reading
   c. "By doing"
      i. Practice multiple choice questions
      ii. Group study
      iii. During your practice

Strategies for Taking Multiple Choice Tests

1. Know the test
2. Answer the question first
3. If you know the answer...
4. If you don't know the answer…
   a. And can limit the options to 2
   b. And don't have a clue
5. Answer as you go

American Board of Plastic Surgery Electronically Administered Tests

1. Will it affect your performance?
2. What will it be like?
   a. Electronically administered.
   b. Window format mock up test
3. Grading
4. Historical Pass/Fail rates

STRATEGIES FOR STUDYING

TAKING AN INVENTORY: What SHOULD I know vs. what DO I know?

High stakes examinations are made from blue prints. Within the American Board of Medical Specialties (ABMS), each specialty board sets forth the content of the specialty's examination in a format which emphasizes the importance of the material and then a test committee then creates questions to fit the blue print. The American Board of Plastic Surgery (ABPS) provides a partial blue print to you. They tell you the topics, but don't tell you the weight of each topic on the examination. The ABPS leaves it to you to intuit how much emphasis they will place on each of the topics outlined.

The partial blue print of the exam available to the test taker (from the ABPS website http://www.abplsurg.org/written_examination_informatio.html)

1. Gross and functional anatomy, and embryology.
2. Basic knowledge of pathology, e.g., the biologic behavior of neoplasms, inflammation, and repair.
3. Basic techniques, wound healing, microsurgery, transplantation.
4. Burns, sepsis, metabolism, trauma, resuscitation, nutrition, endocrinology, shock, hematology.
5. Pre- and postoperative care, anesthesia, cardiorespiratory care, complications, and clinical pharmacology.
6. Cosmetic and Breast Surgery.
7. Tumors of the head and neck, skin, and breast; including treatment by radiation therapy, immunotherapy, chemotherapy, and surgery.
8. Trunk, lower extremity, musculoskeletal system, pressure ulcers, rehabilitation.
9. Hand, peripheral nerves, rehabilitation.
10. Maxillofacial and craniofacial surgery and microsurgery.
11. Congenital anomalies, genetics, teratology, facial deformity, speech pathology, gynecology, and genitourinary problems.
12. Psychiatry, and legal medicine.

How do I figure out what is important?

Each residency training experience is unique, making the generalization of importance of topics somewhat difficult for an individual to determine. For example, if you went to a program with a burn unit, you probably had lots of burn experience and think it is pretty important in the national curriculum but if your program did not have a burn unit you might think that burn care is fairly insignificant. Look at how national sources value topics – how much time and how many pages are devoted to the various topics? Some sources for an idea of the national curriculum in plastic surgery education include Selected Readings in Plastic Surgery, the PSEF Core Curriculum and general plastic surgery texts.

PLANNING YOUR ATTACK

Now that you have decided what you should know, ask yourself how well you know it. One way of organizing things is to create a table with what you know against what you need to know, like the one below. Rank importance from one (not so important) to thirteen (very important) in the how important (first) column. Rank how good you feel about the topic from one (I don't know much) to thirteen (I know this cold). Subtract the second column from the first and a rank list for study should appear.

	How important is it? (Positive Points)	How well do I know it? (Negative Points)	How much should I study? (Relative Rank)
Anatomy & Embryology			
Pathology/Wound healing			

Basic Techniques			
Burns &Critical Care			
Peri-op & Anesthesia			
Cosmetic &Breast			
Skin/H&N/breast tumors			
Trunk/Lower Extremities/ Pressure			
Hand/Rehab/Nerves			
Craniofacial/Micro			
Congenital/GU/Gyn			
Psych/Legal			

For example, if you decided that basic techniques were very important (13) and you knew very little (3) then the number for that topic would be 10. If you decided psych/legal medicine was not important (1) but you were a psych major in college and know a lot (13) the rank would be a very low negative 12. By assigning a rank and deciding what to study in this manner, you will avoid the pitfalls of studying too much minutia and studying what you like to study at the exclusion of what you need to study.

If you are repeating the examination, review your last test performance and see in which areas you scored well and poorly. Use this information to help you fill in the above table.

SETTING YOUR GOALS

You know the date of the examination, you know what you need to study, you know yourself and your ability to take tests, so decide that your goal is to pass them examination. No extra points are noted on the ABPS board certificate for high scores. If you do not think you can get all of your studying down before the test, do not expect to pass. If you do, great, but do not blame the test or the Board for your failure to accomplish your goal. If you were present and studying throughout your residency, much of the test information should already be incorporated into your plastic surgical soul. The qualifying examination should be a matter of reminding yourself of the details and brushing up on areas that present rarely or that were not the forte of your program.

SET ASIDE TIME TO STUDY

Time is the most valuable commodity of the practicing surgeon. Many things are competing for your time: learning to manage your practice, preparing for your cases, taking call, building a reputation, finding a spouse and raising a family, keeping your health and sanity. Setting aside a routine time to study for the boards is helpful. Small amounts of routine time add up. They decrease the need to cram for the boards in the month preceding the test. They decrease the amount of last minute stress and acid build up.

Taking the boards is a professional activity. Set time aside in your professional calendar for board review. You can spend the time away from your practice for an entire week at a board review course. That will cost you the registration, airfare and hotel and a week's time off of work. You can accomplish a similar amount of study without leaving your practice, by setting aside 3 or 4 hours weekly in your schedule. Have your secretary PUT IT ON THE CALENDAR. Come into the office an hour before your staff. Come in on Saturday morning or Sunday morning. Just don't try this at the end of the day when you have a pile of paperwork on your desk! Once you establish the study routine and have this time firmly carved into your schedule, you can use it after the boards for reading your journals, doing paper work or writing papers.

As important as putting the study time on the schedule is respecting that time. You're not likely to double book your obligations during operating time – don't double book your study time. Don't allow your study time to become a convenient time to book meetings, add an extra case or schedule a pedicure. It's study time…

MAKE YOUR STUDY EFFECTIVE

Some hints you probably know but ignore anyway…

-turn off the television – you can't watch the football game or the HBO movie and actually concentrate on your surgery material. The other material is inherently easier (and let's face it, more fun) for your mind to assimilate.

-turn off your phone and let the answering machine do its job during your study periods.

-don't study in bed or on a comfortable couch – the nap will win every time – use your desk or the kitchen table/counter.

-don't study with someone else until you are comfortable with what you know and then ask someone else for help – spoon-fed information doesn't stay with you.

-learn vicariously – listen to what other people say at meetings, in the hallway and at M & M.

STUDY TECHNIQUES

HOW DO YOU STUDY?

An entire section on learning styles is beyond the scope of a short review session. Suffice it to say that different students learn material differently. Most educators would assume that at the stage of certification for a profession that Adult Learning Styles would be the appropriate techniques. Some of that may be true. I personally have found certification exams to be more like an old fashion carrot and stick. The carrot – if you pass, you're done for 10 years and the stick – if you don't pass, it's another few thousand dollars, agony and time off of work. We are all inclined to study what we like, what we do and become good at it – that's what professionals do. The microsurgeons in the room are unlikely to want to study the Tessier classification of facial clefts and the craniofacial surgeons are unlikely to want to study about the effects of the new anti-coagulants on microsurgical flap salvage and complication.

HOW DO YOU LEARN?

For a test such as the qualifying board examination, you just have to study what's on the list. There are ways to make that easier for yourself. If you spend a little time reflecting on the ways that you learn easily you can apply the same learning/teaching style to your studying. Layering of information or repeating it helps cement that information in your mind. How to reinforce your reading depends on the individual. Ask yourself honestly how you learn best?

-when you *hear* material – plan your study schedule around a conference schedule (such as your residents' conference schedule or a review conference such as this one) so that the presentations will reinforce your reading, also look for things on tape/disc and keep the Walkman/Disc player near by. Also, take advantage of Grand Rounds and conference presentations at the closest plastic surgery residency– most offer an hour of CME credit for free – and some one else can organize the esoteric information for you.

-when you *write* information – outline the material, even if you never intend to read your notes; writing out information will help and you can use the scrap paper for the bird cage

-when you *get the wrong answer* and feel stupid – use review books and do the questions right after your reading; don't write in the book so you can use it again to refresh your memory just before the test.

-when you *see* material – invest in the PSEF video series

-when you *verbalize* material to other people – take advantage of your surgical assistants and residents – review with them whatever topic you are reviewing in your studies. Quiz them.

Explain the answer to them. Draw it out for them. Write little cheat sheets with them. Do this on rounds, in the cafeteria and in the OR. It benefits you and it benefits them.

STRATEGIES FOR TAKING MULTIPLE CHOICE TESTS

KNOW THE TEST

The ABPS gives you a very clear description of the test you will take.

> The Written Examination will consist of the following format:
> * 15-minute optional tutorial
> * 400 multiple-choice questions formatted in four blocks of 100 questions. Each block is one hour and 40 minutes in length
> * Total break time of 35 minutes (optional)
> * Total testing time is six hours and 40 minutes. Total time at the test center is no longer than seven hours and 30 minutes.
>
> All candidates will have the same number of questions and the same time allotment. Within each block, candidates may answer questions in any order and review and/or change their answers. When exiting a block, or when time expires, no further review of questions or changing of answers within that block is possible.
>
> Candidates will have 35 minutes of total break time, which may be used to make the transition between blocks and for a break. A break may only be taken between each block of questions.

A summary of that information boils down to having one minute to answer each question, potty breaks are only allowed between blocks of tests and lunch is as long or short as you wish it to be. A minute per question is a generous amount of time for multiple choice questions with a single correct answer, which is the format the Board continues to use.

When you start each section, scroll through the examination briefly to see what you are expected to do and then start.

ANSWER THE QUESTION FIRST

All multiple choice questions have a stem and responses. One of the responses is correct and the other responses are called (appropriately) distracters. Don't allow the distracters to do their job. Read the stem and answer the question. If the stem isn't a question but rather an unfinished sentence, ask yourself what you know about the topic. This mini organization of thoughts will help diminish the confusion that distracters can cause. If you know the answer, record it and move on. Save time for questions that you might not know the answer.

IF YOU DON'T KNOW THE ANSWER…

The first step is to eliminate answers you know to be incorrect. If you can limit your options to two responses, pick one of the two and move on.

Some ways to limit your options to two responses include using the test to your advantage, when possible. Well written stems should not confuse you nor should they give hints to the answer. Not all questions are well written…

-if three of the distracters are the same and one if different, pick the different one. For example if a question about prophylactic antibiotics appears and the answers include 3 macrolides and one first generation cephalosporin, pick the cephalosporin. The other three options are morally equivalent to one another.

-if two distracters are mutually exclusive, exclude one.

-look for congruence in verb and noun forms between the stem and the responses.

If you still don't have a clue…

If you're spending more than a minute or two on the question, THEN you don't know the answer. Don't waste time on something you don't know when you could be answering questions you do know. When in doubt, pick A or B, but pick the same answer consistently so you don't waste time or energy.

ANSWER AS YOU GO

Answer as you go and record those answers. Don't second guess yourself. Answer the question and don't change it. Don't skip around on the exam. Go from front to back.
Never leave a blank, you can count on no credit from a blank spot.

AMERICAN BOARD OF PLASTIC SURGERY ELECTRONICALLY ADMINISTERED EXAMINATIONS

WILL IT AFFECT YOUR PERFORMANCE?

While new to the ABPS, electronically administered examinations are not new to certification. In the health professions, nursing has been very proactive in adopting this technology. Repeat studies in their literature suggest there is no difference in the pass rates between pencil and paper and electronic examination.

WHAT WILL IT BE LIKE?

In order to help you with the new format the board has released multiple old board examination questions in a tutorial format. The tutorial is for a Windows platform but can work with Virtual PC or other windows simulations for the Mac platform. Download this tutorial and use it now. First, it will save you 15 minutes time on the day of the examination, if you don't have to take the tutorial then. Second, it will give you an idea of what the real board questions are like – it's not the In-Service examination all over again. Third, it will give you some practice.

GRADING

Grading of ABMS examinations is generally done with an absolute rather than a relative cut point. That is to say, you must have a certain score to pass. The failure rate is not set at a certain number of standard deviations below the mean. The Board keeps track of its questions performance. When the test is assembled, they have a good idea of how many people will answer correctly or incorrectly. Based on that information a cut point is chosen. This type of grading means that theoretically, every test taker can pass if they have the knowledge. On the curve, the lower 15 percentile or so must fail, even if they know a lot.

HISTORICAL PASS/FAIL RATES

Here are the recent pass and failure rates for the qualifying examination.

Failure Rates ABPS Qualifying Examination
2000: 23.0%
2001: 21.2%
2002: 23.1%
2003: 23.0%

References

Al-Rawahi, Zahra. Cognitive Styles and Medical Students' Learning. Association for the Advancement of Computing in Education (AACE), P.O. Box 3728, Norfolk, VA 23514. Tel: 757-623-7588; e-mail: info@aace.org; Web site: http://www.aace.org/DL/. October 2002.

While a number of systems have been developed based on cognitive styles, and a significant body of research has been carried out about learning with multiple representations, little is known about the effectiveness of systems based on multiple intelligences (MI). To address this, a prototype was built based on Gardner's theory of MI and experiments were performed to study the effectiveness of the system on medical students' learning. The results showed that medical students accomplish deeper understanding of a topic when it is taught in a way that matches their cognitive styles. Moreover, the results indicated that providing students with a rich environment in which they can learn a topic via their chosen modality seems not to be as an effective teaching method as automatically adapting the material.

Gorney B, Maury M. Relationship of Scores and Times of Test Administration via Computer. April 2001.

The purpose of this study was to determine if a relationship exists between scores and the times that medical students choose to take a computer-administered test. The results indicate that students who choose to take a test later within a given time period tend to perform less well than students who take the test earlier. Although the magnitude of the relationships was slight, a negative association was found for both high-stakes national examinations and weekly quizzes associated with a medical school course. Second-year students are required to take the U.S. Medical Licensing Examination (USMLE) Step 1 in March or April, and third-year students are required to take Step 2 between April and July. Students, who are required to attain a national passing score on both examinations in order to progress, may schedule their examinations from several weeks to several months in advance. Data from the Step 1 examination were studied for 2 cohorts of 111 and 102 students. Although the magnitude of the associations found was slight, the negative direction persisted across cohorts and type of test, whether high-stakes national tests or weekly quizzes for second-year students. (SLD)

Pisacano, Nicholas J. Classifying the Content of Board Certification Examinations. Academic Medicine. v64 n3 p149-54 Mar 1989.

A system of medical classification based on the dimensions of body system, etiology, and stage of disease was evaluated by classifying the content of one specialty board's examinations. This classification system may allow a board to define the content of its examinations, monitor requirements for certification, and communicate its standards. (Author/MLW)

Swanson, David B. Setting Content-Based Standards for National Board Exams: Initial Research for the Comprehensive Part I Examination. Academic Medicine. v65 n9 suppl pA1.

This study is the National Board of Medical Examiners exploration of content-based techniques (standard-setting techniques in which pass/fail decisions are based upon the performance of examinees in relation to test content). Two content-based techniques (Angoff and Ebel) and three methods of evaluating examinee performance were studied. (MLW)

Vaughn L, del Rey JG, Baker, R. Microburst Teaching and Learning. Medical Teacher. 23 (1):39-43 Jan 2001.

Introduces Microburst Teaching and Learning, a strategy for combining various teaching styles and methods in 'bursts' with different learning styles to enhance the learning process. The model accommodates adult learning theory, adult attention span, learner motivation, the variety of learning styles found in learners, and the need for efficiency. (Contains 23 references.) (Author/ASK)

AESTHETIC SURGERY

PERIORBITAL REGION

Julius Few, MD

○ **What is analogous to the levator palpebrae superioris aponeurotica, in the lower eyelid?**

Capsulopalpebral fascia.

○ **What is the cause of senile ptosis?**

Attenuation of the levator aponeurosis.

○ **What is the cause of classic congenital ptosis?**

Inadequate/nonexistent levator function.

○ **What is the most appropriate procedure for congenital ptosis?**

Frontalis sling.

○ **In senile ptosis, what happens to the supratarsal crease?**

The crease becomes cephalically displaced due to adhesion between the levator aponeurosis and dermis. The superior crease moves with attenuation of the aponeurosis.

○ **What is the classic treatment of senile ptosis?**

Levator advancement/re-insertion.

○ **What is the most common cause of post surgical lower ectropion?**

The combination of lower eyelid laxity with scarring/traction on the capsulopalpebral fascia-septum interface.

○ **What is the preferred treatment of lower eyelid ectropion?**

Canthoplasty with capsulopalpebral spacer graft (i.e. Alloderm, autologous dermis, palate mucosa, etc.).

○ **The most commonly injured muscle in a blowout fracture?**

Inferior oblique muscle, the only extra-ocular muscle to insert onto bone directly.

○ **Where is the apex of the brow?**

The lateral limbus of the eye in forward gaze.

○ **What is considered an abnormal Schirmer's test?**

Less than 10mm.

○ **What does correction of ptosis in one eye do in a bilateral case?**

Correction will make the non-corrected side *more* ptotic, due to dual innervation- Herring's Law.

○　**How much of the eyelid can be sacrificed and primarily closed?**

Up to 25% total lid loss can be primarily closed.

○　**What nerve travels in the floor of the orbit?**

Infra-orbital nerve.

○　**What muscles are responsible for medial brow retraction?**

Corrugator, depressor supercili, and to lesser extent, orbicularis oculi.

○　**How many fat compartments are in the upper lid?**

Two.

○　**How many fat components are in the lower eyelid?**

Three.

○　**What separates the lower eyelid central and nasal fat pads?**

Arcuate extension of Lockwood's ligament.

○　**What nerve opens the eye?**

Cranial nerve 3.

○　**What nerve closes the eye?**

Cranial nerve 7.

○　**What findings make up a Horner's syndrome?**

Blepharoptosis, pupil miosis, and facial anhidrosis.

○　**What is lagophthalmos?**

Inability to close the eye.

○　**What is chemosis?**

Edema of the conjunctiva.

○　**What is the mucous spot test?**

A subjective measure of dry eye, absence of a film layer on the eye surface indicating chronic dry eye.

○　**What nerve can be found adjacent to the sentinel vein?**

Temporal branch of the facial nerve.

○　**Should the lacrimal gland be excised if ptotic?**

No.

○ **What reconstructive technique is typically used for a central (full thickness) upper eyelid 50% defect?**

Semi-circular skin/muscle flap rotation or Tenzel flap.

○ **What flap is commonly used for total lower eyelid loss?**

Mustarde flap-large skin muscle cheek rotation flap.

○ **What is the most common skin cancer on the eyelid?**

Basal cell cancer.

○ **What is a Hughes flap?**

A tarso-conjunctival flap from the upper eyelid, used to reconstruct >50% lower lid defects, for posterior lining only.

○ **What is the second most common eyelid cancer?**

Squamous cell cancer.

○ **What is the third most common eyelid cancer?**

Sebaceous cell carcinoma.

○ **What is the recovery rate for Bell's palsy?**

Around 84%.

○ **What is the arcus marginalis?**

Periosteal thickening at the orbital rim, where the orbital septum attaches.

○ **What is the lymphatic drainage for the eyelid?**

Medial-submaxillary lymph nodes, lateral-parotid lymph nodes.

○ **What is the function of the procerus?**

The muscle is continuous with the frontalis and inserts into the nasal bone to create horizontal wrinkles of the glabella.

○ **What are the oil secreting glands of the eyelid?**

Meibomian and zeis.

○ **What produces the aqueous layer of the eyelid?**

Lacrimal gland.

○ **What is the anterior lamellae?**

The skin and orbicularis.

○ **What is the posterior lamellae?**

Conjunctiva and Mueller's muscle in the upper eyelid. Conjunctiva and capsulopalpebral fascia in the lower eyelid.

❍   **What branches of the external carotid artery supply the lid?**

Facial, internal maxillary, and superficial temporal.

❍   **What is the vascular supply to the eyelid, from the internal carotid system?**

Dorsal nasal, supratrochlear, supraorbital, lacrimal, and terminal branch of the ophthalmic artery.

❍   **What is SOOF?**

Suborbicularis oculi fat pad.

❍   **What is ROOF?**

Retro-orbicularis oculi fat pad.

❍   **What autologous structure is useful in reconstruction of the posterior lamellae?**

Hard palate mucosal graft.

❍   **What fascia is commonly used to perform frontalis sling?**

Tensor fascia lata.

❍   **How many bones make up the orbit?**

Seven.

❍   **What is the distance from the orbit rim to the apex?**

40-45 mm.

❍   **Where does the nasolacrimal duct drain?**

Beneath the inferior turbinate.

❍   **What is the globe malposition associated with orbital blowout?**

Enophthalmos.

❍   **What sites are involved in a zygomaticomaxillary complex (ZMC) fracture?**

(1) Zygomaticofrontal, (2) Zygomaticomaxillary, (3) Zygomatic arch, (4) Inferior orbital floor, and (5) Anterior wall of the maxilla.

❍   **What is an entropion?**

Inward rotation of the eyelid margin.

❍   **What is a cause of pseudoptosis?**

Enophthalmos.

❍   **If myasthenia gravis is suspected, what test should be ordered?**

Tensilon test- edrophonium injection leading to short term improvement of ptosis.

O   **When are symptoms of ptosis worse in myasthenia?**

Later in the day.

References

Chen,W,P.(ed). Oculoplastic Surgery; The essentials. New York Thieme Publishing, 2001.

McCord, C.D. (ed). Eyelid Surgery; Principles and techniques. Lippinocott-Raven Publishers. Philadelphia. 1995.

Nesi, F.A, Lisman, R.D, Levine, M.R. Smith's: Ophthalmic Plastic and Reconstructive Surgery (2nd ed). St. Louis, Mosby. 1998.

Covington D: Changing patterns in the epidemiology and treatment of zygoma fracture: 10-year review, J Trauma 37(2):243,1994.

Ellis E, Kittidumkerng W: Analysis of treatment for isolated zygomaticomaxillary complex fractures, J Oral Maxillofac Surg 54:386, 1996.

Zingg M: Classification and treatment of zygomatic fractures: a review of 1,025 cases, J Oral Maxillofac Surg 50:778, 1992.

Lemke BN: Anatomic considerations in upper eyelid retraction, Ophthal Plast Reconstr Surg 7:158, 1991.

Lemp MA, Hamill JR: Factors affecting tear film break-up in normal eyes, Arch Ophthalmol 89:103, 1973.

Liu D, Stasior OG: Lower eyelid laxity and ocular symptoms. Am J Ophthalmol 95:545, 1983.

Mathers WD: Ocular evaporation in meibomian gland dysfunction and dry eye, Ophthalmology 100:347, 1993.

Meyer DR and others: Anatomy of the orbital septum and associated eyelid connective tissues: implications for ptosis surgery, Ophthal Plast Reconstr Surg 7:104, 1991.

Ousterhout DK, Weil RB: The role of the lateral canthal tendon in lower eyelid laxity, Plast Reconstr Sur 69:620, 1982.

Goldberg RA and others: Physiology of the lower eyelid retractors: tight linkage of the anterior capsulopalpebral fascia demonstrated using dynamic ultrafine surface coil MRI, Ophthal Plast Reconstr Surg 10:87, 1994.

Jo A, Rizen V, Nikolic V, Banovic B: The role of orbital wall morphological properties in the etiology of "blow-out" fractures, Surg Radiol Anat 11:241, 1989.

Abad JM, Alvarez F, Blazquez MG: An unrecognized neurological syndrome: sixth-nerve palsy and Horner's syndrome due to traumatic intracavernous carotid aneurysm, Surg Neurol 16:140, 1981.

Aiche AE, Ramirez OH: The suborbicularis oculi fat pads: an anatomic and clinical study, Plast Reconstr Surg 95:37, 1995.

Anderson RL, Beard C: The levator aponeurosis attachments and their clinical significance, Arch Ophthalmol 95:1437, 1977.

Eggers HM: Functional anatomy of the extraocular muscles. In Jakobiec F, ed: Ocular anatomy, embryology, and teratology, New York, 1982, Harper and Row, p 783.

Doucett TW, Hurwitz JJ: Canaliculodacryocystorhinostomy in the treatment of canalicular obstruction. *Arch Ophthalmol* 1982;100:306-309.

Wesley RE, McCord CD Jr: Reconstruction of the upper eyelid and medial canthus. In: McCord CD Jr, Tanenbaum M, Nunery WR, eds: *Oculoplastic Surgery*, 3rd ed. New York: Raven Press, 1995: 99-117.

Bergin DJ, McCord CD Jr: Reconstruction of the upper eyelid major defects. In: Hornblass A, ed: *Oculoplastic, Orbital and Reconstructive Surgery*. Baltimore: Williams & Wilkins, 1988: 605-623.

Dryden RM, Wulc AE: Reconstruction of the lower eyelid: major defects. In: Hornblass A, ed: *Oculoplastic, Orbital and Reconstructive Surgery*. Baltimore: Williams & Wilkins, 1988: 630-642.

McCord CD Jr, Nunery WR, Tanenbaum M: Reconstruction of the lower eyelid and outer canthus. In: McCord CD Jr, Tanenbaum M, Nunery WR, eds: *Oculoplastic Surgery,* 3rd ed. New York: Raven Press, 1995: 119-144.

Hilovsky JP: Lid lesions suspected of malignancy. *J AM Optom Assoc* 1995;66(8):510-515.

Arlette JP, Carruthers A, Threlfall WJ, et al: Basal cell carcinoma of the periocular region. *J Cutan Med Surg* 1998;2(4):205-208.

Esmaeli B, Chung H, Pashby RC: Long-term results of frontalis suspension using irradiated, banked fascia lata. *Ophthalmic Plast Reconstr Surg* 1998;14:159-163.

Older JJ: Ptosis repair and blepharoplasty in the adult. *Ophthalmic Surg* 1995;4:304-308.

Berlin AJ, Vestal KP: Levator aponeurosis surgery. *Ophthalmology* 1989;96:1033-1037.

Sires BS, Lemke BN, Dortzbach RK. Characterization of human orbital fat and connective tissue. *Ophthalmic Plast Reconstr Surg* 1996;14(6):403-414.

Hamra S: Arcus marginalis and orbital fat preservation in midface rejuvenation. *Plast Reconstr Surg* 1995;96:354-362.

Aiache AE, Ramirez OH: The suborbicularis oculi fat pads. *Plast Reconstr Surg* 1995;95:37-42.

McCord CD, Tanenbaum M, Dryden RM, Doxanas MT. Eyelid malpositions: entropion, eyelid margin deformity and trichiasis, ectropion and facial nerve palsy. In: McCord CD Jr, Tanenbaum M, eds. *Oculoplastic Surgery*. 2nd ed. New York: Raven Press;1987:279-324.59.

Cogan DG. Myasthenia gravis: a review of the disease and a description of lid twitch as a characteristic sign. *Arch Ophthalmol* 1965;74:217-221.

Maloney WF, Younge BR, Moyer NJ. Evaluation of the causes and accuracy of pharmacologic localization in Horner's syndrome. *Am J Ophthalmol* 1980;90:394-402.

Leone CR. The treatment of entropion andectropion. *Ophth Forum* 1983;1(5):16-24.

Jordan DR, Anderson RL. The lateral tarsal strip revisited: the enhanced tarsal strip. *Arch Ophthalmol* 1989;107:604-606.

McCord Cd, Ellis DS. The correction of lower lid malposition following lower lid blepharoplasty. *Plast Reconstr Surg* 1993;92:1068-1072.

BLEPHAROPLASTY

Hisham Seify, MD, Clinton McCord, MD, and Mark A. Codner, MD, FACS

○ **What are the goals of modern blepharoplasty?**

Correction of brow position and midfacial descent, preservation of upper orbital fullness and a defined upper lid crease, and identifying/treating lower eyelid laxity and upper eyelid ptosis.

○ **What is blepharochalasis?**

A rare inherited disorder characterized by repetitive episodes of eyelid edema and subsequent levator dehiscence and ptosis.

○ **What is dermatochalasis?**

Loosening of the eyelid skin with fat protrusion.

○ **Discuss the anatomy of the eyelid in terms of lamellar structure.**

The eyelid is a bilamellar structure consisting of an anterior lamella and a posterior lamella. The anterior lamella consists of skin and orbicularis oculi muscle, the posterior lamella includes the tarsoligamentous sling, the capsulopalpebral fascia, and the conjunctiva. The septum originates at the arcus marginalis along the orbital rim and separates the two lamellae.

○ **Discuss the tarsoligamentous structure of the eyelid.**

The tarsoligamentous sling creates the support structure for the posterior lamella.
The tarsal plates constitute the connective tissue framework of the upper and lower eyelids. The tarsal plates of the upper and lower eyelid are attached to the orbital rim by the medial and lateral canthal tendons and retinacular support structures.

○ **What is the function of the lateral canthal tendon?**

The lateral canthus consists of a complex connective tissue framework that functions as an integral fixation point for the lower lid.

○ **Discuss the anatomy of the lateral canthus.**

The lateral canthal tendon is formed by the fibrous crura and connects the tarsal plate to Whitnall's lateral orbital tubercle within the lateral orbital rim.

○ **What forms the lateral retinaculum?**

Ligamentous structures from the lateral horn of the levator aponeurosis, lateral rectus check ligaments, Whitnall's suspensory ligament, and Lockwood's inferior suspensory ligament which converge at the lateral canthal tendon.

○ **What is the suspensory ligament of the lower lid ligamentous system?**

The lower eyelid has an analogous inferior suspensory ligament, Lockwood's ligament.
Lockwood's ligament arises from the medial and lateral retinaculum and fuses with the capsulopalpebral fascia inserting on the inferior tarsal border.

○ **What is Clifford's ligament?**

The arcuate expansion of Lockwood's ligament, Clifford's ligament, inserts into the inferolateral orbital rim and fuses with the interpad septum between the central and lateral fat compartments of the lower eyelid.

○ **What are the fat compartments of the lower lid?**

Three fat pockets in the lower eyelid: central, nasal, and lateral.

○ **What is the color of the fat in the nasal compartment?**

The nasal compartment in the lower eyelid is similar in makeup to the nasal compartment of the upper eyelid with more fibrous, pale fat.

○ **What separates the nasal and central fat compartments in the lower lid?**

The inferior oblique muscle separates the nasal and central fat compartments.

○ **What separates the central and lateral fat compartments?**

The central and lateral fat compartments are also separated by an interpad septum as well as a fascial extension from Lockwood's ligament, the arcuate expansion.

○ **What are the key elements for preoperative blepharoplasty evaluation regarding the forehead?**

Brow position, bony brow prominence or retrusion, fat excess or deficiency, glabellar/forehead furrows

○ **What are the key elements for preoperative blepharoplasty evaluation regarding the orbit?**

Visual acuity, visual fields, EOM movement, eye prominence, canthal tilt, upper/lower eyelid laxity, lower eyelid malposition, orbicularis oculi hypertrophy, lacrimal gland ptosis, upper eyelid ptosis, skin quality/excess, postseptal fat herniation

○ **What are the considerations in the preoperative blepharoplasty evaluation regarding the midface region?**

Vector analysis, tear trough deformity, malar bags, cheek ptosis, skin quality and excess

○ **Describe the markings for upper blepharoplasty.**

1. The upper eyelid crease is marked at the level of the mid pupillary line. (8-10 mm superior to the lash margin in women and roughly 7 mm above the lash margin in men.)
2. At the lateral canthus, the lateral marking should be 5-6 mm above the lash line.
3. The superior margin of the planned excision is determined by using utility forceps to pinch and identify the quantity of excess skin and muscle.

○ **Describe the difference in markings for asian eyelids.**

1. When defining the desired location of the crease this is typically lower than in the Caucasian upper eyelid. A distance of 4-6 mm above the lid margin is usually used depending on the patient's desires.
2. Limit the amount of skin and preaponeurotic fat excision since to prevent a high crease and supratarsal hollowness.
3. Preserve the epicanthal fold unless change is specifically requested by the patient.

○ **Describe the markings for lower blepharoplasty.**

From the level of the lateral canthus, a line is extended inferolaterally for approximately 6 to 10 mm within a prominent crow's foot crease. Roughly 10 mm of skin is preserved between the lateral extension of the upper and lower blepharoplasty incisions.

○ **Describe the concepts in approaching fat removal in transconjunctival blepharoplasty.**

The orbital fat can be removed by a transseptal approach which divides the conjunctiva, capsulopalpebral fascia and septum or a retroseptal incision through the conjunctiva and capsulopalpebral fascia leaving the septum intact.

○ **Discuss the objective of canthopexy/canthoplasty.**

Suturing the tarsal plate and lateral retinaculum to the periosteum of the lateral orbital rim to tighten the lower lid tarsoligamentous sling.

○ **What patients will likely require canthoplasty?**

Patients with lid distraction greater than 6 mm require lateral canthotomy and canthoplasty.

○ **Discuss postoperative blepharoplasty care.**

1. Head elevation and the application of ice to the periorbital region is used for 48 hours after surgery
2. Ophthalmic antibiotic ointment is applied along the suture line as well as on the globe to prevent or to reduce evaporative tear film loss.
3. Instruction to avoid the use of eyelid makeup on the suture lines and contact lenses for two weeks following surgery.

○ **Discuss the management of postoperative chemosis.**

Liberal use of ophthalmic ointments and eye drops. More severe chemosis which herniates through the palpebral fissure requires more aggressive management with liberal ophthalmic ointment, patching the eye closed for 24 to 48 hours, and applying gentle pressure from an ace wrap to reduce the swelling. Also, the edematous conjunctiva can be surgically drained.

○ **Discuss the etiology and diagnosis of retrobulbar hematoma.**

Occurs rarely (0.04%) and caused by hemorrhage behind the globe compromising ocular circulation. Symptoms include progressive vision loss and eye pain from increased intraocular pressure.

○ **What is the treatment of retrobulbar hematoma?**

Rapid surgical decompression, administration of mannitol, acetazolamide, and oxygen is advocated as part of the initial management of retrobulbar hematoma.

○ **Discuss the etiology of diplopia following blepharoplasty.**

Usually temporary resulting from edema; permanent diplopia can occur from thermal injury to the inferior oblique or superior oblique muscles from electrocautery.

○ **What treatment exists for postblepharoplasty diplopia?**

Strabismus surgery may be required for patients who do not improve with conservative management.

○ **Discuss the management of lower lid malposition following blepharoplasty.**

Bandage contact lenses to protect the cornea and conservative massage of the lower lid margin for six week postoperative time period. Persistent lid malposition may require surgical intervention including placement of a posterior lamella spacer graft and lateral canthoplasty.

References

Carraway, J.H., Mellow, C.G.: The prevention and treatment of lower lid ectropion following Blepharoplasty. Plast. Reconstr. Surg. 85:971-981, 1990.

Codner, M.A., McCord, C.D., Hester, T.R.: The lateral canthoplasty. Operat. Tech. Plast. Reconstr. Surg. 5:90-98, 1998.

Codner, M.A., Day, C.R., Hester, T.R., Nahai, F., McCord, C.: Management of moderate to complex Blepharoplasty problems. Perspectives in plastic surgery. 15:1, pp. 15-32, 2001.

Fagien S.: Algorithm for canthoplasty: the lateral retinacular suspension: a simplified suture canthopexy. Plast. Reconstr. Surg. 103:2042-2058, 1999.

Flowers, R.S.: Canthopexy as a routine Blepharoplasty component. Clin. Plast. Surg. 20:351, 1993.

Jelks, G.W., and Jelks E.B.: Preoperative evaluation of the Blepharoplasty patient: Bypassing the pitfalls. Clin. Plast. Surg. 20: 213, 1993.

Knize, D.M. The superficial lateral canthal tendon: anatomic study and clinical application to lateral canthopexy. Plast. Reconstr. Surg. 109: 1149, 2002

McCord, C.D.: Lower lid Blepharoplasty. In C.D. McCord (Ed.), *Eyelid Surgery*. Philadelphia: Lippincott-Raven, p. 200, 1995.

McCord, C.D., Codner, M.A., Hester, T.R.: Redraping the inferior orbicularis arc. Plast. Reconstr. Surg. 102:2471-2479, 1998.

Muzaffar, A.R., Mendelson, B.C. and Adams, W.P. Surgical anatomy of the ligamentous attachments of the lower lid and lateral canthus. Plast. Reconstr. Surg. 110: 873, 2002.

CHEMODENERVATION (BOTOX)

Dimitrios Danikas, MD and Mia Talmor, MD

❍ **What is the most common aesthetic procedure in the U.S.?**

Botox injection.

❍ **Where does Botox come from?**

It is the vacuum-dried exotoxin of *Clostridium botulinum* type A.

❍ **What is the mechanism of action of Botox?**

Inhibits acetylcholine release at the neuromuscular junction and may inhibit neuropeptide neurotransmitter release.

❍ **What is the effect of Botox injection in a muscle?**

It induces partial chemical denervation resulting in reduced muscular activity. The muscle may sustain atrophy, axonal sprouting may occur and extrajunctional acetylcholine receptors may develop. Reinnervation of the muscle may occur, thus slowly reversing muscle denervation.

❍ **How many units are in one vial of Botox?**

A vial has 100 units of vacuum-dried neurotoxin.

❍ **What is a unit of Botox?**

One unit of Botox corresponds to the calculated median intraperitoneal lethal dose (LD50) in mice.

❍ **What is the final concentration after reconstitution?**

The powder should be reconstituted with 2.5 or 5.0 ml of <u>non-preserved 0.9% normal saline</u> to a final concentration of 4.0 or 2.0-units/0.1 ml respectively. In reality, physician choice is a factor for how Botox is reconstituted and whether non-preserved saline is necessary.

❍ **How long does Botox retain its potency after reconstitution?**

Prescribing information states that Botox should be used within 4 hours of reconstitution. However, published data suggest that potency can be maintained for up to six weeks with storage at 4°C.

❍ **Do men require a higher dose of Botox?**

Yes, the muscles of men are greater in mass and require higher doses of Botox.

❍ **Can the patient use medications that inhibit clotting before the procedure?**

No. Vitamin E, aspirin and NSAID should be avoided for 2 weeks before treatment. A practical tip is to look for and avoid visible veins when injecting.

❍ **What muscles make the Glabellar Complex?**

Corrugators, procerus and medial orbicularis oculi (depressor supercilii).

❍ **What is the most common site for Botox injection?**

The Glabellar complex.

❍ **What is the function of the corrugator muscles?**

Brow adduction and depression. Move the eyebrow downward and medially, causing <u>vertical wrinkling</u>.

❍ **What is the function of the procerus muscle?**

Brow depression. Depresses the medial head of the eyebrows. Causes <u>transverse lines</u> on nasal dorsum.

❍ **What is the action of the medial orbicularis oculi?**

Brow depression.

❍ **What is the action of the frontalis muscle?**

Brow elevation. Causes horizontal forehead rhytids.

❍ **Can injection of the frontalis result in brow ptosis?**

Yes. All frontalis injections should remain 1 to 2 cm above the orbital rim to reduce the potential for brow ptosis. Injections should avoid the first horizontal line above the brows. Forehead injections should also stay medial to the lateral limbus.

❍ **What is the cause of lateral orbital wrinkles (crow's feet)?**

Muscle activity in combination with photoaging.

❍ **What is the treatment for crow's feet?**

Lateral intradermal or subdermal injection of Botox approximately 1 to 1.5 cm from the orbital rim.

❍ **What are "Bunny lines"?**

Wrinkles on the sides of the nose that radiate downward.

❍ **What is the cause of "Bunny lines"?**

Contraction of the transverse portion of the nasalis muscle.

❍ **What is the treatment for "Bunny lines"?**

Low–dose Botox injection on the upper part of the nasalis.

❍ **How long it takes for muscle paralysis to occur?**

Three to seven days.

❍ **When should the patient be reassessed after treatment?**

Two weeks after the injection. Slight corrections with additional injections can be performed.

❍ **So if a patient returns after 2 days upset that they still have frown lines, what should you tell them?**

An absolute minimum of seven days should pass before considering re-treatment.

○ **What is the cause of vertical perioral rhytids?**

Aging, smoking and orbicularis oris action.

○ **What problems can be caused by over-treatment of the perioral area?**

Difficulty in pursing the lips, speech impairment, difficulty eating, brushing teeth, using a straw and diminished proprioception. Injection of other muscles can cause oral incompetence, drooling and asymmetrical smile.

○ **What is the cause of the dimpled appearance (peau d'orange) of the chin?**

It is the result of the action of the mentalis muscle.

○ **What is the treatment of the Dimpled Chin?**

Botox injection in the midline mass of the mentalis muscle just below the tip of the chin.

○ **What is the action of the platysma?**

Depresses the mandible and pulls the lower lips and corners of the mouth sideways and down, partially opening the mouth.

○ **What patients are candidates for injection of platysmal bands?**

Patients with retained skin elasticity and a minimal descent of submental fat.

○ **What complications can be caused by platysmal band injection?**

Dysphagia, dysphonia and neck weakness. Doses need to be quite high for successful treatment and thus, this application has been slow to gain popularity.

○ **How long do Botox results last?**

The duration of activity for glabellar lines is approximately three to four months.

○ **What is the usual re-treatment interval?**

Three to four months.

○ **What is the most common reported adverse event?**

Headache.

○ **What is the most common cause of complications?**

Diffusion of the toxin to the surrounding musculature.

○ **What can cause eyelid ptosis?**

Diffusion from injection into the corrugator supercilii muscles.

○ **What is the treatment of eyelid ptosis after Botox injection?**

Blepharoptosis is transient and lasts a few weeks. For mild to moderate symptoms reassurance is needed and no further treatment. For symptomatic and severe blepharoptosis ocular decongestants are administered. Alpha-adrenergic agonists antazoline and naphazoline can be prescribed.

○   **How can diffusion be prevented?**

Using a highly concentrated solution, injecting only the involved muscle, instructing the patient to avoid bending or straining after the procedure.

○   **What are the current FDA approved uses of Botox?**

Botox is FDA approved for:
1) the temporary improvement in the appearance of moderate to severe frown lines between the brows in people 18 to 65 years of age
2) the treatment of blepharospasm and strabismus
3) cervical dystonia (a.k.a. spasmodic torticollis)
4) severe primary axillary hyperhidrosis that is inadequately managed with topical agents

○   **How long do Botox results last for the treatment of severe primary axillary hyperhidrosis?**

The median duration of response was 201 days.

○   **What is the recommended dose for the treatment of severe primary axillary hyperhidrosis?**

The recommended dose is 50 units per axilla.

○   **What are the common off-label uses of Botox?**

Cosmetic uses: Forehead horizontal rhytids, lateral orbital wrinkles (crow's feet), vertical perioral rhytids, dimpled appearance (peau d'orange) of the chin and platysmal bands.

Non-cosmetic uses: Migraine headache, chronic low back pain, post-stroke spasticity, traumatic brain injury, cerebral palsy, achalasia, anal fissure and various dystonias.

○   **What are absolute contra-indications to the use of Botox?**

1) infection at the proposed injection site
2) in individuals with known hypersensitivity to any ingredient in the formulation
3) during pregnancy (High doses in pregnant rabbits resulted in abortion or fetal malformations. While no evidence of adverse effects in human fetuses exists, there is insufficient clinical safety data to support the use of Botox in pregnant, cosmetic patients)
4) Patients with peripheral motor neuropathic disorders (amyotrophic lateral sclerosis or motor neuropathy) or neuromuscular junctional disorders (myasthenia gravis or Lambert-Eaton syndrome) may be at increased risk of serious side effects from typical doses of Botox including severe dysphagia and respiratory compromise

○   **What are the relative contraindications to the use of Botox?**

1) diseases of neuromuscular transmission
2) coagulopathy (including therapeutic anticoagulation)
3) nursing mothers
The effect of the toxin may be potentiated with co-administration of aminoglycosides or other agents interfering with neuromuscular transmission (curare-like non-depolarizing blockers, lincosamides, polymyxins, quinidine, magnesium sulfate, anticholinesterases, succinylcholine chloride).

○   **What are the more common adverse reactions to Botox?**

Headache, respiratory infection, flu syndrome, temporary blepharoptosis and nausea.

○ **Is Botox FDA approved as a treatment for migraine headaches?**

No.

○ **What is the evidence that Botox works as a treatment for migraine headaches?**

Double-blinded, placebo controlled studies have reported reduction in the frequency of migraine headaches, particularly in those patients not taking other medication.

References

Clinical Use of Botulinum Toxin. NIH Consensus Statement Online 1990;8:1-20.

Behmand RA, Tucker T, Guyuron B. Single-site botulinum toxin type a injection for elimination of migraine trigger points. Headache 2003;43:1085-9.

Carruthers J, Fagien S, Matarasso SL. Consensus recommendations on the use of botulinum toxin type a in facial aesthetics. Plast Reconstr Surg 2004;114:1S-22S.

Carruthers J, Fagien S, Matarasso SL. Introduction to the consensus recommendations. Plast Reconstr Surg 2004;114:i-iii.

Fagien S. Botox for the treatment of dynamic and hyperkinetic facial lines and furrows: adjunctive use in facial aesthetic surgery. Plast Reconstr Surg 1999;103:701-13.

Fagien S, Brandt FS. Primary and adjunctive use of botulinum toxin type A (Botox) in facial aesthetic surgery: beyond the glabella. Clin Plast Surg 2001;28:127-48.

Fagien S. Botulinum toxin type A for facial aesthetic enhancement: role in facial shaping. Plast Reconstr Surg 2003;112:6S-18S; discussion 19S-20S.

Fagien S. Temporary management of upper lid ptosis, lid malposition, and eyelid fissure asymmetry with botulinum toxin type A. Plast Reconstr Surg 2004;114:1892-902.

Guyuron B, Tucker T, Davis J. Surgical treatment of migraine headaches. Plast Reconstr Surg 2002;109:2183-9.

Guyuron B, Tucker T, Kriegler J. Botulinum toxin A and migraine surgery. Plast Reconstr Surg 2003;112:171S-173S; discussion 174S-176S.

Hexsel D, Dal'forno T. Type A botulinum toxin in the upper aspect of the face. Clin Dermatol 2003;21:488-97.

Hexsel DM, De Almeida AT, Rutowitsch M, et al. Multicenter, double-blind study of the efficacy of injections with botulinum toxin type A reconstituted up to six consecutive weeks before application. Dermatol Surg 2003;29:523-9; discussion 529.

Hexsel DM, Alencar de Castro I, Zechmeister D, Almeida do Amaral A. Re: Hexsel, et al. Multicenter, double-blind study of the efficacy of injections with botulinum toxin type A reconstituted up to six consecutive weeks before application. Dermatol Surg 2004;30:823.

Rohrich RJ, Janis JE, Fagien S, Stuzin JM. Botulinum toxin: expanding role in medicine. Plast Reconstr Surg 2003;112:1S-3S.

Dodick DW, Mauskop A, Elkind AH, Degryse R, Brin MF, Silberstein SD; BOTOX CDH Study Group. Botulinum toxin type a for the prophylaxis of chronic daily headache: subgroup analysis of patients not receiving other prophylactic medications: a randomized double-blind, placebo-controlled study. Headache. 2005 Apr; 45(4):315-24.

BROW LIFT

Dimitrios Danikas, MD and Lloyd B. Gayle, MD

O **Where should the highest brow peak be positioned in females?**

Between the lateral limbus and lateral canthus.

O **What is the aesthetic position of the male brow?**

Lower than the female brow. It is at the level of the orbital rim, horizontal without peaking.

O **What is the surgical significance of the temporoparietal fascia?**

The frontal branch of the facial nerve crosses over the superficial surface of the midportion of the zygomatic arch and traverses the temporal region on the undersurface of this layer.

O **What muscle is the primary elevator of the eyebrow?**

The frontalis muscle.

O **What muscles are innervated by the frontal branch of the facial nerve?**

The frontalis, corrugator, procerus and depressor supercilii muscles.

O **What is the result of frontalis muscle resection?**

Inability to raise the brows, elimination of the transverse wrinkles of the forehead and inadvertent depression of the brows.

O **What is the result of excessive resection of the procerus and corrugator muscles?**

Central depression at the level of the medial brows and nasal root.

O **Excessive resection of the frontalis muscle can cause what?**

Visible depression of the central forehead.

O **What muscles are the primary depressors of the eyebrow?**

The corrugator supercilii muscles.

O **What is the origin and insertion of the corrugator muscles?**

The **origin** is from the frontal bone near the superomedial orbital rim lateral to the origin of the procerus muscles. The corrugators **insert** into the dermis of the forehead skin above the middle third of the eyebrow.

O **What is the result of division or resection of the corrugator muscles?**

Corrugators pull the brows medially, and cause vertical wrinkling. Division will eliminate vertical wrinkling in the glabellar area.

O **What nerve will be injured by en bloc resection of the medial aspect of the corrugator muscles?**

The supratrochlear nerve.

○   **Where is the origin of the procerus muscle?**

The origin is in a paramedian location over the nasal bones inferior and medial to the origin of the corrugator muscles.

○   **The transverse wrinkles of the lower forehead and root of the nose will be obliterated by resection of which muscle?**

The procerus muscle.

○   **What is the result of division or resection of the orbital portion of the orbicularis oculi muscle?**

The orbital portion of the orbicularis oculi muscle interdigitates with the corrugator muscles medially and surrounds the lateral canthus in the zygomatic area. Contraction results in downward displacement of the lateral brow, while resection decreases lateral brow ptosis.

○   **What are the indications for surgical rejuvenation of the upper face?**

Soft tissue ptosis of the forehead, eyebrow, temporal regions, forehead height disparities and permanent static glabellar and forehead lines.

○   **What are the indications for a temporal lift?**

Lateral brow ptosis, temporal soft tissue ptosis and extensive crow's feet.

○   **What are the indications for an endoscopic brow lift?**

Young to middle age, glabellar frown lines and moderate brow ptosis.

○   **What are the indications for a coronal brow lift?**

Old age with deep glabellar and forehead lines, thick oily corrugated skin, forehead height disparity and moderate to severe brow and temporal soft tissue ptosis.

○   **What ligaments should be released for a brow lift?**

The orbital ligaments and the periosteal zones of adhesion.

○   **What are the orbital retaining ligaments?**

They are true dermal to periosteal retaining ligaments, 6 to 8 mm in length and are centered over the zygomaticofrontal suture.

○   **What is the periosteal zone of adhesion?**

It is a wing shaped 1.5 to 2.5 cm band of adherence of the deep galea to the periosteum. Starts at the nasofrontal junction, extends across the forehead over the supraorbital rims and fuses with the orbital ligaments at the zygomaticofrontal junction.

○   **A patient has a high forehead hairline. What is the best approach for preservation of the hairline?**

An anterior hairline (pretrichal) bicoronal browlift will preserve the already high forehead hairline. The incision heals well and may permit the growth of hair anterior to the incision line. All other techniques will elevate the hairline.

○ **When is a pretrichal approach indicated?**

It is indicated for a high hairline and for patients concerned for even a minimal amount of hair loss.

○ **When is the temporal approach indicated?**

For isolated lateral brow ptosis.

○ **Where should incisions for an endoscopic brow lift be placed?**

Either within the hairline and vertically oriented or pretrichal, along the frontal hairline and horizontally oriented.

○ **Is a central incision necessary for an endoscopic brow lift?**

No, with sufficiently medially placed paramedian incisions adequate medial and central dissection can be accomplished.

○ **Where is the plane of dissection in an endoscopic brow lift?**

Subperiosteal.

○ **What muscles are divided in an endoscopic brow lift?**

Both procerus and corrugators are divided and the galeal fat pad is completely visualized.

○ **What is the most common complaint after endoscopic browlift?**

Undercorrection and relapse of brow ptosis.

○ **What are the options for achieving brow support during an endoscopic brow lift?**

Either sutures with screw fixation or the Endotine® device.

○ **What is the Endotine® device?**

It is a proprietary device that has a post on the cranial side for anchoring it in the skull and five angled tines on the superficial side for engaging the periosteum. It is made of a bioabsorbable co-polymer.

○ **Does the Endotine® device has to be removed?**

Unlike metallic screws the Endotine® device typically does not have to be removed.

○ **Is the frontalis muscle divided in a coronal brow lift?**

The frontalis can be either resected, scored full-thickness, or left intact.

○ **What nerves should be preserved during frontalis myotomy?**

The supraorbital, supratrochlear nerves and the frontal branch of the facial nerve.

○ **Scalp sensibility changes are more common after bicoronal or endoscopic browlift?**

Bicoronal incisions are associated with an increased incidence of postoperative neuralgia and neuromas.

References

Connell BJ, Lambros VS and Neurohr GH: The forehead lift: techniques to avoid complications and produce optimal results. Aethetic Plast Surg. 13:217-37, 1989.

De Cordier BC, de la Torre JI, Al-Hakeem MS, Rosenberg LZ, Gardner PM, Costa-Ferreira A, Fix RJ and Vasconez LO: Endoscopic forehead lift: review of technique, cases, and complications. Plast Reconst Surg. 110: 1558-68; discussion 1569-70, 2002

Evans GR, Kelishadi SS and Ho KU: "Heads up" on brow lift with Coapt Systems' Endotine Forehead technology. Plast Reconstr Surg. 113: 1504-5, 2004

Freund RM and Nolan WB, 3rd: Correlation between brow lift outcomes and aesthetic ideals for eyebrow height and shape in females. Plast Reconstr Surg. 97: 1343-8, 1996.

Isse NG: Endoscopic forehead lift. Evolution and update. Clin Plast Surg. 22: 661-73, 1995.

LaTrenta G: *Atlas of aesthetic face and neck surgery*. Philadelphia, Saunders, 2004.

Ramirez OM: Endoscopic subperiosteal browlift and face lift. Clin Plast Surg. 22: 639-60, 1995.

FACE LIFT

Arian Mowlavi, MD

O   **What are the factors that result in the aging face?**

1.   External influence (UV light)
2.   Endogenous factors (genetics)

O   **Please explain UV light damage?**

UV induces photoaging through generation of reactive oxygen species (ROS) that damage enzymes after being absorbed by chromophores. Alpha tocopherol-a superoxide scavenging antioxidant-may counter these effects; Mechanism of dermal damage occurs via induction of three metalloproteinases capable of degrading the dermal collagen matrix.

UVB causes direct damage; wavelength: 280 to 315; responsible for most of DNA damage of skin.

UVA acts through other active molecules; wavelength: 315-400 nm; causes damage if get 100 to 1000X dose of UVB (unfortunately there is considerably more UVA light making it through the ozone).

O   **What are the endogenous changes that occur with aging?**

1. Glycosaminoglycans and proteoglycan: decrease with age
Rational: for use of Restylane and Hyalaform
2. Collagen: decrease by 6 % per decade; results in dermal thinning; results from decrease of Type I collagen. Of interest Type I: III ratio actually increases.

O   **Discuss various disorders and whether surgery would be contraindicated?**

a) **Ehlers-Danlos Syndrome (Cutis Hyperelastica):**
   - hypermobile joints
   - very thin, friable, and hyperextensible skin
   - subcutaneous hemorrhage
   - may stretch skin up to 15 cm or more and it will shrink back
   - posttraumatic bleeding
   - poor wound healing (due to inadequate production of enzyme lysyl oxidase)
   - Surgery-not recommended

b) **Cutis Laxa:**
   - degeneration of elastic fibers in dermis
   - skin does not spring back into position
   - no hyperextensible joints
   - Autosomal dominant or autosomal recessive or X-linked forms all exist
   - recessive form worst of disease presenting with systemic signs
   - Surgery: can be performed.

c) **Pseudoxanthoma elasticum:**
   - occurs in 2 dominant and 2 recessive forms
   - recessive form(Type II)-entire skin is loose fitting
   - diagnose by biopsy to differentiate from cutis laxa
   - Surgery: indicated if do not have severe systemic symptoms.

d) **Progeria(Hutchinson-Gilford Syndrome):**
- rare
- unknown etiology
- autosomal recessive genetic pattern
- craniofacial disproportion(due to premature closure of epiphyses)
- baldness
- pinched nose
- protruding ears
- micrognathia
- internally-loss of subcutaneous fat, arteriosclerosis, and cardiac disease
- do not live long enough to reproduce
- Surgery: not indicated.

e) **Werner's Syndrome(Adult Progeria):**
- autosomal recessive
- patches of skin
- baldness
- aged facies
- hypo and hyperpigmentation
- short stature
- high pitched voice
- cataracts
- mild DM
- muscle atrophy
- osteoporosis
- premature arteriosclerosis
- various neoplasm
- Exhibit severe microangiopathy like DM
- Surgery-Not recommended.

f) **Meretoja Syndrome:**
- systemic form of amyloidosis
- excessively lax skin in persons 20 years or older
- facial polyneuropathy
- amyloid deposits in perineurium and endoneurium of peripheral nerves
- facial neuropathy helps differentiated this disease

g) **Idiopathic skin laxity:**
- patchy areas of mid-dermal elastolysis
- localized fine wrinkling
- without systemic abnormalities
- etiology of disorder has not been elucidated, although
- antecedent inflammatory event such as urticaria suspected

O **Discuss the difference between facial soft tissue perfusion over the lateral versus the anterior or central face?**

Anterior face-perfused by numerous small musculocutaneous perforators;
Lateral face-perfused by relatively few but large fasciocutaneous perforators;

By virtue of elevating facial flaps a significant portion of the fasciocutaneous perforators are disrupted so that the soft tissue must rely on the central musculocutaneous perforators. Medial dissection thus must be performed more conservatively in order to avoid blood flow compromise.

O **What is the cause of the hollowed out look in the cheek region following a face lift during which the malar fat was confidently transposed to its natural pre-ptotic state?**

The malar fat pad itself may atrophy due to disruption of its blood supply thus resulting in the hollowed out look of the cheek. This is because the malar fat pad is perfused preferentially by the angular artery musculocutaneous perforators. If this fat is mobilized in the skin layer and aggressively translocated (> 2 cm), it may be prone to atrophy and thus this deformity. It is advised to keep the malar fat pad with the SMAS layer and thus preserve its musculocutaneous perforators if requiring greater than a 2 cm lift.

O **What is the endpoint to each of the described dissection layers in the cheeks.**

Skin elevation: release of the nasolabial fold.
SMAS elevation: upturning of the modiolus.
Midface lift: elevation of the malar fat pad.

O **Describe the SMAS layer?**

The SMAS was first described by Mitz and Peyronie by 1976. The SMAS becomes attenuated centrally and more fascial over the parotid fascia and over the zygoma region. The SMAS should be dissected off of not only the parotid capsule but also the parotid fascia proper. This will protect all facial nerve branches as they exit the parotid gland.

SMAS is continuous with the following:
a)the risorius, platysma, depressor anguli oris, and the superficial orbicularis oris; a pull on an elevated SMAS should raise the modiolus but will deepen the nasolabial fold (hence the independent skin elevation);

b) zygomaticus major muscle-actually enveloped by the SMAS. This anatomical envelop is the premise for the deep plane lift described by Hamra that involves separation of the anterior SMAS fascia off of the zygomaticus major muscle so that the SMAS dissection can be carried medial to this muscle in an attempt to mobilize the malar fat pad.

O **Describe the retaining ligaments and their significance?**

a) osseocutaneous ligaments: include the zygomatic and mandibular ligaments; zygomatic ligaments are responsible for malar fat descent and nasolabial fold deepening;

b) soft-tissue cutaneous ligaments- include the masseteric cutaneous ligaments stretch from anterior border of masseter to skin and are responsible for jowling;

c) parotid cutaneous ligaments;

d) orbicularis oculi cutaneous ligaments-stretched with herniation of orbital fat pad and loss of malar fat pad support following its descent; stretch of this ligament is associated with development of festoons.

O **Describe the various facial nerves and their significance to face lift?**

a) buccal branch: if injured not typically symptomatic since it demonstrates collateral innervation in 70 % of patients;

b) frontal and mandibular branches: collateral innervation observed in only 15 % patients;
Frontal branch-found on Pitanguy line from 0.5 cm below tragus to 1.5 cm to above lateral eyebrow and accompanied by anterior branch of temporal artery; Ishikawa-noted that frontal branch may course as high as 4cm above lateral canthus; Gosain showed that frontal branch may have up to 2-3 branches posterior to this along the hairline and. Must nick 2 of 3 branches to get major functional deficit; above the zygoma, the nerve runs on the undersurface of temporoparietal fascia or in the subcutaneous plane; if dissecting in temporal hairline- then must dissect either under superficial layer of deep temporal fascia or stay cognizant that the nerve lies in the superficial fat pad just below the superficial temporal fascia. Note two layers of deep temporal fascia separated by superficial

temporal fat pad; rhytidectomy dissection plane: sub-SMAS- dissection up to zygomatic arch then in subcutaneous dissection above zygomatic arch to avoid injury to the frontal branch as it travels cephalad;

c) marginal mandibular branch: travels along mandible angle; Dingman studying cadavers: noted posterior to facial artery-81 % travel above border of mandible vs. 19 % below body of mandible; anterior to facial artery-the nerve travels above inferior edge of mandible (may limit submental liposuction to anterior to facial artery in order to avoid potential injury to this branch); note: facial artery hooks around anterior border of anterior masseter; dynamic studies during rhytidectomy-demonstrated that the nerve may dip 3-4 cm below inferior border of mandible; 50 % of time innervates upper and anterior portions of platysma, while descending cervical branch of facial nerve innervates main body of platysma; if damage this nerve: lose depressor anguli oris and depressor labii inferioris function–responsible for full denture smile; if these are out, the platysma can compensate for their function;

d) Greater auricular nerve (GAN): McKinney's point refers to locating the GAN at 6.5 cm caudal to external auditory canal with the head turned 45 degrees at which point it crosses the anterior belly of the sternocleidomastoid muscle; the nerve runs in close proximity to the external jugular vein lying just beneath the skin and SMAS; Safest place to penetrate the SMAS platysma during face lift is at a point immediately in front of (anterior to) the anterior border of the sternocleidomastoid muscle;

e) lesser occipital: 58 % of cases innervates superior 1/3rd; 21 % of cases innervates superior 2/3rd; in 5 % of cases innervates a majority of the ear except the earlobe; travels over SCM and under SMAS but may be more superficial and vulnerable to injury.

○   **Discuss the complications one might expect after a face lift?**

a) hematoma: most common complication; 2x more common in men; averaging 8 %; a/w systolic blood pressure of 150 or greater preop;

b) nerve injury: buccal branch most often injured but is asymptomatic; GAN: second most common nerve injury (the most common symptomatic nerve injury); Marginal mandibular nerve is injured more often than frontal branch nerve due to advent of platysmal slings that has resulted in an increase incidence of transient marginal mandibular deficits; with platysmal excisions pseudoparalysis observed in 16.5 % of patients and permanent lower lip dysfunction in 0.9 % of patients;

c) Skin dehiscence: over retroauricular region most common; a/w cigarette smoking; nicotine known to trigger release of epinephrine and increase platelet adhesion; nicotine retards wound healing on days 6 to 10 POD;

d) alopecia: due to placement of temporal incision, depth of undermining, and most importantly the tension of the closure (remember this is a redraping more than an excision procedure);

e) postoperative hypertension: this is really a complication! To avoid this, may prophylax with chlorpromazine 25 mg 1 hr before completing surgery and again 3 hours after surgery; repeat dose at 4 hr intervals for 24 hours if SBP > 150; may consider clonidine transdermal patch;

f) Infection (Staph): rare in the face
Minor complications: small hematoma, hypertrophic scars, pigment changes, earlobe traction deformity, i.e. "pixie" ear deformity, and salivary cysts.

RHINOPLASTY

Karol A. Gutowski, MD, FACS

○ **How is the skin of the upper nose different from the skin of the lower nose?**

The skin of the upper two-thirds is thinner and more mobile while that of the lower third is thicker and more adherent.

○ **What is the blood supply to the nasal tip?**

The facial artery supplies the nasal tip via the superior labial artery which gives rise to the columellar branch, and the angular artery which gives rise to the lateral nasal branch.

○ **Name the three nasal vaults?**

Bony, upper cartilaginous and lower cartilaginous.

○ **What is the "keystone area"?**

The junction of the upper lateral cartilages with the septum and the nasal bones.

○ **What is the "scroll area"?**

The overlap of the upper and lower lateral cartilages.

○ **Which muscle is responsible for opening the external nasal valve (nasal flaring)?**

Levator labii alaeque nasi.

○ **Which muscle can shorten the upper lip and decrease nasal tip projection on animation?**

Depressor septi nasi

○ **Which structures provide support for nasal tip projection?**

Lower lateral cartilages, medial crural ligaments, fibrous connections between the upper and lower lateral cartilages, anterior septal angle, and the domal suspensory ligament

○ **Which structures form the nasal septum?**

Quadrangular cartilage, vomer, palatine bone, maxillary crest, and the perpendicular plate of the ethmoid

○ **Which nasal structures form the internal nasal valve?**

The junction of the upper lateral cartilage and the nasal septum.

○ **Which is the normal angle of the internal nasal valve?**

10 to 15 degrees. If the internal nasal valve is narrowed, airflow may be impaired.

○ **Which area of the nasal airway contributes the most to airway resistance?**

The internal nasal valve accounts for 1/2 to 2/3 of airway resistance.

❍   **Describe the location of the ideal nasofrontal angle.**

The deepest part of the nasofrontal angle should be between the upper eyelash line and the supratarsal fold.

❍   **What are the three methods to determine the ideal nasal tip projection?**

1. Fifty to 60 percent of the nasal tip (the distance from the alar-cheek junction to the nasal tip) should lie anterior to a vertical line running adjacent to the most anterior projecting part of the upper lip.
2. The nasal tip should be two-thirds of the ideal nasal length.
3. The length of the nasal tip should equal the alar base width.

❍   **What is the ideal amount of tip rotation (nasolabial angle)?**

In women, 95 to 100 degrees; in men, 90 to 95 degrees

❍   **What is the ideal columellar-lobular angle?**

30 to 45 degrees

❍   **What are the common incisions used in rhinoplasty?**

Marginal incision, intercartilaginous incision, infracartilaginous incision, intracartilaginous (cartilage-splitting) incision, transfixion and hemitransfixion incision, and the transcolumellar incision

❍   **Describe the Tripod Concept of the nasal tip.**

The cartilage of the tip forms a tripod on its side, with the lower limb being the two medial crura and each upper limb being one of the lateral crura. If the base of the tripod is fixed, an increase or decrease in the length of the upper or lower limbs will result in a change in tip position.

❍   **In terms of the tripod concept, what happens when the medial and lateral crura are shortened/weakened?**

If the medial crura (lower limb) are weakened or shortened, the tip will rotate down and back. If the lateral crura and weakened or shortened, the tip will rotate up and back.

❍   **How can tip projection be increased?**

Suturing the tip of the domes to each other, placing a columellar strut, advancing the lateral crura medially onto a columellar strut, and/or placing a tip graft.

❍   **How can tip projection be decreased?**

Use of a complete transfixion incision, cephalic margin resection (or intercartilaginous incision), vertical transection of the lower lateral cartilage, or vertical transection of the medial crura

❍   **After decreasing tip projection, what may happen to the alar base?**

The alar base may flare laterally (widen)

❍   **How can alar base flaring be corrected?**

Alar base resection

○ **How can tip fullness be corrected?**

Cephalic margin resection of the lower lateral cartilages and/or placement of sutures in the dome of the lower lateral cartilages

○ **How much cartilage should be preserved after a cephalic margin resection of the lower lateral cartilages?**

At least a 5 mm strip of the lower lateral cartilages must be preserved

○ **What is an "open roof"?**

Removal of the dorsal hump may result in a space between the medial portion of nasal bones and the bony septum and between the upper lateral cartilage and the septum. This space is referred to as an "open roof" and may result in a postoperative deformity.

○ **How can an "open roof" be corrected?**

Nasal bone osteotomies, dorsal graft, spreader grafts

○ **What are the indications for nasal bone osteotomies?**

Narrowing wide nasal bones, repositioning deviated or deformed nasal bones, closing an open roof deformity

○ **What are the indications for dorsal spreader grafts?**

Recreating dorsal aesthetic lines, restoring the internal nasal valve, buttressing a dorsal septal deviation, or correcting an open roof after dorsal reduction

○ **What are dorsal spreader grafts?**

Dorsal spreader grafts are unilateral or bilateral strips of cartilage placed dorsally between the septum and upper lateral cartilages

○ **What are the dorsal aesthetic lines?**

On frontal view, an imaginary smooth curving line which runs from the supraciliary ridge, medial to the medial canthus, along the lateral nasal wall, and to the tip defining points. These lines define an ideal aesthetic appearance of the nasal structures.

○ **Describe the thickness of the nasal bones.**

The nasal bones are thick at the radix and thin distally towards the tip

○ **What is the nasal cycle?**

The nasal cycle is the normal cyclic alteration between the left and right nasal airway which results in alternating dilatation and constriction of the air passage. When one side is dilated, the other side is constricted and vise versa.

○ **What are 5 anatomic causes for nasal airway obstruction?**

External nasal valve (alar rim) collapse, narrow internal valve, septal deviation, inferior turbinate hypertrophy, masses (tumors, polyps, etc)

○ **What is a supratip break?**

The supratip break is the point, in a profile view, where the dorsal line rises to the tip defining points.

○ **What is the ideal supratip break?**

In profile view in females, the ideal dorsal line is 1-2 mm posterior to a parallel line from the tip defining points. In males, there should not be a supratip break as it may feminize the nose.

○ **How can a supratip break be created during rhinoplasty?**

By creating a difference in projection between the dome projecting points and the dorsal septum, a supratip break can be achieved. In thin skinned patients, a difference of 6 mm may be sufficient while in thick skinned patients, up to 10 mm be needed.

○ **What are the 3 common sources of cartilage grafts?**

Septal, auricular, and rib cartilage

○ **Where is septal cartilage used best?**

Septal cartilage is long and straight, making it very useful for dorsal grafts, spreader grafts and columellar struts. It may also be used for tip grafts and alar support grafts

○ **Where is auricular cartilage used best?**

Ideal for alar cartilage grafts because of its contour. It may also be used for dorsal and tip grafts but because of its weakness, it should not be used when structural support is required.

○ **Where is rib cartilage used best?**

Present in large amounts and provides strong structural support but may result in an unfavorable donor site scar and the graft may be more prone to warping. It may be used in any of the previously described uses.

○ **What is a SIMON?**

Single, Immature, Male, Overly expectant, Narcissistic. Patients who request rhinoplasty and fit this description may be more problematic with regard to satisfaction after surgery.

○ **After harvesting septal cartilage, how much of the septum should remain to provide adequate support for the nose?**

An L-shaped strut of dorsal and caudal septal cartilage, at least 8-10 mm in width, should remain to provide support.

○ **What is the sequence of interventions to control hemorrhage after rhinoplasty?**

Anterior packing, intranasal balloon, posterior packing;
Exploration in operating room with application of hemostatic agents, epinephrine (1:100,000) injections, cauterization;
Angiography and vessel embolization of internal maxillary artery;
Transantral internal maxillary artery ligation;
Anterior ethmoid vessel ligation (Embolization of ethmoid arteries absolutely contraindicated due to risk of blindness)

○ **What are the next steps in evaluating and treating an otherwise healthy patient, who presents four days after a septorhinoplasty, with fever (103.2 F), rash and hypotension.**

Toxic Shock Syndrome may be present; rare but potentially fatal complication caused by *Staph. aureus* and associated with nasal packing or nasal splints. The nasal packing and splints must be removed immediately and cultures should be obtained to look for *Staph. aureus*. Intravenous antibiotics and fluid resuscitation must be promptly initiated.

❍ **What are the functions of the nose?**

Filtration, humidification, conduit for respiration, protection from viruses and bacteria, and temperature regulation

❍ **What is a Cottle sign?**

Improved nasal airflow with lateral cheek traction, which opens the internal nasal valve, is considered a positive Cottle sign and suggests that dorsal spreader grafts may increase the internal valve angle and improve airflow.

❍ **What are the common findings in African-American patients requesting rhinoplasty?**

Wide dorsum, poorly defined tip, wide alar base (flaring), low set radix, short nasal length, acute columellar-labial angle, thick skin and fibrofatty layer

❍ **What is the correct sequence of techniques in rhinoplasty?**

Depends on the deformity to be addressed, use of open versus closed technique, and surgeon experience. Generally, injection of local, incision, and dissection. There is mixed opinion on the sequence of dorsal hump reduction, septal work, tip work, osteotomies, and graft placement. Closure, alar base modifications and dressings are done at the end of the procedure. A common sequence is to set and refine the tip, lower the dorsum, perform osteotomies and then place tip grafts if needed.

❍ **As one example, what is the operative order of the Sheen endonasal rhinoplasty?**

1. Inject local/shave vibrissae/place cocaine pledgets
2. Transfixion incision of columella, anterior third only
3. Widely skeletonize the soft tissues of the nose; make intercartilaginous incision, skeletonize nasal envelope over upper lateral cartilage, then over dorsum, septal incision, use Joseph elevator to elevate to radix (also can use right angled Joseph across radix to detach the final attachment of skin), and then complete transfixion incision
4. Modify dorsum with rasp or #11 blade
5. Develop spreader graft pockets/septal submucous resection to harvest graft material if needed
6. Place bruised cartilage grafts at the root/place spreader grafts
7. Trim caudal edges of upper lateral cartilages
8. Augment lateral bony arch, bilaterally
9. Modify nasal tip as needed (alar resection, lobular, and vestibular excision, and place tip graft)
10. Osteotomies as needed

❍ **What is the response of cartilage to being cut based on Gibson's and Davis's principal?**

Gibson and Davis observed that if cartilage is cut or incised on one side, it would tend to warp towards the opposite side. Therefore, when shaping cartilage, particularly rib grafts, equal amounts must be removed from both sides to prevent warping.

❍ **When should rhinoplasty revision be done?**

Because wound maturation takes about 1 year to complete, revisions should not be done before that time in most cases. Minor revisions can be considered at 6 months postop. With excessive scarring and edema, may need delay up to 2 years

❍ **What is an inverted V deformity and how can it be treated?**

A visible separation between the middle vault and nasal bones on frontal view with an appearance of an inverted "V". It may have an associated middle vault collapse; may be treated with a dorsal graft or spreader grafts.

❍ **What is a supratip (parrot's beak or pollybeak) deformity?**

A persistent fullness in the supratip area following rhinoplasty.

References

Gunter JP, Rohrich, RJ, Adams WP (Eds): Dallas Rhinoplasty - Nasal Surgery by the Masters. St. Louis, Quality Medical Publishing, 2002.

Johnson CM, To WC. A Case Approach to Open Structure Rhinoplasty. Philadelphia, Elsevier Saunders, 2005.

Daniel RK. Rhinoplasty, in McCarthy J (Ed): Grabb and Smith's Plastic Surgery. Philadelphia, Lippincott-Raven Publishers, 1997, 651-667.

Tebbetts JB. Primary Rhinoplasty – A New Approach to the Logic and the Techniques. St. Louis, Mosby, 1998.

Rohrich RJ, Sheen JH. Secondary Rhinoplasty, in Grotting JC (Ed): Reoperative Aesthetic and Reconstructive Plastic Surgery. St. Louis, Quality Medical Publishing, 1995, 401-510.

SKIN RESURFACING

Brian S. Glatt, MD

○ **What are the three most common skin resurfacing modalities?**

1) Lasers 2) Chemical Peels 3) Dermabrasion

○ **Skin resurfacing procedures are particularly good to treat what 2 conditions?**

1) Facial wrinkles 2) Blotchy facial skin pigmentation changes

○ **What is the Fitzpatrick skin type classification?**

Skin Type	Skin Color	Reaction to First Summer Exposure
Fitzpatrick I	White	Always burns/never tans
Fitzpatrick II	White	Usually burns/rarely tans
Fitzpatrick III	White	Occasionally burns/average tans
Fitzpatrick IV	White/Lt Brown	Rarely burns/usually tans
Fitzpatrick V	Brown	Rarely burns/always tans
Fitzpatrick VI	Black	Never burns

○ **What is the significance of Fitzpatrick skin type in preop evaluation for facial resurfacing?**

Fitzpatrick skin type helps predict the risk of hyperpigmentation changes following a skin resurfacing procedure.

○ **What Fitzpatrick type of skin has the lowest risk of hyperpigmentation following skin resurfacing?**

Fitzpatrick I, II, and III

○ **What is the "Grenz Zone"?**

A subepidermal region of dermis where neocollagen formation by fibroblasts occurs after wounding or actinic damage.

○ **What is the relevance of the "Grenz Zone"?**

The thickness of fibroplasia within the Grenz Zone is directly proportional to the strength of the wounding agent. In addition, this area is thought to be responsible for the regenerative changes in the skin seen after resurfacing treatments.

○ **How long should one wait to perform full facial resurfacing after a face lift?**

Classically, at least 3 months to allow the skin to fully heal prior to additional vascular insult.

○ **Why should one stop Accutane (Isotretinoin) prior to any kind of resurfacing procedure?**

Accutane causes atrophy of pilosebaceous glands and therefore impaired re-epithelialization and wound healing.

○ **How long should one stop Accutane (Isotretinoin) prior to any kind of resurfacing procedure?**

At least one year should pass after stopping Accutane in order to give the adnexal structures (epithelial cells, hair follicles) a chance to regrow and reactivate so proper healing (re-epithelialization) can occur after resurfacing.

○ **When can the patient begin wearing make-up following skin resurfacing?**

After full healing, or re-epithelialization, is well under way. Typically 7-10 days after treatment.

○ **Should patients scrub their faces after resurfacing to get rid of old, dead skin?**

Absolutely not. While gentle cleansing is essential; flaky, peeling skin should be left alone after a treatment and allowed to slough naturally. Any interference by picking or peeling could result in severe scar formation or poorly healed wounds.

○ **What are contraindications to skin resurfacing procedures?**

Active facial/oral herpes simplex infection or zoster
Skin disorders which affect healing (e.g. scleroderma, cutis laxa)
Planned future excessive sun exposure
History of extensive electrolysis or laser hair removal to the area
History of keloid/hypertrophic scarring
Recent facial procedures (relative contraindication)
Documented hypersensitivity to peeling agents
Accutane (Isotretinoin) use within 1 year
Pregnancy
Immunodeficiency
Prior radiation therapy to the area
Recent chemotherapy
Unrealistic expectations

○ **What is a chemical peel?**

A process by which different chemical agents are applied to the skin in order to cause a caustic injury and chemical necrosis of the skin to variable depths in order to remove variable amounts of skin to effect healing and subsequently, a more youthful appearance.

○ **What factors may affect the depth of chemical peeling?**

Presence of skin surface oils
Skin water content
Temperature of the room, skin, and solution
Humidity of the air
Length of time the solution is in contact with the skin or number of applications
Use of occlusive or nonocclusive dressings
Inherent thickness of epidermis and dermis
Batch of peel reagent

○ **Which is the most "predictable" peeling agent?**

Phenol

○ **What products are typically used for a "pre-peel regiment"?**

Hydroquinone (bleaching agent), Retin-A (tretinoin), Alpha hydroxy acid cream (Glycolic acid), sunscreen, moisturizers for at least 2-6 weeks. In addition, most patients (depending on their history) should be immediately pretreated with an oral antiviral agent for prophylaxis against HSV infection. Many practitioners also administer antibiotics beforehand.

○ **What effect does Retin-A have on the epidermis?**

Thins the stratum corneum, suppresses melanocytes, melanocyte granules are more evenly distributed, cellular portion thickens, increased vertical polarity of basal layer

❍ **What effect does Retin-A have on the dermis?**

Increased collagen synthesis (Type III) secondary to fibroblast activation, increased elasticity, and increased angiogenesis

❍ **What is the most common side effect of Retin-A?**

Erythema

❍ **Why is hydroquinone used in a pre-peel regiment?**

Its bleaching action (by suppressing melanocyte activity) helps to maintain uniform pigmentation after resurfacing and prevent post-procedure (postinflammatory) hyperpigmentation.

❍ **What are alpha hydroxy (AHA) acid peels?**

The mildest type of common peel formulation, AHA peels are derived from a variety of nontoxic organic acids.

❍ **What are the most common types of alpha hydroxy acid peels?**

Glycolic acid, Lactic acid, Citric acid, Malic acid, and Tartaric acid

❍ **What is the advantage of alpha hydroxy acid peels?**

Produce a mild effect but without extended downtime of more invasive treatments. Can also be used on any patient, regardless of skin color and can also be utilized on areas other than the face.

❍ **Which type of AHA peel is most commonly used in practice?**

Glycolic acid peels, between 35-75%

❍ **How does one increase the penetration of an AHA peel?**

Increase the concentration and/or increase the time of exposure.

❍ **When are alpha hydroxy acid peels indicated?**

For help treating fine, superficial wrinkles or sun damage

❍ **What is a Jessner's Peel?**

A medium-depth, mild peel designed to treat more extensive damage than what can be treated with conventional AHA peels. Typically used as a primer for a definitive TCA peel due to its excellent ability to disrupt the barrier function of the epidermis.

❍ **What does a Jessner's Peel consist of?**

Salicylic acid, lactic acid, and resorcinol mixed in ethanol

❍ **What is the classic agent used to achieve a medium-depth peel?**

Tricholoracetic acid (TCA), typically used at 35%

❍ **How does one increase the strength of a TCA peel?**

Increase the concentration, apply multiple coats, use pretreatment agents (Retin-A)

❍ **What is the Obagi Blue peel?**

A type of superficial TCA peel, it is performed in "cookbook-like" 1-4 steps and can be used on persons of almost any Fitzpatrick skin type

○ **What is a common side effect of the Obagi Blue Peel?**

A blue discoloration of the treated area may remain for up to 10 days

○ **What is a phenol peel?**

Phenol is the prototypical standard agent for a deep chemical peel. It is a skin keratocoagulant, and acts to cause a rapid and irreversible denaturation and coagulation of surface keratin. It causes a predictable, partial-thickness chemical burn injury that results in the formation of a new stratified collagen layer of smoother, more youthful appearing skin. Phenol causes an all-or-none response, and as such, it is difficult to vary peel depth by region.

○ **What are the advantages of a phenol peel?**

It is extremely reliable and has the most consistent depth of penetration, which is into the upper reticular dermis. The histological changes are permanent and the effect is extremely long lasting (>20 years).

○ **How does one increase the penetration of a phenol peel?**

Use a **lower** concentration of phenol, use of an occlusive dressing (taping). Recent evidence suggests that varying the amount of croton oil in the preparation may also serve to vary the depth of peel.

○ **Why does using a higher concentration of phenol penetrate less than lower concentrations?**

Traditionally, it was thought that higher concentrations of phenol are thought to cause more extensive denaturation of superficial proteins in the skin and therefore lead to a greater extent of non-permeability to the remainder of the peel. Lower concentrations of phenol are actually therefore more dangerous to use as they penetrate more deep into the skin. There is, however, some controversy over this issue at present.

○ **How is the treatment area dressed after a phenol peel?**

Either by an occlusive (taping, Flexan, Vigilon) or a non-occlusive (petroleum jelly) dressing

○ **What ingredients make up the Baker/Gordon phenol peel?**

3 cc phenol 88%, 2 cc water, 8 drops liquid soap (Septisol), 3 drops croton oil

○ **Why is croton oil added? Why is Septisol used?**

Croton oil is thought to act as a skin irritant, which acts to deepen the peel; Septisol causes a deeper penetration of the peel, likely secondary to its tension-lowering (surfactant) properties.

○ **Can phenol be used anywhere else besides the face?**

No. Phenol peels used on non-facial areas can result in severe scarring.

○ **What is the most common long-lasting side effect of phenol peels?**

Hypopigmentation, which can be permanent.

○ **Why does hypopigmentation occur after phenol peeling?**

While epidermal melanocytes are still present following phenol peeling, they become unable to synthesize normal amounts of melanin.

○ **What is the most serious medical potential side effect of phenol peels?**

Cardiotoxicity. The risk is significantly increased when phenol is applied to >50% of the facial surface in less than 30 minutes.

❍   **What does laser stand for?**

Light amplification by stimulated emission radiation

❍   **How does a laser cause skin resurfacing?**

Light emitted by a laser is absorbed by tissue (different types of tissue depending on the wavelength of the specific laser). The kinetic energy then turns into heat which coagulates or ablates tissue, depending on laser type and wavelength utilized.

❍   **What property of tissue determines which wavelength will be absorbed?**

Different chromophores (e.g. hemoglobin, water) within the tissue absorb different wavelengths of light

❍   **What are the most important non-skin safety concerns when using a laser?**

Proper eye care and the avoidance of O.R. fires.

❍   **Which types of lasers are most commonly used for cosmetic skin resurfacing?**

The CO2 and Er:Yag lasers

❍   **How does the CO2 and Er:Yag work to resurface the skin?**

The CO2 laser (10,600 nm) gets absorbed by water and creates a *photothermal* effect to increase collagen remodeling and contraction of the skin, but causes greater collateral injury which leads to increased recovery time as well as an increased risk of pigment changes.

The Er:Yag (2940 nm) laser also gets absorbed by water, however due to its wavelength is 10x more efficient than CO2 and works via a *photomechanical* effect. This does cause an increased amount of transudate and less control of bleeding, however this laser type results in less hyperemia, less coagulation necrosis, a shorter healing time, and minimal pigment changes.

❍   **How does one increase the penetration of a laser treatment?**

Increase the pulse energy and/or increase the number of passes.

❍   **Is a pretreatment regiment necessary before laser treatment?**

A pretreatment regiment is not absolutely necessary, however is extremely important in order to maximize results. Typical protocols are the same for chemical peeling, which include Retin-A, hydroquinone, glycolic acid cream, sunscreens, and moisturizers as well as antivirals/antibiotics.

❍   **What is the most common problem following laser resurfacing?**

Hyperpigmentation

❍   **What are the best ways to avoid significant hyperpigmentation following laser resurfacing?**

Use of a bleaching agent (hydroquinone) pre-procedure, discontinuation of hormone therapy, avoidance of sun exposure postoperatively, treating appropriate Fitzpatrick skin type patient population.

❍   **What is the most common type of laser used for hair removal?**

The Nd:Yag laser. It destroys about 90% of hair in the anagen phase with each treatment.

○ **What is dermabrasion?**

A procedure that involves a controlled, mechanical skin injury, typically to the level of the papillary dermis, using a hand-held abrading rotating tip. Different types of abrading tips may include burrs, diamond fraises, and sandpaper.

○ **What are the advantages of dermabrasion over other skin resurfacing techniques?**

It is less costly, easy to learn, and simple to perform; those that taut its effectiveness also claim that the depth of wounding can be more precisely controlled than with other methods.

○ **What are the best conditions treated by dermabrasion?**

It is most commonly used to treat perioral lines/wrinkles, acne scars, traumatic scars, and surgical scars. In addition, rhinophyma has also been successfully treated utilizing dermabrasion.

○ **How does one control the depth of dermabrasion?**

Coarseness of the abrading tip, number of strokes, pressure on the tip during strokes, contact time with skin, altering rotational speed.

○ **Which areas of the face respond best to dermabrasion for skin resurfacing?**

Lines in the perioral region

○ **What is microdermabrasion?**

A superficial ablation of the epidermis only. This is a variation of dermabrasion, however less abrasive crystals are used and less suction applied to the skin, so that there is a more subtle overall response; however, safety is increased. This procedure can be performed in spas and non-medical centers (e.g. hair salons) due to the use of more gentle instrumentation which causes less skin injury compared to traditional dermabrasion.

References

Baker TJ, Stuzin JM, Baker TM. Facial Skin Resurfacing. St. Louis: Quality Medical Publishing, Inc., 1998.

Baker TJ, Stuzin JM. Chemical Peeling and Dermabrasion. In: McCarthy JG, ed. Plastic Surgery. Philadelphia: WB Saunders, 1990:748-786.

Halaas YP. Medium depth peels. Facial Plast Surg Clin N Am 2004; 12:297-303.

Hetter GP. An examination of the phenol-croton oil peel: Part I. Dissecting the formula. Plast Reconstr Surg 2000; 105(1):227-239.

Hirsch RJ, Daya SH, Shah AR. Superficial skin resurfacing. Facial Plast Surg Clin N Am 2004; 12:311-321.

Lynch, SA. Chemical Peeling and Dermabrasion. In: Weinzweig J, ed. Plastic Surgery Secrets. Philadelphia: Hanley & Belfus, Inc., 1999:318-321.

Perkins SW, Castellano R. Use of combined modality for maximal resurfacing. Facial Plast Surg Clin N Am 2004; 12:323-337.

CHEMICAL PEELS

Alberto S. Gallerani, MD

❍ **What is chemical peeling?**

The use of exfoliating agents to destroy portions of epidermis and/or dermis resulting in new epidermal and dermal tissue.

❍ **What are the indications for chemical peeling?**

Rhytids, actinic keratosis, lentigines, melasma, acne vulgaris, rosacea, milia, superficial scarring

❍ **What effect does chemical peeling have on the dermis?**

Decrease in nonlamellar collagen

❍ **How are the exfoliants categorized? Provide examples.**

According to depth of wounding they produce:
Superficial: involves the papillary dermis (TCA 10-20%, Jessner's solution, Salicylic acid, solid CO_2, alpha-hydroxy acids, tretinoin)

Medium depth: to upper reticular dermis (TCA 35-50% + combination, Phenol, Pyruvic acid)

Deep depth: to midreticular dermis (TCA 51-75%, Baker's phenol)

❍ **Name the most common agents used for chemical peeling, and their mechanism.**

Phenol: a keratocoagulant (denatures and coagulates surface keratin)
TCA: Trichloroacetic acid (depth of action dependent on strength)
Croton oil: skin irritant enhancing phenol's action
Soap: surfactant action enhances penetration
Water: slows down keratocoagulation and improves absorption

❍ **What is the Baker formula?**

Phenol (3 ml of 88% USP), Croton oil (3 drops), Liquid soap (8 drops), Water (2 ml)

❍ **What is another name for Phenol?**

Phenol (C6H5OH), also known as carbolic acid, is an aromatic hydrocarbon derived from coal tar.

❍ **Why do some believe that Croton oil and not Phenol is the most important ingredient?**

Because Spira and coworkers found that a 50% phenol solution was as effective as stronger solutions, without increased toxicity. Minute concentration differences in croton are critical to the outcome.

❍ **What is Jessner's Solution?**

Resorcinol 14 g, salicylic acid 14 g, lactic acid 14 mL, ethanol 100 mL

❍ **How is the depth of peeling controlled with Jessner's Solution?**

By the number of coats of solution that are applied.

○ **How is the depth of peeling controlled with Phenol Solution?**

Carrier concentration (croton) or contact time (taping)

○ **How is the depth of peeling controlled with TCA Solution?**

Strength of solution

○ **How is the depth of peeling controlled with Salicylic Acid?**

Number of coats applied

○ **What are the advantages and disadvantages of using Jessner's Solution over TCA?**

The advantages of improved results compared with lower concentration of TCA, no need to neutralize the solution, and therefore no need to time the duration of applications. A disadvantage is the limitation of its use only to the face.

○ **What is Salicylic Acid (SA)?**

Salicylic acid (30%) is a beta hydroxy acid and was the original peeling agent. Used for single or multiple resurfacing of moderately photodamaged facial skin.

○ **How does SA compare to Jessner's solution in strength?**

The SA peel solution is comparable in strength to Jessner's solution—that is, it causes significantly more desquamation than a 70% glycolic acid peel but with the minimal downtime of an AHA peel (unlike TCA).

○ **When does clinical evidence of peeling begin?**

Clinical evidence of peeling usually begins on the second post-peel day and can extend up to 7 days.

○ **What interval between treatments is recommended of Salicylic Acid (SA) peels?**

An interval of 4 weeks is recommended between peels to allow for epidermal regeneration.

○ **What are the advantages of Salicylic Acid (SA) peels?**

1) uniformity of application, producing a white frost visible to the naked eye
2) no risk of overpeeling because the vehicle volatizes in under 3.5 minutes,
3) may also be useful for the treatment of comedonal and inflammatory acne.

○ **What is the Fitzpatrick's Classification of Sun-reactive Skin Types, and how can it be used?**

A classification system based on color and response to sunlight. Types I-III are usually good candidates for chemical peeling, the exception being red haired freckled.
Types V-VI are at risk for unwanted pigmentation changes.

Fitzpatrick Skin Types:

Skin Type	Color	Characteristics
I	White	Always burns/Never tans
II	White	Usually burns/tans with difficulty
III	White	Sometimes mildly burns/usually tans

IV	Medium Brown	Rarely burns/Tans easily
V	Dark Brown	Rarely burns/Tans very easily
VI	Black	Never burns/tans very easily

○ **What role does taping have for phenol and TCA peels?**

Taping will allow for the phenol to last longer and increase the depth of treatment. However, taping will not increase TCA penetration.

○ **What are the advantages to pretreatment?**

Pretreatment with tretinoin and 4% hydroquinone 4 to 6 weeks before treatment with TCA will decrease the thickness of the stratum corneum resulting in a deeper penetration, and the hydroquinone prevents hyperpigmentation by suppressing melanocyte activity.

○ **Which peel should not be used in blacks?**

Phenol and TCA has limited effect on melanocytes.

○ **Is the incidence greater for hypertrophic scaring and hyperpigmentation following phenol than for TCA?**

No, they are the same.

○ **How many months after discontinuing isotretinoin treatment can you skin resurface?**

12-24 months.

○ **How long to delay chemical peels s/p meloplasty?**

3 months

○ **What is a feared complication of TCA peeling while the patient is on oral isotretinoin treatment?**

Hypertrophic scarring

○ **Which is the first sign of phenol toxicity?**

Cardiac arrythmias

○ **What effects does Tretinoin (Retin-A) have on the skin?**

Causes regression of many premalignant lesions of the epidermis
Decreases corneocyte cohesion and thus, thinning of stratum corneum
Thickening of the epidermal layer
More organized vertical cellular polarity
Dispersion of melanocyte granules

○ **What is the mechanism of action of retinoids on skin?**

Decreased activation of metalloproteases resulting from inhibition of AP1 transcription.

○ **What is the long term effect of Retin-A treatment of sun-damaged skin:**

Premalignant lesions regress

○ **What histologic finding is seen with long term use of tretinoin?**

Formation of type III embryonic collagen

○   **What percentage of glycolic acid and how minutes of topical application is used in the setting of melasma?**

50% glycolic acid and 2-4 minutes

○   **What percentage and number of minutes of glycolic acid is used for wrinkles, actinic keratoses, and solar lentigines?**

70% glycolic acid at 4-6 minutes

Integument

○   **What effect does Vitamin A have on fibronectin and monocyte activation?**

Decreases fibronectin production and decreases monocyte activation

○   **What is the most common type of collagen in hypertropic scars?**

Type I: there is also an increase in glycolytic enzyme activity, fibronectin deposition, and production of collagen mRNA

○   **How do deficiencies of vitamin C and iron affect collagen?**

Decreased hydroxylation of proline and lysine

○   **What are the three primary components of dermal connective tissue?**

Glycosaminoglycans, elastic fibers, and collagen—show progressive diminution or disruption with age

○   **What happens to the total amount of *ground substance* (composed of glycosaminoglycans and proteoglycans) with age?**

Decreases with age

○   **What are elastic fibers composed of?**

Two distinct proteins: elastin and microfibrillar components

○   **How much of dermal volume do elastic fibers occupy?**

2% to 4%

○   **What role do elastic fibers have, and how does age affect it?**

They contribute to the structure of the collagen bundles, and with age, disruption of the elastic fibers results in loss of the physiologic recoil and laxity of the skin.

○   **What are oxytalan fibers, and how does age affect it?**

Fine fibers that normally extend perpendicularly through the papillary dermis and into the epidermis. After age 30 they are depleted or lost altogether.

○   **What is the predominant tissue component of normal human dermis?**

Collagen, which comprises 70% to 80% of dermal dry weight.

○   **In adults what is the ratio of Type I to Type III collagen?**

6:1 ratio

○   **How is this ratio affected by age?**

This ratio becomes smaller as the proportion of Type III collagen increases, perhaps reflecting impaired synthesis of Type I collagen in aged skin.

○   **How much per decade does dermal thickness decrease?**

6% per decade of life in both men and women.

○   **How long must one wait to observe patient for allergic reactions after bovine collagen injection:**

1 month

○   **What is the difference between Group III and Group II in Glogau's classification of photoaging groups?**

Group III (usually age 50-65 years) has actinic keratoses (with obvious yellow skin discoloration) with telangiectasia, wrinkling at rest, moderate acne scarring, and patients always wear makeup.

○   **What defines Group IV Glogau photoaging?**

Actinic keratoses and skin cancers have occurred, wrinkling of actinic, gravitational, and dynamic origin, severe acne scarring, and application of makeup that is typically "caked" on.

LASERS

John B. Hijjawi, MD and Samuel J. Lin, MD

Basic Laser Concepts

○ **What does the acronym LASER stand for?**

Light **A**mplification by **S**timulated **E**mission of **R**adiation.

○ **What are three unique properties of laser light as opposed to natural light?**

1. Coherent-laser light is coherent (all waves are spatially and temporally in phase)
2. Monochromatic-the delivered light is of a single spectral color and of a single precise bandwidth
3. Intense-laser light delivers the greatest number of photons per unit area

○ **What is "thermal relaxation time"?**

Time required for a tissue to absorb and diffuse the thermal energy to surrounding tissue.

○ **What is "pulse energy"?**

The energy of one pulse.

○ **So why do these last two facts matter?**

The pulse duration of a laser should be set for LESS time than the thermal relaxation time of the target tissue if you want the target tissue to be heated and destroyed. If the pulse duration is MORE than the thermal relaxation time, the tissue will absorb and diffuse the energy before it is destroyed.

○ **Therefore what is the optimal pulse duration time?**

A time that is LESS than the thermal relaxation time of the target tissue, but MORE than the thermal relaxation time of the surrounding epidermis.

○ **What is "energy"?**

The capacity to do work in joules.

○ **What is "power"?**

The energy delivered divided by the time of application.

○ **What is "power density" (irradiance)?**

The rate of energy delivered per unit area measured in watts per square centimeter.

○ **What is fluence?**

Total laser energy delivered per unit area expressed as joules per square centimeter. The volume of tissue removed is a function of the amount of energy applied.

○ **What is a continuous wave (CW) laser?**

Lasers producing a constant flow of laser energy and, thus, resulting in significant thermal tissue damage. They can be "gated" by using a physical shutter to interrupt the flow of energy.

○ **What is a pulsed laser?**

These lasers produce high-energy, short pulses without the use of a physical shutter.

○ **What is a Q-switched laser?**

Q-switching produces particularly high-energy, short pulse duration beams.

○ **What is the difference between pulsed-dye, tunable-dye and flash lamp-pumped pulsed dye lasers?**

There is no major difference! They are all used to treat vascular anomalies.

○ **Lasers are selected based on their ability to be selectively absorbed by target tissues. These target tissues in the skin are knows as?**

Chromophores.

Clinical Applications

○ **Name three primary chromophores in the skin.**

- hemoglobin
- water
- melanin

○ **What is selective photothermolysis?**

Selective thermal damage of a pigmented target when sufficient fluence at a wavelength is delivered during a time equal to or less than the thermal relaxation time of the target. More simply, energy is delivered to the target more quickly than the target can dissipate it.

○ **What are the advantages of Q-switched lasers?**

They are highly selective in targeting tattoo pigments rather than the actual tissue (skin) holding the pigment.

○ **What are the disadvantages of Q-switched lasers?**

They are associated with transient hypopigmentation.

○ **The Q-switched ruby laser is absorbed by which chromophores?**

- melanin
- carbon in tattoo pigments

○ **What are the clinical applications of the Q-switched ruby laser?**

- pigmented cutaneous lesions (nevus of Ota, café-au-lait spots)
- purple, violet and black ink in professional and amateur tattoos
- traumatic tattoos (embedded carbon)

○ **What are the results of café-au-lait spot treatment with Q-switched ruby lasers?**

While lightening of spots is evident in many patients after about 4-6 treatments, recurrence of the spots is the rule in most cases.

○ **A patient comes to you with a dark rectangle on their upper arm. They tell you a local surgeon used a Q-switched <u>ruby</u> laser to try removing a tattoo of the Canadian flag. What happened and will it get better?**

Q-switched ruby lasers are <u>contraindicated</u> for red, white and skin-colored pigments because they can convert the iron in <u>ferric oxide to ferrous oxide,</u> darkening the pigment <u>irreversibly</u>.

○ **What is the ideal laser for removing a blue-green tattoo?**

•   <u>Q-switched alexandrite laser.</u>
•   Remember, the <u>blue-green</u> waters of the Nile were right outside our hotel window when we visited <u>Alexandria</u>, Egypt.

○ **What is the ideal laser for removing red, orange or brown tattoos?**

•   The Q-switched Nd:YAG laser.
•   Remember going to the <u>N</u>otre <u>D</u>ame (<u>Nd</u>:YAG) football game in the fall, when the leaves were turning <u>red, orange and brown</u>.

○ **Your tattoo removal patient comes in after his second treatment with a Q-switched laser furious that his tattoo is still visible. What do you tell him?**

•   tattoo removal typically takes 3-10 treatments
•   more for professional tattoos
•   fewer for amateur and traumatic tattoos
•   good results are reported in 75-95% of patients

○ **The carbon dioxide laser is absorbed by which chromophores?**

•   Water

○ **What are clinical applications of the carbon dioxide laser then?**

CO_2 lasers are highly absorbed by water in skin. This makes them highly effective for:
•   <u>skin resurfacing of fine rhytids</u>
•   cutting
•   coagulation

○ **Is tretinoin or isotretinoin used for skin preparation before dermabrasion?**

<u>Tretinoin is used</u>. <u>Isotretinoin (Accutane) is contraindicated</u> for 1 year before laser or dermabrasion due to risk of scarring and delayed healing.

○ **Your patient returns to the office with a painful vesicular rash around her mouth 4 days after a CO2 resurfacing treatment. What should you do?**

Treat this <u>HSV outbreak with Acyclovir</u>. Consider prophylactic treatment in any future patient with a history of cold sores.

○ **The tunable-dye laser is absorbed by which chromophores?**

oxyhemoglobin

○ **What are the clinical applications of the tunable-dye (or pulsed-dye) laser then?**

Cutaneous vascular lesions such as:
- port-wine stains
- capillary malformations
- telangiectasias
- spider angiomas

○ **What chromophore is absorbed by the Erbium:YAG laser?**

Water; and it does so 10 times more efficiently than a CO_2 laser.

○ **What is the process by which an Er:YAG laser results in ablative resurfacing?**

A photomechanical process rather than a photothermal process.

○ **What are the primary applications of the Er:YAG laser?**

Ablative resurfacing of the skin.

○ **What are the advantages of the Er:YAG laser over the CO_2 laser in terms of skin resurfacing?**

- less thermal damage to surrounding tissue
- more rapid re-epithelialization
- 5-10% risk of hypopigmentation vs. 40% with CO_2 lasers

○ **What disadvantage do erbium lasers have?**

- they result in a transudative wound
- less dramatic skin tightening than CO_2 lasers

○ **What laser is used for treating lymphatic malformations?**

Erbium laser at 2910 nm.

References

Wittenberg, G. P., Fabian, B. G., Bogomilsky, J. L., Schultz, L. R., Rudner, E. J., Chaffins, M. L., Saed, G. M., Burns, R. L., Fivenson, D. P. (1999). Prospective, Single-blind, Randomized, Controlled Study to Assess the Efficacy of the 585-nm Flashlamp-Pumped Pulsed-Dye Laser and Silicone Gel Sheeting in Hypertrophic Scar Treatment. *Arch Dermatol* 135: 1049-1055.

Utley DS, Koch RJ, Egbert BM: Histologic analysis of the thermal effect on epidermal and dermal structures following treatment with the superpulsed CO_2 laser and the erbium: YAG laser: an in vivo study. *Lasers Surg Med* 1999; 24(2): 93-102.

Grossman MC, Anderson RR, Farinelli W, Flotte TJ, Grevelink JM. Treatment of cafe au lait macules with lasers. A clinicopathologic correlation. *Arch Dermatol.* 1995 Dec;131(12):1416-20.

Ashinoff R, Geronemus RG: Q-switched ruby laser treatment of labial lentigos. *J Am Acad Dermatol* 1992 Nov; 27(5 Pt 2): 809-11.

Alster TS: Cutaneous resurfacing with CO2 and Erbium: YAG lasers: preoperative, intraoperative, and postoperative considerations. *Plast Reconstr Surg* 1999 Feb; 103(2): 619-32.

INJECTABLE FILLERS

Brian S. Glatt, MD

○ **What are the most desirable characteristics of a soft tissue filler?**

- Long lasting
- High use potential
- Easily obtainable
- Biocompatible
- Nonresorbable
- Nonallergenic
- Nonteratogenic
- Noncarcinogenic
- Nonmigratory
- Versatile
- Inexpensive
- Reproducible
- Easily stored
- Minimal side effects

○ **Which kind of filler is considered the "gold standard" by which others are judged?**

Collagen (Zyderm)

○ **What are the most common autologous materials used as injectables?**

Fat, Isolagen, Autologen

○ **What are advantages to using autologous tissue for soft tissue augmentation?**

It is theoretically the ideal filler. It is safe, nontoxic, easily obtainable, and there is no risk of allergic reaction or tissue rejection.

○ **What are disadvantages to using autologous tissue for soft tissue augmentation?**

Potentially limited availability and requires additional surgical procedure.

○ **In what facial areas are fat grafts most effective and long lasting?**

While fat has been used to inject almost every area of the face, certain areas respond better (i.e. the effect lasts longer) to fat grafting. These are more static areas or areas rendered more static by pre-treatment with Botox. Dynamic areas of the face, such as the lips, do not respond as well to fat grafting.

○ **How should fat be injected to ensure maximal effect?**

To maximize fat graft survival, vascularity of the grafts must occur. This is optimized by injecting in a "chain of pearls" technique where small fat droplets are injected in rows into several different planes so each graft can be adequately individually revascularized. In addition, gentle handling and processing of the fat as well as injection via proper cannulas will all help to improve fat graft take.

○ **What is Isolagen?**

A filler consisting of 1-1.5 cc of the patient's own fibroblasts derived from a prior skin biopsy sent into the company. Culture and processing of the biopsy usually takes about 6 weeks. Patients typically require 2-4 treatments to see any improvement.

O   **Are results immediately seen following injection of Isolagen?**

No, results are usually delayed 3-4 months as this product depends upon production of new collagen by the patient's own fibroblasts to have an effect.

O   **Who can Isolagen not be used on?**

Patients > 60 years old. It is thought that their skin is not capable of producing "hearty" enough fibroblasts for this treatment.

O   **How does Autologen differ from Isolagen?**

Autologen is produced from a sample of the patient's own skin (following some other cosmetic procedure) as well, however following processing, the end product is a suspension of the patient's own collagen. A more significant amount of skin is required for production of Autologen.

O   **What is Zyderm/Zyplast?**

Sterile, purified, fibrillar suspensions of bovine-derived dermal collagen suspended in PBS and lidocaine (0.3%). The collagen is derived from calf skins from a closed herd.

O   **What type of collagen is contained in Zyderm/Zyplast?**

95-98% Type I collagen. The rest is type III.

O   **What is the difference between Zyderm-1 and Zyderm-2?**

The concentration of collagen. Zyderm-2 has almost 2x the concentration of collagen (65 mg/ml) than Zyderm-1 (35 mg/ml).

O   **What is Zyplast?**

Zyderm 2 that has been cross-linked with glutaraldehyde.

O   **What effect does glutaraldehyde cross-linking have on a filler?**

Cross-linking is thought to make a filler more resistant to proteolytic degradation as well as making it more viscous in quality and possibly less immunogenic.

O   **How long does collagen usually last as a soft tissue filler?**

Typically, collagen fillers are thought to completely resorb within 3 months.

O   **When should allergy testing take place prior to injecting bovine collagen?**

Initially at 1 month prior to definitive injection. Skin should be examined for an allergic reaction after 3 days and after 1 month.

O   **What is the rate of allergic reaction to bovine collagen skin testing?**

Approximately 3.5%. In addition, 1-5% of patients may still experience an allergic reaction after one negative test.

❍ **What product is used for allergic skin testing prior to collagen injections?**

A test syringe of 0.3 cc of Zyderm I is the standard testing agent. Only about 0.1 cc is used for the actual test.

❍ **How does Cosmoderm/Cosmoplast differ from Zyderm/Zyplast?**

Cosmoderm/Cosmoplast are analogous to Zyderm/Zyplast, however are human-derived collagen products. In addition, allergy testing is not necessary with Cosmoderm/Cosmoplast due to a low incidence of sensitivity. Allergy testing is ALWAYS required prior to injecting Zyderm/Zyplast.

❍ **What is hyaluronic acid (HA)?**

Hyaluronic acid is a naturally-occurring polysaccharide that makes up a majority of the intercellular matrix in human soft tissues.

❍ **Do you need to perform a skin test prior to using a hyaluronic acid filler?**

No. HA is a polysaccharide which is chemically, physically, and biologically identical in the tissues of all species, therefore it is biocompatible to use animal sources in humans without the risk of hypersensitivity reactions.

❍ **What is the main difference between Hylaform and Restylane?**

While both consist of hyaluronic acid as a filler material, Hylaform is developed from rooster combs (animal based), while Restylane is developed via fermentation of sugar by equine streptococci.

❍ **What level of the dermis should HA fillers be injected?**

The upper reticular dermis.

❍ **Do more concentrated formulations of HA cause a greater effect?**

No, because HA is found in the ground substance, it absorbs water and expands. The less concentrated it is, the more water it can bind, and a theoretically longer-lasting result may be produced.

❍ **How long do HA fillers usually last?**

Originally it was thought that HA fillers show effects up to a year, however recent evidence has shown that the effect probably lasts for 6 months at most.

❍ **What is Perlane?**

A more viscous formulation of Restylane with a much larger gel particle size used in the deeper dermis and typically placed subdermally to treat deeper folds.

❍ **What is Cymetra?**

An injectable particulate form of Alloderm, an acellular human dermal allograft derived from cadaveric skin in which the epidermis is removed via a freeze-drying process.

❍ **If it is processed from human tissue, doesn't Cymetra induce a severe allergenic response upon injection?**

No. The processing of Cymetra produces a cell-free dermal product, and therefore does not produce a specific nor a nonspecific inflammatory response. In fact, there is a notable lack of tissue reactivity after implantation.

❍ **What is Radiance?**

Synthetically processed calcium hydroxyapatite beads in an aqueous based gel carrier. The calcium hydroxyapatite has the chemical composition of the major mineral component of bone.

○   **How does Radiance work?**

Fibrous encapsulation of the hydroxyapatite particles creates a well-formed non scar tissue matrix. The implant site does not ossify and it remains soft and flexible, as small, natural movements prevent hardening.

○   **Is Radiance permanent?**

It is not permanent, however its effect is thought to be long-lasting, at least 3 years. Long-term studies still need to be done.

○   **Is liquid silicone safe for use as a soft tissue filler?**

Liquid Injectable silicone (LIS) is FDA approved only for ophthalmologic use in the U.S.

○   **When injected into the skin, how does liquid silicone produce soft tissue augmentation?**

Inflammatory cell reaction to the silicone induces fibroplasia formation around the material, and thus increased collagen deposition, sometimes excessively so, within the treated area.

○   **How can the fibroplasia response be controlled following silicone injection?**

It cannot; over time in some patients, continued growth can become excessive and result in distortion of the injected area. For this reason, in 1965 the FDA prohibited the use of silicone as an injection into the skin.

○   **What is Artecoll?**

Polymethylmethacrylate (PMMA) microspheres suspended in bovine collagen.

○   **Is Artecoll considered a permanent filler?**

Yes, methylmethacrylate is a permanent substance.

○   **How does Artecoll work as a filler?**

The collagen suspension is thought to provide an immediate effect, while fibrosis around the PMMA leads to long-lasting correction as the bovine collagen dissipates over time.

○   **Is skin testing required prior to injection with Artecoll?**

Yes, due to the collagen in the suspension mixture.

○   **At what level should Artecoll be injected into the dermis?**

Artecoll should not be injected into the dermis as palpable thickening and extrusion of the PMMA beads may occur. It should be injected deeper into a subdermal level.

○   **What is Sculptra?**

Sculptra is composed of injectable poly-L-lactic acid microparticles. Poly-L-lactic acid is a biodegradable, biocompatible synthetic polymer from the alpha-hydroxy-acid family. This agent provides a gradual increase in effect after the initial treatment, so undercorrection should always be performed. Sculptra not only provides volume to facial tissues, but also produces a significant increase in dermal thickness (2-3x baseline values). In addition, 2-3 treatments, spaced several weeks or months apart, are usually necessary to see optimal results.

○ **For what condition(s) should Sculptra be used?**

Sculptra is FDA approved in the U.S. only for the treatment of HIV associated lipodystrophy of the face. All other uses are presently considered "off-label".

○ **What is Botox-A?**

Botox-A is a purified form of the most commonly used, and most potent, serotype of botulinum neurotoxin.

○ **What is the mechanism of action of Botox-A?**

Blockade of presynaptic acetylcholine release by binding to specific cell surface receptors.

○ **What effect does Botox-A have on affected muscle groups?**

Muscle fibers become functionally denervated resulting in muscle fiber atrophy and flaccid paralysis. This causes the disappearance of wrinkles on the skin related to that particular treated muscle's action.

○ **What is the time of onset to see the effects of Botox-A?**

Onset of action is 6-36 hours, however maximal effect takes 7-14 days.

○ **How does muscle function recover following paralysis via Botox-A?**

New neuromuscular junctions form and new axonal sprouting replaces nonfunctional muscle junctions to restore function by 3-6 months.

○ **For what aesthetic use is Botox-A officially FDA approved?**

Treatment of glabellar frown lines. Other indications are still considered "off-label."

○ **What muscle is affected when inadvertent ptosis occurs following Botox to the glabella?**

Paralysis of the levator aponeurosis.

○ **How can the effect of Botox be reversed in the case of inadvertent ptosis?**

Naphcon A Ophthalmic (naphazoline hydrochloride / pheniramine maleate) or with Iopidine Ophthalmic Solution 0.5% (apraclinidine hydrochloride); both eye drops provide adrenergic stimulation of Müellers muscle to counteract lid ptosis.

○ **What is the recommended diluent for Botox-A?**

Unpreserved normal saline.

○ **What are contraindications to the use of Botox?**

Hypersensitivity to ingredients (albumin)
History of neuromuscular disease (e.g. myasthenia gravis)
Pregnancy/lactation
Patients on anticoagulation or aspirin
Phobia of injections
Patients treated with aminoglycosides, penicillamine, quinine, Ca channel blockers (these agents can potentiate the effects of botulinum toxin)
Poor psychological adjustment

References

Ashinoff, R. Overview: Soft Tissue Augmentation. Clin Plast Surg 2000; 27(4):479-487.

Coleman SR. Structural Fat Grafts: The Ideal Filler? Clin Plast Surg 2001; 28(1):111-119.

Ellenbogen R. Fat Transfer: Current Use in Practice. Clin Plast Surg 2000; 27(4):545-556.

Frank P, Gendler E. Hyaluronic Acid for Soft-Tissue Augmentation. Clin Plast Surg 2001; 28(1):121-126.

Glatt BS, Bucky LP. Expert Commentary on Injectable Fillers in Facial Aesthetic Surgery. In: Mauriello JA, ed. Techniques of Cosmetic Eyelid Surgery. Philadelphia: Lippincott, Williams, & Wilkins, 2004:268-276.

Gorssman KL. Facial Scars. Clin Plast surg 2000; 27(4):627-642.

Klein A. Collagen substitutes. Clin Plast Surg 2001; 28(1):53-62.

Matarasso A, Deva AK, et al. Botulinum Toxin. Plast Reconstr Surg 2003; 112 (suppl):55S-61S.

Matarasso A, Chia C, at al. Botulinum Toxin. Plast Reconstr surg 2003; 112 (suppl):62S-65S.

Moyle GJ, Lysakova L, Brown S, et al. A randomized open-label study of immediate versus delayed polylactic acid injections for the cosmetic management of facial lipoatrophy in persons with HIV infection. HIV Med. 2004; 5:82-87.

Rohrich RJ, Janis JE, Fagien S, Stuzin JM. The Cosmetic Use of Botulinum Toxin. Plast Reconstr Surg 2003; 112 (suppl):177S-187S.

HAIR REMOVAL/HAIR TRANSPLANTATION

Dimitrios Danikas, MD and Anthony Labruna, MD

○ **What is the genetic basis of male pattern alopecia?**

A single, dominant, sex-linked autosomal gene. An increased level of 5alpha-reductase activity has been noted in susceptible follicles.

○ **Are testosterone and estrogen levels elevated in patients with male pattern alopecia?**

No, testosterone and estrogen levels are normal as are adrenal and liver functions.

○ **What is the Hamilton system of male alopecia?**

Hamilton's classification system of male alopecia is based on the appearance of hair loss at the anterior hairline and the vertex. It has seven classifications regarding the potential for further hair loss.
1 - no hair loss
2 - mild temporal recession
2A- frontal recession - mild
3 - moderate temporal recession
3A- frontal recession - moderate
3V- moderate vertex loss
4-6 - progressive involvement of the vertex and temporal areas
7 - complete loss of frontal and vertex regions

○ **What is donor site dominance?**

Donor site dominance is the ability of hair graft to maintain the integrity and its characteristics independent of the recipient site. It applies to all patients and all scalp areas with alopecia.

○ **Which is the best donor site area?**

The occipital area. Occipital hairs have the longest life span.

○ **In what areas is androgenic (or androgenetic) alopecia more common?**

Androgenic alopecia is more common in the frontal and crown areas of the scalp.

○ **What is the most common inheritance pattern in male baldness?**

A single X-linked autosomal dominant trait is the most common cause of alopecia in men.

○ **What affects the expressivity of the alopecia gene?**

A normal adult male serum androgen level and age.

○ **What are the phases of the hair follicle growth cycle?**

Anagen, catagen and telogen.

❍   **What are the characteristics of the phases of the hair growth cycle?**

The anagen phase lasts 3 years and is the time of active hair growth, about 90% of the scalp's hair are in this phase at any given time. The catagen phase lasts 2 to 3 weeks and is the time of hair loss. The telogen phase lasts 3 to 4 months and there is no hair growth. About 10% of the scalp's hair is in this phase.

❍   **What phase is associated with male pattern alopecia?**

It is associated with a prolonged telogen (no growth) phase and a shortened anagen (active growth) phase.

❍   **What enzyme is associated with male alopecia?**

Genetically susceptible follicles have increased 5alpha-reductase activity.

❍   **What is the action of 5alpha-reductase?**

Converts testosterone into dihydroxytestosterone.

❍   **What is the mechanism of action of finasteride (Propecia)?**

Inhibition of 5alpha-reductase activity.

❍   **Where are the hair follicles located?**

They are indentations of the epidermis located in the subcutaneous layer of the scalp.

❍   **Can a hair grow without the hair bulb?**

The hair bulb is not necessary for hair growth. If the upper two thirds of the hair follicle are transplanted 30% of them will produce new hair.

❍   **What is a micrograft?**

A micrograft contains one or two hair follicles.

❍   **What is a minigraft?**

A minigraft contains three or four hair follicles. A large minigraft contains 5 to 6 hair follicles.

❍   **What is a standard hair graft (a.k.a. punch graft)?**

A round graft 3.5 or 4.5 mm or larger with 8 to 30 hair follicles.

❍   **Where standard grafts should be used?**

In areas where maximum hair density is desired.

❍   **What is the disadvantage of standard grafts?**

Multiple procedures. Patients with dark hair and fair skin may have a "doll" like appearance.

❍   **How long should you wait before repeat placement of standard punch grafts for treatment of male pattern alopecia?**

The surgeon should wait four months because the transplanted hair grows for up to one month and then enters the telogen phase, which lasts another two to three months.

○ **What is the pattern of hair growth after punch grafting?**

Hair growth for one month, then hair loss and normal hair growth after three months.

○ **What is the rate of hair growth six months after a punch graft?**

Normal permanent hair growth at 1 cm monthly.

○ **What is the best technique for anterior hairline and vertex restoration in a patient with dark hair and fair scalp?**

Micrografts and minigrafts.

○ **Why is this?**

Large "punch" grafts of dark hair against the scalp of a light-skinned patient are particularly obvious and susceptible to a "doll" like appearance. Micrografts or minigrafts can be:
1) placed into slit like incisions avoiding scars
2) placed at irregular intervals mimicking the natural hairline
3) have a more acceptable appearance during healing than punch grafts

○ **What is the treatment of a slightly elevated hair graft?**

Light electrodesiccation.

○ **What is the treatment of a slightly depressed hair graft?**

Excision and replacement with a new graft at the same level as the recipient area.

○ **What is the indication for scalp reduction?**

The patient with a stable bald area in the crown or vertex region of the scalp and reasonably dense hair in the temporal and occipital regions. This procedure can significantly reduce the amount of grafting that needs to be done.

○ **What are some common pitfalls of scalp reduction?**

Anterior undermining should be avoided to avoid elevation of the eyebrows. Serial excision is often required as each excision is limited to approximately 4cm depending on the patient's scalp elasticity.

○ **What are some disadvantages of scalp reduction?**

1) If alopecia is unstable, scars can become obvious as more hair is lost. Z-plasties or hair grafts can be used to camouflage such scars.
2) Landmarks such as the eyebrows can be distorted.
3) It is not indicated in patients with residual central hair requiring reconstruction of the anterior hairline.

○ **What is the disadvantage of tissue expansion?**

Multiple procedures and anterior scars. During the expansion process the patient is not pleased with their appearance.

○ **What is the main advantage of tissue expansion for treatment of alopecia?**

The hair follicles will be oriented correctly and as much as 50% of the skull can be covered.

○ **When is excision and primary closure indicated?**

For defects measuring less than 5 cm.

Hair Removal

○ **What does the acronym LASER stand for?**

<u>L</u>ight <u>A</u>mplification by <u>S</u>timulated <u>E</u>mission of <u>R</u>adiation.

○ **What are three unique properties of laser light as opposed to natural light?**

1) <u>Coherent</u>-laser light is coherent (all waves are spatially and temporally in phase)
2) <u>Monochromatic</u>-the delivered light is of a single spectral color and of a single precise bandwidth
3) <u>Intense</u>-laser light delivers the greatest number of photons per unit area

○ **What is "thermal relaxation time"?**

Time required for a tissue to absorb and diffuse the thermal energy to surrounding tissue.

○ **What is "pulse energy"?**

The energy of one pulse.

○ **So why do these last two facts matter?**

The <u>pulse duration</u> of a laser should be set for LESS time than the <u>thermal relaxation time</u> of the target tissue if you want the target tissue to be heated and destroyed. If the pulse duration is MORE than the thermal relaxation time, the tissue will absorb and diffuse the energy before it is destroyed.

○ **Therefore what is the optimal pulse duration time?**

A time that is LESS than the <u>thermal relaxation time</u> of the hair follicle, but MORE than the <u>thermal relaxation time</u> of the surrounding epidermis.

○ **What is "energy"?**

The capacity to do work in joules.

○ **What is "power"?**

The energy delivered divided by the time of application.

○ **What is "power density" (irradiance)?**

The rate of energy delivered per unit area measured in watts per square centimeter.

○ **What is fluence?**

Total laser energy delivered per unit area expressed as joules per square centimeter. The volume of tissue removed is a function of the amount of energy applied.

○ **Lasers are selected based on their ability to be selectively absorbed by target tissues. These target tissues in the skin are knows as?**

Chromophobes.

○ **Name three primary chromophobes in the skin.**

Hemoglobin, water, melanin

○ **What are you targeting in laser hair removal?**

The melanin in the hair follicle.

○ **Who are the ideal patients?**

Those with dark hair and light skin.

○ **What if the patient has light hair?**

Some centers offer a carbon suspension that can be rubbed into the follicle enhancing absorption.

○ **What are some contraindications to laser hair removal?**

1) Current use of photo-sensitizing agents (i.e. Accutane, Retin-A, tetracycline)
2) Patients with grey hair-no current lasers are effective at removing grey hair
3) Patients with a significant tan at the time of treatment
4) Patients with a history of herpes simplex virus should have the possibility of reactivation discussed and be placed on antiviral medication if treatment is pursued

○ **What is selective photothermolysis?**

Selective thermal damage of a pigmented target when sufficient fluence at a wavelength is delivered during a time equal to or less than the thermal relaxation time of the target. More simply, energy is delivered to the target more quickly than the target can dissipate it.

○ **How does selective photodermolysis work?**

Removes hair that has melanin and is in the anagen (growth) phase. Therefore, repeat treatments are usually needed. Also it prolongs the telogen (inactive) phase. Usually there is hair re-growth after a year.

○ **What technique should be used?**

Non-overlapping or minimally overlapping laser pulses delivered with a predetermined spot size. The largest spot size and the highest tolerable fluence will give the best results.

○ **How long should be the treatment interval?**

Laser hair removal requires the presence of a pigmented hair shaft. Therefore, repeat treatment can be performed as soon as regrowth appears. Regrowth is based on the natural cycle, which varies by anatomic location, but the average time is one month.

○ **Is laser hair removal a painless procedure?**

No, hair removal is not a painless procedure. Patients experience discomfort during treatment. A local anesthetic should be applied before treatment.

References

Argenta LC, Marks MW and Pesky KA: Advances in tissue expansion. Clin Plast Surg. 12: 159-71, 1985.

Bell ML: Scalp reduction. Clin Plast Surg. 9: 269-78, 1982.

Derrick C: Laser-Assisted Hair Removal, emedicine.com, 2004.

Oren Reich N and Dorr NP: Biology of scalp hair growth. Clin Plast Surg. 9: 197-205, 1982.

Price VH: Treatment of hair loss. N Engl J Med. 341: 964-73, 1999.

Umbel CO: Micrografts and minigrafts: a new approach for baldness surgery. Ann Plast Surg. 27: 476-87, 1991.

Unger W: Treatment for Baldness, in Aston S, Beasley R and CHM Thorne: Grabb and Smith's Plastic Surgery. Philadelphia, Lippincott-Raven, 1997, pp 569-85.

Vales C: Hair replacement surgery, in JG M: Plastic Surgery. Philadelphia, WB Saunders Co, 1990, vol. 2, pp 1519.

Voigt W, Castro A, Covey DF and Robinson CH: Inhibition of testosterone 5 alpha-reeducates by and antiandrogenicity of allenic 3-keto-5,10-secosteroids. Acta Endocrinol (Copenh). 87: 668-72, 1978.

BODY CONTOURING

Ajaipal S. Kang, MD

○ **Outline the blood supply zones of unoperated abdomen.**

Zone I is the midabdomen, supplied by deep epigastric arcade.
Zone II is the lower abdomen, supplied by external iliac artery system.
Zone III is the flanks and lateral abdomen, supplied by intercostal, subcostal, and lumbar arteries.

○ **What zone is responsible for blood supply to abdominoplasty flap?**

Zone III with some minor collateral flow from zone II

○ **What is the major blood supply to the abdominoplasty flap?**

The lateral intercostal vessels.

○ **What nerve is responsible for numbness of anterolateral thigh after abdominoplasty?**

The lateral femoral cutaneous nerve of the thigh

○ **Name the nerves that are at increased risk for entrapment or injury during abdominoplasty.**

Iliohypogastric, ilioinguinal and intercostal nerves are at an increased risk of injury.

○ **What kind of previous abdominal scar can cause postoperative healing problems in an abdominoplasty patient?**

A supraumbilical scar may hinder dissection and impair blood supply and thus, can lead to wound healing problems.

○ **What is the difference between mini vs. full abdominoplasty?**

Mini-abdominoplasty removes mild amount of lower abdominal skin and fat. The position of umbilicus remains unchanged and the length of the scar is limited. Full abdominoplasty removes excess skin and fat from lower abdomen, plicates the rectus fascia and relocates umbilicus through an elongated scar.

○ **What is the optimal treatment for an obese male with a massive pannus?**

The best treatment is simple, transverse, elliptical wedge resection i.e. panniculectomy.

○ **In a post-abdominoplasty patient, what area has the most tenuous blood supply?**

The suprapubic and lower midline region is at greatest risk for ischemia and necrosis.

○ **What is the most common complication of combined abdominoplasty and liposuction?**

Seroma formation is the most common complication in this situation. The risk is higher in smokers and diabetics.

○ **What operative technique is considered critical in long-term success of body contouring procedures?**

The repair of superficial fascial system provides lasting support.

○ **What is the common location of incision in a massive weight loss patient with redundancy of arm skin?**

The skin should be excised through a medial elliptical incision from medial epicondyle to axillary dome.

○   **What is the most common long-term unfavorable result in a patient undergoing posterior belt lipectomy?**

The common unfavorable results are hypertrophic scarring and asymmetry and flattening of the buttocks.

○   **What operative technique can decrease the incidence of scar widening and ptosis in a patient undergoing medial thigh lift?**

Superficial fascial system should be suspended to Colles' fascia to decrease scar widening and ptosis.

○   **What is the mechanism of arm ptosis and what is appropriate management?**

The mechanism is by loosening of connections of superficial fascial system to the axillary fascia. The operative treatment is brachioplasty.

○   **What is the most common long-term complication of brachioplasty?**

Wide scar is the most common long-term complication.

○   **What is the infiltrate-to-aspirate ratio in superwet suction lipectomy?**

In this case, an equal volume of fat is removed, i.e. infiltrate-to-aspirate ratio of 1:1.

○   **Name the "zones of adherence" of lower extremity as it pertains to liposuction.**

The five zones of adherence are: Inferolateral iliotibial tract, gluteal crease, lateral gluteal depression, distal posterior thigh and middle medial thigh.

○   **What volume of aspirate constitutes "large volume"?**

Lipoaspirate greater than 5 L is considered "large" volume and warrants closer observation and monitoring.

○   **What is the composition of typical tumescent solution?**

The tumescent formula combines 1 L of 0.9% normal saline with 50 cc of 1% lidocaine, 1 cc (1 amp) of 1:1000 epinephrine, and 2.5 cc of 8.4% sodium bicarbonate.

○   **Name the different types of subcutaneous infiltration techniques.**

Dry, wet, superwet and tumescent are the four commonly described techniques.

○   **What is the typical blood loss in superwet technique?**

1%.

○   **What is the most common postoperative complication of liposuction?**

The most common complication is contour irregularities.

○   **What are the main determinants that help to select the optimal procedure for body contouring?**

The optimal procedure is based on the patient's skin tone, abdominal wall musculature, and fat distribution.

○   **Are the fat cells removed during liposuction permanently lost?**

Yes, the cells once removed will never be replaced. However, the remaining fat cells may hypertrophy.

○ **What is the most common cause of death following liposuction?**

Thromboembolism. The rate is one in 5000 procedures in the outpatient setting. Most of the deaths occur during the first 24 hours.

○ **Are liposuction and abdominoplasty considered weight loss operations for obese patients?**

No, these are body contouring operations and should not be confused with weight loss operations, such as gastric bypass.

○ **What is the mechanism of action of ultrasound-assisted liposuction?**

Intense ultrasonic energy disrupts adipocyte cell membranes. It does not disrupt the fibrous connective tissue that surrounds fat cells.

References

Huger WE Jr. The anatomic rationale for abdominal lipectomy. Am Surg. 1979;45:612-617.

Mladick RA. Body contouring of the abdomen, thighs, hips, and buttocks. In: Georgiade GS, Riefkohl R, Levin LS, eds. Textbook of Plastic, Maxillofacial and Reconstructive Surgery. 3rd ed. Baltimore, Md: Williams & Wilkins; 1997:674-684.

Floros C, Davis PK. Complications and long-term results following abdominoplasty: a retrospective study. Br J Plast Surg. 1991;44:190-194.

Matarasso A. Abdominoplasty. In: Achauer BM, Eriksson E, Guyuron B, et al, eds. Plastic Surgery: Indications, Operations, and Outcomes. Saint Louis, Mo: Mosby Ð Year Book, Inc; 2000;5:2783-2821.

de Castro CC, Aboudib JHC, Salema R, et al. How to deal with abdominoplasty in an abdomen with a scar. Aesthetic Plast Surg. 1993;17:67-71

Grazer FM. Abdominoplasty. In: McCarthy JG, ed. Plastic Surgery. Philadelphia, Pa: WB Saunders Co; 1990;6:3929-3963.

Lockwood T. Contouring of the arms, trunk, and thighs. In: Achauer BM, Eriksson E, Guyuron B, et al, eds. Plastic Surgery: Indications, Operations, and Outcomes. Saint Louis, Mo: Mosby Ð Year Book, Inc; 2000;5:2839-2857.

Baroudi R, Kleppke BM, Carvalho CG. Mammary reduction combined with reverse abdominoplasty. Ann Plast Surg. 1979;2:368.

Matarasso A. Liposuction as an adjunct to a full abdominoplasty. Plast Reconstr Surg. 1995;5:829-836.

Lockwood TE. Superficial fascial system (SFS) of the trunk and extremities: a new concept. Plast Reconstr Surg. 1991;87:1009-1018.

Grazer FM. Body contouring. In: McCarthy JG, ed. Plastic Surgery. Philadelphia, Pa: WB Saunders Co, 1990;6:3964.

Lockwood T. Lower body lift with superficial fascial system suspension. Plast Reconstr Surg. 1993;92:1112-1125.

Lockwood T. Brachioplasty with superficial fascial system suspension. Plast Reconstr Surg. 1995;96:912-920.

Klein JA. Tumescent technique for local anesthesia improves safely in large-volume liposuction. Plast Reconstr Surg. 1993;92:1085-1100.

Grazer FM, de Jong RH. Fatal outcomes from liposuction: census survey of cosmetic surgeons. Plast Reconstr Surg. 2000;105:436.

Zocchi ME. Ultrasonic assisted lipoplasty: technical refinements and clinical evaluations. Clin Plast Surg. 1996;23:575-598.

GYNECOMASTIA

Christine Fisher and Ned Snyder IV, MD

○ **What is gynecomastia?**

An increase in ductal tissue and stroma that occurs during periods of hormonal change.

○ **When does gynecomastia most commonly occur?**

Infancy, adolescence, and old age.

○ **What is the incidence and cause of newborn gynecomastia?**

60%, transplacental passage of estrogens.

○ **What is the incidence, peak age, and average duration of pubertal gynecomastia?**

75%, peak age 14-15 years old, 1-2 year duration.

○ **What is the typical size of male pubertal breasts?**

2-2.5 cm

○ **In what percentage of adolescent males does pubertal gynecomastia resolve within 2 years?**

75%

○ **What is the prevalence of gynecomastia in middle aged men?**

30%

○ **What is the prevalence of gynecomastia by the seventh decade?**

>60%

○ **What are the potential etiologies of gynecomastia?**

Physiologic, pathologic, pharmacologic

○ **What are common causes of physiologic gynecomastia?**

Increased estrogens, decreased androgens, decreased androgen receptors, testicle malfunction, familial, idiopathic, debilitating disease (such as burns).

○ **What are common pathologic causes of gynecomastia?**

Hepatitis, cirrhosis, malnutrition, hypogonadism, Kleinfelter's, neoplasms, renal disease, thyroid disease.

○ **What are common neoplastic causes of gynecomastia?**

Testicular (leydig or sertoli cell tumors, choriocarcinoma) adrenal tumors, pituitary adenomas, lung carcinomas, colon or prostate cancer, carcinoma of the breast.

O   **Name some common pharmacologic causes of gynecomastia.**

<u>S</u>ome (spironolactone) <u>M</u>en (marijuana) <u>C</u>an (cimetidine) <u>D</u>evelop (diazepam) <u>R</u>ather (reserpine) <u>E</u>xcessive (estrogens) <u>T</u>horacic (theophylline) <u>D</u>iameters (digoxin)

O   **What causes bilateral increase in breast size as a result of fat deposition without hyperplasia of breast tissue?**

Pseudogynecomastia

O   **What are the three types of gynecomastia?**

Florid, fibrous, intermediate

O   **What is the tissue type and duration of florid gynecomastia?**

Vascular and ductal tissue, usually less than 4 months in duration.

O   **What is the tissue type and duration of fibrous gynecomastia?**

Acellular fibrous stroma with few ducts, <12 months in duration.

O   **Are true acinar lobules seen in the breasts of men with gynecomastia?**

No.

O   **On what areas should the review of systems focus when interviewing a man with gynecomastia?**

Organ changes in the liver, testes, prostate, adrenal, pituitary, lungs, thyroid.

O   **If the testicles are asymmetric in a man with gynecomastia what test should be ordered and why?**

Ultrasound to rule out a testicular tumor.

O   **In a man with gynecomastia and small testicles what test should be ordered?**

Chromosome study for Kleinfelter's

O   **What is the incidence of breast cancer in patients with Kleinfelter's?**

The incidence is 20 to 60 times higher than men with a normal karyotype.

O   **Is there an increased incidence of breast cancer in 46XY men with gynecomastia?**

No.

O   **What labs should be ordered in the evaluation of a man with gynecomastia?**

Liver function tests, urine 17-ketosteroids, gonadotropic hormones, HCG, testosterone, and estrogen.

O   **If estradiol is elevated what is the next test that should be ordered?**

CT scan of the adrenal glands to evaluate for tumors.

O   **If human chorionic gonadotropin (HCG) is elevated what is the next test that should be ordered?**

Ultrasound for testicular tumor

○ **If testosterone is low and LH/FSH are elevated, what is the next test that should be ordered?**

Karyotype to evaluate for Kleinfelter's

○ **What are the indications for gynecomastia surgery?**

Adolescents with gynecomastia for more than 18-24 months, fibrotic or symptomatic male breasts, men at risk for carcinoma of the breast (Kleinfelter's)

○ **What are the surgical classifications of gynecomastia?**

Grade 1: Button of tissue >0.5cm localized to the areola
Grade 2A: Moderate breast enlargement only
Grade 2B: Moderate enlargement with skin redundancy
Grade 3: Very enlarged breasts with redundant skin

○ **For which types of gynecomastia might liposuction be adequate?**

Grade 1 or 2A.

○ **Where should an incision be placed to maximize the cosmetic outcome of male mastectomy?**

Periareolar incision: at the junction of the areola and the skin.

○ **Why are incisions in the areola avoided?**

Scars in the pigmented areolar skin are white.

○ **What is the concern about incisions into the skin lateral to the areola?**

Increased likelihood of hypertrophic scarring

○ **How deep should the periareolar tissue be incised and undermined to avoid nipple inversion?**

A 5-10mm deep incision with 1cm tissue left beneath the areola prevents an inverted nipple final outcome.

○ **How can chest concavity be avoided following male mastectomy?**

Leave a layer of subcutaneous fat over the pectoralis fascia.

○ **What local anesthesia should be used during male mastectomy and why?**

Bupivacaine 0.25% with 1:800,000 epinephrine is used to aid hemostasis and reduce pain on waking.

○ **When is general anesthesia warranted in male mastectomy?**

Grade 2B or higher gynecomastia correction

○ **What is the most common complication following mastectomy for gynecomastia?**

Hematoma or seroma.

○ **Where should drains be placed for best cosmetic result?**

Through the axilla or through a periareolar incision.

O   **How can the best result be obtained in mastectomy for grade 2 gynecomastia?**

Combination of physical resection of glandular tissue and liposuction tapering.

O   **Is skin excision typically necessary for male mastectomy?**

No. Excess skin will resolve within a year of mastectomy in most men with gynecomastia.

O   **For men with severe grade 3 gynecomastia, should tissue removal and liposuction tapering be done as a separate procedure from skin excision?**

Yes. Following the removal of breast tissue, the skin should be allowed a period of time to contract naturally before excess skin is incised.

O   **Following skin excision in mastectomy of grade 3 gynecomastia where anatomically should nipple areola graft be placed?**

On the dermis overlying the fifth rib.

BREAST

BREAST ANATOMY/EMBRYOLOGY

Alvin Cohn, MD and Jayant Agarwal, MD

○ **When do the mammary ridges develop in an embryo?**

Fifth or sixth week of gestation

○ **What is the path of the mammary ridge along the ventral aspect of an embryo?**

Base of the forelimb (future axilla) to the base of the hindlimb (inguinal area)

○ **What is the result of incomplete involution of the mammary ridge?**

Accessory breast tissue and supernumerary nipples

○ **Is amastia more commonly unilateral or bilateral?**

Unilateral

○ **What is the cause of unilateral amastia?**

Arrested mammary ridge development during the sixth week of fetal development

○ **Where is the most common site of aberrant breast tissue?**

Axilla

○ **Where is the most common site of a supernumerary nipple?**

Inframammary area

○ **The breast overlies which ribs?**

2nd-6th

○ **Each cluster of alveoli leads to a milk duct that empties into a lactiferous sinus. Each lactiferous sinus drains one lobe of the breast. How many lobes are in the breast?**

15-25 lobes per breast

○ **What is the most common bacteria cultured from breast tissue?**

Staphylococcus epidermidis

○ **Which vessel provides the dominant blood supply to the breast?**

Internal mammary artery

○ **The internal mammary artery is branch from which artery?**

Subclavian artery (left) /Brachiocephalic artery (right)

❍ **Usually, what vessel is the largest artery entering the pectoralis major muscle and overlying breast parenchyma?**

The second intercostal internal mammary perforator

❍ **Name three branches of the axillary artery (from medial to lateral) that serve as blood supply to the breast.**

Thoracoacromial, lateral thoracic, thoracodorsal arteries

❍ **When dissecting the axilla, if you clip the intercostobrachial nerve, where will you lose sensation?**

Upper medial aspect of arm and axilla

❍ **The intercostobrachial nerve is a branch of what nerve?**

Lateral branch of the 2nd intercostal nerve

❍ **Axillary nodes are noted as level I, level II, or level III. What anatomic structure determines their "level"?**

Pectoralis minor muscle

❍ **Where are level I axillary lymph nodes located?**

Lateral/below the lower border of pectoralis minor

❍ **Where are level II axillary lymph nodes located?**

Behind pectoralis minor

❍ **Where are level III axillary lymph nodes located?**

Medial/above the upper border of pectoralis minor

❍ **What is the primary innervation to the nipple-areola complex?**

Lateral branch of the fourth intercostal nerve

❍ **What is the course of the lateral branch of the fourth intercostal nerve?**

It pierces the deep fascia in the midaxillary line and takes an inferomedial course within the pectoral fascia. On reaching the midclavicular line, it turns 90 degrees and continues through the glandular tissue toward the posterior surface of the nipple.

❍ **What is the normal diameter of the areola complex?**

35-45 mm

❍ **What is the function of the Montgomery glands?**

They are sebaceous glands that produce a waxy substance to assist with lubrication and protection of the NAC

❍ **The suspensory ligaments of Cooper attach which structures?**

Deep pectoralis fascia to the dermis of the breast

○ **What is the lateral margin of the breast parenchyma?**

Lateral margin of the latissimus dorsi

○ **What is the superior margin of the breast parenchyma?**

The clavicle

○ **What is the medial margin of the breast parenchyma?**

Lateral sternum

○ **What is the major component of the anterior axillary fold?**

Pectoralis major

○ **What is the origin of the pectoralis major muscle?**

Medial sternal half of the clavicle and lateral aspect of the sternum/costochondral region, from the sternal notch down to the 6th or 7th costal cartilages

○ **The insertion of the pectoralis major tendon lies between which two muscles?**

Coracobrachialis (posterior) and deltoid (anterior)

○ **Which nerve provides motor innervation to the lateral and inferior pectoralis major muscle?**

Medial pectoral nerve

○ **The serratus anterior originates from costal attachments of the anterolateral aspects of the first through the eighth ribs. Where does this muscle insert?**

Deep medial surface of the scapula

○ **What is the innervation to the serratus anterior muscle?**

Long thoracic nerve

○ **What is the clinical manifestation of injury to the long thoracic nerve?**

Winged scapula

○ **How can one locate the long thoracic nerve?**

Positioned laterally, superficial to the external surface of the serratus anterior muscle in the midaxillary line

○ **If the thoracodorsal artery is proximally occluded/ligated, which vessel is capable of providing a significant portion of blood supply to the latissimus dorsi?**

Serratus branch of the thoracodorsal artery

○ **Which nerves supply innervation to the medial breast?**

The 2nd-6th medial intercostal nerves

❍   **Which condition is associated with a congenital absence of the pectoralis major muscle, usually the sternal component, as well as breast and areolar hypoplasia?**

Poland's syndrome

❍   **Following efferent lymphatic drainage into the deep pectoral nodes and subscapular nodes, which nodes are next in the lymphatic drainage pathway of the breast?**

Central axillary nodes and apical axillary nodes

❍   **Following efferent drainage into the axillary nodes, which nodes are next in the lymphatic drainage pathway of the breast?**

Supraclavicular nodes

❍   **If lymphatic drainage takes a medial pathway (vs. draining into the axilla), which nodes are the primary drainage basin?**

Internal mammary nodes/parasternal nodes

❍   **What aspect of the breast parenchyma supplies lymph to the internal mammary/parasternal nodes?**

The entire gland

❍   **In the youthful, non-ptotic breast, where should the NAC be located?**

Above the IMF

❍   **In the youthful, non-ptotic breast, what is the normal distance between the sternal notch and the nipple?**

17-21 cm

❍   **In the youthful, non-ptotic breast what is the normal distance between the nipple and the IMF?**

7-8 cm

References

Michelow, BJ, Nahai, F. Mastopexy. In: Achauer, BM, Eriksson, E, Guyuron, B, Coleman, JJ, Russell, RC, Vander Kolk, CA, eds. Plastic Surgery: Indications, Operations, and Outcomes. 1st Edition. St. Louis, Missouri: Mosby, 2000: 2769-2770.

Picha, GJ, Batra, MK. Breast Augmentation. In: Achauer, BM, Eriksson, E, Guyuron, B, Coleman, JJ, Russell, RC, Vander Kolk, CA, eds. Plastic Surgery: Indications, Operations, and Outcomes. 1st Edition. St. Louis, Missouri: Mosby, 2000: 2743-2744.

Schlenz I, Kuzbari R, Gruber, H, et al. The sensitivity of the nipple-areolar complex: An anatomic study. PRS, 2000; Volume 105 (3): 905-909.

Bland, KI, Vezeridis, MP, and Copeland, EM, III. Breast. In: Schwartz, SI, G. Shires, T, Spencer, FC, Daly, JM, Fischer, JE and Galloway, AC, eds. Schwartz: Principles of Surgery, 7th Edition. USA: McGraw-Hill Incorporated, 1999: 533-600.

Bostwick, John III. Anatomy and Physiology In: Plastic and Reconstructive Breast Surgery. Second Edition. Volume 1. St. Louis: Quality Medical Publishing, Inc, 2000: 77-120.

BREAST AUGMENTATION

Benjamin D. Eskra, MD

○ **What are the disadvantages of an augmentation performed in the subglandular plane as compared with subpectoral?**

Higher rate of capsular contracture, less satisfactory for mammography, and a higher risk of visibility, palpability and a sharp transition in the upper pole.

○ **What are the disadvantages of an augmentation performed in the subpectoral plane as compared with subglandular?**

Inferior lower-pole shape and inframammary fold definition. Also, late superior migration of the implants or pseudoptosis of the breast are possible.

○ **In which patients should subpectoral implantation be used with caution? Why?**

Patients with significant postpartum atrophy, glandular ptosis, and significant native tissue volume. Higher risk of double-bubble deformity.

○ **What is a "dual plane" augmentation?**

A variation of the subpectoral augmentation designed to reduce the risk of double-bubble deformity.

○ **How is a dual plane augmentation performed?**

Subpectoral dissection is combined with a partial subglandular dissection the extends a variable distance above the inferior border of the pectoralis major muscle.

○ **What makes the dual plane augmentation so versatile?**

The extent of subglandular dissection can be tailored to the degree of looseness, ptosis, or size of the overlying breast soft tissue, extending as far superiorly as the superior border of the areola allowing for implant placement and soft-tissue redraping that results in an aesthetic lower pole.

○ **Describe the four Baker grades of capsular contracture?**

Grade I: No palpable capsule. Grade II: Minimal firmness with palpable, but not visible, implant. Grade III: Moderate firmness with easily-palpable implant and visible implant or distortion. Grade IV: Severe contracture with breast that is hard, tender, painful, and cold, with marked distortion.

○ **What are the two prevailing theories of the etiology of capsular contracture formation?**

Hypertrophic scar formation (e.g. hematoma, granuloma, and hereditary factors), and an *infectious* event.

○ **What should the implant pocket be irrigated with to decrease the incidence of infection and capsular contracture?**

Mixture of 50,000 units of Bacitracin, 1 g Ancef, 80 mg gentamicin, and 500 mL saline.

○ **What is the rate of capsular contracture for subglandular breast augmentation with smooth, saline-filled implants? Subpectoral?**

23-40%; 1%.

O   **What is the rate of capsular contracture for subglandular breast augmentation with textured, saline-filled implants? Subpectoral?**

2-29%; 1%.

O   **What is the ideal patient for a textured, saline-filled implant?**

Patients with adequate soft tissue for whom subglandular positioning of the implant is desired.

O   **Which patients have a greater risk of excessive upper-pole fullness and distortion?**

Thin patients, patients with a high inframammary crease, patients with a vertically or horizontally deficient chest, and ptotic patients.

O   **What is the most important factor in placing an anatomic implant?**

Meticulous attention must be made not to overdissect the implant pocket, which would make rotation more likely.

O   **What factors should be evaluated prior to performing an augmentation that can help to choose the proper implant size, reduce the reoperation rate and produce a more predictable outcome?**

Base width (BW), nipple to inframammary fold distance (N:IMF), soft tissue pinch thickness of the upper pole (STPTUP), and the anterior pull skin stretch (APSS).

O   **What are the common locations for incisions for placing breast implants?**

Periareolar, inframammary, transaxillary, and periumbilical incisions.

O   **Which incision is the most versatile?**

Periareolar.

O   **In which patients should the periareolar incision be used with caution?**

Patients with small areolar diameters (<3cm), and patients with areolas that are lightly colored with indistinct margins.

O   **Patients that undergo a periareolar approach may be at somewhat higher risk for which complications?**

Changes in nipple sensation and difficulty with breast-feeding.

O   **Which incision allows for the simplest and most straightforward approach to breast augmentation?**

Inframammary.

O   **In which patients should the inframammary incision be used with caution?**

Patients with poorly-defined inframammary folds, constricted breasts, or an inframammary fold too close to the areola.

O   **What are the advantages of a transaxillary incision?**

Scar is well-concealed and the dissection does not violate the breast parenchyma.

❍ **Where are the disadvantages of a transaxillary approach?**

Less control and accuracy as compared with a more direct approach, theoretically increasing the risk of implant malposition or asymmetry. Also, it may be difficult or impossible to use the same incision for secondary procedures.

❍ **In which patients should the transaxillary approach not be used?**

Patients with tuberous breast deformity, patients requiring parenchymal rearrangement, or patients in whom an anatomic or large silicone implant have been chosen.

❍ **What are the advantages of a transumbilical approach?**

Inconspicuous scar and lower risk of implant extrusion.

❍ **What are the disadvantages of a transumbilical approach?**

Potential for inaccuracy increases the risk for implant malposition, particularly for textured or shaped implants. Difficult to place implant in subpectoral position, and difficult or impossible to place a silicone gel implant of any significant size.

❍ **What are the legal problems with the transumbilical approach?**

Not approved by the Food and Drug Administration and is thus officially "off-label," making it more difficult to defend an unsatisfactory result.

❍ **What are the long-term changes seen in the breast tissue and chest wall in an augmented patient?**

Breast parenchymal atrophy and costal cartilage remodeling that results in a concave shape of the ribs.

❍ **What is the reported rate of hematoma formation?**

3%.

❍ **What is the reported infection rate?**

0-2.2%.

❍ **What is the most common aerobic pathogen? Anaerobic?**

Staphylococcus aureus. Propionibacterium acnes.

❍ **On average, what is the reported rate of decreased nipple sensation?**

15%.

❍ **What is the rupture rate of saline-filled implants over 5 years? 10 years?**

3-5%. 5-10%.

❍ **What is the reoperation rate for implant-related complications during the first 5 years?**

24-33%.

❍ **What factors increase the risk of rupture of saline-filled implants?**

Underfilling the implant by > 25 mL, intraluminal antibiotics, and intraluminal steroids.

○ **What is the sensitivity of ultrasound in diagnosing silicone implant rupture? Negative predictive value?**

32-74%. 80%.

○ **What is the most accurate imaging modality for evaluating implant integrity?**

MRI.

○ **What is the "linguine" sign?**

A consistent MRI finding of implant rupture seen on T2-weighted images that represents infolding of the collapsed implant shell.

References

Adams WP Jr, Conner WCH, Barton FE Jr, Rohrich RJ: Optimizing breast-pocket irrigation: the post-Betadine era. *Plast. Reconstr. Surg.* 107:1596, 2001.

Berg WA, Caskey CI, Hamper UM, et al: Single- and double lumen silicone breast implant integrity: prospective evaluation of MR and US criteria. *Radiology* 197:45, 1995.

Biggs, T. M., and Yarish, R. S. Augmentation mammaplasty: A comparative analysis. *Plast. Reconstr. Surg.* 85: 368, 1990.

Brown SL, Silverman BG, Berg WA: Rupture of silicone-gel breast implants: causes, sequelae, and diagnosis. *Lancet* 350:1531, 1997.

Burkhardt BR: Capsular contracture: Hard breasts, soft data. *Clin. Plast. Surg.* 15:521, 1988.

Caskey CI, Berg WA, Anderson ND, et al: Breast implant rupture: diagnosis with US. *Radiology* 190:819, 1994.

Chilcote WA, Dowden RV, Paushter DM, et al: Ultrasound detection of silicone gel breast implant failure: a prospective analysis. *Breast. Dis.* 7:307, 1994.

Courtiss EH, Goldwyn RM: Breast sensation before and after plastic surgery. *Plast. Reconstr. Surg.* 58:1, 1976.

Courtiss EH, Goldwyn RM, Anastasi GW: The fate of breast implants with infections around them. *Plast. Reconstr. Surg.* 63:812, 1979.

DeBruhl ND et al: Silicone breast implants: US evaluation. *Radiology* 189:95, 1993.

Gabriel SE, Woods JE, O'Fallon WM, et al: Complications leading to surgery after breast implantation. *N. Engl. J. Med.* 336:677, 1997.

Gayou R, Rudolph R: Capsular contraction around silicone mammary prostheses. *Ann. Plast. Surg.* 2:62, 1979.

Grazer FM, Heinrichs HL: Augmentation mammaplasty: Survey of 200 consecutive implants. *In: Owsley JQ, Peterson RA (eds), Symposium on Aesthetic Surgery of the Breast. St Louis, Mosby,* 1978, Vol 18.

Hakelius, L., and Ohlsen, L. A clinical comparison of the tendency to capsular contracture between smooth and textured gel-filled silicone mammary implants. *Plast. Reconstr. Surg.* 90: 247, 1992.

Hetter GP: Satisfactions and dissatisfactions of patients with augmentation mammaplasty. *Plast. Reconstr. Surg.* 64:151, 1979.

Hidalgo, D. A. Breast augmentation: Choosing the optimal incision, implant, and pocket plane. *Plast. Reconstr. Surg.* 105: 2202, 2000.

Hurst, N. M. Lactation after augmentation mammaplasty. *Obstet. Gynecol.* 87: 30, 1996.

Khouri, R. K., Schlenz, I., Murphy, B. J., and Baker, T. J. Nonsurgical breast enlargement using an external soft-tissue expansion system. *Plast. Reconstr. Surg.* 105: 2500, 2000.

LeRoy J, Given KS: Wound infection in breast augmentation: The role of prophylactic perioperative antibiotics. *Aesthetic Plast Surg* 15:303, 1991.

Marotta JS, Widenhouse CW, Habal MB, Goldberg EP: Silicone gel breast implant failure and frequency of additional surgeries: analysis of 35 studies reporting examination of more than 8000 explants. *J. Biomed. Mater. Res. (Appl. Biomater.)* 48:354, 1999.

McGrath MH, Burkhardt BR: The safety and efficacy of breast implants for augmentation mammaplasty. *Plast. Reconstr. Surg.* 74:550, 1984.

Mladick, R. A. "No-touch" submuscular saline breast augmentation technique. *Aesthetic Plast. Surg.* 17: 183, 1993.

Nahas FX: Breast implants: some considerations about volume *(letter). Plast. Reconstr. Surg.* 107:1918, 2001.

Neifert, M., DeMarzo, S., Seacat, J., Young, D., Leff, M., and Orleans, M. The influence of breast surgery, breast appearance, and pregnancy-induced breast changes on lactation sufficiency as measured by infant weight gain. *Birth* 17: 31, 1990.

Ohlsen L, Ponten B, Hambert G: Augmentation mammaplasty: A surgical and psychiatric evaluation of the results. *Ann Plast Surg* 2:42, 1979.

Pollack, H. Breast capsular contracture: A retrospective study of textured versus smooth silicone implants. *Plast. Reconstr. Surg.* 91: 404, 1993.

Pound, E. C., III, and Pound, E. C., Jr. Transumbilical breast augmentation (TUBA): Patient selection, technique, and clinical experience. *Clin. Plast. Surg.* 28: 597, 2001.

Rohrich RJ: Safety of silicone breast implants: scientific validation/vindication at last. *Plast. Reconstr. Surg.* 104:1786, 1999.

Reynolds HE, Buckwalter KA, Jackson VP, et al: Comparison of mammography, sonography, and magnetic resonance imaging in the detection of silicone-gel breast implant rupture. *Ann. Plast. Surg.* 33:247, 1994.

Rudolph R et al: Myofibroblasts and free silicon around breast implants. *Plast. Reconstr. Surg.* 62:185, 1978.

Silverstein, M. J., Handel, N., and Gamagami, P. The effect of silicone gel-filled implants on mammography. *Cancer* 68: 1159, 1991.

Smahel J: Histology of the capsules causing constrictive fibrosis around breast implants. *Br. J. Plast. Surg.* 30:324, 1977.

Spear, S. L., and Beckenstein, M. The periareolar approach to augmentation mammaplasty. In S. L. Spear (Ed.), *Surgery of the Breast: Principles and Art.* Philadelphia, Pa.: Lippincott-Raven, 1998.

Spear, S. L., and Beckenstein, M. The inframammary approach to augmentation mammaplasty. In S. L. Spear (Ed.), *Surgery of the Breast: Principles and Art.* Philadelphia, Pa.: Lippincott-Raven, 1998.

Spear, S. L., Elmaraghy, M., and Hess, C. Textured surface saline-filled silicone breast implants for augmentation mammaplasty. *Plast. Reconstr. Surg.* 105: 1542, 2000.

Spear, S. L., and Bulan, E. J. The medial periareolar approach to submuscular augmentation mammaplasty under local anesthesia: A 10-year follow-up. *Plast. Reconstr. Surg.* 108: 771, 2001.

Tebbetts JB: Patient evaluation, operative planning, and surgical techniques to increase control and reduce morbidity and reoperations in breast augmentation. *Clin. Plast. Surg.* 28(3):501, 2001.

Tebbetts, J. B. Dual plane breast augmentation: Optimizing implant–soft-tissue relationships in a wide range of breast types. *Plast. Reconstr. Surg.* 107: 1255, 2001.

Tebbetts JB: The greatest myths in breast augmentation. *Plast. Reconstr. Surg.* 107:1895, 2001.

Thornton JW, Argenta LC, McClatchey KD, Marks MW: Studies on the endogenous flora of the human breast. *Ann. Plast. Surg.* 20:39, 1988.

Williams JE: Experiences with a large series of silastic breast implants. *Plast. Reconstr. Surg.* 49:253, 1972.

BREAST IMPLANT EFFICACY/SAFETY

Benjamin D. Eskra, MD

Breast Implants

○ **What is the shell of all modern implants composed of?**

Silicone elastomer.

○ **What is silicone?**

A highly pure polymer of dimethylsiloxane.

○ **What factors affect the viscosity of the silicone?**

The length of the polymer and the degree of cross-linking. Longer chains are more viscous as are more highly-crosslinked chains.

○ **Which implant type has been shown to lower the rate of capsular contracture?**

Textured.

○ **What are the disadvantages of textured implants?**

More visible rippling, greater palpability, and higher cost.

○ **What is the risk in underfilling a saline implant?**

Increased risk of shell folds, visible rippling, and possibly early device failure.

○ **What are the advantages of an anatomically-shaped implant?**

Diminished tendency towards upper-pole fullness, roundness, or distortion and greater volume support for the lower breast.

○ **What is the link between silicone gel-filled breast implants and systemic disease, such as autoimmune diseases, connective tissue disorders, and cancer?**

None.

○ **What changes have been made, during the last ten years, to improve the safety and efficacy of silicone gel-filled implants?**

Low-bleed silicone elastomer shells, more cohesive silicone gels, and implant shell surface texturing.

○ **Does the presence of breast implants affect the early diagnosis of breast cancer?**

No. Several studies have shown that implants do not affect the early diagnosis of breast cancer or the pathological stage at diagnosis.

○ **How does the mammographic imaging of augmented patients differ from nonaugmented patients?**

It is more difficult to compress the augmented breast with standard mammographic techniques. To adequately visualize the augmented breast, Eklund displacement views must be performed.

○ **Does the presence of an implant decrease the amount of breast that can be visualized?**

Yes. One study showed that only 85% of the breast could be visualized as compared with 90% and above in nonaugmented patients.

○ **Does this decrease in breast visualization create a significant difference in the mammographic detection of breast cancer?**

No.

○ **What is the best implant position for mammographic visualization of the breast?**

Subpectoral.

○ **What factor can cause a reduction in mammographic visualization of the augmented breast?**

Capsular contracture.

○ **Is there a difference on mammography between saline and silicone implants?**

No. Silicone and saline have the same mammographic density.

References

Angell, M. Shattuck lecture: Evaluating the health risks of breast implants: The interplay of medical science, the law, and public opinion. *N. Engl. J. Med.* 334: 1513, 1996.

Asplund, O., Gylbert, L., Jurell, G., Ward, C. Textured or Smooth Implants for Submuscular Breast Augmentation: A Controlled Study. *Plast. Reconstr. Surg.* 97: 1200, 1996.

Barnard, J. J., Todd, E. L., Wilson, W. G., et al. Distribution of organosilicon polymers in augmentation mammaplasties at autopsy. *Plast. Reconstr. Surg.* 100: 197, 1997.

Deapen, D. M., Pike, M. C., Casagrande, J. T., et al. The relationship between breast cancer and augmentation mammaplasty: An epidemiologic study. *Plast. Reconstr. Surg.* 77: 361, 1986.

Gumucio, C. A., Pin, P., Young, V. L., et al. The effect of breast implants on the radiographic detection of microcalcification and soft-tissue masses. *Plast. Reconstr. Surg.* 84: 772, 1989.

Hakelius, L., and Ohlsen, L. A clinical comparison of the tendency to capsular contracture between smooth and textured gel-filled silicone mammary implants. *Plast. Reconstr. Surg.* 90: 247, 1992.

Hamas, R. S. The postoperative shape of round and tear drop saline-filled breast implants. *Aesthetic Surg. J.* 19: 369, 1999.

Hammond, D. C. Breast augmentation using anatomic implants. *Oper. Tech. Plast. Reconstr. Surg.* 7: 125, 2000.

Hidalgo, D. A. Breast augmentation: Choosing the optimal incision, implant, and pocket plane. *Plast. Reconstr. Surg.* 105: 2202, 2000.

Heden, P., Jernbeck, J., and Hober, M. Breast augmentation with anatomical cohesive gel implants. *Clin. Plast. Surg.* 28: 531, 2001.

Hurst, N. M. Lactation after augmentation mammaplasty. *Obstet. Gynecol.* 87: 30, 1996.

Jakubietz, M. G., Janis, J. E., Jakubietz, R. G., and Rohrich, R. J. Breast Augmentation: Cancer Concerns and Mammography—A Literature Review. *Plast. Reconstr. Surg.* 113: 117e, 2004.

Muzaffer, A. R., and Rohrich, R. J. The silicone gel-filled breast implant controversy: An update. *Plast. Reconstr. Surg.* 109: 742, 2001.

Neifert, M., DeMarzo, S., Seacat, J., Young, D., Leff, M., and Orleans, M. The influence of breast surgery, breast appearance, and pregnancy-induced breast changes on lactation sufficiency as measured by infant weight gain. *Birth* 17: 31, 1990.

Pollack, H. Breast capsular contracture: A retrospective study of textured versus smooth silicone implants. *Plast. Reconstr. Surg.* 91: 404, 1993.

Rohrich, R. J., Hollier, L. H., and Robinson, J. B. Determining the safety of the silicone envelope: In search of a silicone antibody. *Plast. Reconstr. Surg.* 98: 455, 1996.

Silverstein, M. J., Handel, N., and Gamagami, P. The effect of silicone gel-filled implants on mammography. *Cancer* 68: 1159, 1991.

Spear, S. L., Elmaraghy, M., and Hess, C. Textured surface saline-filled silicone breast implants for augmentation mammaplasty. *Plast. Reconstr. Surg.* 105: 1542, 2000.

Spear, S. L. Breast augmentation with reduced-height anatomic implants: The pros and cons. *Clin. Plast. Surg.* 28: 561, 2001.

Spear, S. L., and Mardini, S. Alternative filler materials and new implant designs: What's available and what's on the horizon? *Clin. Plast. Surg.* 28: 435, 2001.

Su, C. W., Dreyfuss, D. A., Krizek, T. J., et al. Silicone implants and the inhibition of cancer. *Plast. Reconstr. Surg.* 96: 513, 1995.

BREAST CANCER

Alvin Cohn, MD and Jayant Agarwal, MD

○ **What is the average woman's lifetime risk of developing breast cancer?**

12%

○ **What is the lifetime risk of developing breast cancer if you have either the BRCA-1 or BRCA-2 gene?**

85%

○ **Do women with breast cancer caused by inherited genetic abnormalities (i.e. BRCA-1) have more aggressive cancers than women without abnormal genes?**

No

○ **Is BRCA-1 or BRCA-2 affiliated with the development of male breast cancer? What is that male's lifetime risk?**

BRCA-2; 6-7%

○ **Does gynecomastia predispose the male breast to the development of cancer?**

No

○ **Name a syndrome affiliated with male breast cancer.**

Klinefelter's syndrome (47 XXY genotype, hypogonadism, eventual infertility)

○ **What are current American Cancer Society's guidelines for mammography?**

Baseline exam at age 35, annual screening mammogram starting at 40 yrs of age

○ **What are current American Cancer Society's guidelines for mammography in women from high-risk families (i.e. mutation carriers)?**

Screening to begin at 25 years of age, or 5-10 years earlier than the earliest age at which breast cancer was diagnosed in a family member

○ **In women over the age of 50, screening mammography and clinical examination result in what percentage decrease in mortality due to breast cancer?**

25-30%

○ **What is the standard method for pre-operatively confirming the diagnosis of breast cancer?**

Fine-needle aspiration or core needle biopsy

○ **Is Mondor's disease a benign or malignant condition?**

Benign; superficial thrombophlebitis of anterior chest and breast

○   **Classify each of the following regarding their relative risk for the development of invasive breast cancer as either:**
a.   **no increased risk**
b.   **slightly increased risk (1.5-2X)**
c.   **moderately increased risk (4-5X)**
d.   **high risk (8-10X)**

i.	ductal ectasia	[no increased risk]
ii.	papilloma	[slightly increased risk]
iii.	atypical ductal hyperplasia	[moderately increased risk]
iv.	sclerosing adenosis	[slightly increased risk]
v.	epithelial hyperplasia	[no increased risk]
vi.	DCIS	[high risk]
vii.	LCIS	[high risk]
viii.	atypical lobular hyperplasia	[moderately increased risk]

○   **Is there an associated risk of breast cancer associated with fat necrosis?**

No.

○   **Why do fibroadenomas occur predominantly in women aged 20-30?**

Tumors are highly estrogen sensitive

○   **What is a phyllodes tumor? Are they malignant by definition?**

A tumor derived from the stroma/connective tissue of the breast (vs. ductal elements); no, though they can have aggressive/uncontrolled local growth

○   **Which is NOT a risk-factor for the development of breast cancer: obesity, late menopause, or multiparity?**

Multiparity (other risk factors include: increasing age, family history of breast cancer, early menstruation, use of hormone replacement therapy, heavy alcohol consumption, prior use of diethylstilbestrol (DES), heavy radiation exposure)

○   **Which of the following variables confers the lowest increased risk of developing breast cancer: old age, North American descent, African-American ethnicity, or a family h/o breast cancer?**

African-American ethnicity (only increases risk 2x. the other variables increase risk 4x)

○   **What is the most relevant risk factor for the development of breast cancer?**

Family history (first-degree relatives)

○   **Name three syndromes affiliated with familial breast cancer syndromes?**

Breast-ovarian cancer syndrome, Li-Fraumeni syndrome, and Cowden's disease

○   **What is the etiology of peau d'orange appearance of breast skin?**

Tumor invasion of the parenchyma and shortening of Cooper's ligaments due to fibrosis + skin edema

○   **What is the most important prognostic factor regarding overall survival following the diagnosis of breast cancer?**

Nodal status

❍ **What is the incidence of relapse for node-negative vs. node-positive breast cancer patients?**

20-25% vs. 50-75%

❍ **What is the most common site of disseminated disease?**

Bone

❍ **In women who receive appropriate therapy, what is the 5-year disease-free survival for stage I disease?**

85%

❍ **In women who receive appropriate therapy, what is the 5-year disease-free survival for stage II disease?**

66%

❍ **In women who receive appropriate therapy, what is the 5-year disease-free survival for stage III disease?**

41%

❍ **In women who receive appropriate therapy, what is the 5-year disease-free survival for stage IV disease?**

10%

❍ **Regarding the TNM staging for breast cancer, define a T1 lesion.**

Tumor diameter $\leq$ 2 cm

❍ **Regarding the TNM staging for breast cancer, define a T2 lesion.**

Tumor $\leq$ 5 cm but > 2 cm

❍ **Regarding the TNM staging for breast cancer, define a T3 lesion.**

Tumor > 5 cm

❍ **Regarding the TNM staging for breast cancer, define a T4 lesion.**

Any size lesion with direct extension into the chest wall or skin

❍ **According to 2002 AJCC staging guidelines: Does cancer in the ipsilateral supraclavicular nodes affect the N status or the M status?**

N status [N_3] (previously affected M status)

❍ **What is the clinical TNM status of a patient with a 1.5 cm lesion, two mobile, ipsilateral nodes, and no evidence of metastatic disease? What stage is this?**

T1N1M0 (Stage II)

❍ **What is the clinical TNM status of a patient with a 1.5 cm lesion, two fixed, ipsilateral nodes, and no evidence of metastatic disease? What stage is this?**

T1N2M0 (Stage III)

❍ **Does DCIS or LCIS occur more frequently? What is their occurrence ratio?**

DCIS; 3:1

○ **Is there a racial predilection for LCIS?**

Yes; it occurs 12x more frequently in white women

○ **Why does LCIS most commonly present as a non-palpable mass?**

Originates in the lobules and proliferates to the point of filling the lobular lumina while maintaining overall lobular architecture

○ **How do microcalcifications develop?**

Cellular growth outstrips blood supply. Calcium deposition occurs in areas of necrosis

○ **Is DCIS or LCIS more likely to have clinical signs?**

DCIS

○ **Is DCIS or LCIS more likely to be affiliated with microcalcifications?**

DCIS

○ **Does DCIS or LCIS have a predisposition toward bilaterality?**

LCIS

○ **Does DCIS or LCIS have a predisposition toward multicentricity?**

DCIS

○ **What percent of breast cancers are found in the upper, outer quadrant?**

50%

○ **Why does Paget's disease have a better prognosis than other malignancies?**

Visible nipple changes promote earlier consultation

○ **Is Paget's disease more associated with invasive cancer or DCIS?**

DCIS

○ **What percentage of invasive breast cancers are ductal in origin? What percent are lobular in origin?**

80% ductal; 10% lobular

○ **What dreaded complication has been associated with chronic, longstanding, ipsilateral lymphedema following radical mastectomy?**

Lymphangiosarcoma (Stewart-Treves syndrome)

○ **What is the incidence of ipsilateral lymphedema following radical mastectomy?**

15-25%

○ **What is the incidence of ipsilateral lymphedema following modified radical mastectomy?**

15-20%

○ **Why does inflammatory carcinoma portend a poorer prognosis?**

Implies the presence of both lymphatic and vascular invasion, thus, it has a higher frequency of metastatic disease

○ **What is the only surgical option for the treatment of LCIS?**

Bilateral mastectomy

○ **Which variable is affected by the administration of post-op XRT: overall survival, distant recurrence, or local recurrence?**

Local recurrence (improved by 50-75%)

○ **What are two treatment options for a microscopic DCIS tumor (<0.5 cm)?**

Lumpectomy vs. lumpectomy + XRT

○ **What are two treatment options for small DCIS tumors (0.5 -1.9 cm)?**

Lumpectomy + XRT vs. mastectomy

○ **What are two treatment options for large DCIS tumors (>2.5 cm)?**

Lumpectomy + XRT vs. mastectomy + SLNB

○ **What benefit does post-op XRT confer following excisional treatment for DCIS?**

Fourfold relative reduction in both recurrent DCIS and subsequent invasive tumor growth in the ipsilateral breast (local disease control)

○ **What is the treatment of choice for unifocal, invasive breast cancer that can be excised with clear margins (1 cm surrounding the tumor)?**

Breast conservation therapy (lumpectomy) + SLNB (sentinel lymph node biopsy) + XRT

○ **Name two indications for XRT following mastectomy.**

Presence of four or more positive axillary lymph nodes; Primary tumor > 5.0 cm, regardless of axillary status

○ **What is the positive predictive value of a successful SLNB?**

100%

○ **What is the negative predictive value of a successful SLNB?**

95%

○ **Which nodes are typically sampled during an axillary lymph node dissection?**

Level I and II

○ **What are two common indications for performing an ALND following SLND?**

1. If sentinel node is +: ALND performed for staging (prognostic) and local axillary control (therapeutic); 2. If SLND is unsuccessful (no node found): ALND performed for staging

❍   **Name three common combinations of chemotherapy used to treat patients with breast cancer.**

- FAC: fluorouracil, doxorubicin, and cyclophosphamide
- AC: doxorubicin and cyclophosphamide
- CMF: cyclophosphamide, methotrexate, and fluorouracil

❍   **Does preoperative chemotherapy offer any apparent survival advantage compared with postoperative chemotherapy?**

No

❍   **Provide a rationale for the occasional use of preoperative chemotherapy in a patient with an operable breast tumor.**

A significant number of primary tumors will be downstaged, making lumpectomy a possibility for patients who might otherwise require mastectomy

❍   **In a patient with negative axillary nodes and an invasive breast tumor, when is adjuvant chemotherapy indicated?**

If the invasive cancer is >1 cm in largest diameter or if the primary tumor is >3 cm and has favorable histologic findings (pure tubular, mucinous, or papillary)

❍   **In a patient with positive axillary nodes and an invasive breast tumor, should all tumors, regardless of size or histologic findings, be treated with adjuvant therapy?**

Yes

❍   **T/F: Chemotherapy has been shown to improve substantially the long-term relapse-free and overall survival in both premenopausal and postmenopausal women up to age 70 years with lymph node-positive and lymph node-negative disease.**

True

❍   **What is the goal of hormonal therapy?**

To prevent breast cancer cells from receiving stimulation from estrogen

❍   **Name three mechanisms by which estrogen deprivation (i.e. hormonal therapy) can be achieved.**

- Blocking estrogen receptors (i.e. tamoxifen)
- Suppressing estrogen synthesis (i.e. aromatase inhibitors [anastrozole] in post-menopausal women or luteinizing hormone-releasing hormone agonists [goserelin] in pre-menopausal women
- Destruction of the ovaries via surgery or XRT

❍   **Which sub-group of breast cancer patients are not candidates for treatment with tamoxifen?**

Patients with estrogen receptor-negative breast cancer

❍   **Do pre- or post-menopausal women have a higher incidence of ER+ breast tumors?**

Post-menopausal

○ **Because of tamoxifen's association with a slight but definite increased risk of endometrial cancer and venous thromboembolism, are transvaginal ultrasounds or endometrial biopsies indicated in asymptomatic women taking tamoxifen?**

No

○ **Which patients are recommended to utilize tamoxifen in the adjuvant setting?**

Patients with ER+ cancer, independent of menopausal state or lymph-node status (duration of therapy = 5 years)

○ **Is the combination of tamoxifen and chemotherapy more effective than either agent alone?**

Yes

○ **The administration of adjuvant tamoxifen for five years after primary therapy reduces the incidence of contralateral breast cancer by what percent?**

47%

○ **Does overexpression of the HER-2/neu oncogene play a role in patient management?**

Yes; patients with metastatic disease and significant overexpression of HER-2/neu oncogene proteins have a survival benefit from Herceptin (trastuzumab)

References

Fisher B, Costantino J, Redmond, C, et al. Lumpectomy compared with lumpectomy and radiation therapy for the treatment of intraductal breast cancer. N Engl J Med, 1993; Volume 328 (22): 1581-1586.

Goldhirsh A, Glick JH, Gelber RD, et al. Meeting highlights: International consensus panel on the treatment of primary breast cancer. Journal of the National Cancer Institute, 1998; Volume 90 (21): 1601-1608.

Hortobagyi, GN. Treatment of breast cancer. N Engl J Med, 1998; Volume 339 (14): 974-984.

Mincey BA, Palmieri FM, Perez EA. Adjuvant therapy for breast cancer: Recommendations for management based on consensus review and recent clinical trials. The Oncologist, 2002; Volume 7: 246-250.

Eifel P, Axelson JA, Costa J, et al. National Institutes of Health consensus development conference statement: Adjuvant therapy for cancer, November 1-3, 2000. Journal of the National Cancer Institute, 2001; Volume 93 (13): 979-989.

Bland, KI, Vezeridis, MP, and Copeland, EM, III. Breast. In: Schwartz, SI, G. Shires, T, Spencer, FC, Daly, JM, Fischer, JE and Galloway, AC, eds. Schwartz: Principles of Surgery, 7th Edition. USA: McGraw-Hill Incorporated, 1999: 533-600.

Singletary SE, Allred C, Ashley P, et al.: Revision of the American Joint Committee on Cancer staging system for breast cancer. J Clin Oncol 20 (17): 3628-36,

Slamon DJ, Leyland-Jones B, Shak S, et al. Use of chemotherapy plus a monoclonal antibody against HER2 for metastatic breast cancer that overexpresses HER2. N Engl J Med, 2001; Volume 344 (11):783–792.

(Special thanks to Dr. Nora Jaskowiak for editorial assistance with this chapter.)

EXPANDER-IMPLANT AND NIPPLE-AREOLAR RECONSTRUCTION

Karen M. Horton, MD, MSc, BScH

○ **What factors are important in selecting the most appropriate procedure for breast reconstruction?**

1.   Laxity and thickness of the remaining chest skin
2.   condition of the pectoralis and serratus anterior muscles
3.   size of the opposite breast
4.   availability of flap donor sites

○ **What are the benefits of immediate breast reconstruction?**

1.   Decreased psychosocial morbidity
2.   superior aesthetic outcome (inframammary fold and skin envelope maintained)
3.   decreased surgical morbidity (single general anesthetic and recovery period)
4.   reduced overall cost

○ **What are potential disadvantages of immediate breast reconstruction?**

1.   Higher patient expectations
2.   higher risk mastectomy skin flap necrosis (10%)
3.   delay in determination of final margins and need for additional surgery and/or radiation therapy

○ **Who are candidates for immediate breast reconstruction?**

Patients in good general health with stage I or II disease, determined by the size and location of the tumor. Reconstruction has also been described for selected stage III patients with good prognosis.

○ **When should delayed breast reconstruction be considered?**

1.   If tumor clearance is uncertain
2.   patients with extensive stage III or IV disease in whom <u>immediate</u> postoperative chemotherapy and radiation is expected.

○ **Who first described tissue expansion for breast reconstruction?**

Radovan in 1982.

○ **What types of tissue expanders are available for breast reconstruction?**

Tissue expanders differ in their
1.   shape (round, oval, tear drop, anatomic, crescentic)
2.   surface (smooth, textured)
3.   duration (temporary, permanent)
4.   fill characteristics (uniform, differential)
5.   filling ports (internal port, remote external valve)

6.   size or fill volume
7.   number of chambers (single-chamber, dual-chamber)

O   **What are advantages of tissue expansion in breast reconstruction?**

1.   Creates new donor tissue of similar texture, color, sensation
2.   no additional scar
3.   no additional donor site
4.   decreased operating time
5.   shorter recovery period
6.   technical ease

O   **What are the indications for tissue expansion and implant reconstruction?**

1.   Small or medium sized breast
2.   patient not obese and chest wall not irradiated
3.   patient not opposed to implant use
4.   patient prefers not to undergo more extensive surgery
5.   medical contraindications to a more lengthy operation
6.   patient objection to scars of flap reconstruction
7.   patient not a candidate for autogenous reconstruction (multiple scars, limited donor tissue)
8.   bilateral reconstructions

O   **What are the contraindications to expander/implant reconstruction?**

1.   Prior or anticipated chest wall irradiation
2.   morbid obesity
3.   atrophic, tight skin with poor/no pectoralis muscle
4.   mastectomy skin flaps of questionable viability
5.   active infection at the expansion site
6.   residual gross tumor

O   **What are potential problems with expander/implant reconstruction?**

1.   Pain/discomfort/pressure with expansion
2.   infection +/- prosthesis removal
3.   skin erosion or extrusion
4.   skin flap necrosis
5.`   leakage or deflation
6.   malposition
7.   remote injection port malfunction or kinking
8.   internal valvular failure
9.   capsular contracture
10.   hematoma
11.   seroma
12.   implant folds, "knuckles" or wrinkling
13.   indistinct inframammary fold
14.   longer reconstruction period (up to 1 year)
15.   need for multiple operative procedures +/- additional revisional surgeries
16.   rounder appearance without natural ptosis

O   **Where should the tissue expander be placed within the mastectomy pocket?**

The expander should ideally be placed under muscle, and may be either <u>completely submuscular</u> (under pectoralis major, serratus anterior, and the fasciae of rectus abdominis and external oblique), or may be <u>partially submuscular</u> (covered by pectoralis major at its upper pole alone).

Smooth expanders should be placed slightly below the level of the inframammary fold, <u>as they tend to rise upwards with expansion</u>. Textured tissue expanders can be placed at the level of the inframammary fold, as their adherent surface prevents migration and enables lower pole expansion and subsequent ptosis.

○ **What is a "totally submuscular" placement of a tissue expander/implant?**

The implant is placed in a pocket beneath the pectoralis major and serratus anterior muscles, +/- the fascia of the external oblique and rectus abdominis muscles. The implant lies on top of the pectoralis minor muscle. A partially submuscular placement indicates that the lower pole is subcutaneous, with muscle coverage superiorly.

○ **What are potential advantages and disadvantages of complete submuscular coverage?**

Potential advantages include lower incidence of infection, exposure and extrusion. Disadvantages may include ineffective expansion of the lower pole of the breast mound. Complication rates have been found to be equal between these methods.

○ **When does the expansion process begin after surgery?**

At the time of closure, 50-200 cc of sterile saline is added to the expander, or as much will allow tension-free closure without skin blanching. At two weeks, 50-100 cc is injected at weekly or twice weekly intervals. Endpoints for inflation volume include blanching of the skin over the expander and/or patient discomfort; saline is removed until these conditions are reversed.

○ **By how much should the breast pocket be overexpanded once the ideal size has been reached, and how long should overexpansion be maintained for?**

Overexpansion is generally 20% to 30% above the final desired volume. The pocket and capsule are allowed to mature for 3-6 months in the overexpanded state before removal of the expander and replacement with a permanent prosthesis.

○ **What types of implants are available for breast reconstruction?**

All breast implants have a silicone-based shell. In North America, implants are either saline-filled or silicone-filled. Silicone implants may be cohesive gel (firm) or liquid/responsive gel (more viscous).

○ **Which dimensional features must be considered when selecting an implant type?**

1. base diameter
2. height
3. projection
4. volume
5. surface characteristics
6. shape
7. fill material

○ **Which implant types are associated with formation of a fibrous capsule?**

All foreign bodies induce a foreign body reaction and formation of a discrete fibrous shell. Certain factors are <u>associated</u> with a higher incidence of capsular contracture, including:
1. older-generation silicone implants
2. subglandular rather than submuscular/subpectoral placement
3. postoperative hematoma
4. postoperative infection
5. smooth rather than textured surface

○ **What is the Becker implant?**

A permanent combined expander-implant for breast reconstruction or augmentation. This double-lumen prosthesis contains an outer silicone gel-filled lumen surrounding an inner expandable saline-filled lumen with removable filler tube. After achieving overexpansion, the saline reservoir can be deflated to its final desired volume and the filler tube removed under local anaesthesia at the time of nipple reconstruction.

❍   **Do breast implants interfere with chemotherapy or radiation postoperatively?**

No. Chemotherapy may proceed as usual postoperatively, although tissues are usually allowed to heal for 4 weeks before starting therapy. Implants neither block nor enhance the absorbed radiation dose.

❍   **How does radiation affect tissue expansion and skin flap viability?**

Radiation treatment given before skin expansion:
1.   decreases the tissue expansion rate
2.   decreases the total area of expanded skin
3.   decreases the viability of skin flaps raised on expanded skin

Radiation during implant reconstruction results in:
1.   a higher rate of capsular contracture
2.   possible implant extrusion
3.   possibly an unacceptable aesthetic outcome

Nearly half of radiated breasts with saline implants require the addition of, or replacement by a flap for salvage of the reconstruction.

❍   **When may a tissue expander require premature removal?**

Causes for premature removal include infection, exposure, skin necrosis, patient dissatisfaction or persistent breast cancer.

❍   **What techniques may be used to recreate or reconstruct an indistinct inframammary fold?**

1.   External suturing, with direct incision and advancement of a deepithelialized thoracoepigastric flap to the prethoracic wall fascia
2.   Internal suturing, using sutures from the deep dermis or anterior capsule to the prethoracic fascia.

❍   **List the three main techniques described for nipple reconstruction?**

1.   Composite autogenous grafts (contralateral nipple, ear lobule, toe or finger pulp, labia minora, umbilicus, cartilage, dermal-fat grafts
2.   local tissue flaps
3.   alloplastic implants

❍   **Which local flaps have been described for nipple reconstruction?**

1.   Maltese cross flap
2.   skate flap
3.   star flap
4.   C-V flap
5.   S flap
6.   T flap
7.   mushroom flap
8.   double opposing tab flap
9.   H flap
10.   double opposing pennant flap
11.   propeller flap
12.   inchworm flap

13.   fishtail flap
14.   quadrapod flap
15.   pinwheel flap
16.   bell flap

○   **What is the potential risk of banking the ipsilateral nipple-areolar complex (NAC) at the time of mastectomy for later reconstruction?**

Autotransplantation of malignant cells.

○   **What complications are associated with nipple sharing?**

1.   Cicatricial distortion
2.   loss of pigmentation
3.   loss of at least 50% height of the donor nipple
4.   decreased sensation of the contralateral nipple

○   **What techniques are available for areolar reconstruction?**

<u>Skin grafting and tattooing</u>. Skin graft donor sites include the contralateral areola, groin, labia minora, or other redundant skin folds. Tattooing is used to exactly match the contralateral side.

References

Disa JJ, Ad-El DD, Cohen SM et al. The premature removal of tissue expanders in breast reconstruction. Plast Reconstr Surg 1999; 104:1662-1665.

Dvali LT, Dagum AB, Pang CY, et al. Effect of radiation on skin expansion and skin flap viability in pigs. Plast Reconstr Surg 2000; 106(3):624-629.

Georgiade GS. Nipple areola reconstruction. In: Georgiade GS, Riefkohl R, Levin LS, eds. Georgiade Plastic, Maxillofacial and Reconstructive Surgery. 3rd ed. Baltimore: Williams & Wilkins, 1997:817-819.

Georgiade GS, Sundine MJ. Breast reconstruction after mastectomy: overview and implant reconstruction. In: Georgiade GS, Riefkohl R, Levin LS, eds. Georgiade Plastic, Maxillofacial and Reconstructive Surgery. 3rd ed. Baltimore: Williams & Wilkins, 1997::777-782.

Goodman CM, Miller R, Patrick CW et al. Radiotherapy: effects on expanded skin. Plast Reconstr Surg 2002; 110:1080-1083.

Hoover SJ, Kenkel JM. Breast Cancer, Cancer Prevention, and Breast Reconstruction. Selected Readings in Plastic Surgery, 9(30):1-40.

Miller MJ. Immediate breast reconstruction. Clin Plast Surg 1998; 25:145-156.

Shusterman MA. Microsurgical breast reconstruction. In: Aston SJ, Beasley RW, Thorne CHM, eds. Grabb and Smith's Plastic Surgery. 5th ed. Philadelphia: Lippincott-Raven, 1997, 785-790.

Spear SL, Onyewu C. Staged breast reconstruction with saline-filled implants in the irradiated breast: recent trends and therapeutic implications. Plast Reconstr Surg 2000; 105:930-942.

Spear SL, Spittler CJ. Breast reconstruction with implants and expanders. Plast Reconstr Surg 2001; 107:177-187.

Strauch B, Vasconez LO, Hall-Findlay EJ eds. Breast, Chest Wall, and Trunk Reconstruction. In: Grabb's Atlas of Flaps. 2nd ed. Philadelphia: Lippincott-Raven, 1998; 3:1259-1372.

Tyrone JW. Nipple areola reconstruction. Breast Dis 2002; 16:117-122.

BREAST RECONSTRUCTION – AUTOGENOUS TISSUE

Lawrence Iteld, MD, and Jules Feledy, Jr, MD

I. General Principles and Anatomy

❍ **What is the innervation to the nipple-areolar complex?**

Primarily the fourth anterolateral and anteromedial intercostal nerve, often with some contribution from T3 and T5.

❍ **What is the blood supply to the breast?**

Internal mammary perforators (2/3), axillary artery, 3rd-5th intercostal arteries.

❍ **What is the primary lymphatic drainage of the breast? The secondary basin?**

Axillary. Internal mammary.

❍ **What are Cooper's Ligaments?**

Suspensory ligaments that extend from the deep fascia through the breast parenchyma to the dermis of the overlying skin.

❍ **What is amazia?**

Congenital lack of breast development.

❍ **What is amastia?**

Lack of glandular tissue.

❍ **What is athelia?**

Lack of a nipple.

❍ **What are the breast features of Poland Syndrome?**

Hypoplasia/ absence of the ipsilateral sternal head of the pectoralis major.
Hypoplasia/ aplasia of the unilateral breast.
Hypoplasia/ absence of the unilateral ribs.

❍ **What is the timing for reconstruction in Poland Syndrome based upon?**

Development of the contralateral normal breast.

❍ **What are characteristics of Tuberous Breast Syndrome?**

Constricted vertical height, breast hypoplasia, and areolar hypertrophy.

❍ **What is the standard grading of breast ptosis?**

Grade I- Nipple is above or at the inframammary fold level.
Grade II- Nipple is below the IMF.
Grade III- Nipple is below the IMF and below the horizontal lower pole (down-pointing).

○   **What is pseudoptosis?**

The breast mass descends below the inframammary fold while the nipple remains above the IMF.

○   **The 'forbidden triangle' for making scars on the breast is?**

The xiphoid through the nipples up to the acromion.

○   **What is the innervation of the pectoralis major muscle?**

The medial and lateral pectoral nerves. The clavicular portion is supplied by C5-C6 and the sternal muscle fibers are supplied by C7-C8.

II. Patient Selection

○   **What are the major advantages of immediate autologous breast reconstruction?**

Immediate autologous reconstruction, on average, achieves the best cosmetic match to the native, mature breast. The reconstructed breast has ptosis that is determined by the native skin envelope, and a soft feel provided by the transplanted fat. Autologous tissues are more resistant to infection and not subject to capsular contracture. Finally, after the initial reconstruction and necessary revisions, autologous reconstructions require less late interventions and will change in size with patient weight gain and loss. Overall, this is the preferred reconstructive procedure in women who are appropriate candidates.

○   **What are the major disadvantages of immediate autologous reconstruction?**

Compared with implant-based reconstruction, the recovery time, surgical time, and time off of work is increased. In patients with advanced carcinoma who may (stage II) or will (stage III, IV) receive adjuvant radiotherapy, there is risk of compromise to the final reconstruction (see below). Finally, after unilateral reconstruction with lower abdominal tissue, if the woman develops contralateral carcinoma, alternative options must be entertained.

○   **What are the major advantages of delayed autologous reconstruction?**

Patients with advanced carcinoma can receive adjuvant chemo-radiotherapy without delay from reconstructive complications. Additionally, patients with advanced carcinomas, unfavorable histology, or inflammatory disease are at high risk for recurrence and require unimpeded monitoring. Delayed reconstruction will allow for easier monitoring in the first 12-24 months and then follow with reconstruction. Finally, immediate reconstruction may not be feasible because of sub-optimal donor sites and these may become available with weight loss or gain.

○   **What are the major disadvantages of delayed autologous reconstruction?**

Loss of the native skin envelope, need to recreate the inframammary fold, exploration of recipient vessels in previously operated field.

○   **What are some of the major radiation therapy issues that must be considered in autologous breast reconstruction?**

Radiation effects on tissue are permanent and progressive. They include fibrosis, fibroblast dysfunction, local tissue hypoxia, myointimal fibrosis and atherosclerosis, and impaired leukocyte migration. Together these factors predispose radiated tissues to being less elastic, subject to impaired wound healing and infection. Also, the cosmetic outcome of radiated breast is, on average, less supple, more contracted, and worse color match than non-radiated controls.

Immediate autologous reconstructions that are secondarily radiated have variable changes that are unpredictable. Some breasts undergo minimal change while some experience significant volume loss and envelope contracture. Nevertheless, the effects of radiation on autologous reconstruction are better tolerated than prosthetic reconstructions. Implants that are placed in radiated beds or are secondarily radiated are at increased risk of significant capsule contracture, infection, and exposure.

❍   **What reconstruction should be employed if radiation is necessary or has been in the past?**

In general, autologous techniques are recommended in the setting of XRT.

❍   **What is the definition of overweight? Obese?**

Overweight- body mass index (kg/height in m^2) >25
Obese- BMI > 30
In 2000, 65% of Americans are overweight and 30% are obese.

❍   **What are the effects of obesity on autologous breast reconstruction?**

The overall complication rate is increased in obese patients compared to normal weigh controls. These include wound healing delay, total and partial flap loss rates.

❍   **Compared with non-smokers, smokers have an increased risk of which complications following TRAM reconstruction?**

Mastectomy skin flap necrosis, abdominal flap necrosis, and abdominal bulge and hernia.

❍   **What are relative contraindications to autologous reconstruction?**

Obesity (morbid), active nicotine use, connective tissue disease, hypercoagulable disorders, unexplained previous failed reconstruction, inability to withstand the surgical stress of a 6-12 hour operation, inability to comprehend or emotionally accept the donor site complications, unrealistic expectations.

❍   **Indications for latissimus dorsi flap harvest include?**

A thin body habitus with an insufficient pannus for autologous reconstruction, primary musculocutaneous coverage of an implant, and salvage of implant coverage, especially in the irradiated patient.

❍   **What maneuvers can be performed preoperatively in the clinic to determine if the thoracodorsal pedicle is intact?**

The back is examined with the patient standing with hands on her hips and shoulders and elbows adducted to see if the latissimus muscle is intact.

❍   **Which costs more: implant based reconstruction or autologous reconstruction?**

Initially autologous-based reconstructions are more expensive and are largely due to longer intra-operative times and longer hospitalization times. However, over time implant-based reconstructions become more expensive due to need for revision procedures and implant related complications.

III. Autologous Flaps

❍   **What is the most common donor site for autologous breast reconstruction?**

The lower abdomen.

O   **The dominant source vessels to the lower abdominal angiosomes are from which vessels?**

Deep inferior epigastric artery (DIEA)

O   **What is the origin of the DIEA? Pedicle length? Vessel diameter?**

The DIEA originates from the external iliac artery. On average, the pedicle is 7.5 cm long from the origin to the lateral border of the rectus abdominis muscle. This can be significantly lengthened (15cm) with intramuscular dissection. The external diameter of the artery averages 3.5 mm and the confluent vena commitans 4.0 mm at the iliacs.

O   **How does the DIEA supply the lower abdominal skin?**

The DIEA most often splits into medial and lateral branches that give off a variable number of muscular perforators that pass through the rectus abdominis muscle to supply the overlying skin.

O   **What is a TRAM flap?**

Transverse Rectus Abdominis Musculocutaneous flap.

O   **What is the blood supply to the rectus abdominis muscle?**

It is a class III muscle with a dual blood supply. The deep inferior system and the deep superior system.

O   **What is the anatomic orientation of the blood supply of the pedicled TRAM, the superior epigastric artery, as it enters the rectus abdominis muscle?**

It enters at the junction of medial and middle thirds of the rectus muscle.

O   **What are the zones of a TRAM flap? Which are reliable?**

Zone I- Ipsilateral to the blood vessel, medial to the lateral border of the rectus muscle (reliable)
Zone II- Contralateral, medial to the lateral border of the rectus. (Reliable)
Zone III- Ipsilateral, lateral to the lateral rectus border (variable)
Zone IV- Contralateral. Lateral to rectus (unreliable)

O   **Why delay a TRAM flap?**

While the rectus abdominis muscle has a dual blood supply, the lower abdominal skin is preferentially supplied by the inferior system (65%). After division of the deep inferior system and significant increase in vessel diameter and blood flow through the superior epigastric artery is seen. This may reduce fat necrosis compared to standard pedicled TRAM flaps.

O   **Delay of a TRAM flap is optimal after how long?**

10-14 days

O   **What are the two main disadvantages of delayed flaps?**

Additional surgical procedure with attendant surgical morbidity; failure of the technique to completely protect the far contralateral TRAM flap zones

O   **What is supercharging a flap?**

Anastomosing a second blood supply to a flap. In this setting of breast reconstruction, the deep inferior system of a pedicled TRAM is anastomosed to the mammary or thoracodorsal vessels.

What is a muscle-sparing TRAM flap?

The lower abdominal skin is harvested with either the lateral or the medial row of perforating vessels with a cuff of rectus muscle.

What is a DIEP flap?

Perforating vessels are identified and dissected from between the fibers of the rectus muscle down to the proper deep inferior system.

What is the primary advantage of the DIEP flap over the TRAM flap?

Preservation of the rectus abdominis muscle integrity and limited sacrifice of anterior rectus sheath fascia.

What is a PUP flap?

Many authors use this term differently. In general it refers to harvesting the lower abdominal tissues based on a single large peri-umbilical perforator. The perforator is either divided at the fascia level or is traced around the medial edge of the rectus muscle for a short distance.

What is a SIE flap? What are the advantages? Disadvantages?

The superficial inferior epigastric artery originates from the common femoral artery pass above the inguinal ligament and enters the lower abdominal skin above or below Scarpa's fascia. The veins drain into the saphenous bulb. When present and large enough for transfer (~20% of cases), complete preservation of the abdominal wall is possible. However, perfusion does not reliably cross the midline.

What are the most common recipient vessels for a microvascular (free) TRAM?

Internal mammary vessels and thoracodorsal vessels.

What are the advantages to using the internal mammary vessels?

Reliable and avoids an axillary dissection to find the thoracodorsal vessels, which is an important consideration with the increased use of Breast Conservative Therapy (BCT). Preserves the thoracodorsal vessels for use in salvage procedures.

What are the disadvantages to using the internal mammary vessels?

Technically more difficult dissection, left side tend to be smaller than right (controversial data), may be in radiation field of delayed reconstructions, risk for pneumothorax.

What is the incidence of microvascular thrombosis and total flap loss in breast reconstruction?

< 2-5%

What is the most common complication specific to a TRAM flap?

Fat necrosis

What are other common complications of which patients should be aware?

Mastectomy flap necrosis, asymmetry, contour abnormalities, seroma, hematoma, disruption of the inframammary fold, effacement of anterior axillary fold, donor site complications (see below).

○　**How does one inset a lower abdominal flap?**

Every surgeon has their own opinion about the best technique to inset their reconstruction. In general, a narrow breast is inset with the flap vertically or obliquely oriented, whereas a wide breast is inset transversely. Coning the flap provides a useful way to increase lower pole projection.

○　**How does one perform an innervated breast reconstruction?**

The lower abdominal skin is harvested with a sensory nerve (usually 10th intercostal), which is coapted to the 4th intercostal sensory stump. Authors who advocate this procedure feel that erogenous reinnervation can be achieved. Data is still preliminary.

○　**What salvage maneuvers can be performed for a venous-congested pedicled TRAM flap?**

Leeches, supercharging, conversion to a free flap.

○　**What is the blood supply to the latissimus dorsi muscle flap?**

The latissimus dorsi is a Class V muscle with the thoracodorsal (TD) artery being the dominant system. The TD is a terminal branch of the subscapular system. The vessel is approximately 5.5 cm long from the circumflex scapular branch to the intramuscular bifurcation to the descending and transverse branches. In general a pedicle arc of 8 cm can be harvested without difficulty. This allows transposition to the anterior chest for breast reconstruction.

○　**What other important vessel originates from the thoracodorsal system? Why is this important?**

The serratus anterior branch. In the event the thoracodorsal system is utilized for microvascular transfer, if preserved, the serratus branch can provide retrograde perfusion to the latissimus muscle that can be used in salvage procedures.

○　**How can a latissimus dorsi reconstruction be utilized without an implant?**

The "extended" latissimus dorsi flap is usually harvested with a transversely oriented skin paddle that averages 8 cm wide and up to 22 cm long. The adipose layer of the back is harvested over the entire latissimus muscle by beveling outward from the skin island.

○　**What is the next most common donor site for autologous breast reconstruction?**

The gluteal region, i.e. "GAP" flaps

○　**What is the blood supply to the S-GAP? The I-GAP?**

The superior and inferior gluteal arteries respectively.

○　**What are the major advantages of the GAP flaps?**

They provide a donor site for autologous reconstruction in patients without adequate abdominal tissue, especially if bilateral reconstruction is considered.

○　**What are the major disadvantages of the GAP flaps?**

Technically more challenging dissection, shorter pedicles, more fibrous fat, risk of injury to the sciatic nerve with the I-GAP, and need for position changes. Also the donor site can be problematic in unilateral harvest requiring contralateral symmetry procedures.

○ **What is the blood supply the Rubens flap is based upon?**

Deep circumflex iliac artery and vein.

○ **What other donor sites have been advocated in the past 10 years?**

Transversely oriented gracilis musculocutaneous flap, anterolateral thigh musculocutaneous or fasciocutaneous flap.

○ **What options are available for the partial mastectomy defect?**

Local tissue rearrangement, latissimus dorsi muscle or musculocutaneous flap, completion mastectomy and immediate reconstruction.

○ **What is the size limit that can be reliably be fixed with local tissue rearrangement?**

~25%

○ **How can one reconstruct an inferior pole defect?**

Mastopexy or mammaplasty techniques.

○ **What is the preferred technique for lateral partial mastectomy defects?**

Latissimus dorsi flap.

○ **What is the problem with implant reconstruction for the partial mastectomy defect?**

Often can exacerbate asymmetries.

○ **What partial mastectomy defects are best reconstructed with total mastectomy and autologous tissue?**

Large defects of the medial quadrant.

IV. Donor Site Issues

○ **What is the blood supply to the umbilicus?**

Perforating vessels of the deep inferior epigastric artery, small vessels of the ligamentum teres and medial umbilical ligament

○ **What is the most common abnormality of the abdomen after breast reconstruction with lower abdominal tissue?**

Abdominal bulge.

○ **What is the incidence of bulge formation after TRAM flap reconstruction? Hernia?**

Bulge: 5-20%; Hernia: 1-2%

○ **How can abdominal bulges and hernia risk be minimized?**

Reconstruction with prosthetic meshes. In-lay techniques are stronger than on lay.

○ **What are the functional consequences of unilateral rectus abdominis muscle harvest?**

On strict biomechanical testing there is a noticeable decrease in anterior abdominal muscle weakness after muscle harvest. However, most patients do not state that this is a problem in daily activity.

○   **Which patients experience significant compromise from rectus abdominis harvest?**

Athletes, heavy laborers, bilateral muscle harvest, and patients with significant antecedent lower back pain.

○   **What factors contribute to abnormal abdominal function and contour in unilateral breast reconstruction?**

Preservation of rectus abdominis musculature and laterally based intercostals perforators and nerve supply.

○   **Can abdominal weakness result from a DIEP flap harvest?**

Yes.

○   **Does abdominal weakness result from SIEF harvest?**

No.

○   **What considerations need to be given to patients with prior surgery?**

Midline- medial perforators may be divided, inability to perfuse across midline with unilateral harvest.

Open cholecystectomy- unable to utilize right pedicled TRAM.

Low transverse (Pfanensteil)- medial perforators may be divided. Deep inferior epigastric vessels may be injured.

Umbilical hernia- Risk for umbilical necrosis.

CABG- Internal mammary vessels, and subsequently the superior epigastric vessels, may be unavailable.

○   **What is the most common donor site complication with latissimus dorsi flaps?**

Seroma, occurring in up to 30% of patients.

BREAST RECONSTRUCTION – ALTERNATIVE FLAPS

Karen M. Horton, MD, MSc, BScH

○ **List considerations in selecting an appropriate method for breast reconstruction.**

1.   laxity and thickness of remaining breast skin
2.   condition of the pectoralis major and serratus anterior muscles
3.   size of the opposite breast
4.   availability of flap donor sites
5.   patient wishes
6.   surgeon training and preference.

○ **List the advantages of autogenous tissue breast reconstruction.**

(1) More natural shape than implants, (2) normal consistency, (3) less need to alter the contralateral breast, (4) reconstruction is permanent, (5) reconstruction ages with the patient.

○ **What are indications for autogenous tissue breast reconstruction?**

(1) Patient preference, (2) mastectomy site tissue deficiency, (3) recurrent capsular contracture with implant reconstruction, (4) recurrent periprosthetic infection, (5) coverage of implants at risk for extrusion, (6) salvage of ruptured silicone implants and granuloma formation, (7) history of collagen vascular disease, (8) previous chest wall irradiation.

○ **What are contraindications of autogenous tissue breast reconstruction?**

(1) Inadequate donor site soft tissue and skin, (2) injury to donor or recipient vessels, (3) uncontrolled hypertension or diabetes, (4) morbid obesity, (5) heavy smoking, (6) severe pulmonary, cardiac or renal disease, (7) autoimmune disease, (8) anticoagulation therapy.

○ **What are the best aesthetic subunits of the breast?**

(1) Nipple, (2) areola, (3) expanded areola, (4) inferolateral crescent, (5) inferior half, (6) total breast. Autogenous reconstruction using these perceived subunits for skin paddles may improve the overall aesthetic appearance of the breast mound. Less aesthetic subunits include the upper inner quadrant, medial half, inferomedial quadrant, and random patch of flap skin.

○ **Which pedicled flaps have been described for breast reconstruction?**

(1) Pedicled latissimus dorsi, (2) pedicled TRAM/VRAM flap, (3) thoracoepigastric flap, (4) omental flap, (5) external oblique flap, (6) lateral abdominal skin flap.

○ **Which random flaps have been described for breast reconstruction?**

(1) Sliding skin flap from the abdomen, (2) composite cone ("dog-ear") flap, (3) midabdominal skin flap, (4) contralateral breast flap, (5) deepithelialized arm flap, (6) tubed abdominal flap, (7) adipofascial anterior rectus sheath flap.

○ **List the free flaps that have been described for breast reconstruction.**

(1) Free TRAM flap, (2) VRAM flap, (3) DIEP flap, (4) SIEA flap, (5) Rubens (DCIA) flap, (6) TFL (lateral transverse thigh) flap, (7) ALT flap, (8) omental flap, (9) groin flap, (10) adipofascial / anterior rectus sheath flap, (11) inferior or superior gluteal flap, (12) S-GAP flap, (13) I-GAP flap, (14) vertical gracilis flap, (15) TUG flap (transverse upper gracilis), (16) free LD flap, (17) TAP flap, (18) intercostal artery perforator flap.

○   **What is the blood supply and classification of the latissimus dorsi (LD) flap?**

The main pedicle is the thoracodorsal artery and vein, which arises from the third part of the subscapular artery, and enters the undersurface of the muscle 8-12 cm from its insertion. In 86% of cases, it divides into a vertical descending branch and a transverse horizontal branch within the muscle. The LD is a type V flap, with secondary segmental pedicles from the posterior intercostal and lumbar artery perforators.

○   **Describe the origins and insertion of the LD muscle?**

Origins include: (1) lower 6 thoracic spines and supraspinous ligaments, (2) posterior layer of lumbar fascia, (3) tendinous attachments to posterior iliac crest, (4) interdigitations with external oblique muscle, (5) lower 3-4 ribs, (6) scapula. It inserts via a 10 cm long tendon into the floor of the bicipital/intertubercular groove of the humerus, behind the tendon of the long heard of biceps brachii.

○   **Which variations of the LD flap have been described for breast reconstruction?**

(1) LD muscle only flap (+/- implant), (2) LD myocutaneous flap (+/- implant), (3) "extended" LD flap (no implant), (4) "total autogenous" LD flap (no implant), (5) endoscopically-harvested LD flap, (6) free LD flap.

○   **Which configurations of skin paddles have been described for the LD flap?**

Transverse, vertical, crescentic, oblique, fleur-de-lis pattern. Approximately 8-10 cm of back skin can be harvested with the flap, with primary closure of the donor site.

○   **How can the LD pedicle be lengthened?**

By (1) dividing the tendinous insertion to the humerus, (2) dividing the serratus anterior branch, or (3) dividing cutaneous branches to the lateral chest wall. The tendon may be transposed anteriorly and repositioned to recreate an absent anterior axillary fold.

○   **What are the advantages and disadvantages of the LD flap for breast reconstruction?**

Advantages include (1) reliable vascular pedicle, (2) large diameter vessels (artery 2.5 mm, vein 3.5 mm), (3) favorable geometry for breast reconstruction, (4) well-vascularized tissue to prevent radiation-related complications. Disadvantages include (1) implant required for projection in most cases, (2) large, visible scar on the back, (3) frequent postoperative seroma.

○   **What is done with the thoracodorsal nerve upon transposition of the latissimus muscle to the anterior chest?**

The motor nerve may be divided primarily upon flap transposition to the chest in order to avoid involuntary muscle contraction. The nerve may also be preserved to preserve muscle bulk, and secondarily divided if problems with movement occur.

○   **How has the LD flap been successfully harvested when the main thoracodorsal pedicle was damaged/unavailable?**

By retrograde flow from the collateral serratus anterior branch to the lateral thoracic artery. The thoracodorsal artery gives off 1-2 branches to the serratus muscle prior to entering the LD muscle.

○   **What are the advantages of microvascular free tissue transfer over conventional pedicled transfer of autogenous tissue?**

(1) Enhanced vascular perfusion/reliability, (2) ability to transfer large volumes of tissue and perform shaping manoeuvres without tethering from pedicle, (3) easier flap insetting without pedicle, (4) no tunnel or deformity from transposed pedicle, (5) occasionally improved donor site morbidity, (6) greater choice of donor sites, with ability to tailor flap to body habitus of patient, (7) less risk of complications from smoking or diabetes on larger, higher-flow vessels.

○   **What are disadvantages of free flap breast reconstruction?**

Requirements of microsurgical training and potential for complete flap loss.

○   **What are the indications for free flap reconstruction of the breast?**

(1) Large chest wall defects following radical mastectomy +/- radiation, where regional flaps will not suffice, (2) previously failed regional flaps, (3) desire to minimize donor site morbidity, (4) inadequate TRAM tissue, (5) violation of TRAM flap pedicle, previous TRAM or abdominoplasty, (6) surgeon's preference for free tissue transfer, (7) patient risk factors such as tobacco use or obesity.

○   **What are potential benefits of immediate breast reconstruction with free tissue transfer?**

(1) Psychologic benefit – immediate return of body image, (2) soft, uncontracted skin envelope of skin-sparing mastectomy unaffected by scar tissue and contracture, (3) remaining breast skin easily assumes the normal breast contour once volume restored, (4) only skin removed during mastectomy requires replacement, (5) inframammary fold and other breast landmarks are preserved and used, (6) exposed recipient vessels in axilla or nearby in the vicinity of the mastectomy defect, (7) fewer revisional and contralateral procedures to improve symmetry, (8) single hospitalization, (9) less time away from home or work, (10) less overall cost.

○   **List some specific contraindications to free flap breast reconstruction?**

(1) Previous division of microvascular pedicle, (2) significant medical morbidity (COPD, hepatic dysfunction, renal failure), (3) endocrine abnormalities (pheochromocytoma, uncontrolled hyperthyroidism), (4) Raynaud's phenomenon with refractory vasospasm.

○   **Which recipient vessels have been described for microvascular breast reconstruction?**

(1) Internal mammary vessels, (2) internal mammary perforators, (3) thoracodorsal vessels, (4) axillary vessels, (5) subscapular vessels, (6) circumflex scapular vessels, (7) lateral thoracic vessels, (8) thoracoacromial vessels, (9) serratus branches, (10) transverse cervical vessels, (11) gastroepiploic vessels, (12) branches of the external carotid vessels.

○   **What are the advantages and disadvantages of the internal mammary vessels over the thoracodorsal vessels for microvascular anastomosis?**

Advantages include: (1) more versatile and medial insetting of breast flap, (2) vascular pedicle free from arm and shoulder movement, (3) avoidance of brachial plexus complications, (4) vessels available despite previous axillary surgery or radiation, (5) excellent arterial flow from proximity to heart and large caliber, (6) surgeon and assistant comfort operating over center of chest, (7) good size match with DIEA system.

Disadvantages include: (1) requires medial chest scar exposure in delayed reconstruction, (2) additional time and dissection for rib cartilage removal, (3) delicate, thin walled, fragile internal mammary veins, (4) compromise of future availability of IMA for coronary bypass surgery, (5) risk breaching parietal pleura with hemothorax or pneumothorax, (6) movement of the thorax in and out of microscopic focus with respirations, (7) vein may be single or diminutive on the left side, (8) risk of contour depression with rib cartilage harvest in thin patients with significant ptosis.

○   **What are potential advantages and disadvantages of internal mammary artery perforating vessels for microsurgical breast reconstruction?**

Advantages include sparing of the IMA for possible future cardiac surgery, thoracic deformity with rib removal avoided, limited dissection decreases operative time. Disadvantages include limited surgical exposure, caliber incompatibility with flap vessels (0.5- 0.8 mm), and technical challenge.

○ **When would free flaps other than the TRAM, DIEP or SIEA flaps be considered for breast reconstruction?**

(1) Inadequate abdominal fat, (2) high-risk abdominal scars, (3) patient preference, (4) previous abdominal flap harvest/failure, (5) previous abdominoplasty, (6) lifestyle choice, (7) pregnancy plans – although normal pregnancies have been reported after TRAM flap surgery.

○ **Which scars are safe in harvesting abdominal tissue for breast reconstruction?**

(1) Appendectomy, (2) hysterectomy, (3) C-section, (4) laparoscopic cholecystectomy, (5) other laparoscopic scars.

○ **In which situations would abdominal tissue be inappropriate for breast reconstruction?**

(1) Inadequate abdominal fat, (2) high risk abdominal scars (paramedian, abdominoplasty, colostomy, ileostomy), (3) patient preference, (4) previous TRAM flap failure, (5) previous abdominoplasty, (6) pregnancy plans.

○ **What is a "perforator"?**

A vessel that has its origin in one of the axial vessels of the body, and that passes through structures besides interstitial connect tissue and fat before reaching the subcutaneous fat layer. Perforators may be direct (piercing the deep fascia without traversing any other structural tissue), or indirect, running first through muscle, septum or epimysium.

○ **Is the SIEA flap a "perforator flap"?**

By definition, no. The SIEA is a type A fasciocutaneous axial flap, supplied directly from the superficial inferior epigastric artery (SIEA), superficial to Scarpa's fascia. The SIEA arises from the femoral artery halfway between the pubic tubercle and the anterior superior iliac spine, 2-3 cm inferior to the inguinal ligament in the femoral triangle.

○ **What are the anatomic variations of the SIEA origin?**

The SIEA and superficial circumflex iliac artery (SCIA) share a common origin from the femoral artery 48% to 79% of the time, the SIEA and SCIA arise independently in approximately 17%, and the SIEA is absent in up to 35% of cases.

○ **What are the advantages and disadvantages of the SIEA flap for breast reconstruction?**

Advantages include: (1) same abdominal tissue as in TRAM or DIEP flaps, with zero risk of abdominal wall hernia, bulge or weakness, (2) can design flap more inferiorly with resultant low and inconspicuous scar, (3) shorter recovery time and less postoperative pain. Disadvantages include: (1) absent or diminutive vessels in 30% to 40% of cases, (2) short pedicle (2-6 cm), (3) small diameter vessels (artery 1.5-2.5 mm, vein 2-3 mm) with challenging vascular anastomosis, (4) vascular territory only reliable to midline (can only harvest a hemi-abdomen).

○ **What are advantages and disadvantages of perforator flaps over traditional musculocutaneous flaps?**

Advantages include: (1) less donor site morbidity, (2) muscle sparing, (3) versatility in design to include as little or as much tissue as required, (4) improved postoperative recovery. Disadvantages include: (1) require meticulous dissection of perforators through underlying tissue, (2) increased operative time, (3) variability in position and size of perforator vessels, (4) if sufficiently traumatized, perforators have tendency to stretch, kink or twist, causing vasospasm or thrombosis.

○ **What are features of and contraindications to commonly used perforator flaps?**

Acceptable perforator flap donor sites have: (1) predictable and consistent blood supply, (2) at least one large perforator of diameter >0.5 mm, (3) sufficient pedicle length for the procedure, (4) primary donor site closure without wound tension. Common contraindications to perforator flap procedures include: 1) patients with insufficiently small perforators (<0.5 mm), (2) excessive scarring at donor site, (3) heavy smokers.

O   **What are the I-GAP and S-GAP flaps?**

Perforator flaps supplied by branches pf inferior and superior gluteal artery, respectively. The gluteal arteries are terminal branches of the internal iliac artery and are codominant pedicles of the gluteus maximus muscle, separated by the piriformis muscle.

O   **Which nerve innervates the entire gluteus maximus muscle?**

The inferior gluteal nerve.

O   **What are the advantages and disadvantages of the S-GAP flap for breast reconstruction?**

Advantages include: (1) abundant adipose tissue for breast mound reconstruction, (2) can lengthen vascular pedicle by intramuscular dissection, (3) easily concealed donor site scar, (4) excellent projection of stiff adipose tissue, (5) preserves entire gluteus maximus muscle, (6) avoids exposure and retraction of the sciatic nerve.

Disadvantages include: (1) technically demanding flap harvest with steep learning curve, (2) difficult hemostasis, (3) short vascular pedicle (3-5 cm), (3) increased size discrepancy between diameter of donor and recipient vessels as the pedicle is lengthened, (4) postoperative contour deformity with unilateral flap harvest, (5) smaller skin paddle available, (6) frequent donor site seroma.

O   **How is the S-GAP blood supply identified?**

The superior gluteal artery (SGA) emerges from the edge of the sacrum through the suprapiriform foramen, 1/3 the distance along a line drawn from the posterior superior iliac spine (PSIS) to the greater trochanter tuberosity. The skin paddle is designed as a horizontal ellipse centered over perforators which are detected by preoperative Doppler ultrasound. The flap can be safely raised on a single perforator.

O   **What structures exit the sciatic notch and may be encountered when raising an I-GAP flap?**

(1) Inferior gluteal artery and vein, (2) sciatic nerve, (3) pudendal nerve, (4) inferior gluteal nerve, (5) posterior cutaneous nerve of thigh, (6) pudendal artery and vein.

O   **How may the gluteal artery perforator flap be made sensate?**

By anastomosis of the nervi clunium superioris, which provides sensation to the buttock region, to the 4th intercostal nerve of the chest. These sensory nerves originate from dorsal branches of the lumbar segmental nerves and perforate the deep fascia just above the iliac crest, lateral to the PSIS.

O   **Which structures are key to identifying the vascular pedicle of the I-GAP flap?**

The posterior cutaneous nerve of thigh and accompanying posterior thigh vessels, which arise from the inferior gluteal artery. These vessels can be traced superiorly under the inferior border of the gluteus maximus muscle, toward the sciatic notch and over the belly of the piriformis muscle. The sciatic nerve lies just deep to this plane.

O   **What are the advantages and disadvantages of the I-GAP flap for breast reconstruction?**

The I-GAP flap shares the advantages of the S-GAP flap. Specific disadvantages include: (1) risk of postoperative sciatica with sciatic nerve exposure, (2) tender scar in gluteal crease, (3) obligate sacrifice of sensory posterior cutaneous nerve of thigh, (4) potential posterior thigh neuroma.

O   **Describe the ideal patient for gluteal artery perforator flap breast reconstruction?**

Thin patient, nulliparous, high-risk abdominal scars or otherwise not a TRAM candidate, with insufficient volume in alternative donor sites. Bilateral reconstructions are best performed staged to limit operative time, repositioning intraoperatively, blood loss and surgeon fatigue.

○   **What is the blood supply of the Rubens flap?**

Cutaneous perforators from the descending branch of the deep circumflex iliac artery (DCIA) and vein. The Rubens flap is the cutaneous component of the DCIA osteocutaneous flap, described by Taylor. This redundant fat collection over the iliac crest was named for the 16th century painter Peter Paul Rubens' depiction of this area in the female form.

○   **Who is the ideal patient for the Rubens flap?**

A "gynecoid" (pear-shaped) female of normal weight, who has had a previous abdominoplasty or TRAM flap and desires autogenous breast reconstruction.

○   **What are the dimensions of the DCIA flap vascular pedicle?**

The pedicle averages 5-6 cm in length. The DCIA diameter is 2-3 mm, and the DCIV is 2.5-4.0 mm. Subperiosteal dissection and inclusion of a small muscular cuff around the pedicle protects the vessels are they travel over the iliac crest.

○   **What are potential complications of the Rubens flap?**

(1) Detailed donor site closure – the abdominal wall muscles must be reattached firmly to the iliac crest, using drill holes and sturdy sutures or bone anchors, (2) risk of hernia with insufficient donor site repair, (3) significant postoperative pain, (4) sensory nerve deficits (paresthesias, anaesthesia, neuroma), (5) significant donor site seroma, (6) donor site deformity necessitating contralateral procedure for symmetry.

○   **What is the blood supply of the lateral transverse thigh (TFL) flap?**

The transverse branch of the lateral femoral circumflex artery (LFCA) and venae comitantes. The LFCA (2-3 mm) arises from the profunda femoris artery. The LFCV (2-4 mm) enters the femoral vein, rather than the profunda femoris system. The TFL pedicle averages 7-8 cm.

○   **How is the TFL flap innervated?**

By the superior gluteal nerve (motor) and the lateral cutaneous branch of T12 / lateral femoral cutaneous nerve (sensory).

○   **What are the variations of the TFL flap?**

The skin paddle can be oriented transversely, obliquely, or vertically. Lateral orientation allows harvest of the skin and fat of the "saddlebag" region of the female hip. Vertical orientation allows a large skin area and facilitates primary closure in a "vest-over-pants" fashion.

○   **What are potential complications of the TFL flap?**

(1) Femoral nerve injury, (2) donor site seroma, (3) donor site deformity with a hollowed-out thigh contour.

○   **Which nerves are at risk in dissection of thigh and buttock area flaps?**

The femoral nerve is at risk with the TFL (lateral thigh) flap harvest. The sciatic nerve is at risk with the I-GAP flap. The cutaneous branch of T12 (lateral femoral cutaneous nerve of thigh) is at risk during the DCIA (Rubens) flap harvest.

○   **What is the blood supply of the anterolateral thigh (ALT) flap?**

Perforators from the descending branch of the lateral circumflex femoral artery, roughly located at the midpoint of a line linking the ASIS and the superolateral border of the patella.

○   **What are advantages and disadvantages of the ALT flap for breast reconstruction?**

Advantages include a long vascular pedicle (7-15 cm) with large vessel diameter (2-3mm), availability of a large amount of skin, ability to innervate the flap using the lateral femoral cutaneous nerve. Potential disadvantages include the visible donor scar and contour defect, need to skin graft donor defects wider than 8 cm, and variability of vessels that may require conversion to an ipsilateral anteromedial thigh flap, ipsilateral TFL flap, or contralateral ALT flap.

○   **Describe the TAP flap for breast reconstruction?**

The thoracodorsal artery perforator (TAP) flap may be transferred pedicled or free to the chest for breast reconstruction. The lateral branch of the thoracodorsal artery supplies perforators to skin and fat overlying the latissimus dorsi muscle.

○   **What are the advantages of the TAP flap?**

(1) Improved aesthetic appearance with intact latissimus dorsi muscle, (2) preservation of muscle function aids with rehabilitation, (3) vasculature – possibility of flow-through anastomosis, (4) anastomosis – reliable, wide diameter vessels, (5) follow-up T1-weighted MRI facilitates postoncologic follow-up, if required, (6) pedicle – average 20 cm, out of the zone of injury/radiation, (7) sensation – neurorrhaphy for sensation with intercostal nerves, (8) low incidence of seroma – no dead space.

○   **What are potential disadvantages of the TAP flap?**

(1) Size – limited to 10-12 cm x 25-30 cm, (2) perforators variable, (3) steep learning curve for experience, (4) requires lateral decubitus positioning for harvest, (5) may not enable two-team surgery, (6) interposition nerve grafts often required for neurorrhaphy.

○   **What is the TUG flap for breast reconstruction?**

The free transverse upper gracilis (TUG) myocutaneous flap, supplied by the ascending branch of the medial circumflex femoral artery. Pedicle length averages 6 cm, and vessel diameter, 1.6 mm. Vascular studies reveal the main cutaneous perforating vessels supply a transverse orientation of skin and subcutaneous tissue reliably approximately 10 cm distal to the pubic tubercle. Donor site closure creates a medial thigh lift.

○   **How does cigarette smoking affect flap blood flow?**

(1) Nicotine activates the sympathetic nervous system and produces cutaneous vasoconstriction, leading to compromise of tissue capillary blood flow, (2) carbon monoxide binds to hemoglobin and shifts the oxygen-hemoglobin saturation curve to the left, causing tissue hypoxia, (3) increased platelet aggregation from increased plasma fibrinogen levels, potentiating vascular thrombosis, (4) decreased endothelial synthesis of nitric oxide that impairs endothelium-dependent vasodilation of arteries.

○   **How does smoking affect the results of autogenous tissue breast reconstruction?**

Smoking interferes with wound healing and is associated with a significantly higher rate of mastectomy skin flap necrosis, abdominal wound dehiscence, postoperative infection, and fat necrosis. Nicotine slows blood flow to flaps and increases platelet adhesiveness. Smoking has not been found to increase complications with microvascular anastomoses or to increase the rate of free flap loss.

○   **What mammographic changes may be visible following breast reconstruction with autologous tissue?**

(1) Reconstructed breast composed of muscle, fat, vascular structures and skin in no orderly arrangement, (2) no remaining parenchymal structures, ducts, or Cooper's ligaments, (3) vascular clips may be present at or near the

muscle flap, (4) areas of skin thickening (5) patchy tissue densities or fat necrosis, (6) lucent oil cysts +/- calcified walls, (7) implant, if used.

○ **Which additional steps may further delineate a mammographic finding post-reconstruction?**

(1) Eklund displacement views, (2) spot views, (3) magnification films, (4) correlation with clinical examination, (5) fine needle aspiration cytology or core biopsy to rule out malignancy.

References

Allen RJ. The superior gluteal artery perforator flap. Clin Plast Surg 1998; 25:293-302.

Arnez ZM, Khan U, Pogorelec D et al. Breast reconstruction using the free superficial inferior epigastric artery (SIEA) flap. Br J Plast Surg 1999; 52:2760279.

Arnez ZM, Pogorelec D, Planinsek F et al. Breast reconstruction by the free transverse gracilis (TUG) flap. Br J Plast Surg 2004; 57:20-26.

Beckenstein MS, Grotting JC. Breast reconstruction with free-tissue transfer. Plast Reconstr Surg 2001; 108:1345-1353.

Blondeel PN, Van Landuyt KHI, Monstrey, SJM et al. The "Gent" consensus on perforator flap terminology: preliminary definitions. Plast Reconstr Surg 2003; 112:1378-1382.

Blondeel PN. The sensate free superior gluteal artery perforator (S-GAP) flap: a valuable alternative in autologous breast reconstruction. Plast Reconstr Surg 1999; 52:185-193.

Chevray PM. Breast reconstruction with superficial inferior epigastric artery flaps: a prospective comparison with TRAM and DIEP flaps. Plast Reconstr Surg 2004; 114:1077-1983.

Elliott LF, Hartrampf Jr. CR. The Rubens flap. The deep circumflex iliac artery flap. Clin Plast Surg. 1998; 25:283-291.

Elliott LF, Beegle PG, Hartrampf Jr CR. The lateral transverse thigh free flap: an alternative for autogenous-tissue breast reconstruction. Plast Reconstr Surg 1990; 85:169-178.

Fisher J, Bostwick III J, Powell RW. Latissimus dorsi blood supply after thoracodorsal vessel division: the serratus collateral. Plast Reconstr Surg 1983; 72:502-509.

Geddes CR, Morris SF, Neligan PC. Perforator flaps: evolution, classification, and applications. Ann Plast Surg 2003; 50:90-99.

Germann G, Steinau HU. Breast reconstruction with the extended latissimus dorsi flap. Plast Reconstr Surg 1996; 97:519-526.

Guerra AB, Metzinger SE, Bidros RS et al. Breast reconstruction with gluteal artery perforator (GAP) flaps. A critical analysis of 142 cases. Ann Plast Surg 2004; 52:118-125.

Guerra AB, Metzinger SE, Lund KM et al. The thoracodorsal artery perforator flap: clinical experience and anatomic study with emphasis on harvest techniques. Plast Reconstr Surg 2004; 114:32-41.

Hartrampf Jr CR, Noel RT, Drazan L et al. Ruben's fat pad for breast reconstruction: a peri-iliac soft tissue free flap. Plast Reconstr Surg 1994; 93:402-407.

Hartrampf Jr CR, Anton MA, Bried JT. Breast reconstruction with the transverse abdominal island (TRAM) flap. In: Georgiade GS, Riefkohl R, Levin LS, eds. Georgiade Plastic, Maxillofacial and Reconstructive Surgery. 3rd ed. Baltimore: Williams & Wilkins, 1997:786-797.

Hidalgo DA. Aesthetic refinement in breast reconstruction: complete skin-sparing mastectomy with autogenous tissue transfer. Plast Reconstr Surg 1998; 102:63-70.

Hokin JAB, Silfverskiold KL. Breast reconstruction without an implant: results and complications using an extended latissimus dorsi flap. Plast Reconstr Surg 1987; 79:58-64.

Hoover SJ, Kenkel JM. Breast cancer, cancer prevention, and breast reconstruction. Selected Readings in Plastic Surgery, 9(30):1-40.

Kaplan JL, Allen RJ, Guerra A et al. Anterolateral thigh flap for breast reconstruction: review of the literature and case reports. J Reconstr Microsurg 2003; 19:63-68.

Leibman AJ, Styblo TM, Bostwick III J. Mammography of the postreconstruction breast. Plast Reconstr Surg 1997; 99:698-704.

Maxwell GP, Hammond DC. Breast reconstruction following mastectomy and surgical management of the patient with high-risk breast disease. In: Aston SJ, Beasley RW, Thorne CHM, eds. Grabb and Smith's Plastic Surgery. 5th ed. Philadelphia: Lippincott-Raven, 1997, 763-784.

Munhoz AM, Ishida LH, Montag E et al. Perforator flap breast reconstruction using internal mammary perforator branches as a recipient site: an anatomical and clinical analysis. Plast Reconstr Surg 2004; 114:62-68.

Oslin BD, Grotting JC. Microsurgical breast reconstruction. In: Georgiade GS, Riefkohl R, Levin LS, eds. Georgiade Plastic, Maxillofacial and Reconstructive Surgery. 3rd ed. Baltimore: Williams & Wilkins, 1997:798-806.

Papp C, McCraw JB. Autogenous latissimus breast reconstruction. Clin Plast Surg 1998; 25:261-266.

Rizzuto RP, Allen RJ. Reconstruction of a partial mastectomy defect with the superficial inferior epigastric artery (SIEA) flap. J Reconstr Microsurg 2004; 20(6):441-446.

Shaw WW. Discussion: The internal mammary artery and vein as a recipient site for free-flap breast reconstruction: a report of 110 consecutive cases. 1996; 98:690-692.

Shaw WW, Watson J, Ahn CY. Alternatives in autologous free-flap breast reconstruction. In: Georgiade GS, Riefkohl R, Levin LS, eds. Georgiade Plastic, Maxillofacial and Reconstructive Surgery. 3rd ed. Baltimore: Williams & Wilkins, 1997:807-816.

Spear SL, Davison SP. Aesthetic subunits of the breast. Plast Reconstr Surg 2003; 112:440-447.

Strauch B, Vasconez LO, Hall-Findlay EJ eds. Breast, Chest Wall, and Trunk Reconstruction. In: Grabb's Atlas of Flaps. 2nd ed. Philadelphia: Lippincott-Raven, 1998; 3:1259-1372.

Wei FC, Suominen S, Cheng MH et al. Anterolateral thigh flap for postmastectomy breast reconstruction. Plast Reconstr Surg 2002; 110:82-88.

BREAST RECONSTRUCTION – MICROSURGERY

Charles K. Lee, MD, Mark W. Kiehn, MD, Rudolf Buntic, MD, and Gregory M. Buncke, MD

○ **In what percentage of patients is the TRAM flap not available for autologous breast reconstruction?**

25%. This is secondary to previous history of abdominal surgery or inadequate bulk of abdominal tissue.

○ **What is the dominant blood supply to the TRAM flap?**

Deep inferior epigastric vessels

○ **What are the 4 main functions of the rectus abdominis muscles?**

The rectus abdominis muscles are involved in the first 30° of lumbar spine flexion, stabilize the upper body, provide the site of insertion for the oblique and transversus abdominis muscles and assist in raising intraabdominal pressure.

○ **What other muscles are involved in torso flexion?**

Iliopsoas muscles (strongest upper body flexors) and the vertically oriented fibers of oblique muscles (lesser role)

○ **What is the "usual" relationship between the DIEA (deep inferior epigastric artery) perforators and the SIEA?**

Inverse — When the DIEA perforators are large or abundant, the SIEA is usually small and vice versa.

○ **How much abdominal wall fascia is taken with the SIEA flap?**

None.

○ **Where is the SIEA vessels found in relation to the inguinal ligament?**

2-3 cm below the ligament.

○ **Is the SIEA usually deep or superficial to Scarpa's fascia BELOW the inguinal ligament?**

Deep.

○ **Is the SIEA usually deep or superficial to Scarpa's fascia ABOVE the inguinal ligament?**

Superficial

○ **How do you design an S-GAP (Superior Gluteal Artery Perforator) flap?**

The flap is designed along a central axis formed by origin of the SGA at 5 cm inferior to posterior iliac spine and the dome of maximum lateral fullness. Dissection is carried over gluteus maximus from lateral to medial. The medial origin of the muscle is taken down to expose the pedicle.

○ **What flap dimensions can be obtained with the SGAP Flap?**

Skin: width 6-13 cm; length 20 – 33 cm. Pedicle length 8cm.

○ **What is a substantial disadvantage of the SGAP flap?**

Harvest requires prone or lateral repositioning during surgery.

○ **Can the SGAP flap be sensate?**

Yes, by the repairing the dorsal branches of the lumbar segmental nerves to the T4 intercostal nerve.

○ **Which nerve is sacrificed in the harvest of an Inferior Gluteal Flap?**

Posterior cutaneous nerve of thigh

○ **What is the vascular supply to the Ruben's Flap?**

Deep circumflex iliac system

○ **What is the average pedicle length of the Ruben's flap?**

7 cm

○ **What is a common donor site complication with this flap?**

Hernia due to inadequate repair of the abdominal wall at the iliac crest.

○ **Why perform the DIEP flap with its difficult dissection?**

Minimize donor site morbidity.

○ **How many perforators does this flap require to succeed?**

One good perforator.

○ **Will a perforator from the medial or lateral row provide better perfusion to zone 4?**

Medial row

○ **Which system – deep or superficial inferior epigastric – reliably supplies a greater area of the lower abdominal wall?**

Superficial inferior epigastric

○ **Which orientation (horizontal or transverse) of the skin paddle is most reliable when harvesting a gracilis musculocutaneous flap?**

Transverse.

○ **What is an advantage of this flap?**

Medial thigh lift, hidden donor scar, and minimal patient repositioning.

○ **At what level is the skin paddle centered for the TUG flap?**

Level of the pedicle – also level of major perforator

○ **Which vessels have become the most preferred recipient vessels in microsurgical breast reconstruction?**

The internal mammary vessels (internal thoracic).

○ **What are the advantages of the IM Vessels?**

Good size match with DIE vessels, improved positioning of the flap on the chest (more medial), avoid axillary dissection need for thoracodorsal vessels, preserves the dominant pedicle for the lattissimus dorsi muscle (lifeboat for reconstruction).

○ **The IMV is usually smaller on the Left or Right side?**

Left

○ **What are the advantages to the use of an IMA perforator as a recipient vessel?**

The IMA is preserved for future cardiac surgery, reduces the possibility of thoracic deformities, and simpler dissection

○ **What vessels are available as recipients for microsurgical breast reconstruction?**

Thoracodorsal, IMA, IMA Perforators, Thoracoacromial artery, Lateral Thoracic, Circumflex scapular arteries (branch of subscapular Artery)

○ **How many branches does the thoracoacromial artery usually have?**

4 main branches: Pectoral, Deltoid, Clavicular, Acromial

○ **How many centimeters lateral the sternal border are the Internal Mammary Vessels?**

1.5 cm

○ **At which intercostal interspace is anastomosis to the IM vessels usually performed in breast reconstruction?**

3rd

○ **What are two lifeboat veins in microsurgical breast reconstruction?**

Cephalic vein and external jugular. Both can be transposed and have been used successfully in problem venous anastomosis.

References

Arnez ZM et al, "Breast Reconstruction by the Free Transverse Gracilis Flap," British Association of Plastic Surgeons 2004: 57: 20-26.

Arnez ZM et al, "Breast Reconstruction using the SIEA flap," Br. Jo of Plastic Surgery Jan 1999: 276.

Blondeel PN, "The sensate free S-Gap flap," Br. Jo. of Plastic Surgery 1999: 52: 185.

Buncke HJ Microsurgery: Microsurgery: Transplantation and Replantation 1991.

Harris JR, "The Thoracoacromial/Cephalic Vascular System for Microvascular Anastomosis in the Vessel Depleted Neck," Arch Otolaryngology Head and Neck Surgery Vol 128 March 2002: 319.

Lantieri LA, et al, "Use of Circumflex Scapular Vessels as Recipient for Autologous Breast Reconstruction," PRS December 1999: 2049

Mehrara BJ, et al, "Alternative Venous Outflow Vessels in Microvascular Breast Reconstruction," PRS August 2003: 448.

Munhos AM, et al, "Perforator Flap Breast Reconstruction Using IM Perforator Branches as Recipient Site," PRS July 2004: 62.

Schoeller T, et al, "Medial Thigh Lift Free Flap for Autologous Breast Augmentation after Bar iatric Surgery," Obesity Surgery 12: 2002: 831.

Vandervoort M et al, "Perforator Topography of the Deep Inferior Epigastric Perforator Flap in 100 Cases of Breast Reconstruction," PRS May 2002: 1912.

Weschedlberger G and Schoeller T, "Traverse Myocutaneous Gracilis Free Flap, " PRS July 2004: 69.

Weschelberger G, et al, "Surgical technique and clinical application of the transverse gracilis myocutaneous free flap," Br. Jo. of Plastic Surgery (2001)54: 423.

Yousif NJ, et al, "The Traverse Gracilis Musculocutaneous Flap," Annals of Plastic Surgery Vol 29, December 1992: 482.

GYNECOMASTIA

Daron C. Hitt, MD

○ **Define gynecomastia.**

Glandular enlargement of the male breast.

○ **What is pseudogynecomastia?**

Enlargement of male breast due to fatty tissue.

○ **What are the three peaks in age distribution of gynecomastia?**

Neonatal, pubertal, and adult.

○ **What is the incidence of gynecomastia in each age group?**

60-90% neonates, 4-69% pubertal, and 35-65% adults.

○ **What is the Simon classification of gynecomastia?**

I: Small but visible breast development no skin redundancy.
IIa: Moderate breast development no skin redundancy.
IIb: Moderate breast development with skin redundancy.
III: Severe breast development with large skin redundancy.

○ **Name the hallmark location of gynecomastia?**

Directly beneath the nipple, eccentric masses may be malignant.

○ **What is symptomatic gynecomastia?**

Breast pain and tenderness.

○ **What are the clinical characteristics of pubertal gynecomastia?**

Glandular tissue greater than 4cm in diameter, resembles early female breast development.

○ **What is pubertal macrogynecomastia?**

Resembles Tanner stage IV development, greater than 5cm, will not regress.

○ **What is pathologic gynecomastia?**

Gynecomastia secondary to underlying disease or drug effect.

○ **Name the four categories of clinical etiologies of gynecomastia?**

Physiologic, pathologic, pharmacologic, familial.

○ **How is familial gynecomastia genetically transmitted?**

X-linked recessive or sex-limited autosomal dominant.

O   **What is the normal average areolar diameter in the male nipple areola complex?**

25-30mm.

O   **What is the pathogenesis of pubertal gynecomastia?**

Increased conversion of androgens to estrogens in tissue sites. Decreased daytime secretion of testosterone

O   **What is the pathogenesis of senescent gynecomastia?**

Primary testicular failure and increased adipose tissue leading to increased aromatase activity.

O   **What is the pathogenesis of drug induced gynecomastia?**

Administration of exogenous estrogens   e.g. Marijuana.
Reduction of androgen effect   e.g. Ketoconazole.
Direct testicular effect   e.g. Alkylating agents.
Blockade of androgen action   e.g. cimetidine.

O   **Elevated levels of which gonadotropins leads to gynecomastia?**

LH and HCG.

O   **How does primary testicular failure lead to increased estrogen to androgen ratio and gynecomastia?**

Reduced androgen production and increased aromatase activity in Leydig cells resulting in increased estrogen levels.

O   **By what mechanism do testicular tumors increase estrogens?**

Steroid producing tumor cells and paraneoplastic production of HCG.

O   **What mechanism is thought to cause gynecomastia associated with hyperthyroidism?**

Increased production of androstenedione.

O   **What two mechanisms result in gynecomastia in liver tumor patients?**

Increased HCG secretion and increased aromatization of circulating adrenal androgens.

O   **What endocrinopathies lead to gynecomastia?**

Hypogonadism, hyperthyroidism, and adrenal disorders.

O   **What tumors are associated with pubertal gynecomastia?**

Endocrine (pituitary, adrenal, and testicular), liver, and breast.

O   **What chronic diseases are associated with gynecomastia?**

Ulcerative colitis, cystic fibrosis, AIDS, liver disease, and malnutrition.

O   **What congenital form of primary testicular failure has gynecomastia as a common finding?**

Klinefelter's syndrome.

○ **What percentage of testicular tumors present with gynecomastia?**

5-10%.

○ **What radiographic modalities are used to diagnose gynecomastia?**

Ultrasound and mammography.

○ **Describe the mammographic patterns seen with gynecomastia?**

Nodular, dendritic/fibrous, and diffuse glandular patterns.

○ **What should be suspected with an eccentric breast mass?**

Malignant mass.

○ **When should mammography be used to evaluate gynecomastia?**

To rule out malignancy.

○ **Which laboratory tests should be obtained in pubertal gynecomastia?**

No routine tests. Test if abnormalities are suspected from history and physical.

○ **Which laboratory tests should be obtained in adult onset gynecomastia?**

Electrolytes, LFTs, TFTs, BUN, creatinine, testosterone, estradiol, FSH, LH, HCG.

○ **What is the typical serum prolactin level in patients with gynecomastia?**

Normal.

○ **Which conditions cause elevated prolactin levels in association with gynecomastia?**

Prolactin-secreting pituitary neoplasms, and hypothyroidism.

○ **What physical exam findings help differentiate gynecomastia from breast cancer?**

Gynecomastia is characterized by symmetric mobile disc subareolar tissue. Breast cancer is usually an ill-defined subareolar eccentric mass, hard, painless, ulcerated, immobile, has nipple retraction, and exhibits discharge.

○ **What historical information is important in the gynecomastia patient?**

Onset, duration, decreased libido, erectile dysfunction, infertility, medication history, and history of chronic disease.

○ **What medical treatments have shown to be effective for gynecomastia?**

Danazol, Tamoxifen, and Testosterone.

○ **What percentage of patients experience reduction in breast size with danazol use?**

60% with marked reduction, 25% moderate reduction.

○ **What effect does tamoxifen have on gynecomastia?**

Reduction in breast pain, and a small decrease in breast size.

○ **What common gender chromosome disorder is associated with gynecomastia?**

Klinefelter's Syndrome.

○ **Name the modalities for treating gynecomastia?**

Pharmacologic treatment, surgery, and radiation.

○ **How successful is radiation in reducing gynecomastia?**

Incidence of gynecomastia decreased to 28% if radiation was given prophylactically before use of flutamide.

○ **What surgical options are available to treat gynecomastia?**

Liposuction, subcutaneous mastectomy through various approaches, or combination therapy.

○ **What technique is most useful for gynecomastia without skin excess?**

Ultrasound-assisted liposuction (UAL).

○ **How is standard liposuction useful in gynecomastia?**

Reduces bulk of breast fullness when high percentage of breast tissue is fat. Aids in contouring.

○ **What suctioning technique has proven useful for hypertrophied fibrous breast tissue?**

UAL

○ **What are the complications associated with surgical resection?**

Inversion of nipple or areola, necrosis of nipple areolar complex, contour deformity, poor scarring, skin redundancy, inadequate excision, asymmetry, hematoma, seroma, and infection.

○ **What is the "doughnut" or "saucer" deformity?**

Overresection beneath nipple causing a concave appearance.

○ **How do you avoid the saucer deformity?**

Maintain adequate thickness on the nipple areolar flap.

○ **What is the most common complication with direct excision?**

Over resection and hematoma.

○ **What technique can be used with severe gynecomastia?**

Free nipple graft with crescent excision.

References

Beckenstein MS, Windle BH, and Stroup RT. Ann Plast Surg. 1996; 36:33-36.

Daniels IR and Layer GT. Gynaecomastia. Eur J Surg. 2001; 167:885-892.

Glass AR. Gynecomastia. Endo Met Clin North Am. 1994; 23:825-837.

John Bostwick III Aesthetic Problems. In: Plastic and Reconstructive Breast Surgery. Second Edition. St. Louis: Quality Medical Publishing, Inc. 2000:584-607.

Mahoney CP. Adolescent gynecomastia. Ped Clin North Am. 1990; 37:1389-1401

Riefkohl R, Zavitsanos GP, Courtiss, EH. Gynecomastia. In: Georgiade GS, Riefkohl R, Levin LS, eds. Plastic, Maxillofacial and Reconstructive Surgery. Third Edition. Baltimore: Williams & Wilkins, 1987:820-828

Rohrich RJ, Ha RY, Kenkel J, and WP Adams. Classification and management of gynecomastia: defining the role of ultrasound-assisted liposuction. Plast Reconstr Surg. 2003; 111: 909-923.

Volpe CM, Rafetto JD, Collure DW, Hoover EL, and Doerr RJ. Unilateral male breast masses: cancer risk and their evaluation and management. Am Surg. 1999; 65: 250-253.

Wise GJ, Roorda AK, and Kalter R. Male breast disease. J Am Coll Surg. 2005; 200:255-269.

BREAST REDUCTION AND MASTOPEXY

Robert Oliver, MD

❍ **Where does the nipple-areolar complex (NAC) get its innervation from?**

Predominately from the <u>lateral cutaneous branches of the 4th intercostal sensory nerve</u>. These fibers course deep within the pectoralis fascia before rising to innervate the NAC from its posterior surface in 93% of cadaveric specimens.

❍ **What is the sensory innervation to other areas of the breast?**

The upper pole is innervated by the supraclavicular nerves, which come from the third and fourth branches of the cervical plexus. The medial and lateral breast is innervated by the anterior and lateral cutaneous branches of intercostals nerves two thru seven.

❍ **What is the dominant vessel in the arterial supply to the breast?**

The major blood supply comes from the <u>internal mammary artery (IMA) perforators</u> (estimated 60% total), with significant collaterals from the <u>lateral thoracic artery</u>, the <u>thoracoacromial trunk</u>, the <u>thoracodorsal artery</u>, as well as numerous <u>intercostal</u> perforators from interspaces 3-5.

❍ **What are some relative preoperative indications that a free nipple graft may be required during reduction mammoplasty?**

- estimated 1500 gm or more reductions
- nipple transpositions > 25cm
- smokers
- diabetic patients

❍ **What determines the cup size of bra?**

Cup size is a common reference point when patients describe their goals for breast reduction and describes the relationship of breast girth to chest girth. If breast girth exceeds chest girth by 1 inch, the cup size is an A; 2 inches is a B; 3 inches is a C, 4 inches is a D, and 5 inches is a DD.

❍ **What is Regnault's correlation between chest girth and the amount of glandular resection required to approximate bra cup size?**

Chest Circumference (inches)	Amount to remove for each cup size reduction
32-34	100 gm
36-38	200 gm
42-44	300 gm
44-46	400 gm

❍ **What is the management of the dusky post-op NAC?**

1. Release the sutures holding the NAC to make sure there is not a tension-related problem.
2. If no brisk change in appearance, the flap should be opened in the operating room to check for pedicle-kinking or hematoma which could explain the ischemia.

3.   If neither of those is apparent, a free-nipple graft should be performed on a de-epithelialized bed.

4.   There are several case-reports of salvage of ischemic NAC's with hyperbaric oxygen.

❍   **Why does a free-nipple graft survive when a NAC on a dermal-glandular pedicle won't?**

The metabolic demands of the NAC as a skin graft are less.

❍   **What is the aesthetic appearance of a free-nipple graft?**

There is always some degree <u>of hypo-pigmentation</u> which may require tattooing, especially in dark-skinned patients.

❍   **In the rare cases requiring a repeat reduction mammoplasty, what should be done when the previous pedicle type is unknown?**

Strong consideration should be given to a planned free nipple graft. If you do know the previous pedicle design, the same pedicle should ideally be used to minimize the risk of devascularizing either the NAC or even the pedicle itself.

❍   **Is a de-epithelialized dermal pedicle required to maintain NAC viability?**

No, although it theoretically provides a greater margin for error. The NAC can clearly survive on a well designed glandular pedicle alone in favorable patients.

❍   **What's the advantage of a closed (versus open) design with a Wise inverted-T pattern-type flap design?**

A closed design, one in which the NAC opening is not initially precut in the incision, allows much greater flexibility for placing the nipple at the proper projecting part of the breast as well as allowing adjustments for symmetry with the contra-lateral breast.

❍   **What's the key difference between the classic Strömbeck and McKissock techniques?**

Both are inverted-T style designs with bipedicled dermoglandular flaps. They differ in the pedicle orientation with the Strömbeck oriented horizontally, while the McKissock "bucket handle" is folded on itself and oriented vertically.

❍   **What are the odds of finding an occult breast cancer in a breast reduction specimen?**

Retrospectively, this has been <u>estimated between a 0.16 to 0.4% incidence</u> on several recent studies.

❍   **What is the effect of reduction mammoplasty on breast cancer risk?**

In peri and post-menopausal women (age 40 +) there was consistent reduction in relative risk (0.2 versus 0.7 in controls) for developing breast cancer.

❍   **What is the reduction in breast cancer risk after prophylactic mastectomy?**

The reduction in risk for developing breast cancer is 90% for bilateral prophylactic mastectomy. A unilateral prophylactic mastectomy after developing breast cancer in the contra-lateral breast approaches a 95% risk reduction.

❍   *What are some medical conditions associated with gynecomastia?*

- obesity
- renal or liver dysfunction
- adrenal tumors
- hypo/hyperthyroidism
- testicular tumors
- Kleinfelter's syndrome

O **What are some common medicines that can cause gynecomastia?**

- Amphetamines
- H2 blockers
- proton pump inhibitors
- digoxin
- haldol
- isoniazid
- methyl-dopa
- spironolactone
- TCA's

O **Where is the most common place for keloid scarring to occur with breast reductions?**

At the medial edge of the transverse incision.

O **What are the recommendations for mammograms post-reduction?**

A post-reduction mammogram 6-12 months after reduction should be performed to establish a new baseline image for future comparison.

O **What is the result of overly long IMF-NAC vertical limbs with Wise-pattern inferior pedicle procedures?**

As the length of the vertical limb increases much beyond 5cm, premature bottoming-out of the tissue has been frequently observed.

O **Who are the best candidates for good results with suction assisted lipectomy (SAL) breast reductions?**

The best candidates are breasts with little to no ptosis and a higher fatty composition.

O **What is the effect of SAL on breast mammography?**

A number of small clinical series have not produced the feared post-operative calcification which can necessitate further work-up to rule out malignancy in the short term follow-up.

O **What percentage of people may be able to successfully breast feed after reduction mammoplasty?**

Up to 68% in some studies. This is nearly equivalent to the rate of successful attempts at breast-feeding in women who have never had breast reduction.

O **What is virginal (juvenile) hypertrophy?**

The abrupt development of unilateral or bilateral gigantomastia in adolescent girls presumably secondary to estrogen hypersensitivity. Treatment includes reduction mammoplasty with the addition of Tamoxifen postoperatively to lower the risk of recurrence. Reduction alone has high recurrence rates.

O **What are the differential diagnoses when considering virginal hypertrophy?**

- fibroadenoma
- cystosarcoma phyllodes
- breast hamartoma
- post traumatic phenomena

O **What are the characteristics of the vertical breast reduction technique as described by Dr. Madeline Lejour?**

The Lejour technique includes:
- superior based NAC pedicle
- a "mosque" shaped skin excision pattern
- aggressive liposuction sculpturing prior to glandular resection
- liberal lower pole parenchymal resection
- plication of medial/lateral parenchymal "pillars" to attain projection
- a short vertical limb that does not violate the IMF

An important conceptual change from previous reduction procedures is the avoidance of relying on the skin brassiere alone to maintain shape.

❍ **How doe the Hall-Findlay reduction differ from the Lejour technique?**

The Hall-Findlay procedure uses a medial or superior-medial pedicle with a liberal lateral-inferior glandular resection. Liposuction is used for final contouring and addressing residual axillary fullness rather then early and often in the procedure as in the Lejour technique.

❍ **What is the conceptual advantage of many of the medial and superior pedicles to the inferior pedicle?**

The resection of the dependent inferior glandular is maximized while the upper pole fullness is maintained.

❍ **What is the upper size limit of reductions that Dr. Lejour believes can be done satisfactorily with a VBR technique?**

1000 gm. Of note, many surgeons feel aesthetic outcome starts to be compromised at 400-500 gm with VBR.

❍ **What is the immediate post-operative shape characteristic of the VBR?**

Frequently it's described as looking like "an upside-down breast" with exaggerated upper pole fullness, a hollow inferior pole, downward-projecting nipples, and a bunched vertical limb with a puckered appearance. This predictable shape settles out into a pleasing appearance over several months with a low incidence of revisions of the puckered scar required.

❍ **How is breast ptosis graded?**

1st degree- nipple position <u>at the IMF</u>
2nd degree- nipple position <u>below the IMF</u> but above the lowest level of the breast
3rd degree- nipple position has descended <u>below the lowest level of the breast</u>

❍ **What is pseudoptosis?**

Where the breast mass descends behind the NAC, but the nipple position remains above the IMF.

❍ **What's the most common planning error with breast reduction or mastopexy procedures?**

Placing the nipple position too high, resulting in an uncorrectable deformity many times.

❍ **What are some rough guidelines for deciding nipple position?**

A sternal notch-to-nipple distance between 21-23 cm and an inferior limb length of 5-7 cm are the most commonly recommended. Transposition of the nipple to the IMF ("Pitanguay's Point") along the breast meridian establishes a pleasing grade I ptosis.

❍ **When might you commonly have to place a nipple above IMF during a reduction or mastopexy?**

When performing a unilateral symmetry procedure to a contra-lateral reconstructed breast, which frequently have higher NAC's from the rounded shape and capsular contraction of implant reconstruction.

○ **What are stereotypical changes to the IMF produced by inferior pedicle procedures versus superior or medial pedicle designed?**

The classic inferior pedicle tends to lower the IMF, while the superior, medial, and superior-medial procedures of Lejour and Hall-Findlay predictably raise the IMF.

○ **How do you account for the IMF position when doing a vertical reduction to avoid crossing it with the vertical limb?**

The lower border of the mosque design will need to terminate several centimeters above the existing IMF. Recommendations are a 2cm distance for small reductions and mastopexies, and up to a 6 cm for the larger reductions (800 gm+).

○ **Relaxation of what structure allows breast ptosis?**

Cooper's ligaments specifically, combined with atrophy of the glandular tissue.

○ **What usually determines the need for mastopexy after implant explantation?**

The level of ptosis preoperatively, as it usually is not changed significantly post-removal.

○ **What are some relative contraindications to circumareolar ("doughnut") mastopexy techniques?**

- >24cm sternal notch-NAC distance
- Grade 2 or greater ptosis
- Skin laxity
- When breast implants are being significantly downsized or removed at the same operation

○ **What are the most common problems with the periareolar mastopexy procedures?**

Unpredictable scarring and widening of the NAC over time due to tension. In addition the purse-string effect has the effect of flattening the breast and decreasing projection.

○ **How does the Benelli "Round Block" technique for periareolar mastopexy address problems with the scarring?**

By transmitting the tension away from the NAC and onto the deeper dermal layer of the surrounding skin with a permanent circumferential suture that establishes the new areolar width.

○ **What are the principles of addressing the tuberous breast deformity?**

- Augmentation of the hypoplastic breast tissue (may require tissue expansion prior)
- Lowering of the IMF
- Radial scoring of the parenchyma to allow redraping
- Circumareolar reduction of the oversized NAC

○ **When combining breast augmentation and mastopexy procedures, what are some general recommendations for placing the NAC in relation to the sternal notch?**

The lift achieved from the augmentation can reduce the distance necessary to elevate the NAC. Some guidelines espoused for predicting this relationship include:
- 225cc or less implants => NAC should be placed at ~21cm
- 250-325cc implant => NAC placed at 22cm,

- 350cc+ implants => NAC placed at 23cm

○   **When should a staged mastopexy/augmentation procedure be considered?**

When much more then 3cm of nipple elevation is required, the predictability of the combined procedure starts to get more difficult and has been suggested by some to be guideline for separating the procedures for best results.

○   **What is the unique feature of the Goes mesh mammoplasty technique?**

Support of the breast mound with an internal Vicryl-polyester mesh tacked down to pectoralis fascia, which maintains the shape postoperatively in part due to scarring around the mesh.

References

Benelli, L. A New Periareolar Mammaplasty: The "Round Block" Technique. *Aesthetic Plast. Surg.* 14:93, 1990.

Courtiss, E.H., and Goldwyn, R.M. Reduction Mammaplasty by the Inferior Pedicle Technique. *Plast. Reconstr. Surg.* 59: 500, 1977.

Hall-Findlay, E.J.: A Simplified Vertical Reduction Mammaplasty: Shortening the Learning Curve. *Plast. Reconstr. Surg.* 104:748, 1999.

Hester, T.R., et al: Breast Reduction Utilizing the Maximally Vascularized Central Breast Pedicle. *Plast. Reconstr. Surg.* 76:890, 1985.

Hidalgo, D. Improving Safety and Aesthetic Results in Inverted Scar Breast Reduction. *Plast. Reconstr. Surg.* 103:874, 1999.

Lassus, C. A 30-year Experience with Vertical Mammaplasty. *Plast. Reconstr. Surg.* 97:373, 1996.

Lejour, M. Vertical Mammaplasty and Liposuction of the Breast. *Plast. Reconstr. Surg.* 94: 100, 1994.

HAND AND EXTREMITIES

ANATOMY/EMBRYOLOGY

Hanif Ukani, MD, FRCSC and Matthew M. Hanasono, MD

Nail

○ **Where does the nail grow from?**

90% from the germinal matrix, and 10% from the sterile matrix, which is also involved in adherence of the nail plate to the nailbed.

○ **What is the hyponychium?**

The junction between the nail bed and the skin at the most distal aspect of the finger. This area, loaded with lymphocytes, is considered a barrier to infection.

○ **What is the perionychium?**

The tissue that extends along the lateral edge of the nail and the eponychium.

○ **What is the lunula?**
T
he white area of proximal nail, where the cell nuclei are still present.

Finger

○ **What is Camper's chiasm?**

A reunion of FDS tendon after splitting around FDP tendon (after the chiasm, the FDS again splits into radial and ulnar slips that insert into the middle 3/5th of the middle phalanx).

○ **What is the function of the instrinsic flexors of the hand?**

The lumbricals extend the IPJ and simultaneously flex the MPJ. This puts your fingers into an **"L"** position which stands for **L**umbrical.

○ **What are the origin and insertion of the lumbricals?**

- They originate on the radial side of the FDP tendons
- Pass volar to the transverse metacarpal ligaments
- Insert on the radial lateral band of the extensor mechanism

○ **Where are Cleland's and Grayson's ligaments located with respect to the digital neurovascular bundles?**

- Cleland's ligaments are dorsal
- Grayson's ligaments are volar
- (C-ceiling, G-ground)

○ **What are the attachments of Cleland's and Grayson's ligaments?**

- **C**leland's-attach **B**one to skin (A**BC**D...)

-       <u>G</u>rayson's-attach <u>F</u>lexor sheath to skin (…E<u>FG</u>)

◯   **How many pulleys comprise the flexor sheath of the digits?**

There are 5 annular and 3 cruciate pulleys.

◯   **Where are the A2 and A4 pulleys located?**

Proximal-proximal phalanx (A2) and middle-middle phalanx (A4).

◯   **What is the clinical significance of the A2 and A4 pulleys?**

They need to be preserved in order to <u>prevent bowstringing</u> of the flexor tendons.

◯   **What is the clinical significance of bowstringing?**

The loss of mechanical advantage and tendon excursion results in a flexion lag and loss of power.

◯   **What are the pulleys in the thumb?**

2 annular pulleys and 1 oblique pulley
A1: at MCP joint
O: over proximal phalanx
A2: at PIP joint

◯   **Which of these are most important?**

The oblique pulley.

◯   **What are the proximal and distal attachments of the Oblique Retinacular Ligament of Landsmeer?**

Proximal: distal metaphysis of the proximal phalanx, and the A2 pulley
Distal: The lateral conjoint tendon, which forms the conjoined extensor tendon

◯   **What is the function of the Oblique Retinacular Ligament of Landsmeer?**

Coordinated combined flexion and coordinated combined extension of the PIP and DIP joints

◯   **What are the attachments of the Transverse Retinacular Ligament of Landsmeer?**

Volar Attachment: volar plate and flexor tendon sheath in the region of the A2 pulley
Dorsal Attachment: Lateral Bands

◯   **Describe the sources of flexor tendon nutrition**

A. Blood supply
    1. bony insertion
    2. muscle belly
    3. Vincular system
B. Diffusion from the synovium within the flexor tendon sheath

◯   **Where do the dorsal digital nerves originate?**

From the volar digital nerves at the level of the PIP, thus the fingernails receive sensory input from the volar nerves.

Hand

○ **What bones make up the "fixed unit" of the hand?**

- 2nd metacarpal
- 3rd metacarpal
- trapezoid
- capitate

○ **What is the relationship of the EIP to the EDC to the 2nd digit?**

EIP and EDM are both ulnar to their respective EDC tendons (note: radial and supernumerary may occur).

○ **Where are the four insertions of the extrinsic extensor tendons?**

1. Base of the proximal phalanx
2. Base of the middle phalanx
3. Base of the distal phalanx (via slips to the lateral bands)
4. Transverse metacarpal ligament and volar plate

○ **What are the thenar muscles and their motor innervations?**

1. Opponens pollicis (median nerve)
2. Abductor pollicis brevis (median nerve)
3. Flexor pollicis brevis (dual innervations: recurrent branch of the median nerve [superficial head], deep motor branch of the ulnar nerve [deep head])

○ **What are the hypothenar muscles and their motor innervations?**

1. Opponens digiti minimi (ulnar nerve)
2. Abductor digiti minimi (ulnar nerve)
3. Flexor digiti minimi (ulnar nerve)

○ **How many fascial spaces exist in the hand?**

Nine.
1. Thenar space
2. Midpalmar space
3. Hypothenar space
4. Subfascial web space in the palm and interdigital area ("collar button")
5. Dorsal subcutaneous space
6. Dorsal subaponeurotic space
7. Radial bursa
8. Ulnar bursa
9. Parona's space-potential space between the flexor tendons and pronator quadratus

○ **What are the junctura tendinae?**

Interconnections between the common digital extensors on the dorsum of the hand which prevent independent finger extension.

○ **What are the 3 vascular arches of the hand**

Superficial palmar arch: ulnar artery origin, leads to digital vessels
Deep palmar arch: radial artery origin, leads to volar MC arteries

Dorsal carpal arch: origin radial and ulnar dorsal carpal arteries, leads to dorsal MC arteries
Remember <u>DR</u>. <u>SU</u>ess-Deep Radial, Superficial Ulnar.

❍   **What are the flexor tendon zones?**

Zone 1: Distal to the insertion of FDS
Zone 2: From the A1 Pulley to the insertion of FDS
Zone 3: From the Carpal Tunnel to the A1 pulley
Zone 4: Carpal Tunnel
Zone 5: Proximal to the Carpal Tunnel

❍   **What are the extensor tendon zones?**

Zone 1: DIP joint
Zone 2: Middle phalanx
Zone 3: PIP joint
Zone 4: Proximal Phalanx
Zone 5: MCP joint
Zone 6: Metacarpal
Zone 7: Extensor Retinaculum
Zone 8: Proximal to Extensor Retinaculum

❍   **What are the extensor tendon zones of the thumb**

Zone 1: IP Joint
Zone 2: Proximal Phalanx
Zone 3: MCP joint
Zone 4: Metacarpal
Zone 5: CMC joint

❍   **What are the natatory ligaments?**

Transverse fibers of fascia located at the distal palmar crease.
Their contracture in Dupuytren's causes adduction contracture limiting digit abduction

❍   **What is the most mobile joint in the hand?**

The first CMC joint between the trapezium and the thumb metacarpal

Wrist

❍   **What are the boundaries of the carpal tunnel?**

- Transverse carpal ligament
- Scaphoid tubercle
- Crest of the trapezium
- Pisiform and hamate

❍   **What are the contents of the carpal tunnel?**

- 10 structures
- FDS x 4
- FDP x 4
- FPL
- median nerve

○ **How are the FDS tendons arranged within the carpal tunnel?**

3   4 (volar)
2   5 (dorsal)

○ **What are the boundaries of Guyon's canal?**

- Transverse carpal ligament (floor)
- Volar carpal ligament (roof)
- Pisiform(laterally)
- Hook of the hamate (medially)

○ **What are the contents of the extensor compartments?**

1.   APL, EPB
2.   ECRL, ECRB
3.   EPL
4.   EDC, EIP
5.   EDM
6.   ECU

○ **What bony structure separates the 2nd and 3rd extensor compartments?**

Lister's tubercle.

Forearm

○ **In what percentage of patients is the palmaris longus tendon absent?**

Approximately 15%.

○ **Which muscles make up the "mobile wad"?**

1.   Brachioradialis
2.   ECRL
3.   ECRB

○ **Where do the ECRL and ECRB insert?**

Into the bases of the 2nd and 3rd metacarpals respectively.

○ **Where is the radial artery located in the forearm?**

In the volar forearm between brachioradialis and FCR.

○ **Where is the posterior interosseous artery located in the forearm?**

In the dorsal forearm, between ECU and EDQ

Nerve

○ **What is a Martin-Gruber anastomosis?**

It is a motor anastomosis present in 10-25% of people between the median (or AIN) and ulnar nerves <u>in the forearm</u> that may lead to underestimation of ulnar nerve injury

○   **What is a Riche-Cannieu anastomosis?**

A motor anastomosis between the median and ulnar nerve <u>in the hand</u>.

○   **How many roots, trunks, divisions, cords, and terminal branches comprise the brachial plexus?**

- 5 Roots (ventral rami of C5-8, T1; occasional contributions from C4 and T2)
- 3 Trunks (upper, middle, lower)
- 6 Divisions (anterior and posterior for each trunk)
- 4 Cords (posterior, lateral, and medial, named for position relative to axillary artery)
- 5 Terminal branches (musculocutaneous, axillary, radial, median, and ulnar nerves)
- Mnemonic: "Rob Taylor Drinks Cold Beer"

○   **What muscles in the hand are innervated by the median nerve?**

- index and long finger lumbrical muscles
- abductor pollicis brevis
- opponens pollicis
- superficial head of the flexor pollicis brevis. (1/2 LOAF)

○   **Where does the motor branch of the median nerve arise with respect to the transverse carpal ligament?**

The origin of the motor branch is variable with 46% extraligamentous, 31% subligamentous, and 23% transligamentous.

○   **What does the anterior interosseous nerve supply?**

It is a branch of the median nerve and supplies:
1. FPL
2. FDS to index and middle fingers
3. pronator quadratus

○   **Where is the origin of the palmar cutaneous nerve?**

- A sensory branch of the medial nerve
- Arises 6 cm proximal to the flexor retinaculum
- Runs between the FCR and PL

○   **What are the potential sites of median nerve compression in pronator syndrome?**

1. under the lacertus fibrosus (bicipital aponeurosis)
2. under the Ligament of Struthers (attaches pronator teres to humerus)
3. between the humeral and ulnar heads of pronator teres

○   **What are the potential sites of ulnar nerve compression in cubital tunnel syndrome?**

1. The Arcade of Struthers
2. Medial Head of Triceps (Hypertrophy)
3. Ligament of Osborne
4. FCU

○   **How can I remember the difference between the Arcade and Ligament of Struthers?**

Remember that the M.L.S. or Major League Soccer (Median Ligament of Struthers) is here in the U.S.A. (Ulnar-Struthers Arcade).

Embryology

○ **When is the critical period of embryologic development for the upper limb?**

The upper limb develops mainly during the fourth to eighth weeks after fertilization.

○ **What is the function of the apical ectodermal ridge (AER)?**

The apical ectodermal ridge (AER) is responsible for proximal to distal differentiation.

○ **What happens if the AER is destroyed?**

Loss of the AER leads to limb truncation and congenital amputation. (Failure of the AER to separate is the most common cause of syndactyly.)

○ **What is the function of the zone of polarizing activity (ZPA)?**

The zone of polarizing activity (ZPA), which resides in the posterior margin of the limb bud, is responsible for anterior-posterior development

○ **What is the sonic hedgehog compound?**

It is a signaling molecule produced in the ZPA.

○ **What happens if the ZPA is duplicated?**

Duplication of the ZPA results in a mirror hand deformity.

○ **What is the Wnt (wingless type) pathway?**

The Wnt (wingless type) pathway occurs in a third signaling center in the dorsal ectoderm. The Wnt pathway is responsible for dorsal-ventral differentiation.

○ **What happens to the limb if the Wnt pathway is lacking?**

If the 3rd signaling center is lacking, palm duplication occurs.

○ **What cellular mechanism has to fail in development for syndactyly to occur?**

Apoptosis.

References

Gellman H, Botte MJ, Shankwiler J, Gelberman RH: Arterial patterns of the deep and superficial palmar arches. Clin Orthop 2001 Feb; (383): 41-46.

Green, DP, Hotchkiss, RN, Pederson WC, Wolfe SW., MD, Roselius, E: Green's Operative Hand Surgery, : 5th ed. Churchill Livingstone, 2005

Lister G: Injury. In: Lister's The Hand: Diagnosis and Treatment. 4th ed. Edinburgh, Scotland: Churchill Livingstone; 1999: 18.

Moore KL: Clinically Oriented Anatomy. 2nd ed. Baltimore, Md: Lippincott Williams & Wilkins; 1985.

Moore KL, Persaud TVN: The limbs. In: The Developing Human: Clinically Oriented Embryology. 5th ed. Philadelphia, Pa: WB Saunders; 1993: 375-83.

Tickle C: Embryology. In: Gupta A, Kay SPJ, Scheker LR, eds. The Growing Hand: Diagnosis and Management of the Upper Extremity in Children. 1st ed. London, UK: Mosby; 2000: 25-32.

Williams PL, Warwick R: Gray's Anatomy. 37th ed. Edinburgh: Churchill Livingstone; 1989.

ANESTHESIA

Michel Saint-Cyr, MD and Hanif Ukani, MD

I Basic Nerve Cell Physiology

○ **What is the resting potential value of a nerve cell membrane?**

All cells have a resting potential: an electrical charge across the plasma membrane with the interior of the cell negative with respect to the exterior. The size of the resting potential can vary but in excitable cells is about -70 mill volts (mv).

○ **What determines the resting potential of a nerve cell?**

The resting potential arises from 2 activities:

1.   The sodium/potassium ATPase, which moves 3 sodium ions outside the cell for every 2 potassium ions inside the cell, produces a net loss of positive charges and results in a negative intracellular charge.
2.   Facilitated diffusion of potassium outside the cell

○ **Describe the ionic relations in the cell for sodium, potassium, chloride and calcium ions.**

1.   The sodium/potassium ATPase produces:
    a.   A concentration of Na^+ outside the cell that is some 10 times greater than that inside the cell
    b.   A concentration of K^+ inside the cell some 20 times greater than that outside the cell
2.   The concentrations of chloride ions (Cl^-) and calcium ions (Ca^{2+}) are maintained at greater levels outside the cell.

○ **Describe the depolarization of a nerve cell membrane.**

Before an action potential can be formed the nerve cell membrane is depolarized by either a mechanical stimulus (sound, stretch etc) or a neurotransmitter (ex: acetylcholine). This allows the facilitated diffusion of sodium into the cell, which reduces the resting potential at that area on the cell and creates an excitatory postsynaptic potential or EPSP.

○ **Describe the formation of an action potential.**

If the initial depolarization stimulus reaches a threshold voltage of –50 mv, then an action potential will be generated from that area of the cell membrane. This opens hundreds of voltage-gated sodium channels and creates a massive influx of sodium. The sudden complete depolarization of the membrane opens up more of the voltage-gated sodium channels in adjacent portions of the membrane. In this way, a wave of depolarization sweeps along the cell. This is the action potential, or nerve impulse.

○ **Why is the action potential an *all-or-nothing* event?**

If the critical threshold of –50 mv membrane depolarization is reached then an action potential will be produced, if not, then no action potential will result. Strong stimuli produce no stronger action potentials than weak ones.

○ **How is membrane repolarization re-established?**

1. Diffusion of potassium ions out of the cell.
2. Closure of sodium channels.

○ **What is the refractory period?**

A second stimulus applied to a neuron less than 0.001 second after the first will not trigger another impulse. The membrane is depolarized, and the neuron is in its **refractory period**. Not until the -70 mv polarity is reestablished will the neuron be ready to fire again.

○ **How long does the refractory period last?**

Varies, in some human neurons the refractory period lasts only 0.001-0.002 seconds. This means that the neuron can transmit 500-1000 impulses per second.

○ **What is the node of Ranvier?**

Myelinated neurons are encased in a fatty sheath called the myelin sheath, which is the expanded plasma membrane of an accessory cell called the Schwann cell. Where the sheath of one Schwann cell meets the next, the axon is unprotected. This area is called the node of Ranvier.

○ **Why is conduction in myelinated neurons faster then in unmyelinated ones?**

Voltage-gated sodium channels of myelinated neurons are confined to the nodes of Ranvier. The inflow of sodium ions at one node creates just enough depolarization to reach the threshold of the next. In this way, the action potential jumps from one node to the next. This results in much faster propagation of the nerve impulse than is possible in unmyelinated neurons.

II Action of Local Anesthetics

○ **What is a conduction block?**

It is the reversible interruption of conduction within a neural structure by a local anesthetic.

○ **When does conduction block occur?**

It occurs when local anesthetic molecules occupy enough sodium channels within an axon to interrupt its activity.

○ **How does conduction block by a local anesthetic occur?**

Local anesthetics act by binding to open gated sodium channels causing them to remain inactive, thus preventing subsequent depolarization.

○ **Why do local anesthetics have a higher potency for nerves with a higher frequency of stimulation?**

Nerve that have a higher frequency of stimulation have more activated open sodium channels which are more susceptible to the action of local anesthetics.

○ **Why are myelinated nerves easier to block then unmyelinated ones?**

In myelinated nerves only the nodes of Ranvier need to be exposed to local anesthetic for conduction block to occur. In unmyelinated fibers, the full length and circumference of the nerve must be exposed to local anesthetic.

○ **What three structures make up the anesthetic molecule?**

1. Aromatic ring (hydrophobic)
2. Tertiary amine (hydrophilic)
3. Intermediate chain (contains either an amide or ester bond)

○ **Local anesthetics are classified into which two groups?**

1. Esters
2. Amides

○ **What is the pH of local anesthetic solutions?**

Local anesthetics are weak bases with a pKa ranging from 7.7 to 9.1. Commercially prepared solutions are prepared as hydrochloride salts of the cation with a pH of 5.0 to 6.0 without epinephrine and a pH of 2.0-3.0 with epinephrine. This is why they burn so much.

○ **The pharmacological activity of local anesthetics is determined by which three physiochemical properties?**

1. Lipid solubility
2. Protein binding
3. pKa

○ **How does lipid solubility affect the action of local anesthetics?**

Increased lipid solubility of a local anesthetic will increase its potency because nerve cell membranes are highly hydrophobic. Increased nerve block will occur because of facilitated entry across the nerve cell membrane.

○ **How does protein binding affect the action of local anesthetics?**

Local anesthetics with a higher protein binding will have greater contact with the nerve membrane and thus a longer duration of action.

○ **How does the pKa affect the action of local anesthetics?**

The pKa of a local anesthetic determines the speed of onset of the nerve conduction block.

Fifty percent of the anesthetic will exist in its basic and cationic form at a given pKa. The non-ionized basic form has the highest lipid solubility and hence highest speed of onset. Because local anesthetics are prepared as hydrochloride salts with a pH of 5.0-6.0 some delay in onset will occur due to physiological buffering which is required to establish a significant base form concentration.

○ **What two ways can the onset of local anesthetics be accelerated?**

Preparation of the local anesthetic solution as a hydrocarbonate salt instead of a hydrochloride salt.

Addition of sodium bicarbonate to the local anesthetic prior to injection.

○ **List four ester local anesthetics.**

1. Procaine
2. Tetracaine
3. Benzocaine
4. Cocaine

O   **List three amide local anesthetics.**

1.   Lidocaine
2.   Bupivacaine
3.   Prilocaine
4.   Note that these all have an "i" before the "-aine".

O   **How are esters metabolized?**

Esters are rapidly hydrolyzed by <u>plasma</u> pseudocholinesterase.

O   **How are amides metabolized?**

<u>Liver cells</u> metabolize amides intracellularly. Because of this longer process, an accumulation of repeated doses can cause systemic toxicity. Patients with poor liver function and congestive heart failure will have a significantly prolonged amide half-life.

III Toxicity of Local Anesthetics

O   **What types of toxicities are related to local anesthetics?**

1.   Direct tissue toxicity (buffers, preservatives, potential for intraneural injection)
2.   Systemic toxicity (CNS, cardiac, methemoglobinemia)

O   **What factors determine the toxicity of a local anesthetic?**

1.   Potency or lipid solubility (increased CNS toxicity)
2.   Total dose delivered
3.   Rate of plasma uptake
4.   Protein binding
5.   Site of injection (highly vascularized tissues increase the rate of uptake)

O   **How does the addition of epinephrine reduce a local anesthetic's toxicity?**

1.   Produces vasoconstriction which:
a.   Decreases vascular uptake
b.   Lowers peak plasma levels
c.   Slows time course to peak level (reduced CNS toxicity)

O   **What toxic effects are associated with the addition of epinephrine?**

1. Hypertension
2. Tachycardia
3. Cardiac arrhythmia
4. Myocardial ischemia

O   **Name three factors, which decrease seizure threshold and increase the risk of CNS toxicity:**

1.   Hypercarbia
2.   Hypoxia
3.   Acidosis

O   **Name two agents, which can be used to treat seizures following CNS toxicity:**

1.   Benzodiazepine (increases seizure threshold and can prevent seizure activity)

2.   Sodium thiopental

○   **Describe the evolution of local anesthesia induced CNS toxicity.**

1.   CNS excitation (occurs first)
     a.   Dizziness
     b.   Light-headedness
     c.   Tinnitus
     d.   Circumoral numbness
     e.   Metallic taste in the mouth
     f.   Loss of consciousness
     g.   Muscular twitching
     h.   Convulsions

2.   CNS depression (occurs later)
     a.   Respiratory depression
     b.   Cardiorespiratory arrest

○   **What are the effects of local anesthetic toxicity on the cardiovascular system?**

1.   Increased sodium channel blockade within the cardiac conduction system causes:
     a.   Decreased Purkinje fiber firing and prolonged conduction time
     b.   Long PR interval
     c.   Widened QRS complex
     d.   Sinus bradycardia and asystole
     e.   Direct myocardial depressant
     f.   Ventricular arrhythmia (increased reentrant pathway activity)

○   **What measures can be used to prevent or minimize systemic reactions to local anesthetics?**

1.   Avoid intravascular injections (frequent aspirations while injecting)
2.   Always use smallest possible dose and concentration
3.   Add epinephrine (avoid in digits and in patients with ischemic heart disease)
4.   Premedication with benzodiazepine (elevates convulsive threshold)
5.   Use a small test dose

○   **What measures can be used to treat toxic systemic reactions to local anesthetics?**

1.   Always follow principles of ACLS
2.   Convulsions:
     a.   Hyperventilation with O_2 to reduce $PaCO_2$
     b.   Diazepam, Midazolam, Pentothal 50-100 mg I/V

○   **What is the estimated adult toxic dose of lidocaine without epinephrine?**

Maximal dose/kg: 5 mg/kg
Maximal single dose: 300 mg

○   **What is the estimated adult toxic dose of lidocaine with epinephrine?**

Maximal dose/kg: 7 mg/kg
Maximal single dose: 500 mg

○   **What is the maximum total dose of epinephrine in a healthy adult?**

0.25 mg

❍   **How is a concentration of 1:200,000 of epinephrine prepared?**

Add 0.05 mg (or 0.05 ml of 1:000 concentration) of epinephrine to each 10 ml of local anesthetic solution used (maximum of 50 ml of local anesthesia).

❍   **What is the onset and duration of 1% lidocaine with and without epinephrine?**

Lidocaine 1%   Lidocaine 1% with epinephrine
Onset: 5-10 min   Onset: 3-5 min
Duration: 45-60 min   Duration: 60-120 min

❍   **Describe the various indications and concentrations for lidocaine.**

1. Local infiltration: 0.5-1 % (45-60 min)
2. Intravenous regional anesthesia (IVRA) 0.5% 40 ml total for upper extremity (45-60 min)
3. Peripheral nerve block 1-2% (1-3 hours)
4. Motor nerve block 2% (60-80 min)

❍   **What common local anesthetics are used for peripheral nerve blocks?**

Agent	Concentration	Duration (min)
2-Chloroprocaine	2-3%	30-75
Lidocaine	1-2%	45-120
Mepivacaine	1-2%	120-300
Bupivacaine	0.25-0.5%	300-720
Etidocaine	0.5-0.75%	300-720

❍   **What causes methemoglobinemia?**

The oxidation of hemoglobin from its ferric to ferrous form by prilocaine and benzocaine. Visible cyanosis can occur when concentrations exceed 4 g/dl and tissue hypoxia and cyanosis can be treated with methylene blue.

❍   **Allergic reactions to local anesthetics are most often associated with which agents?**

A true allergic response to local anesthetics is very rare. Most allergies are associated with ester agents, which are metabolized to para-amino-benzoic acid (PABA), which can also be found throughout the pharmaceutical and cosmetic industries. Allergies to amides are even rarer and have been linked to methylparaben which is a preservative added to multi-dose vials of lidocaine to retard bacterial growth.

Nerve blocks

❍   **What different types of anesthesia are available for the upper extremity?**

1. General
2. Regional
a. Brachial plexus blocks (interscalene, supraclavicular, infraclavicular, axillary)
b. Bier block (IVRA) intra-venous regional anesthesia
c. Peripheral nerve blocks (radial, ulnar and median nerves at elbow and wrist)
d. Metacarpal blocks
e. Digital nerve blocks

❍   **What are the advantages of using regional anesthesia in the upper extremity?**

1. Decreased morbidity in high risk patients

2. Prevention of all afferent stimuli from reaching CNS (prevention of vasoconstriction, vasodilation effect)
3. Post-operative pain relief
4. Decreased post-operative nausea and vomiting
5. Emergency procedures (*full stomach*)
6. Earlier ambulation
7. Outpatient surgery

○ **What are the disadvantages of using regional anesthesia in the upper extremity?**

1. Extra time required for block to be effective
2. Incomplete or failed block
3. Residual numbness or paresthesia
4. Potential infection, hematoma, nerve injury
5. Potential toxicity from intravascular injection

○ **What are some contraindications to using regional anesthesia?**

1. Local sepsis, infection
2. Allergy to local anesthetics
3. Coagulopathy, anticoagulant therapy
4. Uncooperative patient
5. Peripheral nerve damage

○ **Which nerves form the brachial plexus?**

The union of the anterior primary divisions of C5-8 and T1 forms the brachial plexus with variable contributions from C4 and T2.

○ **Briefly describe the organization of the brachial plexus.**

Robert-roots (5 of them, C5-T1)
Taylor-trunks (3 of them, superior, middle and inferior)
Drinks-divisions (6 of them, an anterior and posterior division for each trunk)
Coffee-cords (3 of them, posterior, lateral and medial)
Black-branches or named peripheral nerves

○ **Which peripheral nerve originates from the lateral, medial and posterior cords?**

1. Lateral cord: musculocutaneous nerve and contribution to median nerve
2. Medial cord: ulnar nerve, medial antebrachial and medial brachial cutaneous nerves, contribution to median nerve
3. Posterior cord: radial and axillary nerves

○ **Name the three types of brachial plexus blocks to the upper extremity.**

1. Interscalene block
2. Supraclavicular block
3. Infraclavicular block
4. Axillary blockade

○ **What are the advantages and disadvantages of the interscalene brachial plexus block (ISB)?**

Indications:
Shoulder surgery, upper arm surgery
Advantages:
Effective analgesia for surgery or arthroscopy of the shoulder
Disadvantages:

Frequently misses:
1.   medial cutaneous nerve of the arm
2.   intercostobrachial nerve
3.   ulnar nerve
Not suitable for hand anesthesia (sparing of C8 and T1) ulnar nerve
Failure rate 8.7%
Complications:
100% ipsilateral phrenic nerve block (C3-5)
Horner's syndrome
Hoarseness, dysphagia, blurred vision
Involvement of recurrent laryngeal and cervical sympathetic nerves can occur

O   **What are the advantages and disadvantages of the supraclavicular brachial plexus block (ISB)?**

Indications:
Surgery of the arm, elbow and hand
Advantages:
Well suited for long surgery or prolonged post-operative pain relief.
Complete, prompt, long acting block
Arm can be in any comfortable position (Modified Brown's plumb-bob approach)
Disadvantages:
Pneumothorax 0.4-6%
Ipsilateral phrenic nerve paralysis 60%
Occasional Horner's syndrome

O   **What are the advantages and disadvantages of the infraclavicular brachial plexus block (ICB)?**

Indications:
Surgery of the arm, elbow and hand
Advantages:
Long acting hand and arm anesthesia
Reliable block of musculocutaneous and axillary nerves
Lower risk of pneumothorax compared to supraclavicular block
Uses more obvious landmarks then SCB
Disadvantages:
Increased risk of intravascular puncture as the plexus surrounds the subclavian artery at this level

O   **What are the advantages and disadvantages of the axillary brachial plexus block?**

Indications:
Most widely used brachial plexus block in hand surgery
Advantages:
Simple, safe and reliable technique
Well suited for outpatient surgery
Remote from neck and thorax
Disadvantages:
Can miss the musculocutaneous nerve and thus the lateral antebrachial cutaneous nerve
Complications
Intravascular injection
Soreness or bruising of the axilla, persistent numbness

O   **Describe the relationship of the radial, ulnar and median nerves to the axillary artery.**

1.   The radial nerve is posterior to the axillary artery
2.   The ulnar nerve is inferior to the axillary artery
3.   The median nerve is superior to the axillary artery

○ **What is a Bier block and how is it performed?**

1. An IV catheter is placed as distally as possible in the operated limb and the upper extremity is elevated and exsanguinated with an Esmarch bandage starting from distal to proximal.
2. A <u>dual tourniquet</u> is placed on the operated arm and the proximal cuff is inflated prior to removal of the Esmarch bandage.
3. Lidocaine 0.5% 40-50 ml without preservatives is injected slowly (smaller doses of 30 ml can be used if a forearm tourniquet is used).
4. The proximal tourniquet cuff can be deflated after 20 min **after confirming that the distal tourniquet cuff has been inflated** to avoid escape of intravascular local into the central circulatory system.
5. This distal cuff is inflated over an anesthetized area and can be tolerated for an additional 40 minutes.
6. A minimum occlusion time of 20 minutes is recommended based on peak plasma values of local anesthetics.

○ **What are the advantages and disadvantages of the Bier block?**

<u>Advantages:</u>
Ease of administration
Rapid onset
Rapid recovery of motor function
Suitable for outpatient surgery
<u>Disadvantages:</u>
Tourniquet pain when procedure longer then 1 hour
Accidental or early release of tourniquet can lead to toxic intravascular injection
Loss of anesthesia following cuff deflation
Exsanguinations of a painful extremity
Post-operative pain

○ **What are contraindications to using a Bier block (IVRA)?**

1. Any condition which precludes to use of a tourniquet
   a. Sickle cell anemia
   b. Severe peripheral vascular disease
   c. Established soft tissue infection
   d. Tumors

○ **What are some causes of post-operative neuritis?**

1. Tourniquet pressure above 250 mmHg
2. Limb position during surgery (ex: pressure over ulnar nerve at the elbow)
3. Duration of tourniquet time > 2 hours
4. Regional blocks
   a. Sharp needles instead of bevel block needles
   b. Intra-neural injection
   c. Perineural hematoma
   d. Seeking paresthesia
   e. Higher concentrations than necessary of local anesthetics

○ **Name four types of peripheral nerve blocks.**

1. Elbow block
2. Wrist block
3. Metacarpal block
4. Digital block

○ **Elbow block.**

1. **<u>Rarely performed</u>** because of variations and overlapping of the distribution of the nerves.

2. Only allows for 20-30 minutes of tourniquet time
3. Individual elbow blocks most useful for supplementing anesthesia following incomplete brachial plexus blocks.

○ **Describe the landmarks for performing ulnar, median, radial, and medial and lateral antebrachial cutaneous nerve blocks at the elbow.**

Ulnar: Posterior to the medial epicondyle, 3-5 cm proximal
Median: Medial to brachial artery, medial to biceps tendon, slightly above line between epicondyles
Radial: Anterior aspect of the lateral epicondyle, lateral to the biceps tendon
Medial and lateral antebrachial cutaneous nerves: subcutaneous ring block around the elbow.

○ **What are the advantages and disadvantages of using wrist blocks?**

Advantages:
Simple to perform
Retained motor function (except intrinsics)
Disadvantages:
Surgery time limited because of tourniquet pain after 20-30 minutes

○ **Describe the landmarks for performing ulnar, median, and superficial radial nerve block at the wrist.**

Ulnar: Radial to the flexor carpi ulnaris tendon, at the level of the proximal wrist crease and in the direction of the pisiform bone. (can also inject dorsally at same point to block the dorsal ulnar cutaneous nerve)
Median: Between the palmaris longus and flexor carpi radialis tendons at the level of the proximal wrist crease.
Superficial branch of radial nerve: Base of the extensor pollicis longus tendon and across the anatomical snuffbox, lateral to the radial artery.

○ **How many nerve branches supply the digits?**

Four nerve branches supply digital sensation: 2 volar and 2 dorsal branches along the respective sides of each digit.

○ **How does the ulnar nerve distribution differ form the median nerve distribution distal to the DIP joint?**

In the small finger, the dorsal digital nerve extends up to the end of the finger whereas in the median nerve distribution the volar digital nerve supplies a dorsal branch that comes off distal to the PIP joint. Dorsal branches need to also be blocked for complete finger anesthesia.

○ **What kind of approaches can be used for a digital nerve block?**

1. Volar approach:
    a. Common digital nerve
    b. Proximal to the common digital arterial communications
    c. Skin wheal made over the flexor tendon proximal to the distal palmar crease, 2-3 ml of lidocaine without epinephrine is injected on each side of the flexor tendons.
    d. More painful then the dorsal approach
2. Dorsal approach:
    a. Less painful
    b. Allows simultaneous blockade of dorsal branches without a second stick
    c. Injection to the side of the extensor tendons proximal to the web and then palmarly to block the volar digital nerves.
3. Intrathecal or flexor tendon sheath approach:
    a. Single injection 2 ml into the flexor tendon sheath at the level of the distal palmar crease or metacarpophalangeal flexion crease
    b. Rapid onset

○ **What should be avoided during digital blockade?**

1. Use of epinephrine
2. Circumferential ring blocks
3. Excessive or prolonged digital tourniquet
4. Excessive local anesthetic volume injection

○ **What does a stellate ganglion block interrupt?**

Sympathetic innervation of the upper extremity

References

Tetzlaff JE. The Pharmacology of Local Anesthetics. Anesthesiol Clin North America. 2000 Jun;18(2):217-233.

Gerancher JC. Upper Extremity Nerve Blocks. Anesthesiol Clin North America. 2000 Jun;18(2):297-317.

Lin YC, Krane EJ. Regional Anesthesia and Pain Management in Ambulatory Pediatric Patients. Anesthesiol Clin North America. 1996 Dec;14(4):803-816.

Ben-David B. Complications of Regional Anesthesia: An Overview. Anesthesiol Clin North America. 2002 Sept;20(3):665-667.

Ramamurthy S, Hickey R. Anesthesia. Green's Operative Hand Surgery Fourth Edition, Churchill Livingstone, 1999, pp. 22-47.

HAND TUMORS

Jeffrey B. Friedrich, MD

○ **What is the role of computed tomography in assessing upper extremity tumors?**

Used to evaluate extent of bone destruction, as well as calcified lesions.

○ **What is the role of magnetic resonance imaging in assessing upper extremity tumors?**

Used for evaluation of lesions involving bone and soft tissue.

○ **How is clonality used to differentiate between neoplasms and benign tissue growths (i.e. Dupuytren's disease)?**

Benign and inflammatory conditions are typically polyclonal, whereas neoplasms are monoclonal.

○ **In which direction should the incision be oriented when obtaining a biopsy of an upper extremity mass?**

Longitudinal (rather than transverse or zig-zag) so as to incorporate the biopsy site within the definitive excision or amputation.

○ **When performing a biopsy on a lesion, should one dissect around muscle planes, or split the muscle sharply?**

Split sharply (to avoid seeding other muscle compartments).

○ **What is the staging system for musculoskeletal tumors?**

Stage	Grade	Site
IA	low (G1)	intracompartmental
IB	low	extracompartmental
IIA	high (G2)	intracompartmental
IIB	high	extracompartmental

Benign Tumors

○ **What is the usual etiology of epidermal inclusion cysts?**

Trauma that causes epidermal cells to become imbedded in the dermis.

○ **What is the treatment of epidermal inclusion cysts?**

Complete excision along with the skin puncture wound.

○ **What are the clinical findings seen with a subungual glomus tumor?**

Severe pain, cold sensitivity, tenderness

❍   **What is the likely diagnosis of a patient with a subcutaneous elevation just proximal to the eponychial fold and nail grooving?**

A mucous cyst, or fluid-filled ganglion of the DIP joint associated with bony spurs and nail grooving.

❍   **What is the treatment of mucous cysts?**

Cyst excision and removal of bone spurs.

❍   **What is the treatment of a subungual glomus tumor?**

Removal of nail, excision of tumor.

❍   **What is the name of the lesion that is commonly found on the dorsal hand that is round, elevated, and usually has a central crater. This lesion usually resolves spontaneously, and only occasionally progresses to squamous cell carcinoma?**

Keratoacanthoma

❍   **What is the natural history of keratoacanthomas?**

They all undergo three phases. 1) proliferation 2) maturation 3) involution
The clinical story will usually include the rapid growth of a pre-existing lesion that then gradually gets smaller as the central crater expels a keratin plug.

❍   **What are the first and second most common tumors or masses of the hand?**

Ganglions and giant cell tumors, respectively.

❍   **What is the predominant cell type in giant cell tumors (a.k.a. localized nodular synovitis)?**

Histiocytes.

❍   **What is the usual site of origin of giant cell tumors?**

Flexor tendon sheath.

❍   **What is the treatment of giant cell tumors?**

Excision along with stalk (if present).

❍   **What is the difference between a neurofibroma and a neurilemmoma?**

Neurofibroma: in the substance of the nerve. Neurilemmoma: on the nerve surface.

❍   **How does this difference impact treatment?**

Neurilemmoma can be "shelled out" easily, while neurofibroma requires transection at the proximal and distal fascicles.

❍   **Are these common tumors?**

Neurilemmomas are the most common benign nerve tumors in the upper extremity.

❍   **What is another common name for neurilemmoma?**

Schwannoma.

O   **A patient presents with multiple neurofibromas of the upper extremity and cutaneous café-au-lait spots. What is your diagnosis?**

Von Recklinghausen disease or neurofibromatosis Type 1.

O   **A patient presents with bilateral acoustic schwannomas. What is the likely diagnosis?**

Neurofibromatosis Type 2. Note that these patients rarely have neurofibromas.

O   **What diagnostic studies can be used to differentiate between neurofibroma and neurilemmoma?**

MR and nerve conduction studies.

O   **What is the chief problem seen with desmoid tumors?**

High rate of recurrence (especially in female patients).

O   **In general, what is the treatment of upper extremity arteriovenous malformations (AVMs)?**

Ligation of feeding vessels, complete excision.

O   **What is the most common benign bone tumor?**

Enchondroma

O   **What are the common locations of enchondromas?**

Phalanges and metacarpals.

O   **What is Ollier's disease?**

Multiple enchondromatosis.

O   **What is Maffucci's syndrome?**

Multiple enchondromas and hemangiomas.

O   **What is the lifetime chance of a solitary enchondroma undergoing malignant transformation?**

10%

O   **What do they degenerate into?**

Chondrosarcomas.

O   **What is the treatment of enchondromas?**

Curettage and bone grafting.

O   **What benign cartilaginous tumor is similar to enchondromas and most commonly is found at the metaphyseal-diaphyseal junction of the phalanges?**

Periosteal chondroma

❍ **What is the peak age range of unicameral bone cysts (UBC)?**

5-10 years. In fact it is seen almost exclusively in children.

❍ **What is the typical presentation of UBC?**

An incidental finding on X-ray or a <u>pathologic fracture</u> through the cyst.

❍ **What non-surgical treatment is used for unicameral bone cysts (UBC)?**

Intralesional steroid injection.

❍ **What is the name of a blood-filled cyst that typically occurs in the metaphysis of a metacarpal, and then grows toward the physis?**

Aneurysmal bone cyst (ABC)

❍ **What is the peak age range of aneurysmal bone cysts (ABC)?**

Second decade of life.

❍ **What is the typical presentation of ABC?**

Swelling and pain often following an injury.

❍ **What is the treatment of ABCs?**

Curettage and bone grafting. This is an erosive, although benign, lesion that has to be removed.

❍ **What is the usual structure of an osteochondroma?**

Bone stalk and cartilaginous cap growing from the metaphysis in skeletally immature patients.

❍ **What are the symptoms of an osteoid osteoma?**

Pain at night relieved by NSAIDs.

❍ **How do osteoid osteomas present on imaging studies?**

Sclerotic nidus with a lucent halo, less than 1.0 cm in diameter.

❍ **What is the histology of osteoid osteomas?**

Very vascular nidus of osteoblasts.

❍ **What is the treatment of osteoid osteomas?**

Curettage and bone grafting.

❍ **What is an osteoblastoma?**

Same as an osteoid osteoma, but greater than 1 cm in diameter.

❍ **What is the clinical presentation of a giant cell tumor of bone (GCT)?**

Gradual swelling, pain, sometimes with pathologic fracture, most often in the distal radius.

○ **Why do some classify GCTs as low-grade malignancies?**

They can metastasize and cause death.

○ **Where do GCTs of bone typically metastasize?**

The lung.

○ **How do GCTs look on radiographs?**

Lytic lesion; no new bone formation; encroaches on, but does not penetrate joint surface.

○ **What is the surgical treatment of GCTs?**

Excision, joint reconstruction if necessary.

○ **What is the pathophysiology of fibrous dysplasia?**

Bone marrow of involved bone(s) filled with non-calcified collagen.

○ **What is the X-ray appearance of fibrous dysplasia?**

Ground glass opacity.

○ **Is treatment of fibrous dysplasia of the hands required?**

Not usually.

○ **What is a chondroblastoma?**

Rare epiphyseal bone tumor seen in young adults. It has a "cobblestone" appearance on microscopy.

○ **What is synovial chondromatosis?**

Synovial cells undergo metaplasia to become cartilaginous. These can form nodules which break off within the joint space.

○ **What are some other common soft tissue masses in the upper extremity?**

Ganglia, lipomas, foreign body granulomas, retinacular cysts, palmar fibromatosis or nodules (Dupuytren's)

Malignant Tumors

○ **What is the most common malignant tumor of the hand?**

Squamous cell carcinoma

○ **When treating melanoma of the hand, how is the amputation level determined?**

Amputate proximal to the nearest joint (i.e. for a subungual melanoma, amputation would be through the middle phalanx)

○ **What is the name of a lesion arising in the dermis that presents as a purple-red plaque or nodule?**

Dermatofibrosarcoma protuberans (DFSP)

❍ **Has Mohs' surgery been shown to be effective for DFSP?**

Yes

❍ **What is a strong risk factor for malignant peripheral nerve sheath tumor (MPNST)?**

Neurofibromatosis (von Recklinghausen's disease)

❍ **What is a synovial cell sarcoma?**

High-grade sarcoma that grows in proximity to (but not in) joints. Size of the lesion is proportional to the mortality.

❍ **What is the treatment of synovial cell sarcoma?**

Wide excision, lymph node sampling (and dissection if nodes involved).

❍ **What other sarcoma is similar to synovial cell sarcoma and usually arises from muscle?**

Epithelioid sarcoma.

❍ **What about the spread of epithelioid sarcoma makes it dangerous?**

It moves proximally along fascial planes, tendons, and lymphatics.

❍ **What is the most common malignant primary bone tumor of the hand seen in children and teens?**

Osteogenic sarcoma

❍ **How does osteogenic sarcoma look on plain radiograph?**

Bone growth outside normal skeletal boundaries.

❍ **Is there a role for external beam radiation in treatment of osteogenic sarcoma?**

No

❍ **What is the most common malignant primary bone tumor of the hand in adults?**

Chondrosarcoma

❍ **What is the benign predecessor that can rarely degenerate into a chondrosarcoma?**

Enchondroma

❍ **What is a typical presentation of a Ewing sarcoma of the hand?**

Pain, swelling, soft tissue mass; can also have fever, elevated WBC and/or ESR.

❍ **What is the radiographic presentation of Ewing sarcoma?**

Large lytic lesion of bone with a soft tissue component.

❍ **What are the common sites of Ewing sarcoma of the hand?**

Metacarpals, phalanges

○   **What is the treatment of Ewing sarcoma?**

Surgical excision, systemic chemotherapy, $\pm$ external beam radiation

○   **What percentage of patients with primary cancers in other parts of the body will develop a metastasis to the hands or feet?**

0.3 %

○   **What is the most common primary carcinoma that metastasizes to the hand?**

Bronchogenic carcinoma.

○   **When primary carcinoma metastasizes to the hand, where does it go?**

The distal phalanx.

References

Athanasian EA, Wold LE, Amadio PC. Giant cell tumors of the bones of the hand. J Hand Surg 1997; 22A: 91-98.

Athanasian EA. Bone and soft tissue tumors. In Green DP, Hotchkiss RN, Pederson WC, eds. Green's Operative Hand Surgery. 4th ed. Philadelphia: Churchill Livingstone, 1993: 2223-53.

Bednar MS, Weiland AJ, Light TR. Osteoid osteoma of the upper extremity. Hand Clin. 1995; 11: 211-21.

Enneking WF, Spanier SS. Current concepts review: The surgical staging of musculoskeletal sarcoma. J Bone Joint Surg, Am. 1980; 62(6): 1027-1030.

Floyd WE III, Troum S. Benign cartilaginous lesions of the upper extremity. Hand Clin. 1995; 11: 119-32.

Mankin HJ, Lange TA. The hazards of biopsy in patients with malignant primary bone and soft tissue tumors. J Bone Joint Surg, Am 1982; 64(8): 1121-2.

Scaglietti O, Marchetti PG. The effects of methylprednisolone acetate in the treatment of bone cysts. J Bone Joint Surg, Br. 1979; 61(2): 200-4.

Simon MA, Finn HA. Diagnostic strategy for bone and soft tissue tumors. J Bone Joint Surg, Am 1993; 75(4): 622-31.

Trumble TE, Berg D, Bruckner JD, et al. Benign and malignant neoplasms of the upper extremity. In Trumble TE, ed. Principles of Hand Surgery and Therapy. 1st ed. Philadelphia: W.B. Saunders, 2000: 529-78.

HAND INFECTIONS

César J. Bravo, MD

○ **What organism is commonly found in hand infections?**

Staphylococcus aureus. Seen in 50%-80% of all upper extremity infections.

○ **What is the basic treatment principle when dealing with infections of the hand?**

DICE.

Drainage and **D**ébridement.
Immobilization.
Chemotherapy (antibiotics).
Elevation.

○ **What are the common pathogens found in diabetic patients with hand infections?**

Gram-negative and polymicrobial infections.

○ **How do hand infections in immunocompromised patients behave?**

Hand infections in this population tend to run a more virulent course then in non-immunocompromised patients, e.g., herpetic whitlow will not resolve spontaneously and require antiviral agents.

○ **What characterizes cellulitis in the hand?**

Characterized by erythema, swelling, and tenderness.

○ **What is the most commonly involved organism in cellulitis of the hand?**

Group A β-hemolytic streptococcus.

○ **What other organism is also involved, specifically in less severe cases of cellulitis?**

Staphylococcus aureus.

○ **What are the oral antibiotics of choice in cellulitis of the hand?**

Nafcillin, dicloxacillin, and cephalexin; erythromycin if allergic to penicillin.

○ **How does a subcutaneous abscess typically occur in the hand?**

After a puncture wound or a response to a retained foreign body.

○ **What are the most commonly isolated pathogens in human-bite infections?**

α-Hemolytic *Streptococcus* and *Staphylococcus aureus*.

○ **What organism is commonly isolated in one third of human bite wounds?**

Eikenella corrodens. Cultured in 7%-29% of human bites. Must be cultured in 10% carbon dioxide.

❍ **What organism commonly infects animal-bite and scratch wounds?**

Pasteurella multocida.

❍ **Why do you need an X-ray if the patient had a simple animal bite?**

To rule out a retained foreign body like a broken tooth.

❍ **What are the common cultures requested in hand infections?**

Aerobic cultures, anaerobic cultures, cultures in Löwenstein-Jensen medium for atypical Mycobacterium (*Mycobacterium marinum* at 32°, *Mycobacterium tuberculosis* at 37°)

❍ **What are the common stains needed in hand infections?**

Gram stain, Ziehl-Nielson stain (atyp. Mycobacterium), Tzanck smear (herpes simplex virus)

❍ **When evaluating a hand infection and a fungi is suspected; what preparation should be done for examination?**

Potassium hydroxide preparation.

❍ **What is the most common infection in the hand in human immunodeficiency virus (HIV) positive patients?**

Herpes Simplex infection.

❍ **When using an aminoglycoside (e.g., gentamicin) for gram-negative coverage; what adverse effects are commonly overlooked?**

Nephrotoxicity and ototoxicity.

❍ **What is the antibiotic of choice for *M. marinum*?**

Minocycline.

❍ **What is the drug of choice for methicillin-resistant *S. aureus* (MRSA) infections of the hand?**

Vancomycin.

❍ **The most common hand infection is:**

Paronychia. It is an infection beneath the eponychial fold. Not to be confused with perionychium, which is the skin around the nail margin.

❍ **What is a runaround abscess?**

A paronychial infection that forms an abscess that tracks beneath the entire nail fold superficial to the nail plate.

❍ **In what type of patient population is chronic paronychial infection often seen?**

Patients exposed to constant moisture. Also, children who frequently dig in dirt.

❍ **What organism is commonly implicated in chronic paronychial infection and how is it treated?**

Candida albicans. Marsupialization and nail removal.

❍   **What adjunct treatment for chronic paronychial infections is recommended?**

Topical corticosteroid-antifungal ointment (3% Clioquinol in a triamcinolone-nystatin ointment).{Mycolog}

❍   **What subset of diabetic patients with hand infections have particularly high morbidity?**

Renal transplant patients.

❍   **What is a felon?**

Close space infections of the digital pulp.

❍   **What is the most common organism found in felons?**

Staphylococcus aureus-just like in the rest of hand infections.

❍   **What are the preferred incisions for draining a felon?**

Midvolar and high lateral incisions. NOT fish-mouth incisions.

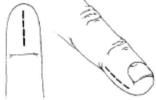

❍   **What type of incision used for draining a felon is associated with vascular compromise of the digital pad?**

Fish-mouth incisions.

❍   **How long does viral shedding and ability to infect others persist in people with herpetic whitlow?**

Until lesion epithelialization is complete.

❍   **What is the natural course of herpetic whitlow?**

A self limiting disease resolving over a period of seven to ten days.

❍   **What is pyogenic flexor tenosynovitis (or suppurative tenosynovitis) of the hand?**

A bacterial infection of the flexor sheath. *Staphylococcus aureus* is again the most common causative organism.

❍   **What are the four signs described by Kanavel characteristic of pyogenic flexor tenosynovitis? (Kanavel's cardinal signs)**

(1)   Flexed resting position of the involved digit.
(2)   Tenderness over the flexor sheath.
(3)   Severe pain with passive extension.
(4)   Fusiform swelling.
Note: all signs may not be present, especially early in the course of infection

❍   **Really?**

Well, no. Originally Kanavel never mentioned fusiform swelling but it has become closely associated with descriptions of flexor tenosynovitis over the years.

O   **What type of bacterial flexor tenosynovitis usually results from hematogenous spread?**

Gonococcal infections.

O   **Which two digital flexor sheaths communicate with bursae in the palm thus can propagate proximal extension of tenosynovial infections?**

The flexor sheath of the thumb (radial bursa) and the small finger (ulnar bursa). The ulnar and radial bursa extend proximally in 50%-80% of persons into the carpal tunnel.

O   **What is a horseshoe abscess?**

Infection of either small finger or thumb flexor sheath with contiguous spread through the communication of the radial and ulnar bursae.

O   **What has happened if a patient with suppurative flexor tenosynovitis of the small finger suddenly develops acute carpal tunnel symptoms?**

Extensive proximal spread of infection into Parona's space (the quadrilateral potential space at the wrist bordered by the pronator quadratus, digital flexors, pollicis longus, and flexor carpi ulnaris).

O   **Can contiguous spread from the index-finger sheath cause infection of thenar space?**

Yes.

O   **How do you treat early infections of suppurative flexor tenosynovitis (within 24 hours)? Late?**

Elevation, splinting, and IV antibiotics. Surgical debridement.

O   **If limited incision and catheter irrigation is used, why is it important to make sure catheter is within digital sheath?**

Digital compartment syndrome can occur as fluid fills the interstitial tissue.

O   **What deep spaces of the hand can be involved in infection?**

Dorsal subaponeurotic, thenar, midpalmar, Parona's quadrilateral, and interdigital subfascial web spaces.

O   **Name the fascial spaces of the hand and the possible contiguously infected area?**

Fascial Space	Infected Area
Middle palmar space	Infection of ring or middle finger
Thenar space	Infection of index flexor tendon sheath
Dorsal subaponeurotic space	Aponeurosis of extensor tendons (deep)
Dorsal subcutaneous space	Entire dorsum of hand

O   **What are the most common infectious agents in deep space hand infections?**

Streptococcus, *S. aureus*, and coliform organisms.

O   **What is the name used when the interdigital subfascial web space is infected?**

Collar button abscess. Treated with incision and drainage/broad spectrum antibiotics.

O   **Why are they called collar button abscesses?**

They typically form two swellings-one volarly and one dorsally with each on one end of a narrower stalk. The shape is like a dumbbell or the collar-buttons used on shirts years ago. Tuxedos still come with collar-buttons frequently.

O   **In contrast to a simple dorsal subcutaneous abscess, a collar button abscess is characterized by:**

Abducted resting posture of the adjacent digits.

O   **An infection of the thenar space, first web space, and dorsoradial aspect of the hand is known as:**

Dumbbell or pantaloon infection.

O   **The boundaries of the thenar space are:**

Volar: Index finger flexor tendon.
Dorsal: Adductor pollicis musculature.
Radial: Insertion of adductor pollicis into the proximal phalanx of thumb and thenar muscle fascia.
Ulnar: Septum extending from palmar fascia to the volar ridge of the third metacarpal (midpalmar septum).

O   **Why is the thumb held in marked abduction in thenar space infections?**

This posture reduces pressure (and thus pain) within the thenar space.

O   **What are the mimickers of hand infection?**

Gout, pseudogout, pyogenic granuloma, pyoderma gangrenosum, and neoplasia.

O   **What is the most common algae infections seen in fisherman?**

Prototheca wickerhamii (Tx: Tetracycline).

O   **What are the recommended incisions for drainage of thenar-space infections?**

Combined dorsal and palmar incisions of the first web-space.

O   **Why are incisions that parallel the first-web commissure not recommended in thenar space infection?**

To avoid web space contracture.

O   **What is the only infection resulting in loss of palmar concavity?**

Midpalmar space infection.

O   **What are the boundaries of the midpalmar space?**

Volar: Flexor tendons and lumbricals.
Dorsal: Middle and ring finger metacarpals and second and third palmar interosseous muscles.
Radial: Midpalmar septum.
Ulnar: Hypothenar muscles.

O   **Exposure to what virus causes Milker's Node in the hand (or granuloma)?**

Poxvirus. Handling a cow's udder.

O   **What is an interdigital pilonidal cyst?**

When a foreign piece of hair enters the web space and becomes secondarily infected. Seen in barbers and sheep shearers.

❍ **What is the usual rate of infections after elective hand surgery?**

1%-7%; 0.47% deep infection rate after carpal tunnel release.

❍ **Name organisms found in hand infections associated with river or sea water?**

Vibrio vulnificus-coastal and brackish water. (Tx: tetracycline, chloramphenicol)
Mycobacterium marinum-fresh water and salt water. (Tx: rifampin, ethambutol, trimethoprim-sulfamethoxazole)
Aeromonas hydrophilia- fresh water (Tx: ciprofloxacin, tetracycline, trimethoprim-sulfamethoxazole)

❍ **What is sporotrichosis?**

A chronic granulomatous infection caused by the saprophytic fungus *Sporothrix schenckii.* Most common subcutaneous fungal lesion in North America seen mostly in the upper extremities.

❍ **What is the treatment of choice for sporotrichosis? If allergic to iodine?**

Oral potassium iodide. Itraconazole.

❍ **What organisms are commonly found in septic arthritis of the hand? Cause?**

Staphylococcus aureus and *Streptococcus. Haemophilus influenza* (young). *Gonococcus* (young adult with <u>monarticular non-traumatic</u> septic arthritis). Penetrating trauma.

❍ **Most common cause of osteomyelitis in the hand?**

Open fractures.

❍ **What is necrotizing fasciitis? Usually caused by?**

Liquefaction necrosis of the fascia with selective spread along fascial planes involving skin and muscle during later stages of infection with bullae formation, myonecrosis, and skin slough. Group A *Streptococcus.*

❍ **Gas gangrene is frequently caused by?**

Clostridium perfringens.

❍ **Are there pathognomonic physical findings in atypical mycobacterial infections of the hand?**

No, but deep infections are frequently associated with abundant tenosynovitis or joint synovitis.

❍ **What unique infection can occur in the hands of patients receiving Taxol?**

Subungual abscess of multiple digits (including the toes) with painful onycholysis or nail plate separation.

References

Hausman MR, Lisser SP: Hand infections. *Orthop Clin North Am* 1992;23:171-185.

Mann RJ, Hoffeld TA, Farmer CB: Human bites of the hand: Twenty years of experience. *J Hand Surg [Am]* 1977;2:97-104.

Chuinard RG, D'Ambrosia RD: Human bite infections of the hand. *J Bone Joint Surg Am* 1977;59:416-418.

Goldstein EJC, Citron DM, Wield B, et al: Bacteriology of human and animal bite wounds. *J Clin Microbiol* 1978;8:667-672.

Arons MS, Fernando L, Polayes IM: Pasteurella multocida: The major cause of hand infections following domestic animal bites. *J Hand Surg [Am]* 1982;7:47-52.

Hurst LC, Amadio PC, Badalamente MA, et al: *Mycobacterium marinum* infections of the hand. *J Hand Surg [Am]* 1987;12:428-435.

Hitchcock TF, Amadio PC: Fungal infections. *Hand Clin* 1989;5:599-611.

Fowler JR: Viral infections. *Hand Clin* 1989;5:613-627.

Glickel SZ: Hand infections in patients with acquired immunodeficiency syndrome. *J Hand Surg [Am]* 1988;13:770-775.

Schecter W, Meyer A, Schecter G, et al: Necrotizing fasciitis of the upper extremity. *J Hand Surg [Am]* 1982;7:15-20.

Reid A, Botte, MJ: Hand Infections: Treatment Recommendations for Specific Types. *J American Academy Orthopaedic Surgeons 1996*;4:219-230.

Canales FL, Newmeyer WL III, Kilgore ES Jr: The treatment of felons and paronychias. *Hand Clin* 1989;5:515-523.

Siegel DB, Gelberman RH: Infections of the hand. *Orthop Clin North Am* 1988;19:779-789.

Kanavel AB: *Infections of the Hand,* 7thed. Philadelphia: Lea & Febiger, 1939.

Neviaser RJ: Infections, in Green DP(ed): *Operative Hand Surgery,* 3rd ed. New York: Churchill Livingstone, 1993,vol 1, pp 1021-1038.

Burkhalter WE: Deep space infections. *Hand Clin* 1989;5:553-559.

Freeland AE, Senter BS: Septic arthritis and osteomyelitis. *Hand Clin* 1989;5:533-552.

DUPUYTREN'S CONTRACTURE

Abdulaziz Jarman MB.BS, FRCSC, Alexander Anzarut, MD, MSc, and Michael Morhart, MSc, MD, FRCSC

○ **What is the cause of Dupuytren's disease?**

It is usually familial disease with multifactorial causes. The tissue-level problem is a proliferative fibroplasias.

○ **What are the diseases associated with Dupuytren's disease?**

1. Diabetes Mellitus.
2. Anti-convulsant therapy and epilepsy.
3. Chronic alcoholism.
4. HIV infection.
5. Tobacco consumption.

○ **Is the disease related to work or trauma?**

The disease has been noticed to increase in heavy manual workers or following injury to the hand.

○ **Who gets this disease?**

Typically Scandinavian or Northern European males (10:1 prevalence over women).

○ **Where do they get it?**

The most common fingers to get Dupuytren's are the ring and small fingers.

○ **What is Ledderhose's disease?**

Plantar fibromatosis.

○ **What is Peyronie's disease?**

Penile fibromatosis.

○ **Do these have anything to do with Dupuytren's diathesis?**

Yes. Dupuytren's diathesis is the presence of a strong family history of Dupuytren's disease associated with knuckle pads, Ledderhose's or Peyronie's disease. The patient often develops aggressive disease at a young age with a high likelihood of recurrence following surgery.

○ **What are the risk factors in developing Dupuytren's disease?**

1. Family history.
2. Other type of fibromatosis.
3. Early and aggressive onset.
4. Severe bilateral disease.

○ **What is Luck's classification of the disease?**

Three phases:
1. Proliferative phase.

2. Involutional phase.
3. Residual phase.

○ **What is the difference between the collagen in normal fascia and that of the disease?**

Normal fascia contains mostly Type I collagen, whereas collagen in Dupuytren's disease contain mostly Type III collagen.

○ **What cell type is implicated in Dupuytren's?**

The myofibroblast.

○ **Name the normal fascia and their pathological forms in Dupuytren's disease?**

Pretendinous band becomes pretendinous cord.
1. Lateral digital sheet becomes lateral cord.
2. Natatory ligament becomes natatory cord.

○ **What other cords contribute to the disease?**

Central and spiral cords.

○ **What forms the spiral cord?**

It is formed by the pretendinous band, spiral band, lateral digital sheet and Grayson's ligament.

○ **What other ligaments in the hand are not affected by the disease?**

Superficial transverse ligament.
1. Deep transverse ligament.
2. Cleland's ligament.
3. Landsmeer's ligament.

○ **What causes MCP joint flexion contracture in Dupuytren's disease?**

Pretendinous cord.

○ **What causes PIP joint flexion contracture in Dupuytren's disease?**

Spiral cord, lateral cord and central cord.

○ **What causes MCP adduction contracture in Dupuytren's disease?**

Natatory cords and the termination of the transverse fibers of the palmar aponeurosis.

○ **Does the DIP got involved in Dupuytren's disease? If so, how?**

Yes, essentially by the retrovascular cord and to some extent by the lateral cord.

○ **What is the key to thing to remember about natatory cords?**

They prevent abduction of the fingers at the MCP joints.

○ **What causes neurovascular displacement in the disease?**

The spiral cord.

○   **What is the histological hallmark of the disease?**

The high cellularity. Notably, polyclonal in nature suggesting that the tissue is not truly neoplastic.

○   **What could it be caused by?**

Local ischemia and production of free radicals.

○   **What are the two forms of the diseased fascia?**

Cord or nodule.

○   **What is the histological feature of the nodule?**

Dense collection of myofibroblasts.

○   **What are the histological features of the cord?**

Contains no myofibroblasts but highly organized collagen as seen in tendons.

○   **What causes cord contracture?**

Myofibroblasts in the nodules account for active contraction.

○   **Where are nodules usually located?**

Usually just distal or just proximal to the distal palmar crease.

○   **What is the differential diagnosis for Dupuytren's disease (including isolated nodules)?**

1.   Ganglion.
2.   Inclusion cyst.
3.   Epithelioid sarcoma.
4.   Camptodactyly.
5.   Trigger finger.

○   **What are the non-surgical treatments for the Dupuytren's disease?**

1.   Steroid injections.
2.   Splinting and skeletal traction.
3.   Ultrasound therapy.
4.   Laser therapy.
5.   Collagenase and enzymatic fasciotomy.

○   **How successful is the non surgical treatment?**

Usually not successful, although there is growing data suggesting that collagenase has significant potential use.

○   **What are the indications for surgery?**

1.   MCP and PIP contracture of 30 degrees or more.
2.   Severe adduction contracture.

○   **What is the table top test?**

Described by Hueston, it simply tests the patients ability to place the palm flat on a table top. Once they cannot, some surgeons recommend surgery.

○ **What are the three aspects to be considered in the surgical treatment of the Dupuytren's disease?**

1. Management of the skin.
2. Management of the fascia.
3. Management of the wound.

○ **What does management of the skin involve?**

It involves the skin incision either transverse or longitudinal (either linear, zig-zag or lazy S).

○ **What does management of the fascia involve?**

Either can be utilized:
1. Incision (fasciotomy).
2. Local excision. (Regional fasciectomy).
3. Wide excision (extensive radical fasciectomy).

○ **What does management of the wound involve?**

The wound is either sutured, left open or skin grafted.

○ **What is dermatofasciectomy?**

Wide excision of the involved palmar and digital skin and fascia combined with skin grafting.

○ **What are possible indications for skin grafting?**

1. Patients with Dupuytren's diathesis.
2. Patients with recurrent PIP joint contracture.
3. Patients with primary, severe PIP contracture resulting in skin deficiency at closure once the joint has been restored to extension.

○ **What is the difference between extension and recurrence of the disease?**

Extension refers to the postoperative appearance of the disease in an area of the hand not involved in the surgery. Recurrence refers to postoperative appearance of the disease in the area of previous surgery.

○ **Mention some complications of the surgery?**

1. Neurovascular bundle injury.
2. Hematoma and skin necrosis.
3. Joint stiffness.
4. Reflex sympathetic dystrophy.
5. Recurrent or uncorrected deformity.

○ **What is the post-operative management?**

1. Operated hand usually splinted in extension.
2. Wound care and frequent dressing changes.
3. Active and passive range of motion exercises post operatively.
4. Splinting varies depending on the surgical technique used.
5. PIP joint usually need 6 weeks of full time splinting and at least 3 months of night splinting.

References

McGrouther DA. Dupuytren's contracture. In: Green DP, Hotchkiss RN, Pederson WC, eds. *Green's Operative Hand Surgery.* Vol one. 4th ed. New York: Churchill Livingstone; 1999:563-591.

Macfarlane RM, Ross DC. Dupuytren's disease. In: Weinzweig J, ed. *Plastic Surgery Secrets.* Philadelphia: Hanley and Belfus; 1999:554-559.

Lubahn JD. Dupuytren's disease. In: Trumble TE, ed. *Hand Surgery Update 3 Hand, Elbow and Shoulder.* Rosemont: American Society for Surgery of the Hand; 2003:393-401.

Hurst LN. Dupuytren's contracture. In: Achauer BM, Ericksson E, Guyuron B, et al, eds. *Plastic Surgery Indications, Operations And Outcomes.* Vol Four. St. Louis: Mosby; 2000:2057-2071.

Benson LS, Williams CS, Kahle M. Dupuytren's contracture. *Journal of the American Academy of Orthopaedic Surgeons.* Jan/Feb 1998;6(1):24-35.

NERVE COMPRESSION SYNDROMES

Jeffrey B. Friedrich, MD

○ **How is nerve conduction in the carpal tunnel reported?**

In terms of "latency", with the unit being milliseconds (msec).

○ **What is "latency"?**

The time it takes for an electrical stimulus to travel along a nerve from the site if stimulation to a recording electrode in a target muscle.

○ **How is nerve conduction at the elbow reported?**

In terms of velocity (meters/second).

○ **What is a clinically significant decrease in velocity at the elbow?**

10 or more m/sec

Ulnar Nerve:

Thoracic Outlet Syndrome

○ **What nerve is affected with thoracic outlet syndrome (TOS)?**

Lower trunk of brachial plexus with symptoms mimicking cubital tunnel syndrome.

○ **What are the contents of the "thoracic outlet"?**

Subclavian vein, subclavian artery, brachial plexus.

○ **TOS is more common in what gender?**

Female

○ **Within the population of patients with cervical ribs, how many are bilateral?**

50%

○ **When do patients with TOS typically get their symptoms (ulnar-sided numbness)?**

When their arms are above their heads.

○ **What is Adson's maneuver?**

Dampening of radial pulse with inhalation, neck extension and head rotation to the affected side in patients with TOS. There are varying descriptions of how to perform this maneuver.

○ **How accurate is an Adson's maneuver?**

False positives are so common that test is thought of in terms of historical interest only.

○ **What is Wright's maneuver?**

Reproduction of TOS symptoms or dampening of radial pulse with arm hyperabducted and head in neutral or turned away from the affected side.

○ **How accurate is Wright's maneuver?**

It is positive in 7% of normal patients and thus should be used only to support a diagnosis of compression in patients with arterial symptoms.

○ **What is Roos' maneuver?**

Both arms are put into 90 degrees of abduction and external rotation and the patient is asked to open and close the hands for three minutes. Many patients will have forearm fatigue, but patients with TOS have reproduction of their symptoms.

○ **How accurate is Roos' maneuver?**

It is the most reliable of the three maneuvers noted. However, some patients with carpal tunnel syndrome and no TOS will develop symptoms limited to the median nerve distribution.

○ **What are the electrodiagnostic testing results seen with TOS?**

Negative EMG for ulnar nerve, positive somatosensory evoked potentials with arm in offending position.

○ **Name the two approaches to the thoracic outlet?**

Supraclavicular and transaxillary

○ **What is similar and what is different about the presentation of TOS and cubital tunnel syndrome?**

Similar: ulnar distribution numbness; different: TOS has medial forearm numbness.

Cubital Tunnel Compression

○ **How do you tell the difference between ulnar nerve compression at the cubital tunnel from compression at the wrist (Guyon's Canal)?**

Sensory changes on the dorsoulnar hand.

The dorsal sensory branch of the ulnar nerve branches from the main ulnar nerve about 7cm proximal to the pisiform, between the cubital tunnel and Guyon's canal, providing sensation to the dorsoulnar hand. Therefore, patients with cubital tunnel compression should have some difference in sensation of the dorsoulnar hand between the affected side and unaffected side.

○ **What is the distribution of motor weakness seen with cubital tunnel syndrome?**

FDS of ring and small fingers, ulnar intrinsic muscles.

○ **Describe Froment's sign.**

With ulnar nerve palsy, patients compensate for lack of adductor pollicis (ulnar innervated) function by flexing the thumb IP joint (pinch power then provided entirely by the median innervated FPL).

○ **Describe the Bunnel "O" sign.**

It is the same as Froment's sign.

○ **What are common sites of ulnar nerve compression?**

1. Arcade of Struthers-a fascial arcade of intermuscular septum through which the nerve passes. Present in 70% of patients.
2. Intermuscular septum between the brachialis and medial head of triceps. Can cause compression even in absence of Arcade of Struthers so they are distinct.
3. Medial head of triceps-whether by hypertrophy (bodybuilders) or anterior subluxation over medial epicondyle.
4. Cubital Tunnel-Osborne's Ligament-a fascial arcade formed between the two heads of the FCU. The most common site of compression.
5. Flexor-pronator aponeurosis-a fascial band between the FDS and FDP.
6. Guyon's canal-at the wrist. Second most common site of entrapment.

○ **Where is the Arcade of Struthers?**

8 cm proximal to the medial epicondyle.

○ **What is the cubital tunnel?**

Floor-medial collateral ligament of elbow (spans from medial epicondyle to olecranon).
Roos-Osborne's Ligament.
Sides-medial epicondyle and olecranon (to which the above two structures attach).

○ **What are implicated as the main compressive structures in cubital tunnel syndrome?**

Arcade of Struthers, intermuscular septum, Osborne's ligament or band (fascia connecting ulnar and humeral heads of FCU), and the flexor-pronator aponeurosis.

○ **Explain why the elbow hyperflexion test elicits symptoms of cubital tunnel syndrome?**

1. Elbow flexion increases the distance the ulnar nerve has to travel to traverse the elbow.
2. Feel your own olecranon and medial epicondyle with your elbow extended. Now flex your elbow and feel how the distance between them grows, tightening Osborne's Ligament and compressing the nerve.

○ **What is a Martin-Gruber anastomosis, and what is its significance in relation to cubital tunnel syndrome?**

Interconnection between the median and ulnar nerve at the level of the forearm; presence of this anomalous interconnection can result in spared intrinsic muscle function with cubital tunnel syndrome (because the median nerve innervates the intrinsics in this situation).

○ **What is a Riche-Cannieu anastomosis?**

Interconnection between the median and ulnar nerve in the hand, typically the deep or motor branch of the ulnar nerve. Again, there may be confusion for the examiner as typically ulnar innervated muscles continue to function.

○ **What are the key steps involved in anterior submuscular ulnar nerve transposition?**

Release of FCU origin, transposition of ulnar nerve anterior to medial epicondyle, resuturing of FCU to epicondyle.

O   **So you have to do at least a sub-muscular transposition of the nerve, right?**

Maybe not. In 1957 <u>Geoffrey Osborne</u>, a British orthopedic surgeon, reported 13 cases of cubital tunnel syndrome in which he released the ligament or band that now bears his name noting that it was tight in elbow flexion but lax in extension. These patients did no differently than those patients having a formal transposition. Several studies since then have supported this treatment.

O   **What is Guyon's canal?**

Roof-volar carpal ligament proximally and palmaris brevis distally.
Floor-transverse carpal ligament.
Ulnar wall-pisiform.
Radial wall-hard to say. Some think of the hamulus (hook of the hamate) but in many specimens the ulnar neurovascular bundle lies palmar or even radial to the hamulus.

O   **Guyon must have been a great hand surgeon to have a canal named after him.**

No. Jean Casimir Félix Guyon was a French Urologist and founding member of the Association Internationale d'Urologie in 1907. In 1861 he described the canal that bears his name and <u>hypothesized</u> that it could compress the ulnar nerve.

O   **What are the usual causes of ulnar tunnel syndrome?**

Ganglions, trauma (hamate fractures), tumors, vascular anomalies, arthritis.

O   **What is the distribution of numbness with ulnar tunnel syndrome?**

Small and ring fingers, but not dorsum of hand (because dorsal sensory branch is not involved).

O   **In general, what is the treatment for ulnar tunnel syndrome?**

Exploration of Guyon's canal, decompression of nerve, removal of space-occupying lesion, ulnar artery reconstruction (if necessary). You have to feel for masses as they are responsible for 30-45% of all cases of ulnar tunnel syndrome.

Median Nerve

O   **What are syndromes associated with median nerve compression?**

Pronator Syndrome
Anterior Interosseous Syndrome-a.k.a Kiloh-Nevin Syndrome
Carpal Tunnel Syndrome

O   **What conditions are associated with an increased incidence of carpal tunnel syndrome (CTS)?**

Most are idiopathic, but can be associated with pregnancy, diabetes, alcoholism, arthritis, amyloidosis or thyroid disorders.

O   **What are the borders of the carpal tunnel?**

Roof-transverse carpal ligament
Floor-carpal bones and their ligaments
Radial wall-trapezium and scaphoid tubercle
Ulnar wall-hook of hamate

○ **What are the classic symptoms of CTS?**

Numbness (index, middle, radial side of ring finger), weakness, nocturnal pain.

○ **What are the structures thought to cause effort-associated CTS (i.e. symptoms seen with repetitive gripping)?**

Lumbrical muscles. They arise from the flexor digitorum profundus (FDP) tendons, and are within the carpal tunnel during gripping activities.

○ **What is Phalen's test?**

Wrist is passively dropped into flexion. If symptoms are seen within 30 seconds, the test is positive.

○ **What electrodiagnostic study results signify median nerve conduction changes?**

Median nerve latency increase of 10% or more above that of the ulnar nerve.

○ **What electrodiagnostic study result signifies muscle denervation with CTS?**

Fibrillation potentials in the abductor pollicis brevis.

○ **What is the success rate of steroid injections for CTS?**

Only approximately 20-22% of patients get long-term (>18 months) relief.

○ **Where is the motor fasciculus of the median nerve at the wrist?**

Radial and palmar.

This should be easy to remember since the recurrent motor branch of the median nerve comes off of the main nerve radially and palmarly.

○ **What is Kaplan's line and how is it used to determine the position of the motor branch of the median nerve?**

Kaplan's line is a line drawn along the ulnar border of the abducted thumb. The intersection of this line and one drawn longitudinally from the index-middle finger web space is the rough approximation of the motor branch.

○ **What are the patterns of the route of the motor branch to the thenar musculature in relation to the transverse carpal ligament?**

Extraligamentous (approximately 50%), subligamentous (30%), and transligamentous (20-25%).

○ **What are the advantages of endoscopic carpal tunnel release when compared with the open technique?**

Less scar tenderness, and earlier restoration of grip and pinch strength. But after three months there are no differences.

○ **What has been demonstrated as the chief disadvantage of endoscopic carpal tunnel release when compared to open?**

Greater incidence of reversible nerve injury (4.3% in endoscopic vs. 0.9% in open).

○ **In what outcomes are endoscopic and open carpal tunnel release equivocal?**

Pain and return to work.

O   **What are sites of median nerve compression in the elbow/forearm?**

1.   Ligament of Struthers-ligament between humeral supracondylar process and medial epicondyle
2.   Lacertus fibrosis-a.k.a. bicipital aponeurosis-a fascial band between the biceps tendon and the fascia of the
        flexor pronator mass
3.   2 heads of the pronator teres
4.   FDS fibrous arch

O   **How can one specifically test for median nerve compression at the ligament of Struthers?**

When flexing the elbow <u>against resistance</u>, the symptoms are exacerbated.

O   **How can one specifically test for median nerve compression at the pronator teres?**

With resisted pronation, symptoms are exacerbated. The elbow must be fully extended to avoid confusion with compression by the bicipital aponeurosis.

O   **How can one specifically test for median nerve compression at the FDS arch?**

<u>Long finger flexion test</u>-with resisted flexion of the long finger, the FDS arch compresses the median nerve and symptoms are exacerbated.

O   **What is a Gantzer's muscle?**

An <u>accessory head of the FPL</u> originating from the medial humeral epicondyle and possibly also the coronoid process of the ulna and found in up to 45% of specimens. It can contribute to <u>compression of the median nerve</u> in pronator syndrome or the anterior interosseous nerve.

O   **What is the chief difference between the pronator syndrome and the anterior interosseus nerve (AIN) syndrome?**

Deficits in pronator syndrome are sensory, deficits in AIN syndrome are motor.

O   **What are the symptoms of the pronator syndrome?**

Pain in forearm, numbness in median nerve sensory distribution (thumb, index midlle fingers).

O   **What muscles are innervated by the anterior interosseus nerve?**

1.   Flexor Pollicis Longus
2.   Pronator Quadratus
3.   FDP to index finger
4.   FDP to middle finger (this varies between the A.I.N. and ulnar nerve depending on the patient)

O   **What are the symptoms of anterior interosseus syndrome (AIN)?**

Loss of precision pinch (can't flex thumb IP or index DIP), pain in the forearm relieved by rest.

O   **What can patients with anterior interosseous syndrome NOT do?**

Make an "OK" sign. They can't flex their thumb IP or index DIP joints.

O   **Is there a difference in the surgical treatment of AIN syndrome and pronator syndrome?**

No; in both cases the nerve is explored completely and released from all compressing structures.

Radial Nerve

○   **What are possible sites of radial nerve compression?**

1.   The lateral humeral intermuscular septum.
2.   Radial head.
3.   Supinator fascia-a.k.a. Arcade of Frohse (Posterior Interosseous Nerve Syndrome)
4.   Vascular Leash of Henry-radial recurrent vessels at the elbow.
5.   ECRB
6.   Between brachioradialis and ECRL-Wartenberg's Syndrome (involves the superficial sensory branch of the radial nerve only).

○   **What is the most common site of radial nerve compression?**

Supinator muscle fascia (a.k.a. the Arcade of Frohse).

○   **Where is the radial tunnel?**

It runs from the radial head to the distal edge of the supinator; the biceps tendon is the medial wall, and the extensor carpi radialis longus (ECRL) and extensor carpi radialis brevis (ECRB) origins form the lateral wall.

○   **What are the symptoms of radial tunnel syndrome?**

Lateral elbow pain, especially with repetitive elbow extension. Motor findings are usually absent.

○   **What physical exam finding differentiates radial tunnel syndrome from lateral epicondylitis?**

Tenderness 4 cm distal to lateral epicondyle is seen with radial tunnel syndrome.

○   **Is there typically a sensory component to posterior interosseus nerve syndrome?**

No; the PIN innervates the extensors, and therefore results in weakness and pain, but not sensory deficits.

○   **What is the difference between radial tunnel syndrome and posterior interosseous nerve compression?**

In radial tunnel syndrome symptoms involve pain over the dorsoradial forearm near the elbow. There is rarely weakness.
In posterior interosseous nerve compression symptoms involve weakness of the thumb and finger extensors AS WELL AS pain.

○   **What is the role for surgery in PIN syndrome and radial tunnel syndrome?**

Radial tunnel syndrome should be initially managed non-operatively (muscle palsy is not seen with this syndrome); PIN syndrome should be treated operatively to prevent permanent muscle palsy.

○   **What is the Vascular Leash of Henry?**

A network of radial recurrent vessels at the elbow which can compress the radial nerve in either its posterior interosseous branch, its superficial sensory branch or both.

○   **What is Wartenberg's syndrome?**

Compression neuropathy of the radial sensory nerve due to trapping between the brachioradialis and ECRL. Other names include superficial radial neuritis or "cheiralgia paresthetica".

○   **What can cause Wartenberg's syndrome?**

External compression (handcuffs), tight watch, surgical scarring, repetitive activities.

○   **What is Wartenberg's *Sign* then?**

Indicates ulnar neuropathy. The patient is unable to hold the small finger against the ring finger with the fingers in extension due to the unopposed action of the <u>radially innervated</u> extensor digiti minimi and the weak <u>ulnarly innervated</u> palmar interossei which are unable to adduct the small finger to the ring finger.

References

Fitzgerald BT, Dao KD, Shin AY. Functional outcomes in young, active duty military personnel after submuscular ulnar nerve transposition. J Hand Surg 2004, 29A(4): 619-24.

Lowe JB, Mackinnon SE. Management of secondary cubital tunnel syndrome. Plas Recon Surg 2004, 113(1): 1e-16e.

Thoma A, Veltri K, Haines T, et al. A systematic review of reviews comparing the effectiveness of endoscopic and open carpal tunnel decompression. Plas Recon Surg 2004, 113(4): 1184-91.

Thoma A, Veltri K, Haines T, et al. A meta-analysis of randomized controlled trials comparing endoscopic and open carpal tunnel decompression. Plas Recon Surg 2004, 114(5): 1137-46.

Trumble TE. Compressive neuropathies. In Trumble TE, ed. Principles of Hand Surgery and Therapy. 1st ed. Philadelphia: W.B. Saunders, 2000: 324-41.

Szabo RM. Entrapment and compression neuropathies. In Green DP, Hotchkiss RN, Pederson WC, eds. Green's Operative Hand Surgery. 4th ed. Philadelphia: Churchill Livingstone, 1993: 1404-47.

Posner MA. Compressive ulnar neuropathies at the Elbow: I. Etiology and Diagnosis. Journal of the American Academy of Orthopedic Surgeons, 1998, 6 (5):282-288.

FRACTURES/DISLOCATIONS

George S. Athwal, MD, FRCSC

O **What three structures provided the greatest stability to the proximal interphalangeal joint?**

The three-sided box configuration of the medial and lateral collateral ligaments and the volar plate

O **What is the classification of Mallet fractures of the finger?**

Type 1: closed tendon avulsion with or without fracture
Type 2: laceration with extensor tendon disruption
Type 3: open injury with loss of skin and tendon substance
Type 4: physeal fracture in children

O **What is the treatment of choice for a displaced fracture of the dorsal base of the distal phalanx comprising over 25% of the articular surface?**

Operative intervention with closed or open reduction and internal fixation

O **What is the treatment of choice for a volar base fracture of the distal phalanx with loss of the flexor digitorum profundus insertion?**

Open reduction and internal fixation

O **What is the acceptable angulation for metacarpal shaft fractures (index, middle, ring and little)?**

Index metacarpal: 10 to 15 degrees
Middle metacarpal: 10 to 15 degrees
Ring metacarpal: 30 to 35 degrees
Small metacarpal: 40 to 45 degrees

O **What is the most likely direction of angulation of an unstable transverse metacarpal shaft fracture?**

Apex dorsal angulation due to the volar directed pull of the interosseous muscles

O **What are some indications for operative fixation of phalangeal and metacarpal fractures?**

- malrotation
- irreducible fractures
- intra-articular fractures
- open fractures
- fractures with bone loss
- fractures with associated tendon, vascular or nerve injury
- polytrauma patients

O **How does one assess for malrotation in phalangeal and metacarpal fractures?**

The hand is assessed with the fingers in extension and flexion. In extension the fingers should be parallel and in flexion they should all point toward the scaphoid tuberosity. Malrotation would present as subtle overlap or scissoring of the fingers.

❍ **What is the #1 complication of operatively treated phalangeal fractures?**

Digital stiffness

❍ **What is the most likely block to reduction in a complex dorsal dislocation of the metacarpophalangeal joint?**

Volar plate

❍ **What two structures act as a noose around the metacarpal head in an irreducible (complex) dorsal dislocation of the index MCP joint?**

The flexor tendons (ulnarly) and the lumbricals (radially) maintain a tight encirclement around the narrow neck of the metacarpal preventing reduction.

❍ **In a Bennett's fracture, what is the deforming force that causes proximal migration of the thumb metacarpal?**

Abductor pollicis longus

❍ **What is a Stener lesion?**

A Stener lesion is formed when the distally avulsed ulnar collateral ligament of the thumb metacarpophalangeal joint comes to lie dorsal to the leading edge of the adductor aponeurosis.

❍ **What are the most reasonable treatment options for a fracture/dislocation of the proximal interphalangeal (PIP) joint with a severely comminuted volar base fracture of the middle phalanx involving 40% of the joint surface?**

Volar plate arthroplasty or Suzuki-type dynamic external fixation/traction

❍ **In volar dislocation of the PIP joint, what commonly associated injury must be examined for?**

Rupture or avulsion of the extensor tendon central slip

❍ **What is the treatment for a 5th metacarpal neck fracture (Boxer's Fracture) with 40 degrees of apex dorsal angulation?**

40 degrees is the maximal angulation acceptable, however, some would suggest attempted closed reduction to improve angulation and ulnar gutter splinting.

❍ **What is the most common carpal bone fractured?**

Scaphoid fractures account for 80% of all carpal bone fractures

❍ **Describe the anatomy of the major blood supply to the scaphoid.**

The major blood supply is from branches of the radial artery that enter the dorsal ridge of the scaphoid (distal to the scaphoid waist). This blood supply accounts for 70 to 80% of the total blood supply of the scaphoid and 100% of the blood supply to the proximal pole.

❍ **What is snuffbox tenderness?**

Tenderness on palpation of the anatomic snuffbox (interval between the tendons of the first and third dorsal compartments distal to the radial styloid), which may indicate fracture of the scaphoid.

○ **What is a scaphoid humpback deformity?**

The apex dorsal angulation seen with a scaphoid waist nonunion or malunion. The distal scaphoid fragment angulates volarly and the proximal scaphoid fragment extends with the lunate.

○ **What type of carpal instability is seen most commonly with a malunited scaphoid (humpback deformity)?**

Dorsal intercalated segment instability (DISI) is visualized on a lateral radiograph as the proximal scaphoid fragment extends with the lunate.

○ **What is the definition of scaphoid fracture displacement or instability?**

- presence of a fracture gap of greater than 1mm on any radiographic projection
- scapholunate angle of greater than 60 degrees
- radiolunate angle of greater than 15 degrees
- intrascaphoid angle of greater than 30 degrees

○ **What is the space of Poirier?**

A palmar area of inherent capsular weakness <u>between the capitate and lunate</u>, which is torn in perilunate injuries creating a capsular rent across the midcarpal joint.

○ **What is Mayfield's progressive sequence of perilunate disruption or dislocation?**

Stage I – disruption of the scapholunate interosseous ligament complex
Stage II – disruption through the Space of Poirier and the lunocapitate interval
Stage III – disruption of the lunotriquetral ligament complex and resultant separation of the entire carpus from the lunate
Stage IV – dislocation of the lunate from its fossa in to the carpal tunnel

○ **What is a "lesser arc" injury?**

This type of injury refers to a purely ligamentous disruption around the lunate.

○ **What is a "greater arc" injury?**

This type of injury refers to disruption around the lunate that involves fractures of some or all of the carpal bones.

○ **What is the most common "greater arc" injury?**

A trans-scaphoid perilunate fracture - dislocation

○ **What is the normal intra-carpal angle between the scaphoid and lunate (scapholunate angle)?**

Between 30 to 60 degrees

○ **What is the most sensitive and specific test for assessment of post-traumatic avascular necrosis of the scaphoid?**

Magnetic resonance imaging-MRI.

○ **What is scaphocapitate syndrome?**

Fracture of the neck of the capitate with rotation of the proximal fragment in association with a scaphoid waist fracture

O   **What is carpal instability dissociative (CID)?**

Refers to intrinsic ligament disruptions that occur between carpal bones of the same carpal row (i.e. scapholunate dissociation caused by a scapholunate ligament tear).

O   **What is carpal instability nondissociative (CIND)?**

Refers to extrinsic ligament disruptions that occur between carpal rows (i.e. midcarpal instability).

O   **What is Watson's scaphoid shift test?**

The test assesses for scapholunate ligament dissociation. The examiner applies dorsally directed thumb pressure over the patient's distal scaphoid tubercle. If the SL ligament is torn, pain is elicited when the proximal pole of the scaphoid subluxates dorsally out of the scaphoid fossa of the radius as the patient's hand is passively moved from ulnar deviation to radial deviation.

O   **What is a Terry Thomas sign?**

Increased gap between the scaphoid and lunate, greater than 3mm, indicative of a scapholunate dissociation.

O   **On a PA wrist radiograph, what are findings of scapholunate dissociation?**

- Terry Thomas sign
- cortical ring sign
- reduced carpal height
- triangular shaped lunate
- foreshortened scaphoid

O   **What are Gilula's lines?**

Gilula et al described three smooth curved lines on a PA projection of the carpus. The first line represents the proximal cortical surfaces of the proximal carpal row. The second line represents the distal cortical surfaces of the proximal carpal row and the third line represents the proximal cortical surfaces of the distal carpal row. A step-off or disruption in any of these lines may indicate carpal malalignment or instability.

O   **What radiographic projection would best visualize a hook of hamate fracture?**

Carpal tunnel profile view

O   **What is the treatment of choice for a symptomatic hook of hamate nonunion?**

Excision of the hamate hook

O   **What is the "safe" position of immobilization for the hand?**

The "safe" position or the intrinsic-plus position of James is 70 degrees of MCP joint flexion and full IP joint extension.

O   **What is the Salter-Harris classification of physeal injuries?**

Salter-Harris Classification
Type I – transverse fracture through the physis
Type II – fracture through the physis with a metaphyseal fragment
Type III – fracture through the physis and in to the epiphysis (intra-articular)
Type IV – fracture through the physis, epiphysis and metaphysis
Type V – crush in jury of the physis

References

Stern PJ. Fracture of the metacarpals and phalanges. In: Green DP, ed. Operative Hand Surgery. 4th ed. New York: Churchill Livingstone Inc., 1999:711-771.

Glickel SZ, Barron OA, Eaton RG. Dislocations and ligament injuries in the digits. In: Green DP, ed. Operative Hand Surgery. 4th ed. New York: Churchill Livingstone Inc., 1999:772-808.

Amadio PC, Taleisnik J. Fractures of the carpal bones. In: Green DP, ed. Operative Hand Surgery. 4th ed. New York: Churchill Livingstone Inc., 1999:809-864.

Garcia-Elias M. Carpal instabilities and dislocations. In: Green DP, ed. Operative Hand Surgery. 4th ed. New York: Churchill Livingstone Inc., 1999:865-928.

Henry M. Fractures and dislocations of the hand. In: Bucholz RW and Heckman JD, ed. Rockwood and Green's Fractures in Adults. 5th ed. Philadelphia: Lippincott Williams and Wilkins, 2001:655-748.

Seitz WH, Papandrea RF. Fractures and dislocations of the wrist. In: Bucholz RW and Heckman JD, ed. Rockwood and Green's Fractures in Adults. 5th ed. Philadelphia: Lippincott Williams and Wilkins, 2001:749-814.

TENDON INJURIES

Steven L. Henry, MD

Anatomy And Physiology

○ **From where do tendons receive their nourishment?**

In the forearm, from vessels in the paratenon.
In the hand, from the vincular vessels (intrinsic system) and from the synovial fluid (extrinsic system) within the tendon sheath.

○ **Which source is more important to the tendons in the hand?**

Synovial fluid.

○ **What are the vincula?**

Folds of mesotendon containing blood vessels. Each tendon (FDS and FDP) has two vincula, a short vinculum distally and a long vinculum proximally, that enter the dorsal surface of the tendons.

○ **What are the source vessels of the vincula?**

The transverse digital arteries, which enter the fibro-osseous tunnel at the levels of the cruciate pulleys.

○ **How is the short vinculum of the superficialis tendon related to the long vinculum of the profundus tendon?**

They cross each other at the distal P1 level.

○ **How many pulleys are there in the fingers?**

Eight (5 annular and 3 cruciate).

○ **What effect do the pulleys have?**

They prevent bowstringing of the flexor tendons in flexion increasing the effective excursion of the tendons and thus the degree of finger flexion.

○ **Which pulleys are the most important in the fingers, and where are they located?**

- A2, at the proximal part of the proximal phalanx
- A4, at the middle part of the middle phalanx

○ **The interval between which annular ligaments has no cruciate ligament?**

Between A1 and A2. The first cruciate ligament lies between A2 and A3.

○ **How many pulleys are there in the thumb?**

Three:
- A1 at the MP level,

- Oblique at the P1 level, and
- A2 at the IP level.

The oblique and A2 pulleys are the most important in the thumb.

○ **What comprises the floor of the fibro-osseous tunnel?**

The periosteum of the phalanges and the volar plates of the MP and PIP joints.

○ **What lies immediately volar to the volar plate of the PIP joint?**

FDS tendon.

○ **Describe the orientation of the FDS tendons within the carpal tunnel.**

The tendons of the index and small fingers are dorsal to the tendons of the long and ring fingers.

Flexor Tendons

○ **Describe the boundaries of the five flexor zones of the fingers.**

Zone I   Distal to the insertion of FDS on P2
Zone II   Within the fibro-osseous tunnel. Out to the FDS insertion).
Zone III   The area of the palm between the carpal tunnel and the fibro-osseous tunnel
Zone IV   Within the carpal tunnel.
Zone V   Proximal to the carpal tunnel.

○ **What are the two main deficits resulting from zone I tendon laceration?**

Loss of DIP flexion and diminution of grip strength.

○ **What provides the stronger repair in Zone I injuries—suturing of tendon ends together or anchoring of tendon end directly to bone?**

Anchoring directly to bone.

○ **What is the farthest the FDP tendon should be advanced to achieve direct anchoring to bone?**

1 cm.

○ **What is a jersey finger?**

Avulsion of the FDP tendon from its insertion on P3, (an injury that might be the result of reaching out to grab an opponents jersey in a rugby match).

○ **What finger is most commonly affected?**

Ring finger.

○ **Describe the three types of FDP avulsion injuries.**

Type I   Tendon retracts into palm.
Type II   Tendon retracts to level of PIP.
Type III   Tendon avulsed with large bony fragment, which catches at A4.

○ **Which type of FDP avulsion is most common? Which has the best prognosis? The worst?**

Most common: type II.
Best prognosis: type III.
Worst prognosis: type I.

○ **Why must type I FDP avulsion be repaired without significant delay?**

Because both the vincular and synovial nutritional supplies have been disrupted.

○ **What holds the FDP tendon at the level of the PIP in a type II FDP avulsion?**

The vincula.

○ **A heavy laborer sustained a type I FDP avulsion 1 month ago. What treatment should be considered?**

DIP fusion, if the joint is symptomatically unstable.

○ **Where is a zone II flexor tendon laceration usually located with respect to the skin laceration?**

Distal (the finger is usually flexed at the time of injury).

○ **If the vinculum is ruptured in a zone II injury, to where will the tendon usually retract?**

To the palm, just proximal to the A1 pulley, held in place by the lumbrical.

○ **How can the tendon be retrieved from the palm?**

A rubber catheter or infant feeding tube is guided down the tendon sheath from the site of injury in retrograde fashion. An incision is made at the distal palmar crease, and the catheter is retrieved from the proximal end of the fibro-osseous tunnel. The tendon is attached to the catheter and pulled back into the tunnel.

○ **What can happen if the FDP tendon is repaired but the FDS is not?**

High risk of rupture of the FDP repair, loss of dexterity and grip strength, and hyperextension deformity at the PIP.

○ **When should flexor tendon lacerations be repaired?**

As soon as possible, but successful tendon healing may be possible after a delay of several weeks if the vincular or synovial nutritional supplies are intact.

○ **What percentage of the total strength of a tendon repair is attributable to the epitendinous suture?**

About 20%.

○ **Following repair, when does tendon rupture most commonly occur?**

Around the tenth post-operative day.

○ **How should the patient be splinted following flexor tendon repair?**

The wrist should be held in approximately 30 degrees of flexion, the MPs in 50-70 degrees of flexion, and the IPs in full extension.

○ **When should passive range of motion exercises be initiated following flexor tendon repair? Active range of motion?**

Passive: as soon as possible.

Active: at 4-6 weeks, depending on the security of the repair (although some protocols call for earlier active motion).

○   **How is a splint commonly constructed to permit active extension and passive flexion?**

A rubber band is attached to the nail of the involved finger and to the splint in the region of the distal volar forearm. The rubber band provides resistance against active IP extension (the MP is blocked at 60-70 degrees of flexion), and passively pulls the finger into flexion.

○   **What is the most important prerequisite to flexor tendon grafting?**

Full passive range of motion.

○   **What are the most common donor sites for flexor tendon grafts?**

Palmaris longus, plantaris, and the long toe extensors.

○   **Where is plantaris with respect to the Achilles tendon?**

Anterior and medial.

○   **In reconstructing a zone II FDP injury with a graft, how can the appropriate length of the graft be determined?**

By matching the cascade of the injured digit with its uninjured neighbors.

○   **What can happen if the graft is too long?**

Lumbrical plus deformity, in which attempts to flex the finger cause paradoxical extension of the interphalangeal joints.

○   **What is quadriga syndrome?**

If one FDP is tethered or shortened following a repair, the others can't shorten enough to achieve full flexion. Try flexing your ring finger DIP while holding your long finger in extension with the other hand. Named by Verdan for the Roman charioteers who controlled teams of four horses with four sets of reins slung over their backs.

○   **What is the most common complication of tendon grafting?**

Adhesions.

○   **Following a zone II flexor tendon repair, a patient has limited active range of motion and has made little progress in therapy. When is the earliest that flexor tenolysis should be considered?**

At least three months of therapy should be attempted prior to performing tenolysis.

○   **What is a Hunter rod?**

A Hunter rod is a flexible silicone implant that is placed within a scarred flexor tendon bed. Formation of a capsule around this implant will create a pseudosheath within which a tendon graft can later be placed.

Extensor Tendons

○   **At what level do the extensor tendons lie within a synovial sheath?**

At the level of the extensor retinaculum. The extensor tendons are surrounded only by paratenon at all other levels.

○ **What tendons are present within each of the six extensor compartments?**

•	First	APL, EPB
•	Second	ECRL, ECRB
•	Third	EPL
•	Fourth	EDC, EIP
•	Fifth	EDQ
•	Sixth	ECU

○ **Which tendon inserts on the 2nd MC? On the 3rd? On the 5th?**

- ECRL on the 2nd
- ECRB on the 3rd
- ECU on the 5th

○ **What is the relationship of the proprius tendons (EIP and EDQ) to the communis tendons at the level of the MPs?**

The proprius tendons lie <u>ulnar</u> to the communis tendons.

○ **The EDC tendon is often missing from which finger?**

The small finger. In these instances, there are often two slips of EDC to the ring finger. There may also be two slips of EDQ to the small finger.

○ **What extends the IPs when the MP is extended? When the MP is flexed?**

The intrinsics when the MP is extended, the extrinsics when the MP is flexed.

○ **A patient sustains a dorsal hand laceration at the mid-metacarpal level, completely transecting the EDC tendon to the long finger. He is able to extend the IPs with the MP blocked in flexion. How is this possible?**

The juncturae tendinae are interconnections between the extensor tendons at the level of the distal metacarpals. The juncturae extend in a distal-oblique direction from the EDC tendon of the ring finger to those of the small finger and long finger, and from the EDC tendon of the long finger to that of the index finger. In this case, the tendon was lacerated proximal to the junctura, which transmits extensile force from the ring finger tendon to the long finger tendon.

○ **Which extensor tendons do not have juncturae?**

The proprius tendons (EIP and EDQ).

○ **What are the sagittal bands?**

The sagittal bands are transverse ligamentous structures that pass from the extensor tendon to the volar plate of the MP. Their function is to hold the extensor tendon in place over the MP. They are somewhat analogous to the A1 pulley of the flexor system, except that the sagittal bands undergo proximal and distal excursion with extension and flexion of the MP, much like a bucket handle.

○ **What is a common option for reconstructing a sagittal band that is not primarily repairable?**

Use of a strip of junctura tendinae.

○ **What holds the extensor mechanism in place over the PIP?**

Transverse retinacular ligament.

○   **Where is the extensor trifurcation?**

Proximal to the PIP, the extensor tendon trifurcates into a central slip and two lateral bands. The central slip inserts on the dorsal base of P2, while the lateral bands bypass the PIP and insert on P3.

○   **Where is the triangular ligament? What does it do?**

The triangular ligament spans the dorsal surface of the middle phalanx, <u>connecting the lateral bands to each other</u>. It helps to prevent the lateral bands from migrating volarly.

○   **What deformity results from laceration of the central slip with preservation and volar migration of the lateral bands?**

Boutonnière deformity.

○   **A patient has sustained a complete laceration of the EPL tendon, yet can still extend the IP joint of the thumb. How is this possible?**

The intrinsics of the thenar eminence insert on the extensor hood and can provide weak extension of the IP. In addition, the EPB can have a superficial division that inserts on the extensor hood. However, only the EPL can extend the entire first ray. Thus, if the patient places the palm flat on a table, he or she will be unable to lift the thumb off the table in the presence of a complete EPL laceration.

○   **Describe the zones of injury of the extensor tendons of the fingers.**

Odd zones are over joints.
Zones I, III, V, and VII overlie the DIP, PIP, MP, and carpal joints, respectively. Zones II, IV, VI, and VIII overlie the P2, P1, MC, and distal forearm, respectively.

○   **What can be done to prevent adhesions in the repair of a zone VII extensor tendon laceration?**

Excision of the portion of the extensor retinaculum that overlies the repair site.

○   **How should a patient be splinted after extensor tendon repair?**

The wrist is splinted in 45 degrees of extension, with the MPs in 10 to 20 degrees of flexion. If the injury is distal to the MPs, the interphalangeal joints should be held in extension; otherwise, the IPs need not be included in the splint. Splinting is continued for 3-4 weeks prior to initiation of protected range of motion therapy.

○   **What is a mallet finger?**

Flexion deformity of the DIP resulting from loss of continuity of the extensor mechanism.

○   **Describe the classification of mallet finger injuries.**

Type I   Closed, with or without a small chip fracture.
Type II   Open laceration.
Type III   Deep abrasion of skin and tendon substance.
Type IV   P3 fracture. This type includes transepiphyseal fracture in children (type IV-A), hyperflexion injuries
            (type IV-B), and hyperextension injuries (type IV-C). Note that these fractures involve significant
            portions of the articular surface and are not to be confused with the largely irrelevant chip fractures
            seen in type I injuries.

○   **How are various types of mallet injuries treated?**

Type I   Splinting of the DIP in slight hyperextension (no more than 5 degrees) for 6-8 weeks, followed by night splinting for 2 weeks.

Type II   Repair of skin and tendon with a single figure-of-eight suture, followed by splinting as above.

Type III   Skin coverage and tendon graft.

Type IV-A   Closed reduction of the fracture, followed by extension splinting for 3-4 weeks.

Type IV-B   Extension splinting, with ORIF reserved for cases in which the fragment is significantly displaced or the distal phalanx has subluxated volarly.

Type IV-C   As above.

References

Britton EN, Kleinert JM. Acute flexor tendon injury: repair and rehabilitation. In: Peimer CA, ed. Surgery of the Hand and Upper Extremity. New York: McGraw-Hill, 1996:1113-1132.

Doyle JR. Extensor tendons--acute injuries. In: Green DP, ed. Operative Hand Surgery. 2nd ed. New York: Churchill Livingstone Inc., 1988:2045-2072.

Lee WAP, Gan BS, Harris SU. Flexor tendons. In: Russell RC, ed. Plastic Surgery: Indications, Operations, and Outcomes, Vol. IV: Hand Surgery. St. Louis: Mosby, 2000:1961-1982.

Pederson WC. Extensor tendons. In: Russell RC, ed. Plastic Surgery: Indications, Operations, and Outcomes, Vol. IV: Hand Surgery. St. Louis: Mosby, 2000:1983-1994.

Schneider LH, Hunter JM. Flexor tendons--late reconstruction. In: Green DP, ed. Operative Hand Surgery. 2nd ed. New York: Churchill Livingstone Inc., 1988:1969-2044.

THE PERIONYCHIUM

Alexander Anzarut, MD, MSc, Abdulaziz Jarman, MB.BS, FRCSC, and Michael Morhart, MSc, MD, FRCSC

Anatomy

○ **Name the labeled structures:**

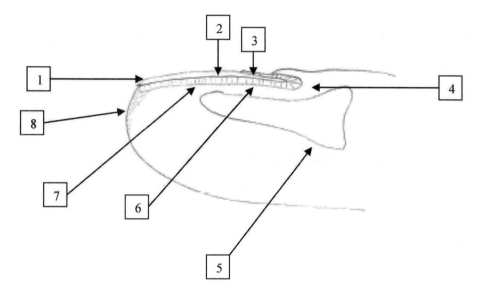

1. Nail plate
2. Lunula
3. Eponychium
4. Nail fold
5. Distal phalanx
6. Germinal matrix
7. Sterile matrix
8. Hyponychium

○ **What is the lunula?**

The curved white opacity representing the visible, distal portion of the germinal matrix.

○ **What is the eponychium?**

The thin membrane over the dorsum of the nail at the nail fold.

○ **What is the nerve supply to the perionychium?**

Dorsal branches from the volar digital nerves.

○ **What is the arterial supply to the nail?**

Two dorsal branches of the volar digital arteries.

○ **What makes up the nailplate?**

Flattened sheets of anuclear keratinized epithelium densely adherent to one another.

○   **What is the perionychium?**

The skin at the lateral nail margin.

○   **What changes occur in the nail plate distal to the lunula?**

The cell nuclei degenerate distal to the lunula. This is the junction of the sterile and germinal matrix.

Physiology

○   **What produces the nailplate?**

The germinal matrix produces 90% of the nail plate volume.

○   **What contributes to nailplate adherence?**

The sterile matrix

○   **What contributes to the smooth shiny surface of the nailplate?**

The roof of the nail fold.

○   **Name 5 functions of the finger nail?**

1) Protection of the fingertip
2) Improved pulp tactile sensation through provision of counterforce to the pulp
3) Assists in picking up objects
4) Self defense (scratching)
5) Regulation of peripheral circulation

○   **What area of the body has the highest concentration of lymphatics?**

The hyponychium

○   **What is the composition of the hyponychium?**

It is a mass of keratin with a large population of lymphocytes and polymorphonuclear leukocytes.

○   **Purpose of the hyponychium?**

Barrier to infection.

○   **At what rate does the nail grow?**

An average of 0.1mm/day or 100 days for complete nail growth, however after an injury distal growth is halted for 21 days as the proximal nail thickens.

Medical Pathology

○   **What is clubbing?**

Exaggerated convex curvature of the nail plate.

○ **What conditions are thought to cause clubbing?**

- Familial clubbing (idiopathic)
- Pulmonary disease-pulmonary fibrosis, sarcoidosis, cystic fibrosis
- Cardiac Disease-cyanotic congenital heart disease, bacterial endocarditis
- GI Disease-Ulcerative colitis, Crohn's, liver cirrhosis
- Cancer-thyroid, thymus, disseminated CML
- Other-acromegaly, pregnancy

○ **What is chromonychia?**

Changes in nail color.

○ **What causes this?**

Renal failure, subungual hemorrhage or medications.

Surgical Pathology

○ **What is onycholysis?**

Premature separation of the nail bed and nail plate.

○ **What causes this?**

Abnormalities of the sterile matrix, often secondary to post-traumatic scarring.

○ **What medications are strongly associated with onycholysis?**

Taxane chemotherapeutics including paclitaxel and docetaxel.

○ **What causes longitudinal splitting of the nail plate?**

Abnormalities of the germinal matrix (ventral nail fold), often secondary to post-traumatic scarring between the nail roof and nail floor.

○ **What causes longitudinal grooving in the nail plate?**

Abnormalities of the nail fold (tumor, bony change, or post-traumatic deformities).

○ **What are nail spikes or remnants?**

Small, often painful, volumes of nail plate that grow through the overlying skin. These usually occur after incomplete removal of the nail matrix following fingertip amputations.

○ **How are these treated?**

Definitive excision.

○ **Which is the most commonly injured finger nail?**

The long finger followed, in order of descending length, by the ring, index, small and thumb.

○ **What is the most common mechanism of injury?**

Doors.

O   **What is the significance of a subungual hematoma?**

There is an underlying nailbed injury.

O   **How are these treated?**

Trephination if the hematoma covers less than 50% of the nail plate. Removal of the nail plate and direct repair of the nail bed is required if the hematoma is > 50% of the nail plate.

O   **What is trephination?**

Creation of a hole in the nail plate to allow drainage of the hematoma, done with a large bore needle. The nail plate should be surgically scrubbed prior to trephination to avoid infection.

O   **When should nail bed injuries be treated and why?**

Acutely because secondary repair will rarely provide satisfactory results.

O   **Do you need an X-Ray of the fingertip?**

Yes, to evaluate the distal phalanx.

O   **What percent of nail bed injuries are associated with a distal phalanx fracture?**

50%.

O   **How are non-displaced fractures treated?**

Repair the nail bed if necessary and replace the nail plate, to act as a splint.

O   **How are unstable displaced fractures treated?**

Fracture reduction, bony fixation with crossed K-wires, repair of the nail bed, and replacement of the nail plate.

O   **What is the treatment for an avulsed nail plate?**

Find the nail plate, replace the nail plate with any attached portions of sterile matrix. If this is not available splint the nail fold open with a piece of Adaptic, the back of a suture pack or portion of a Penrose drain.

O   **After nail plate removal, why is it important to replace the nail plate (or use a substitute replacement)?**

To splint the repair and prevent scarring between the roof and floor of the nail fold.

O   **With severe crush injuries what is done with the nail bed tissue attached to the nail plate after the nail plate is removed?**

Replaced onto the nail bed as free grafts.

O   **When are split free nail bed grafts used?**

To replace large defects in the nail bed.

O   **Where is a split free nail bed graft harvested from?**

Ideally from an undamaged area on the injured finger or from an amputated digit.

○ **What is alternative source for split nail bed grafts?**

The great toe.

○ **What is a hook nail deformity?**

Nail that curves volar sharply at the finger tip.

○ **What causes this?**

Inadequate tip support, usually due to traumatic loss of bone.

○ **What causes nail ridges?**

Scar beneath the nail bed or an irregularly healed distal phalanx fracture.

○ **What is the treatment?**

Excision of the scar and/or smoothing out of the irregularity.

○ **What causes a split nail deformity?**

A ridge or longitudinal scar in the germinal matrix.

○ **What is the treatment?**

Resection of the scar and replacement with a FULL thickness germinal matrix graft (typically from the 2nd toe).

○ **What causes non-adherence of the nail plate?**

A transverse scar in the sterile matrix.

○ **What is the treatment?**

Scar resection and replacement with a split-thickness sterile matrix graft.

○ **What are nail cysts or nail spikes?**

A spike of nail plate growing out from an amputation stump.

○ **What causes this?**

Failure to remove all of the germinal matrix from the nail fold when performing an amputation at the proximal portion of the distal phalanx.

○ **What is the treatment?**

Complete resection of the nail cyst and its wall.

Infectious Diseases

○ **What is an acute paronychia?**

Infection of the skin surrounding the nail plate.

❍ **What is the most common cause?**

Staphylococcus aureus infection.

❍ **What is the treatment?**

Drainage with or without partial nail plate removal.

❍ **What causes chronic paronychia?**

Chronic bacterial or fungal infection. It often occurs among patients with hands that are frequently wet.

❍ **How is it treated?**

It requires systemic anti-fungals or antibiotics with or without nail plate removal.

❍ **What is onychomycosis?**

Chronic fungal infections of the nail.

❍ **How does it present?**

Nail plate discolouration, thickening and onycholysis.

❍ **How is this treated?**

Topical anti-fungals alone are typically unsuccessful. Topical anti-fungal with nail plate removal or systemic antifungal are recommended.

❍ **What is the most common cause of paronychial infections?**

Chronic fungal infections.

❍ **What is the most common bacterial infection of the nail?**

S. aureus paronychium.

❍ **What is the treatment?**

Drain any abscesses by lifting the paronychium with or without partial nail plate removal followed by soapy water soaks 3 – 4 times a day.

Oncology

❍ **Name 3 common benign periungual tumors.**

Mucous cyst, glomus tumor, and pyogenic granuloma.

❍ **What is a mucous cyst?**

A dorsal ganglion of the DIP, they are usually associated with an osteophyte.

❍ **How does it present?**

Dorsal swelling of the DIP with or without longitudinal grooving of the nail plate.

○ **How are they treated?**

Excision of the ganglion and removal of the osteophyte.

○ **What is the key to the treatment of a mucous cyst?**

Removal of the osteophyte.

○ **How do glomus tumors present?**

These are 1-2mm in size and have a classic triad of tenderness, pain, and <u>cold sensitivity</u>.

○ **How can they be diagnosed?**

MRI.

○ **How are they treated?**

Resection with an approach that includes removal of the nail plate.

○ **What is a pyogenic granuloma?**

Exuberant mass of granulation tissue that forms after a relatively minor trauma.

○ **How are they treated?**

Complete excision through curettage or ablation with silver nitrate sticks. Incomplete excision will lead to recurrence.

○ **Differential diagnosis of a pigmented subungual lesion?**

Posttraumatic hemorrhage (most common), benign nevus, subungual melanoma.

○ **What is the differential diagnosis of pigment deposition within the nail plate?**

Melanonychia striate longitudinalis (benign lesions common in black patients), a benign subungual nevus, and a malignant melanoma.

○ **What is Hutchinson's sign?**

Broad pigmented streaks of variegated colour with cuticular pigmentation within the nail plate. It is associated with a subungual melanoma.

○ **How is a subungual hematoma differentiated from a subungual melanoma?**

Mark the nail plate and watch. If it is a hematoma it will migrate distally. Ultimately, a nail bed biopsy is recommended if even minor suspicion of melanoma exists.

References

Zook EG, Brown RE. The perionychium. In: Green DP, ed. *Green's Operative Hand Surgery.* Vol 2. 4th ed. New York: Churchill Livingstone; 1999:1353-1380.

Zook EG, Van Beek AL, Russell RC, Beatty ME. Anatomy and physiology of the perionychium: A review of the literature and anatomic study. *Journal of Hand Surgery.* 1980;5:528-536.

Baden HP. Regeneration of the nail. *Archives of Dermatology.* 1965;91:619-620.

Seaberg DC, Angelos WJ, Paris PM. Treatment of subungual hematomas with nail trephination: A prospective study. *American Journal of Emergency Medicine.* 1991;9:209-210.

Newmeyer WL, Kilgore ES. American Family Physician. *Common injuries of the fingernail and nail bed.* 1977;16:93-95.

Zook EG, Russell RC. Reconstruction of a functional and esthetic nail. *Hand Clinics.* 1990;6:59-68.

Schiller C. Nail replacement in fingertip injuries. *Plastic and Reconstructive Surgery.* 1957;19:521-530.

Kleinert HE, Kutz JE, Fishman JH, McGraw LH. Etiology and treatment of the so-called mucous cyst of the finger. *Journal of Bone and Joint Surgery.* 1972;54A:1455-1458.

Sorene ED, Goodwin DR, Wong CH, et al. Magnetic resonance imaging of a tiny glomus tumour of the fingertip: a case report

Quitkin HM, Rosenwasser MP, Strauch RJ. The efficacy of silver nitrate cauterization for pyogenic granuloma of the hand. *J Hand Surg [Am].* May 2003;28(3):435-438.

Fleegler E, Ziewonwicc RJ. Tumors of the perionychium. *Hand Clinics.* 1990;6:113-134.

Uncommon hand tumours. *Scand J Plast Reconstr Surg Hand Surg.* Dec, Jul 2001;35(4):429-431.

RHEUMATOID HAND

César J. Bravo, MD

○ **What are the three primary goals in treating the rheumatoid hand?**

PRC.
1. **P**ain relief
2. **R**estoration of function
3. **C**osmetic improvement of the hand.

○ **What are the three basic principles in rheumatoid hand surgery?**

1. Synovectomy/soft tissue reconstruction done early in disease.
2. Highly erosive disease (arthritis mutilans) treat early with fusion before bone loss.
3. Correction of deformity which causes loss of motion may severely compromise hand function.

○ **What surgical sequence should be followed in a rheumatoid patient?**

1. Lower extremity addressed first.
2. Proximal joints before distal joints (e.g., elbow before wrist, wrist before metacarpophalangeal joint (MPCJ) and proximal interphalangeal joint (PIPJ)).

○ **What is an essential part of the preoperative evaluation in a rheumatoid patient?**

Cervical spine evaluation. 25%-50% of patients can have atlantoaxial instability (plain cervical radiographs including flexion and extension views is standard).

○ **What is the pathogenesis in rheumatoid arthritis (RA) of the hand?**

Autoimmune disorder resulting in erosive synovitis of the hand and wrist secondary to injury to synovial microvascular endothelial cells triggering an inflammatory reaction causing influx of polymorphonuclear leukocytes (PMNs), monocytes, and macrophages.

○ **Inflammatory cells/mediators produced by macrophages, monocytes, PMNs stimulate which cell type in the rheumatoid hand?**

Osteoclast. These are responsible for subchondral osteopenia.

○ **What are the extra-articular manifestations seen in RA? Which one is most common?**

Vasculitis, pericarditis, pulmonary nodules, episcleritis, subcutaneous nodules.

○ **Which one is most common?**

Subcutaneous nodules (25% of patients with RA).

○ **Manifestation of accumulated inflammatory cells around capillaries of the synovium and tenosynovium is known as?**

Synovitis and tenosynovitis.

❍   **Is pattern of joint involvement in RA different from osteoarthritis (OA) of the hand?**

Yes. In RA metacarpophalangeal joint (MCPJ) and proximal interphalangeal joint (PIPJ) are commonly involved. In OA, distal interphalangeal joint (DIPJ) and basilar joint of thumb are involved.

❍   **What are Bouchard's nodes?**

Enlargement of PIPJ seen mainly in RA. Note: Heberden's nodes are seen in OA and refer to DIP enlargement.

❍   **What is the most frequently affected area about the wrist in RA patients?**

Distal radioulnar joint (DRUJ).

❍   **Decreased active digital flexion in a patient with RA is usually caused by what?**

Synovial nodules within flexor tendons. These nodules within retinacular system reduce active flexion of finger.

❍   **What is the natural course of rheumatoid disease with articular involvement at the metacarpophalangeal joint (MCPJ)?**

Progressive joint erosion and collapse with palmar displacement.

❍   **How is the wrist affected in patients with RA?**

Synovitis begins in ulnar aspect of the wrist with the DRUJ and radiocarpal joint first affected usually sparing the midcarpal joint. Erosive changes seen at the prestyloid recess of the ulnar styloid, sigmoid notch of radius, insertion of radioscapholunate ligament, and the scaphoid waist.

❍   **What is the natural course of wrist deformities with rheumatoid disease?**

Supination, palmar dislocation, radial deviation, and volar-ulnar dislocation of the carpus on the radius.

❍   **What are the treatment options available for the rheumatoid DRUJ/wrist?**

Treatment/Procedure	Benefit
Synovectomy of radiocarpal joint and DRUJ	Pain relief, done after 6 months of medical treatment and no radiographic changes
Partial arthrodesis (radiolunate and scaphoradiolunate fusions)	Prevent progression of collapse. Radiolunate preserves function in patients with ulno-carpal translocation.
Resection hemiarthroplasty of DRUJ	Preserve length of ulna and TFCC attachments. No DRUJ contact on pronation/supination---pain relief.
Darrach procedure (resection of distal ulna)	Easy. Can have radioulnar impingement/instability though.
Sauvé-Kapandji (fusion of DRUJ, osteotomy of ulna at radial metaphyseal flare)	Less cosmetic defect than Darrach. Can have radioulnar impingement. Good for younger patients.
Total wrist arthrodesis	90%-95% good to excellent results (fused in 10°-20° extension and neutral deviation)
Wrist arthroplasty	Motion preserving procedure (good bone stock, minimal deformity, intact extensors)

DRUJ, distal radioulnar joint; TFCC, triangular fibrocartilage complex

❍   **What is the total wrist arthroplasty experience in the USA?**

1967.   Swanson. Silicone hinge.
1972.   Meuli. Ball and trunnion.
1973.   Volz. Dorsopalmar tracking.
1977.   Figgie and Ranawat. Trispherical (hinge).
1982.   Beckenbaugh. Biaxial (ellipsoidal).
1990.   Mennon. Universal (anatomic).
2002.   Adams. Universal 2 (uncemented).

○   **What are current accepted indications for total wrist arthroplasty?**

1.   Painful pancarpal (diffuse) and advance arthritis.
2.   Progressive deformity with advanced arthritis.
3.   Patients who do not use walking aids with affected hand.
4.   Other joints of same extremity have significant limitations.
5.   Personal factors (low-demand activities that require wrist motion).
6.   Contralateral wrist fused.

○   **What are current accepted contraindications for total wrist arthroplasty?**

1.   Previous sepsis.
2.   Rupture and not fully reconstructible wrist extensors.
3.   Resorption of distal carpal row.
4.   Previous wrist arthrodesis (autofusion not a contraindication)
5.   Previously failed silicone implant if fragmented and silicone synovitis.
6.   Progressive deformity with advanced arthritis.

○   **In the rheumatoid hand, are women affected more than men?**

Yes. 2.5:1.

○   **What is a painless dorsal wrist mass distal to the extensor retinaculum typically in RA patients?**

Typical presentation of extensor tenosynovitis and a harbinger of extensor rupture. Tenosynovectomy indicated after 4-6 months of medical treatment to prevent rupture of extensor tendon.

○   **What is the differential diagnosis of a patient with a rheumatoid hand and with inability to extend his fingers?**

1.   Ulnar subluxation of the extensor tendon over MP joints second due to attritional lengthening of the radial sagittal band.
2.   Posterior interosseous nerve palsy (PIN) because of synovitis at the elbow.
3.   MP joint subluxation/dislocation.
4.   Extensor tendon attritional rupture.

○   **When should PIN palsy at the elbow be a prime consideration in RA patients?**

If they have inability to extend all 4 fingers and IP joint of thumb. Also, unable to deviate the wrist ulnarly secondary to extensor carpi ulnaris (ECU) paralysis.

○   **Does a patient with an extensor tendon rupture have the ability to maintain digit extended if passively placed in that position?**

No. They also lose the tenodesis effect of the hand (e.g., finger extension with wrist flexion and vice versa).

○   **In decreasing incidence which extensor tendons are affected by RA?**

•   Extensor digiti minimi (EDM)

- Extensor digitorum communis (EDC) small
- EDC ring
- EPL
- EDC middle

○ **What anatomical landmark contributes to extensor pollicis longus rupture in patients with RA?**

Lister's tubercle. Contributes to attritional rupture while acting as a bone pulley.

○ **What is Vaughn-Jackson syndrome?**

Ischemic rupture of ulnar extensor tendons secondary to prominent irregular ulnar head. Most common cause of tendon rupture in RA patients.

○ **What is Caput-Ulnae syndrome?**

Failure of the ulnar aspect of the wrist and DRUJ secondary to RA resulting in:
1.   Dorsal dislocation of distal ulna.
2.   Supination of carpus on the radius.
3.   Volar subluxation of ECU.

○ **What is the "piano key sign"? What does it signify?**

Elicited when the prominent ulnar head is volarly depressed and rebounds as pressure is released. DRUJ instability, seen in a third of patients with RA.

○ **What is the "scallop sign" in patients with rheumatoid arthritis?**

Erosion of the radial sigmoid notch with formation of a sclerotic border. It is an ominous sign of impending extensor tendon ruptures.

○ **When is extensor tendon surgery indicated in patients with RA?**

1.   Refractory to medical treatment.
2.   Dorsal dislocation of the ulnar head.
3.   A positive scallop sign.
4.   Recurrent dorsal tenosynovitis.

○ **Is surgery needed after an extensor tendon rupture in RA patients to prevent damage to intact tendons?**

Yes. Unchecked tenosynovitis damages outer surfaces of underlying tendons, leads to tendon adhesions and eventual attritional rupture. Surgery should include tenosynovectomy.

○ **What is a *pseudotendon* in patients with RA?**

A thin strand of opaque tissue situated between healthy appearing tendinous material proximally and distally.

○ **Attritional rupture of flexor pollicis longus (FPL) in known as?**

Mannerfeldt-Norman syndrome. Most common <u>flexor</u> tendon rupture in RA.

○ **Where is the most common location for rupture of FPL?**

Scaphoid. Secondary to a spur at the level of STT joint. (If spur not excised will lead to tendon ruptures of the FDP tendons in a radial to ulnar progression.)

○ **The most common location of flexor tenosynovitis?**

The palm. Seen as pain, triggering, and tendon rupture with passive finger flexion that is greater than active flexion.

○ **Should the A1 pulley be preserved in rheumatoid patients?**

Yes! Avoids increasing the lever arm of the tendon and thus potentiating flexion deformity at the MP joints.

○ **Triggering secondary to digital flexor tenosynovitis usually locks the digit in flexion. What is happening if it is instead locked in extension?**

The profundus tendon nodule distally at the A2 pulley is the cause of locking.

○ **What are the commonly used extensor tendon transfers used after rupture?**

Ruptured Tendon	Transfer Recommended
EPL	EIP to EPL or EPB to EPL at metacarpal level
EDM and EDC5, or EDM alone	EIP to EDC5 or EDM, side to side to EDC4
EDM, EDC5, EDC4	EDC4 side to side to EDC3,EIP to EDM or EDC5, tendon grafts
EDC5/EDM, EDC4, EDC3	FDS (long) to EDC4 and EDC5, EDC3 side to side to EDC2/EIP
EDC5/EDM,EDC4,EDC3,EDC2	FDS (long) to EDC2 and EDC3, FDS (ring) to EDC4 and EDC5

EPL, extensor pollicis longus; EDM, extensor digiti minimi; EDC, extensor digitorum communis; FDS, flexor digitorum superficialis.

○ **How is tension adjusted in extensor tendon reconstruction/transfer in patients with RA?**

Wrist in 40° extension the MCP joints are capable of 15° of flexion and wrist in full extension complete MCP flexion should be possible.

○ **What is associated with extension loss of all 4 fingers with absence of all digital extensor and proprius tendon function at surgery?**

Palmar dislocation of the carpus on the radius rather than extensor tenosynovitis.

○ **What is a contraindication in using the superficialis flexor tendon for extensor tendon transfer in RA?**

Presence of swan-neck deformity and significant flexor tenosynovitis.

○ **What is the recommended treatment for loss of wrist extensors in RA?**

Arthrodesis of the wrist.

○ **What is Clayton's procedure in the rheumatoid hand? Prevents what?**

Transfer of the ECRL to ECU. Redistributes wrist forces diminishing radial rotation and volar subluxation of carpus at the wrist.

○ **What are the eight steps leading to metacarpophalangeal joint (MPJ) ulnar drift?**

1. Synovitis leading to stretching of radial sagittal bands.
2. Extrinsic extensors subluxate into intermetacarpal sulcus, become ulnar deviators.
3. Lax MP collateral ligaments from joint synovitis allow ulnar deviation.
4. Synovitis causing further damage to cartilage and bone—destabilizes MPJ.

5. Ulnar intrinsics contract and become ulnar and volar deforming forces.
6. Radial deviation of wrist alters vector pull on the extrinsic extensors toward ulnar direction.
7. Flexor sheath synovitis distends retinaculum allowing the flexors to shift in an ulnar direction.
8. Resultant forces during pinch are in volar and ulnar direction

❍ **What is the Nalebuff classification of MPJ in a rheumatoid hand?**

Stage I: Only synovial proliferation.
Stage II: Recurrent synovitis without deformity.
Stage III: Moderate articular degeneration, ulnar and palmar drift of digits that is passively correctable.
Stage IV: Severe joint destruction with fixed deformities.

❍ **What is the treatment recommendation based on the Nalebuff classification of MPJ?**

Stage I: Medical management and splinting.
Stage II: Synovectomy (after 6 months of medical treatment).
Stage III: Synovectomy plus extensor tendon relocation, intrinsic releases, crossed intrinsic transfers, and radial collateral ligament imbrication.
Stage IV: Silicone spacer combined with relocation of extensors and radial collateral ligament imbrication.

Surgical intervention reserved for patients with pain and functional disability.

❍ **If you have MPJ disease and tendon rupture, which do you treat first?**

Metacarpophalangeal joint(MPJ). Multiple authors recommend treating both at same time.

❍ **What is the reported arc of motion usually achieved after silicone interposition arthroplasty for MPJ in patients with RA?**

40°-60°. Regression of digits ulnarly commonly seen, typically < 10°.

❍ **What is a swan-neck deformity? Causes?**

PIP hyperextension and DIP flexion with a DIP mallet caused by synovitis attenuating volar plate at the PIP, FDS rupture, intrinsic tightness from MPJ disease.

❍ **What is the recommended treatment and classification for rheumatoid swan-neck deformity?**

Classification based on severity of PIP deformity, stiffness, and arthritis:

Type	Description	Treatment
I	PIP flexible in all MCPJ positions	**Proximal** Fowler's tenotomy, flexor PIP tenodesis, SORL reconstruction
II	PIP joint flexion position dependent on MCPJ	Intrinsic release and/or realignment or arthroplasty MCPJ
III	PIP flexion limited in all MCPJ positions	Open capsular release, dorsal skin releases, closed manipulation with/without pinning, lateral band mobilization
IV	Radiographic joint destruction with minimal PIP joint motion	Arthrodesis and arthroplasty

PIP, proximal interphalangeal; SORL, spiral oblique retinacular ligament; MCPJ, metacarpophalangeal joint.

❍ **What is a boutonnière deformity? Causes?**

Hyperflexion of PIP joint and hyperextension DIP joint caused by synovitis leading to attenuated central slip, volar subluxation of lateral bands, tight transverse retinacular ligament, volar plate contracture.

❍   **What is the recommended treatment and classification for rheumatoid boutonnière deformity?**

Classification based on PIP motion and severity of arthritis:

Type	Description	Treatment
I	Mild loss of PIP active extension, full passive PIP extension	Synovectomy, inject PIP and splints, lateral band, or **distal** Fowler's tenotomy
II	Moderate loss of PIP extension, full passive PIP extension	Synovectomy, central slip reconstruction, lateral band reconstruction, or **distal** Fowler's tenotomy
III	PIP not passively correctable, no arthritic changes	PIP injection, serial extension casting, consider Type II treatment if motion restored
IV	Fixed PIP contracture, arthritic changes	Objective is to reduce PIP, PIP fusion or arthroplasty.

PIP, proximal interphalangeal

❍   **What is the most common rheumatoid thumb deformity?**

Boutonnière deformity (MP joint flexion and IP joint hyperextension).

❍   **What is the Nalebuff Classification of rheumatoid thumb?**

Type I: Boutonnière deformity.
Type II: Boutonnière deformity with CMC involvement.
Type III: Swan-neck deformity (stage 1-CMC synovitis, stage2- CMC joint synovitis, MP joint extension deformity
          correctable, stage 3-CMC joint destruction, MP joint extension deformity fixed).
Type IV: Gamekeeper's deformity.
Type V: Swan-neck deformity with MP joint and CMC unaffected.
Type VI: Arthritis mutilans.

❍   **What is the recommended treatment for the first four stages of the rheumatoid thumb?**

	Early Disease	*Moderate Disease*	*Advanced Disease*
Type I	MP synovectomy and EPL rerouting	MP fusion or arthroplasty	IP fusion and MP arthroplasty
Type II	MP synovectomy and EPL rerouting	MP joint fusion and CMC hemiarthroplasty	MP joint fusion and CMC hemiarthroplasty
Type III	CMC partial trapezial/metacarpal base resection CMC implant arthroplasty	MP fusion CMC partial trapezial/metacarpal base resection	MP fusion CMC partial trapezial/metacarpal base resection CMC implant arthroplasty Release 1st web space contracture
Type IV	MP synovectomy, UCL reconstruction	MP fusion	MP fusion Release 1st web space contracture

MP, metacarpophalangeal; EPL, extensor pollicis longus; CMC, carpometacarpal; UCL, ulnar collateral ligament

○   **What is the recommended treatment for the stages V and VI of the rheumatoid thumb?**

Stage V:
a. No articular degeneration of MPJ--- Volar capsulodesis.
Articular degeneration---MPJ fusion.
Stage VI: Fusion and soft tissue balancing when possible.

○   **What are the three major types of juvenile rheumatoid arthritis (JRA)?**

(Based on presentation at onset of diagnosis and during first 6 months of disease.)
1.   Systemic onset (25%).
2.   Polyarticular onset (30%).
3.   Pauciarticular onset (45%).

○   **Name five clinical differences found in JRA not found in the rheumatoid hand?**

1.   Ulnar deviation of wrist and metacarpals.
2.   Radial deviation of metacarpophalangeal joints.
3.   Abnormal ring and small fingers metacarpals secondary to long bone epiphyseal accelerated maturation.
4.   Shortened ulna.
5.   Narrow small tubular bones of the hand.

References

Freiberg RA, Weinstein A. The scallop sign and spontaneous rupture of finger extensor tendons in rheumatoid arthritics. Clin Orthop 1072;83:128-130.

Herren DB, Simmen BR. Limited and complete fusion of the rheumatoid wrist. JAmerican Society for Surg of the Hand 2002;2:21-32.

Lipsky PE. Rheumatoid arthritis. in: Braunwald E, Fauci AS, Kasper DL, Hauser SL, Longo DL, Jameson JL, eds. Harrison'sPrinciples of Internal Medicine. 15th ed. New York:McGraw-Hill, 2001: 1928-1937.

Nalebuff EA: Diagnosis, classification and management of rheumatoid thumb deformities. Bull Hosp Jt Dis 1968;29:119-137.

Nalebuff EA. Surgical treatment tendon ruptures in the rheumatoid hand. Surg Clin North Am 1969;49:811-822.

Millender LH, Nalebuff EA, Holdsworth DE. Posterior interosseous nerve syndrome secondary to rheumatoid synovitis. J Bone Joint Surg 1973;55A:753-757.

Millender LH, Nalebuff EA, Ream AR Jr, Gordon M. Dorsal tenosynovectomy and tendon transfer in the rheumatoid hand. J Bone Joint Surg 1974; 56a: 601-609.

Moore JR, Weiland AJ, Valdata L. Tendon ruptures in the rheumatoid hand: analysis of treatment and functional results in 60 patients. J Hand Surg 1987;12A:9-14.

Stuart PR, Berger RA, Linscheid RL, An K. The dorsopalmar stability of the distal radioulnar joint. J Hand Surg 2000; 25A:689-699.

Sauerbier M, Hahn ME, Fujita M, Neale PG, Berglund LJ, Berger RA. Analysis of dynamic distal radioulnar convergence after ulnar head resection and endoprosthesis implantation. J Hand Surg 2002;27A:425-434. 6A:601-609.

Richards RA, Wilson RL. Management of extensor tendons and the distal radioulnar joint in rheumatoid arthritis. J American Society for Surg of the Hand 2003; 3: 132-144.

Terrono AL. The rheumatoid thumb. J American Society for Surg of the Hand 2001;1:81-90.

Wadstein T. Spontaneous rupture of the long extensor tendon of the extensor pollicis longus. Transplantation of the extensor indicis proprius. Acta Orthop Scand 1946;16:194-202.

Wilson RL. Rheumatoid arthritis of the hand. Orthop Clin North Am 1986;17:313-342.

OBSTETRICAL BRACHIAL PLEXUS INJURIES

Reuben Bueno, MD

❍ **What is the cause of obstetrical brachial plexus palsy?**

Traction injury to the brachial plexus during the birth process

❍ **What is the estimated incidence of obstetrical brachial plexus palsy?**

0.5 to 2 per 1000 births

❍ **What is the rate of complete, spontaneous recovery?**

A wide range has been reported in the literature from 30% to 95%

❍ **What maternal factors may be associated with obstetrical brachial plexus palsy?**

- diabetes
- pre-eclampsia
- long duration of labor
- previous history of delivery problems with earlier pregnancies

❍ **What factors during birth may be associated with obstetrical brachial plexus palsy?**

- vertex or breech presentation
- shoulder dystocia
- difficult delivery with history of meconium or cord around the neck
- forceps or vacuum use during delivery

❍ **What child factors may be associated with obstetrical brachial plexus palsy?**

- large baby for gestational age
- history of humerus fracture or clavicle fracture during birth

❍ **What are the signs of Horner's syndrome?**

- ptosis
- miosis
- anhidrosis
- enophthalmos

❍ **What is the significance of Horner's syndrome in a patient being evaluated for brachial plexus injury?**

The presence of Horner's syndrome suggests disruption of sympathetic fibers proximal to where the pre-ganglionic fibers arise from T1

❍ **Describe the typical posture of Erb palsy.**

The features of upper plexus palsy ("waiter's tip" position) involving C5, C6 , $\pm$ C7 are:
- shoulder adduction and internal rotation
- elbow extension
- forearm pronation
- wrist flexion
- finger flexion

○   **What is the most widely accepted criterion for surgery in obstetrical brachial plexus palsy patients?**

Absence of elbow flexion by 3 months of age

○   **How is the neuroma lesion managed?**

Neuroma resection and grafting has provided better results than neurolysis alone

○   **What are sources for nerve grafting in brachial plexus reconstruction?**

Sural nerve and cervical plexus

○   **If the source root has been avulsed and anatomic grafting cannot be done, innervation must be provided by alternate sources. This can be accomplished from remaining roots (intra-plexal neurotization) or donor nerves outside the plexus (extra-plexal neurotization). What are the options in extra-plexal neurotization?**

Spinal accessory nerve, intercostal nerves, contralateral C7 root

○   **What secondary surgical procedure is used to improve wrist extension after brachial plexus reconstruction?**

Pronator teres to extensor carpi radialis brevis tendon transfer

○   **What secondary surgical procedure is used to improve shoulder external rotation after brachial plexus reconstruction?**

L'Episcopo latissimus dorsi muscle transfer

References

Capek L, Clarke HM, Curtis CG. Neuroma-in-continuity resection: Early outcome in obstetrical brachial plexus palsy. *Plast Reconstr Surg*. 102:1555-62, 1998.

Gilbert A. Long-term evaluation of brachial plexus surgery in obstetrical palsy. *Hand Clin*. 11:583-94, 1995.

La Scala GC, Rice SB, Clarke HM. Complications of microsurgical reconstruction of obstetrical brachial plexus palsy. *Plast Reconstr Surg*. 111:1383-88, 2003.

Marcus JR, Clarke HM. Management of obstetrical brachial plexus palsy: Evaluation, prognosis, and primary surgical treatment. *Clin Plastic Surg*. 30:289-306, 2003.

Michelow BJ, Clarke HM, Curtis CG, et al. The natural history of obstetrical brachial plexus palsy. *Plast Reconstr Surg*. 93:675-80, 1994.

BRACHIAL PLEXUS

Cay M. Mierisch, MD

Demographics

O **What is the most common mechanism for brachial plexus injuries?**

Closed injury (traction, compression or combination of the two)

O **What is the most common location of brachial plexus injuries?**

Supraclavicular, root and trunks

O **What is the typical mechanism of a C8-T1/lower trunk traction injury?**

Forceful abduction of the arm overhead

O **What brachial plexus injury is typically produced by violent lateral bending of the head and neck?**

Traction injury of C5, C6 / upper trunk

O **What is a common site for brachial plexus compression injuries?**

Between clavicle and first rib, near coracoid process

O **What are the demographics of the majority of patients with brachial plexus injuries?**

Male, age 15-25

O **What proportion of brachial plexus injuries occur in motor vehicle accidents?**

70%

O **What type of vehicle is most commonly implicated in brachial plexus injuries?**

The motorcycle (70% of MVA)
Snow mobiles in colder climates

O **At what level do most root avulsions occur?**

Lower roots (C7, C8, T1)

Anatomy

O **How many nerve roots form the brachial plexus?**

Five (C5-8, T1)

O **What term describes a contribution of the C4 nerve root to the brachial plexus?**

Prefixed plexus

O   **What phenomenon is described by the term "post-fixed" brachial plexus?**

T2 contribution to the plexus

O   **What are the five separate sections of the brachial plexus?**

Roots, trunks, divisions, cords, terminal branches
(Robert Taylor Drinks Coffee Black)

O   **What structure is formed by coalescence of the ventral and dorsal rootlets?**

The nerve root

O   **What vascular structure is associated with the C7 root in the exposure of the cervical region of the brachial plexus?**

Transverse cervical artery

O   **The medial cord of the brachial plexus receives contributions from which nerve roots?**

C8 and T1

O   **Where does the nerve root leave the spinal canal?**

Through the neuroforamen

O   **What is contained in the dorsal root ganglion?**

The cell bodies of the sensory nerves

O   **Where do the motor nerves travel?**

In the volar root ganglion. (V-volar, Vroom!!)

O   **What is described by the term pre-ganglionic brachial plexus lesion?**

Lesion proximal to the dorsal root ganglion
Intradural rupture of the rootlets
avulsion from spinal cord

O   **How are the upper, middle and lower trunk typically formed?**

Upper trunk by C5 and C6
Middle trunk by C7
Lower trunk by C8 and T1

O   **What is Erb's point?**

Point where C5 and C6 merge to form upper trunk

O   **What structures join to become the posterior cord?**

All 3 posterior divisions

○ **What is formed by the anterior divisions of the upper and middle trunk?**

The lateral cord
-Imagine a football announcer-"Number 34 runs <u>up</u> (<u>upper</u> trunk) the <u>middle</u> (<u>middle</u> trunk) and throws a <u>lateral</u> (<u>lateral</u> cord)!"

○ **What continues as the medial cord?**

The anterior division of the lower trunk

○ **The cords are named after their location in relation to which structure?**

The axillary artery

○ **What part of the brachial plexus crosses underneath the clavicle?**

The divisions

○ **What muscles are innervated by the dorsal scapular nerve?**

Rhomboid major/minor and levator scapulae

○ **What are the terminal branches of the posterior cord?**

Proximal to distal:
upper subscapular n.
thoracodorsal n.
lower subscapular n.
axillary n.
radial n.

○ **What branches originate at the C5 root level?**

phrenic n. contribution
long thoracic n. contribution
dorsal scapular n. (levator scapulae, rhomboids)

○ **What are the terminal branches of the medial cord?**

4 "medial (or median) structures and the ulnar nerve.
<u>Medial</u> pectoral n.
<u>medial</u> brachial cutaneous n.
<u>medial</u> antebrachial cutaneous n.
contribution to the <u>median</u> n.
ulnar n.

○ **What are the branches of the lateral cord?**

Lateral pectoral n.
contribution to the median n.
musculocutaneous n.

○ **What branches originate from the upper trunk?**

Suprascapular n.
nerve to the subclavius

❍   **Where is the inferior cervical sympathetic ganglion located?**

In proximity of the T1 nerve root

Physical Exam

❍   **What is Horner's syndrome?**

Ptosis
Miosis
Anhydrosis
Enophthalmos

This constellation indicates a lesion of the cervicothoracic sympathetic ganglion (adjacent to C8, T1) disrupting the oculosympathetic pathway.

❍   **How is muscle strength graded?**

By the British Medical Research Council (MRC) Grading System.
M0-No evidence of contractility
M1-Evidence of contractility but no motion
M2-Complete range of motion with gravity eliminated
M3-Complete range of motion against gravity
M4-Complete range of motion against some resistance
M5-Normal power

❍   **Examination of which upper extremity functions will test for the condition of the posterior cord?**

Wrist extension (radial n.)
Elbow extension (radial n.)
Shoulder abduction (axillary n. via deltoid)

❍   **How can the condition of the suprascapular n. be tested?**

Shoulder elevation (supraspinatus)
external rotation (infraspinatus)

❍   **What is a strong indicator for a preganglionic lesion at the C8 and T1 nerve roots?**

Presence of a Horner's syndrome (indicating a lesion of the cervicothoracic sympathetic ganglion (adjacent to C8, T1).

❍   **Dysfunction of which nerve will result in scapular winging with forward elevation of the shoulder?**

Long thoracic nerve via serratus anterior (SALT-serratus anterior long thoracic)

Radiology

❍   **What is the significance of transverse process fractures on the cervical spine x-rays in brachial plexus patients?**

May indicate root avulsion

○ **What findings on a chest x-ray may point towards a brachial plexus lesion?**

Fractures of the first and second rib

○ **What is the significance of pseudomeningoceles on a cervical CT myelogram?**

Indicates root level injury

○ **What finding would be expected on the chest x-rays of patients with phrenic nerve injury?**

Elevation of ipsilateral hemi-diaphragm

Electrical Studies

○ **What do fibrillation potentials in the EMG indicate?**

Denervation of the tested muscles (just like the heart fibrillates when it is dieing).

○ **After acute brachial plexus injury, how soon would muscles exhibit fibrillations in the EMG?**

10-14 days for proximal muscles and 3-4 months for distal muscles

○ **What evidence can be found in electrodiagnostic studies of preganglionic lesions?**

Preservation of sensory nerve action potentials (SNAPs)

○ **What is the significance of the appearance of nascent potentials in follow-up EMGs?**

Early sign of reinnervation

○ **What does the presence of intra-operative nerve action potentials (NAPs) across a lesion indicate?**

Intact axons

○ **How many patients with detectable NAPs across a lesion will make a clinically useful recovery?**

90%

○ **What pattern of NAPs would be expected in a preganglionic plexus lesion?**

Accelerated conduction velocity with increased amplitude

○ **What do motor evoked potentials (MEP) assess?**

Integrity of motor pathway via the ventral root (remember Vroom)

○ **How can the integrity of the sensory pathway via the dorsal roots be tested?**

Somatosensory evoked potentials (SSEP)

Treatment Principles

○ **When is immediate exploration and primary repair of brachial plexus injuries indicated?**

Sharp, open injuries

○   **What is the preferred treatment for low velocity gun shot wounds of the brachial plexus?**

Observation, local would management

○   **What type of nerve injury is typically associated with low velocity gun shot wounds?**

Neuropraxia

○   **What is the recommended time frame for brachial plexus exploration in stretch injuries that fail to recover?**

3-6 months

○   **What is the order of priority for restoration of function to the flail extremity?**

Elbow flexion
shoulder abduction/stability
hand sensibility
wrist extension/finger flexion
wrist flexion and finger extension

○   **What type of injury is preferably addressed with primary nerve repair?**

Sharp laceration, not possible in stretch injuries

○   **What procedure needs to be performed to facilitate intraoperative nerve conduction studies?**

External neurolysis

○   **What is the treatment for electrically silent ruptures or neuromas of the brachial plexus that are electrically silent?**

Interpositional nerve grafting (e.g. sural cable graft)

○   **What upper extremity function should be targeted if interpositional nerve grafting from a functioning C5 nerve root is performed?**

Shoulder abduction (suprascapular, axillary nerves)

○   **What nerve root (when available) should be used to restore elbow flexion by interpositional sural nerve grafting?**

C6 (musculocutaneous n.)

○   **How can triceps function be restored in a patient with a brachial plexus injury at the trunk level?**

By interpositional grafting from C7 across the zone of injury

Nerve Transfer

○   **What type of brachial plexus injuries requires the use of nerve transfer (neurotization) to restore function?**

Preganglionic injuries

○ **How can a nerve transfer accelerate recovery of function?**

By decreasing the distance between the nerve repair site and the end organ (muscle)

○ **What is the Oberlin transfer?**

Transfer of select ulnar nerve fascicles in the upper arm to motor branches of the musculocutaneous nerve to the biceps to restore elbow flexion

○ **What function can be restored by neurotizing the suprascapular nerve with spinal accessory or phrenic nerve?**

Shoulder abduction/external rotation

○ **What nerve can be targeted in addition to suprascapular nerve to further improve shoulder abduction?**

Axillary nerve

○ **What donor nerves are available for neurotization to restore elbow flexion in a "panbrachial" plexopathy without signs of recovery?**

Intercostal nerves,
Spinal accessory via nerve grafts
Phrenic nerve with interpositional grafts

○ **What nerve transfers are commonly used for restoration of biceps function after upper trunk disruption?**

Medial pectoral nerve to musculocutaneous nerve or the biceps motor branch
Oberlin transfer

○ **What is the advantage of the Oberlin transfer over interpositional nerve grafts from C6 to regain biceps function?**

Faster recovery of function

○ **In the Oberlin transfer fascicles of the ulnar nerve transmitting which function should preferably be used?**

Fascicles that stimulate wrist flexion (FCU)

○ **What is the advantage of a vascularized nerve graft?**

Reinnervation at a faster rate (theoretically)

○ **What <u>contralateral</u> nerve root can be used as a donor of large amounts of motor axons?**

C7-usually half of it

○ **What function is addressed by contralateral C7 transfer via vascularized ulnar nerve to the median nerve?**

Finger flexion

○ **What overall success rate can be expected with nerve transfers to the musculocutaneous nerve?**

71% flexion strength > M3, 37% > M4

○ **What is the success rate of the Oberlin transfer?**

97% for >M3, 94%>M4

○ **How much shoulder abduction can be expected in a good result after nerve transfer?**

45 degrees

○ **What options are available for restoration of elbow flexion in patients that present late (>12 months after injury)?**

Free functioning muscle transfer
Tendon transfer of available, expendable muscles
Steindler flexorplasty (transposition of flexor-pronator origin to anterior humerus
Pectoralis major transfer
Latissimus dorsi transfer
Triceps transfer

Obstetrical Brachial Plexus Injury

○ **What are the risk factors for obstetrical brachial plexus palsy?**

increased birth weight
vertex presentation
births that require instrumentation for delivery
shoulder dystocia

○ **What are causes for obstetric brachial plexus injury (Birth palsy)?**

Traction injury secondary to
Fetal malposition
Cephalo-pelvic disproportion
Forceps use

○ **What are the three distributions observed in obstetric brachial plexus palsy?**

Erb's palsy
Panplexus palsy
Klumpke's palsy

○ **What nerve roots are involved in <u>Erb's palsy</u>?**

C5-6-upper roots

○ **What nerve roots are involved in <u>Klumpke's</u> palsy?**

C5-T1-lower roots

○ **What is considered an indication for surgery in obstetric brachial plexus injuries?**

Absent biceps recovery at age three months

○ **What does the Mallet classification assess?**

Upper extremity function

○ **Which root levels are more likely to be affected by root avulsions?**

Lower levels C8, T1

○ **What is the mainstay for treatment of children with partial lesions?**

Conservative treatment
ROM exercises
Prevent contractures

○ **What is the typical pattern of contracture of the shoulder in children with brachial plexus birth palsy?**

Internal rotation
Adduction

○ **What tendon transfer can be used to improve external rotation of the shoulder and prevent the development of internal rotation contracture?**

Transfer of latissimus dorsi and teres major to the humeral greater tuberosity

○ **What deformity of the elbow will frequently develop in children with obstetric brachial plexus palsy?**

Posterior radial head dislocation
Typically by age 5 to 8

○ **What is a typical finding at the forearm in children with obstetric palsy?**

Supination contracture

References

Brandt KE and Mackinnon SE: A technique for maximizing biceps recovery in brachial plexus reconstruction. J Hand Surg 1993;18A:726-733.

Brunelli G and Monini L: Direct muscular neurotization. J Hand Surg 1985;10A:993-997.

Doi K, Muramatsu K, Hattori Y, Otsuka K, Tan SH, Nanda V and Watanabe M: Restoration of prehension with the double free muscle technique following complete avulsion of the brachial plexus. Indications and long-term results. J Bone Joint Surg 2000;82A:652-666

Narakas A: The treatment of brachial plexus injuries. Int Orthop 1985;9:29-

Carvalho GA, Nikkhah G, Matthies C, Penkert G and Samii M: Diagnosis of root avulsions in traumatic brachial plexus injuries: value of computerized tomography myelography and magnetic resonance imaging. J Neurosurg 1997;86:69-76.

Ruch DS, Friedman AH and Nunley JA: The restoration of elbow flexion with intercostal nerve transfers. Clin Orthop 1995;314:95-103.

Oberlin C, Beal D, Leechavengvongs S, Salon A, Dauge MC and Sarcy JJ: Nerve transfer to biceps muscle using a part of ulnar nerve for C5-C6 avulsion of the brachial plexus: anatomical study and report of four cases. J Hand Surg 1994;19A:232-237.

Bertelli JA and Ghizoni MF: Brachial plexus avulsion injury repairs with nerve transfers and nerve grafts directly implanted into the spinal cord yield partial recovery of shoulder and elbow movements. Neurosurgery 2003;52:1385-1390.

TENDON TRANSFERS

Cay M. Mierisch, MD

Principles

○ **What should the patient's joints be assessed for prior to considering a tendon transfer?**

1. Mobility
2. Contracture

○ **What is a prerequisite for successful outcome of tendon transfers?**

Flexibility of the joint to be moved by transferred tendons

○ **So what are the goals of preoperative therapy?**

Maintain passive mobility
Prevent joint contractures

○ **What factors need to be considered when selecting a donor muscle for tendon transfer**

1. Adequate strength
2. Tendon excursion
3. Straight line of pull
4. Synergism of action between the donor and recipient muscles
5. Expendable donor
6. Tissue equilibrium

○ **What geometric feature correlates with the strength of a muscle?**

Cross-sectional area of the muscle

○ **What does the work capacity of a muscle correlate with?**

Muscle volume

○ **What does muscle excursion correlate with?**

Muscle fiber length

○ **How much tendon excursion can be found in wrist flexors and extensors?**

30 mm

○ **What is the amplitude of tendon excursion for finger extensors and flexors respectively?**

1. 50 mm
2. 70 mm
Thus, when wrist tendons are used to restore finger function, there is usually incomplete correction.

○ **How can the effective amplitude of tendon excursion be increased?**

1. Increasing the number of joints the muscle tendon unit crosses
2. Dissection of the muscle from its surrounding fascial attachments

RADIAL NERVE

○   **What is the most significant limb dysfunction after radial nerve palsy?**

Inability to extend the wrist and stabilize for all other hand activities.

○   **What is the effect of restoring active wrist extension on grip strength?**

Grip strength will increase 3-5 fold.

○   **What is the advantage of maintaining active wrist motion?**

Tenodesis effect.

○   **What is the tenodesis effect?**

Finger extension with wrist flexion. Try this on yourself.

○   **What are the indications for tendon transfer?**

Insufficient recovery of function after nerve injury that has been observed for an appropriate length of time.

○   **In general what are the available donor muscles for tendon transfers in radial nerve palsy?**

All extrinsic median and ulnar nerve innervated muscles.

○   **What muscle tendon transfers are included in the Brand Transfer for radial nerve palsy?**

1. PT to ECRB
2. FCR to EDC
3. PL to EPL
Thus, wrist, finger and thumb extension, the critical deficits in radial nerve palsy, are restored.

○   **What is the Boyes tendon transfer?**

A tendon transfer for radial nerve palsy including:
1. PT to ECRB
2. FDS III to EDC
3. FDS IV to EIP and EPL
4. FCR to APL and EPB

○   **What is the advantage of the Boyes Transfer?**

It can be used in patients who do not have a palmaris longus.

○   **What tendon transfers are included in the FCU transfer for radial nerve palsy?**

1. PT to ECRB
2. FCU to EDC
3. PL to EPL

○   **What is the preferred tendon transfer to restore active wrist extension in a radial nerve palsy?**

PT to ECRB

○ **What muscle tendon transfers can be used for restoration of MPJ extension?**

1. FCR to EDC
2. FCU to EDC
3. FDS III to EDC

○ **What is the theoretical advantage of the FDS III to EDC transfer in restoration for MPJ extension?**

1. Straight line of pull
2. Expendable donor
3. Sufficient strength
4. Sufficient excursion
5. Synergism

○ **What are potential disadvantages of the FCU to ECRB transfer?**

Weakness of wrist flexion with wrist radial deviation deformity and unnecessary strength of wrist extension

○ **What is the primary choice for restoration of finger extension?**

FCR to EDC transfer

○ **Why does the FDS III transfer not interfere with the flexor power of the other three FDS muscles?**

Because the FDS III has a separate muscle belly

○ **What are the two functions of the functioning EPL?**

1. Thumb IP extension
2. Thumb adduction

○ **How can the PL to EPL transfer restore thumb abduction in addition to thumb extension?**

Rerouting the EPL from the 3rd dorsal compartment and allowing it to lie along the 1st dorsal compartment will convert it's adduction moment into an abduction moment

○ **Which anatomic route is used for the FDS III to EDC tendon transfer?**

FDS III tendon is rerouted through a large window in the interosseous membrane of the forearm

○ **What is the position of immobilization after tendon transfers for wrist extension, finger extension, and thumb extension?**

1. 90° elbow flexion
2. Neutral forearm rotation
3. 45° wrist extension
4. Full extension of MPJ
5. Thumb abduction and full extension of IP and MPJ

○ **When should dynamic splinting be initiated?**

After 3 weeks of initial immobilization

○ **What does the dynamic splint after tendon transfer for radial nerve palsy entail?**

1. Dynamic extension outrigger
2. 30° wrist extension
3. MP flexion block at 30° increased at weekly intervals
4. Active ROM initiated at 5 weeks post op

○ **How is extensor lag at the MPJ postoperatively addressed?**

1. Delay of passive ROM and dynamic splinting
2. Extension splinting

MEDIAN NERVE

○ **What is the major deficit associated with low median nerve palsy?**

Loss of thumb opposition

○ **What muscles facilitate thumb opposition?**

1. Abductor pollicis brevis
2. Opponens pollicis
3. Superficial head of flexor pollicis brevis

○ **What are conditions leading to loss of thumb opposition?**

1. Median nerve laceration
2. Chronic carpal tunnel syndrome
3. Congenital deficiency of thenar musculature (thumb hypoplasia)
4. Polyneuropathy
5. Thenar trauma

○ **What trapezio-metacarpal joint motions constitute thumb opposition?**

1. Abduction
2. Flexion
3. Pronation-opposes the volar surfaces of the thumb and fingers

○ **What explains maintained ability of thumb opposition after complete median nerve laceration at the wrist?**

Variable ulnar nerve innervation of the superficial head of the flexor pollicis brevis

○ **What are four reliable options for opponensplasty?**

1. EIP
2. ADM (Huber)
3. Palmaris longus (Camitz)
4. FDS of the ring finger

○ **What are the landmarks of the vector line of pull for the most common tendon transfers to restore thumb opposition?**

1. Os pisiform
2. APB insertion

○ **What is the most common tendon transfer used for low median nerve palsy?**

EIP to APB transfer

○ **Where can the EIP tendon be located at the dorsum of the 2nd MPJ?**

Ulnar to the EDC tendon to the index

○ **How is proper tensioning of the opponensplasty assessed?**

1. Full thumb adduction with passive wrist flexion
2. Appropriate thumb opposition with passive wrist extension

○ **What is the Huber transfer?**

Abductor digiti minimi transfer for thumb opposition

○ **What is the classic indication for the Huber transfer?**

Congenital hypoplastic thumb

○ **What is the advantage of the Huber transfer?**

Cosmesis – the muscle bulk restores the hypoplastic thenar eminence

○ **What is the disadvantage of the Huber transfer in thumb hypoplasia?**

Insufficient tendon for thumb MCP reconstruction. The long or ring finger FDS transfer does not have this limitation although it lacks bulk.

○ **What is the position of immobilization after opponensplasty?**

1. Thumb spica with opposition of thumb
2. Slight wrist extension for EIP and ADM transfers
3. Slight wrist flexion for FDS and PL transfers

○ **What additional deficits distinguish the high from the low median nerve palsy?**

1. Inability to bend the thumb IP joint (FPL)
2. Inability to bend the index and long finger (FDS, FDP)

○ **How is the variability in loss of finger flexion particularly of the long finger explained?**

Variable innervation of the FDP of the long finger by the ulnar nerve

○ **What is the preferred procedure to restore a normal finger flexion cascade in high median nerve palsy?**

Side to side tenodesis of long and index finger FDP to the ring and small finger FDP

○ **What donor muscle is most commonly used for restoration of FPL function?**

Brachioradialis

○ **How can the available excursion of the brachioradialis muscle be maximized?**

1. Mobilization of the muscle
2. Freeing it from its fascial envelope up to the proximal forearm
3. Excursion up to 5 cm can be accomplished

❍ **What is the appropriate tension of the BR to FPL transfer?**

1. Full IP extension with 20 of wrist flexion
2. Adequate IP flexion with wrist extension

❍ **How can lack of active forearm rotation be addressed?**

Rerouting of the biceps tendon insertion to the lateral aspect of the proximal radius

❍ **What is the significance of sensory deficits?**

1. Limit the usefulness of tendon transfers
2. Every effort to restore sensation should be made prior to tendon transfer via…
        i. Nerve repair/grafting
        ii. Nerve decompression
        iii. Nerve transfers
        iv. Neurovascular island flaps

ULNAR NERVE

❍ **What is low ulnar nerve palsy as opposed to high ulnar nerve palsy?**

Lesion of ulnar nerve distal to innervation of FDP

❍ **Which fingers will typically be clawing in low ulnar nerve palsy?**

Small and ring finger

❍ **What is the reason for the claw deformity?**

Absent intrinsic muscle function (remember the ulnar innervated lumbricals extend the ring and small finger PIP joints)

❍ **Why do index and long finger typically not develop clawing in isolated ulnar nerve palsy?**

Persistent function of the radial two lumbrical muscles which are median innervated

❍ **What does the claw deformity involve?**

1. Hyperextension of the MPJ
2. Inability to fully extend the PIP and DIP

❍ **Which type of ulnar nerve palsy will demonstrate more significant clawing?**

1. Low ulnar nerve palsy
2. Persistent function of ulnar two FDP in low ulnar nerve palsy will produce deforming force on the PIP joints. These FDPs are not functional in high ulnar nerve palsy.

❍ **What eponym describes the clawing of ring and small finger?**

Duchenne's sign

❍ **What is the Bouvier maneuver?**

Blocking of MP hyperextension which will allow the EDC to fully extend the PIP and DIP

○ **What is the Wartenberg sign?**

Inability to adduct the extended small finger

○ **What is the deforming force for the Wartenberg sign?**

Unopposed pull of the radially innervated EDQ (absent 4th dorsal IO muscle)

○ **What is the Froment's sign?**

Hyperflexion of the thumb IP joint with key pinch to compensate for the deficient thumb adductor

○ **What is the Jeanne's sign?**

Hyperextension of the MPJ of the thumb with attempted key pinch

○ **What tendon transfers are available to restore thumb adduction?**

1. ECRB to thumb adductor via intercalated tendon graft
2. FDS of long or ring to thumb adductor insertion

○ **Which route is used for the ECRB transfer for thumb adduction?**

1. Subcutaneously extracompartmental
2. around the 2nd or 3rd metacarpal neck
3. volar to adductor pollicis
4. deep to flexor tendon and neurovascular structures

○ **What are the general two types of tendon transfers that are performed for correction of claw deformity?**

1. Static transfer
2. Dynamic transfer

○ **What is involved in a static anti-claw transfer?**

Tenodesis of the lateral bands with a tendon graft around the deep transverse metacarpal ligaments providing an internal splint that prevents hyperextension of the MPJ

○ **What does the Zancolli lasso procedure effectively treat?**

Claw deformity

○ **What does the Zancolli Lasso procedure consist of?**

1. FDS is looped back to itself around the A1 pulley
2. Providing a dynamic flexion moment at the MPJ

○ **What tendon transfer to correct claw deformity originates from the dorsal side of the wrist?**

The Bunnell-Stiles tendon transfer

○ **What are the steps of the Bunnell-Stiles tendon transfer?**

1. ECRL transected distally and rerouted dorsally
2. 2 slips of palmaris longus or plantaris graft extension sewn into the ECRL
3. Tendons rerouted through the lumbrical canal (volar to the deep transverse metacarpal ligament)

4. Graft tails attached to radial lateral bands of the ring and small fingers or alternatively to radial side of proximal phalanx (see next question)

○   **What deformity can occur after the Bunnell-Stiles transfer to the radial lateral bands?**

Swan neck deformity

○   **How can the development of swan neck deformity after the Bunnell-Stiles tendon transfer prevented?**

Transfer of the tendon to the proximal phalanx rather than the lateral band

○   **What patient factors lead to a higher likelihood of swan neck deformity after the Bunnell-Stiles transfer into the lateral bands?**

PIP joint hyperextensibility

○   **What additional function is lost in a high ulnar nerve palsy?**

Absent small and ring finger FDP

COMBINED PALSIES

○   **What is the most common mechanism for combined nerve palsies?**

Lacerations - particularly at the wrist

○   **What is the most common combined nerve palsy?**

Low median-ulnar nerve palsy

○   **What are the requirements for restoration of wrist and hand function in low median and ulnar nerve palsy?**

1. Improve key pinch
2. Thumb abduction (to improve opposition)
3. Tip pinch (increase index strength in pinch which has been compromised by 1st dorsal interosseous palsy)
4. Power finger flexion with coordinated MP and PIP motion
5. Sensibility in the distribution involved in key pinch

○   **What is the preferred thumb opposition transfer in combined median-ulnar nerve palsy?**

1. EIP transfer
2. Second choice: PL, FDS

○   **What muscles are preferred for restoration of thumb adduction?**

1. ECRB
2. Long finger FDS

○   **How can the last two transfers use the FDS if these are for combined ulnar-median nerve palsies?**

Because they are for low (wrist level) combined palsies.

○   **What procedures can help to improve thumb-index tip pinch?**

1. Thumb IP fusion
2. Transfer of APL with graft extension to first dorsal interosseous

○ **What type of procedure will help with integration of MP and IP joint motion?**

Intrinsic transfers (e.g. Bunnell-Stiles)

References

Friden J., Lieber RL: Tendon Transfer Surgery: Clinical Implications of experimental studies. Clin. Orthop 2002; 403S: 163-170.

Mc Carroll Hr: Tendon Transfers. In Light TR, ed. Hand Surgery Update 2nd ed. Rosemont, IL American Academy of Orthopaedic Surgeons,1999 161-169.

Green DP: Radial nerve palsy. In Green DP, Hotchkiss RN, Pederson WC, ed. Green's Operative Hand Surgery 4th ed Vol II New York Churchill Livingstone 1999: 1481-1496.

Anderson GA, Lee V, Sundararaj GD: Opponensplasty by Extensor indicis and Flexor digitorum superficialis tendon transfer. J Hand Surg 1992; 17B:611-614.

Goldfarb CA, Stern PJ: Low ulnar nerve palsy JASSH 2003;3:14-26.

Omer, G.: Combined nerve palsies. In: Green DP, Hotchkiss RN, Pederson WC, ed. Green's Operative Hand Surgery 4th ed Vol II New York Churchill Livingstone 1999: 1542-1555.

SLAC WRIST/WRIST KINEMATICS

Thomas Wiedrich, MD

○ **What is the blood supply to the proximal pole of the scaphoid?**

The main blood supply is from the radial artery and enters through small foramina in the dorsal ridge. Fractures proximal to this area may result in avascular necrosis of the proximal pole.

○ **Which extrinsic wrist ligament is felt to be the strongest support in the wrist?**

The radio-scaphocapitate ligament is felt to be the most important ligament for wrist support.

○ **As the wrist moves from ulnar deviation to radial deviation, what happens to the scaphoid?**

The scaphoid moves from an extended position into a palmar flexed position.

○ **What are the major extrinsic ligaments of the dorsal wrist?**

The dorsal radiocarpal ligament and the dorsal intercarpal ligament are the major dorsal extrinsic wrist ligaments.

○ **What does DISI stand for?**

DISI stands for dorsal intercalary segment instability and is related to tears of the scapho-lunate ligament.

○ **What is the Terry Thomas sign?**

The Terry Thomas sign is an abnormal gap between the scaphoid and lunate that occurs in scapho-lunate ligament tears. It is named after the gap-toothed British comedian.

○ **The spilled tea-cup sign is seen in which carpal instability pattern?**

The spilled tea-cup sign is seen in Volar Intercalary Segment Instability (VISI).

○ **What is meant by "progressive perilunar instability"?**

Progressive perilunar instability is a progression of injury, beginning at the scapholunate joint and progressing in severity to total perilunar injury.

○ **What is Stage I perilunar instability?**

Stage I perilunar instability is scaphoid dislocation or a scapholunate interosseous ligament tear.

○ **What is Stage II perilunar instability?**

Stage II perilunar instability is a scapholunate ligament injury with capitate dislocation and a tear through the Space of Poirier.

○ **What is Stage III perilunar instability?**

Stage III perilunar instability is a perilunate dislocation.

○ **What is Stage IV perilunate instability?**

Stage IV perilunate instability is a lunate dislocation.

○   **How does one differentiate a perilunate dislocation from a lunate dislocation?**

In a perilunate dislocation, the lunate remains seated in the lunate fossa of the radius and all other carpal bones are sitting dorsal to their typical position. In a lunate dislocation the lunate is dislocated palmarly into the carpal tunnel and the other carpal bones are in their typical location.

○   **What is the most common fracture in carpal bones?**

The scaphoid is the most commonly fractured carpal bone?

○   **What differentiates a perilunate dislocation and a trans-scaphoid perilunate dislocation?**

In a trans-scaphoid perilunate dislocation, the scaphoid bone is fractured and the scapho-lunate interosseous ligament remains intact.

○   **What radiographic lines in the wrist are used to help determine normal anatomy from certain pathologic states including lunate and perilunate dislocations?**

Gilula's lines show continuity of the radiocarpal and midcarpal joints.

○   **What is the scaphoid shift test?**

The scaphoid shift test is a test looking for scapholunate ligament injury. With the wrist held in ulnar deviation, and the examiner's thumb holding pressure on the scaphoid tubercle, the wrist is passively brought into radial deviation. In patients with scapholunate dissociation, the scaphoid, being held extended by the thumb, shifts dorsally causing pain and a clunk as the scaphoid moves back into the scaphoid fossa.

○   **What is the current treatment for the acute static scapholunate dissociation?**

Most surgeons are currently performing scapholunate ligament repair, supplemented by some form of dorsal wrist capsulodesis.

○   **What is the current treatment for lunate and perilunate dislocations?**

The recommended treatment is ORIF with both volar capsular repair and dorsal ligament repair.

○   **What is the current recommendation for proximal pole fractures of the scaphoid?**

Due to the high rate of non-union ORIF with screw fixation, using a dorsal approach is recommended.

○   **What is ulnar translocation of carpus?**

In individuals where there is tearing of the radioscaphocapitate and long radiolunate ligaments, the carpus will sometimes migrate ulnarly and volarly following the slope of the radius. Translocation can also occur in certain rheumatologic conditions of the wrist.

○   **Which fractures of the radius are frequently associated with scapholunate ligament tears?**

Intra-articular fractures of the radius which are in the vicinity of the scapholunate ligament are frequently associated with scapholunate ligament tears.

○   **What is the appropriate initial treatment for an individual who after a fall onto an outstretched hand has pain in the snuffbox and negative radiographs?**

The appropriate initial treatment is short arm thumb spica splinting or casting with follow-up in 2 weeks. Continued pain in the snuff box in the absence of x-ray findings required additional studies to rule out scaphoid fracture (Bone Scan/MRI/CT Scan).

○ **Scaphoid fractures in which location have the best prognosis?**

Fractures of the distal pole of the scaphoid have the best prognosis. These fractures can be managed by short arm thumb spica splint or short arm thumb spica cast.

○ **What is the second most commonly fractured carpal bone?**

The triquetrum is the second most commonly fractured carpal bone. Most triquetral fractures are dorsal marginal fractures.

○ **What is the most common mechanism for fractures of the hook of the hamate?**

Most fractures of the hook of the hamate occur as the result of a direct blow.

○ **If one suspects a hook of the hamate fracture clinically, what is the best confirmatory study?**

The best confirmatory for hook of hamate fractures study is a CT scan.

○ **In a patient with a hook of hamate non-union, what is the best treatment?**

The best treatment for a hook of hamate non-union is excision of the hook of the hamate.

○ **What imaging modality is used to stage Kienbock's disease?**

Plain radiographs are used to stage Kienbock's disease. MRI is helpful in diagnosing Kienbock's disease.

○ **What are the X-ray findings in Stage I Kienbock's disease?**

X-rays are either normal or you may see linear fractures in the lunate.

○ **What are the X-ray findings in Stage II Kienbock's disease?**

The lunate shows increased density in Stage II Kienbock's disease.

○ **What are the X-ray findings in Stage III Kienbock's disease?**

The lunate shows collapse and/or fragmentation in Stage III Kienbock's disease.

○ **What are the X-ray findings in Stage IV Kienbock's disease?**

Arthritis is present in Stage IV Kienbock's disease.

○ **What X-ray finding of the bones of the forearm is associated with Kienbock's disease?**

Ulnar negative variance has been associated with Kienbock's disease.

○ **What are the measurements of carpal height used for?**

Measurements of carpal height are used as a means of diagnosing scapholunate dissociation. The normal ratio is 0.54. Smaller ratios are indicative of the carpal collapse seen in scapholunate dissociation.

○ **What does the term SLAC wrist refer to?**

The term SLAC refers to scapholunate advanced collapse.

○ **What is the SLAC procedure and what must be normal to consider this procedure?**

The SLAC procedure is a four-corner (C-L-H-T) fusion with excision of the scaphoid and radial styloidectomy. The lunate fossa and proximal articular surface of the lunate must be intact to consider this procedure.

○ **What radiographic findings are usually present in patients with a lunato-triquetral ligament tear?**

Plain radiographs are usually normal in patients with isolated lunato-triquetral ligament tears. VISI deformities can be seen in more complex LT ligament injuries.

○ **What are the components of the triangular fibrocartilage complex?**

The components are the TFC proper, the ulnar collateral ligament, the ECU subsheath, the meniscus homologue, the ulnolunate and ulnotriquetral ligaments, and the dorsal and palmar radioulnar ligaments.

○ **What parts of the scapho-lunate ligament are responsible for the biomechanical behavior of the joint?**

The thick dorsal and volar portions of the ligament are 3mm thick and give strength and integrity to the joint.

○ **What is a Geisler Stage 0 scapholunate instability?**

A Geisler Stage 0 instability is an arthroscopic test done through the mid-carpal joint. In Stage 0 a probe cannot be passed into the S-L joint.

○ **What is a Geisler Stage 1 scapholunate instability?**

A Geisler Stage 1 instability occurs when a probe can be passed into the S-L joint through the midcarpal joint.

○ **What is a Geisler Stage 2 scapholunate instability?**

A Geisler Stage 2 instability occurs when a probe can be twisted in the S-L joint

○ **What is a Geisler Stage 3 instability?**

A Geisler Stage 3 instability occurs when the arthroscope can be passed through the midcarpal joint to the radiocarpal joint. This is also known as the drive-through sign.

○ **What is a Geisler Stage 4 instability?**

A Geisler Stage 4 instability occurs when there is arthritis present.

○ **What percent of arthrograms will show a scapholunate ligament tear in an asymptomatic patient?**

27% of arthrograms will show an S-L tear in asymptomatic patients.

○ **What is the reported accuracy of MR arthrogram for determining S-L ligament tears?**

The reported accuracy of MR arthrography is 95%.

○ **What is the definitive diagnostic test for intercarpal pathology?**

Wrist arthroscopy is the definitive test for intercarpal pathology.

References

Adolfsson L. Arthroscopy for the diagnosis of post-traumatic wrist pain. J Hand Surg. 1992;17B: 46-50.

Barber H. The interosseous arterial anatomy of the adult human carpus. Orthopedics. 1972;5:1-19.

Beckenbaugh RD. Accurate evaluation and management of the painful wrist following injury. Orthop Clin North Amer. 1984;15:289-306.

Berger RA. The gross and histologic anatomy of the scapholunate interosseous ligament. J Hand Surg. 1996;21A:170-178.

Dobyns JH, Linscheid RL, Chao EYS, et al. Traumatic instability of the wrist. AAOS Instructional Course Lectures. 1975;24:182-199.

Fisk GR. Carpal instability and the fractured scaphoid. Ann R Coll Surg Engl. 1970;46: 63-76.

Fisk GR: The wrist. J Bone and Joint Surg. 66:396-407.

Garcia-Elias M, Dobyns JH, Cooney WP, and Linscheid RL. Traumatic axial dislocations of the carpus. J Hand Surg. 1989;14A: 446-456.

Gilula LA, Destout JM, Weeks PM, et al. Roentgenographic diagnosis of the painful wrist. Clin Orthop Relat Res. 1984;187:52-64.

Green DP and O'Brien ET. Classification and management of carpal dislocations. J Bone and Joint Surg. 1980;149:55-71.

Johnson RP. The acutely injured wrist and its residuals. Clin Orthop Relate Res. 1980;149:33-44.

Kirschenbaum D, Sieler S, Solonick D, et al. Arthrography of the wrist J Bone and Joint Surg. 1995;77A:1207-1209.

Lavernia CJ, Cohen MS and Taleisnik J. Treatment of scapholunate dissociation by ligamentous repair and capsulodesis. J Hand Surg. 1992;17:354-359.

Lichtman DM, Schneider JR, Swafford AR, et al. Ulnar midcarpal instability-clinical and laboratory analysis. J Hand Surg. 1981;6:515-523.

Linscheid RL, Dobyns JH. The unified concept of carpal injuries. Ann Chir Main. 1984;3: 35-42.

Lynched RL, Dobbins JH, Be about JW, et al. Traumatic instability of the wrist. J Bone and Joint Surg. 1972;54A:1612-1632.

Mayfield JK, Johnson RP, Kilcoyne RK. Carpal dislocations: Pathomechanics and progressive perilunar instability. J Hand Surg. 1980;5:226-241.

Moneim MS,. Management of greater arc carpal fractures. Hand Clinics. 1988;4:457-467.

Panagis JS, Gelberman RH, Taleisnik J, et al. The arterial anatomy of the human carpus. Part II: The interosseous vascularity. J Hand Surg. 1983;8:375-382.

Ruby LK, Cooney WP III, An KN, et al. Relative motion of selected carpal bones: A kinematic analysis of the normal wrist. J Hand Surg. 1998;13A:1-10.

Taleisnik J. Carpal instability. J Bone and Joint Surg. 1988;70A:1262-1268.

Viegas SF. Midcarpal arthroscopy: Anatomy and Technique. Arthroscopy. 1992;8:385-390.

Watson HK, Ashmead D IV, Maklouf MV. Examination of the scaphoid. J Hand Surg. 1988;13A: 657-660.

Watson HK, Ballet FL. The SLAC wrist: scapholunate advanced collapse pattern of degenerative arthritis. J Hand Surg. 1984;9A: 358-365.

Wiedrich TA. The use of suture anchors in the hand and wrist. Oper Techn in Plas and Reconst Surg. 1997;4:42-48.

Zlatkin MB, Chao PC, Osterman AL, et al. Chronic wrist pain: Evaluation with high resolution MR imaging. Radiology. 1989;173: 723-729.

REPLANTATION

Charles K. Lee MD, Mark W. Kiehn MD, and Gregory M. Buncke MD

DIGITAL REPLANTATION

❍ **What are the current indications for digital replantation?**

- Thumb
- Multiple Digits
- Single Digit Distal to Sublimis
- Hand at the wrist or forearm (sharp amputation)
- Any level amputation in a child

❍ **What is the order for a single digit replant?**

BEFANV
- Bone
- Extensors
- Flexors
- Arteries
- Nerves
- Veins

❍ **What is the order for multiple digit replantations—digit by digit or structure by structure?**

Structure by structure, systemically repairing as above.

❍ **What are the functional deficits associated with ray amputation of the index finger?**

Loss of power grip and key pinch.

❍ **What is the lumbrical plus deformity?**

The FDP tendon and lumbrical muscle migrate proximally after division of the tendon in trauma. With flexion, tension is exerted on the lumbrical via the radial lateral band causing <u>paradoxical extension of the PIP during flexion of the MP joint</u>.

❍ **Treatment?**

Division of the lumbrical insertion.

❍ **What is the treatment of venous congestion after digital replantation?**

1. Removal of dressings
2. Leech therapy
3. Heparin
4. Nail bed bleeding with heparin soaked sponges
5. Revision of the venous anastomosis

❍ **Which tissue is most sensitive to warm ischemia?**

Skeletal muscle.

O   **What is the maximal cold ischemia time reported for digital replantation?**

30-40 hrs.

O   **What is the Quadrigia Effect?**

Weakness in flexion of fingers secondary to excess pull of one FDP tendon of the amputated finger.

O   **What is the maximum nerve gap for use of a neural tube (PGA)?**

2.5cm

O   **What nerves are available for use as donors for nerve grafting?**

- posterior interosseus nerve
- sural nerve
- superficial radial nerve
- superficial peroneal nerve

O   **What is the treatment of choice for a tip amputation through the nailbed without bone exposure?**

Local dressings changes

O   **What is a good option for a thumb tip amputation with exposed bone?**

Moberg flap.

O   **How much advancement can be obtained from a Moberg flap?**

1.5cm

O   **What are contraindications to digital replantation?**

- Severe concomitant injuries
- Severely crushed or mangled
- Multi-level amputations
- Significant co-morbidities
- Prolonged warm ischemia time
- Mentally unstable/ self-mutilation
- Single finger proximal to FDS insertion

O   **How many arteries and veins needed for a digital replantation?**

1 Artery, 1 Vein (2 are preferred)

O   **Is an artery only digital replantation possible?**

Yes. Leeching and/or bleeding of the nailbed can be used to relieve venous congestion.

O   **How many places can you find a digital vein?**

Two. Dorsal and Volar.

O   **What is the concern in avulsion amputation vs. guillotine amp?**

Zone of injury much greater in avulsion injuries.

O   **What is the Chinese Stripe sign or Red Stripe sign?**

A red streak along the artery indicating severe intimal injury along the length of the vessel?

O   **What is the best method for treating the zone of injury of an artery or vein in cases of crush or avulsion injuries?**

Resection of compromised vessel and vein grafting.

O   **Where can veins be reliably found on the hand dorsum?**

Proximal to each web space

O   **What vascular pattern exists in a finger that was crushed and has the appearance of venous congestion and slow capillary refill?**

Loss of proper digital artery inflow, intact venous flow

O   **8 months post digital replantation, what operation would you offer to the patient with minimal passive or active ROM?**

Extensor tenolysis and open capsulotomy.

O   **What operation would you offer for someone with good passive but minimal active ROM?**

Flexor tenolysis.

O   **What is the greatest danger in digital reoperation after replantation?**

Injury to the neurovascular bundle embedded in scar.

O   **What is fluorimetry?**

A method of monitoring tissue perfusion by injecting fluorescein dye intravenously and using a fluorometer to quantitatively measure rise and fall of fluorescein in tissue.

O   **What if there is a 2-3 fold rise but no fall in the numbers?**

Sign of venous congestion

O   **What if the absolute number is very low and remains low, but the digit clinically looks viable?**

Thick skin or dirty skin can alter the numbers.

O   **At the microanastomosis, what is the predominant layer on day 3?**

Platelets

O   **On Day 4-14?**

Pseudointima

O   **On Day 14-onward?**

Intima.

○   **One year post replantation at the PIPJ level with severe arthritis or fusion at the PIPJ. What surgery can you offer the patient?**

PIP joint arthroplasty.

LEECHES & ANTICOAGULANTS

○   **Scientific name for Medical Leeches?**

Hirudo medicinalis

○   **Action of hirudin?**

- Binds activated thrombin (1:1)
- Inhibits conversion of fibrinogen to fibrin
- Blocks activation of factors V, VIII, XI, vWF
- Decreases activation of TPA, protein C, plasmin
- Prolongs thrombin-dependant coagulation tests (PTT, TT, ACT, ECT)
- There is no direct effect on platelets or endothelial cells
- Can monitor by thrombin time and PTT

○   **Excretion of hirudin?**

Renal excretion

○   **Organism to cover while patient is on leech therapy?**

Aeromonas hydrophila—enteric organism which can cause severe soft tissue infection Can cover with third generation cephalosporin (Ceftizox), Bactrim

○   **What is the mechanism of Heparin?**

Action is primarily via activation of serum antithrombin III and lowering of blood viscosity; increases ATIII activity

○   **What is the mechanism of Dextran?**

- Polysaccharide –Molecular weights of 40,000 and 70,000.
- decreases platelet aggregation by imparting a negative charge on the platelets, inactivating vWF,
- modifying structure of fibrin,
- altering rheologic property of blood.
- Possible complications: Antigenic test dose of less than 5cc must be given prior to administration of a full dose.
- Renal failure-volume expansion.

○   **What is the mechanism of Aspirin?**

- Acetylates cyclooxygenase enzyme
- Decreases arachodonic acid, Thromboxane, Prostacyline
- Decreases platelet aggregation and vasoconstriction

○   **What is the mechanism of Thorazine?**

Potent vasodilator.

○ **What is the mechanism of Papaverin?**

Salt of an opium alkaloid. Smooth muscle relaxant especially with cerebral and peripheral ischemia associated w/ arterial spasm.

○ **What is the mechanism of Lidocaine?**

Potent local vasodilatation. Commonly used as a 2% solution

○ **What is the definitive role of anticoagulation in microsurgery?**

Controversial. Not enough randomized controlled trials to definitively characterize its role. Common uses: High does heparin irrigation during the micro anastomosis. IV heparin after a thrombotic event with anastomotic revision.

HYPERCOAGULABLE STATES

○ **What percentage of venous thrombotic events in the human body are caused by genetic factors?**

Inherited deficiencies account for 5-15% of venous thrombosis

○ **Is the Antiphospholipid Antibody associated with arterial or venous thrombosis?**

It is associated with both.

○ **What is Activated Protein C Resistance (APC/Factor V Leiden)?**

- One of the most common hereditary causes of thrombophilia.
- 4% frequency in European population, extremely uncommon in Africans, Asians, Austrailians.
- APC inactivates Factors V and VIII—keeps thrombosis in check

○ **What is a Prothrombin 2021A Mutation?**

- Relative risk of thrombosis with this mutation is 2.8
- Prevalence-2%
- extremely uncommon in nonwhite population
- Treatment: Coumadin 3-6mo; recurrence- indefinitely

○ **What is Hyperhomocysteinemia?**

- Usually an enzyme deficiency in states of chronic renal disease, hypothyroid, malignancy.
- Can be associated with medications.
- Strong correlation between elevated homocysteine levels and arterial and venous disease.
- Arterial-Increased cardiac, cerebral vascular disease; 3X risk.
- Venous-Increased risk of thrombosis

○ **How much does an Elevated Factor VIII cause a hypercoagulable state?**

Levels greater than 1500 IU/L- lead to a 5X increase of thrombosis

○ **Does an Elevated Factor XI cause an increased rate of thrombosis?**

Yes. Relative risk 2.2

❍   **What is the workup for hypercoagulable states?**

Be suspicious when patient has a thrombotic event early in life (age <45), family history, recurrence
Lab studies to order: AntiThrombin III, Protein C &S, antiphospholipid antibody, Factor V Leiden, Prothrombin 2021 A Mutation, homocysteinemia. Involve a hematology oncologist early.
Note: Prot C &S, antithrombin III are decreased in acute thrombosis; Antithrombin III decreased during heparin

❍   **Which Urbaniak class of Ring Avulsion Injury is considered a relative contraindication to replantation?**

III—Complete degloving or complete amputation

❍   **What type of flap can be used if there is a soft tissue defect in a Type II Ring Avulsion Injury?**

Venous flow through flap.

❍   **What is the average 2PD of a replanted thumb?**

9mm-11mm

❍   **What is the average 2PD of a replanted digit?**

8-15mm—depending on sharp vs. avulsion.

❍   **How much time should you tell a patient he will have to wait for cold intolerance symptoms to resolve?**

At least 2 years, possibly a lifetime.

SCALP REPLANTATION

❍   **What is the typical history of a scalp amputation?**

Young female factory worker with long hair, with avulsion of scalp along the supraorbital rim extending to the ears laterally and to the nape of the neck posteriorly.

❍   **Which vessels are commonly used for replantation?**

- Superficial temporal
- Posterior auricular
- Occipital
- Supraorbital
Usually a single artery and vein can be used to replant the scalp. Vein grafts are commonly used.

❍   **What is a common complication after scalp replantation?**

Hematoma.

EAR REPLANTATION

❍   **Which vessels are commonly used in ear replantation?**

Superficial temporal or posterior auricular.

❍   **Venous drainage?**

Veins are extremely difficult to find and most often, the ear has to be leeched.

LIP REPLANTATION

○ **Which arteries to look for in a lip replantation?**

Labial arteries.

○ **Veins in lip replantation?**

Extremely difficult, usually requires leeching.

○ **Most common cause of lip amputation?**

Dog bite.

○ **Can the tongue be replanted?**

Yes. 3 have been reported in the world literature.

LOWER EXTREMITY REPLANTATION

○ **What can you do with the remaining amputated leg if replantation is not possible at a below knee amputation site with significant soft tissue loss?**

Foot fillet flap.

PENIS REPLANTATION

○ **Common cause of penile amputation?**

Self mutilation.

○ **Vessels in penile replantation?**

Dorsal vein and deep arteries in corpora.

References

Alpert BS, Buncke HJ, Mathes SJ, "Surgical Treatment of the Totally Avulsed Scalp," Clinics in PS, Vol 9 No 2, April 1982: 145.

Buncke GM, et al, "Hand Reconstruction with Partial Toe and Multiple Toe Transplants," Clinics in Plastic Surgery October 1992: 859.

Buncke HJ Microsurgery: Microsurgery: Transplantation and Replantation 1991.

Buncke HJ, Chang DW, "History of Microsurgery," Seminars in Plastic Surgery Vol 17, No 1, 2003: 5.

Buncke HJ "Microvascular Hand Surgery-Transplants and Replants- Over the Past 25 Years," The Jo of Hand Surgery, May 2000: 415-428.

Buntic RF and Buncke HJ, "Successful Replantation of an Amputated Tongue," PRS May 1998: 1604

Chalain T, Jones G, "Replantation of the Avulsed Pinna: 100% Survival with a Single Arterial Anastomosis and Substitution of Leeches for a Venous Anastomosis, " PRS June 1995:1275.

Classen DA, "The indications and reliability of Vein Graft Use in Free Flap Transfer," Can J PS Vol 12, No 1 Spring 2004: 27.

Conrad MH, Adams WP, "Pharmacologic Optimization in Microsurgery in the New Millennium," PRS Dec 2001: 2088.

Hammond DC, "Microsurgical Replantation of the Amputated Nose" PRS May 2000

Kay S, et al, "Ring Avulsion Injuries: Classification and Prognosis," Journal of Hand Surgery March 1989: 204.

Pederson WC "Replantation," PRS March 2001: 823-844.

Walton RL et al, "Microsurgical Replantation of the Lip: A Multi-Institutional Experience," PRS August 1998: 358.

Wei FC, "Free Style Free Flaps, " PRS September 15 2001: 910.

TOE-TO-HAND TRANSFER

Christiaan Schrag, BSc, MD, FRCS (C), Fu-Chan Wei, MD, FACS

○ **Which 2 arterial pedicles may supply great toe or second toe transfers?**

The first dorsal metatarsal artery (FDMA) and the first plantar metatarsal artery (FPMA). The FDMA is dominant in 70% of cases, FPMA in 20% and both are of equal caliber in 10%.

○ **Where in the foot is the FDMA located?**

The FDMA lies between the first and second metatarsals, at varying depths from superficial to the interosseous muscle to intramuscular to a position plantar to the interosseous muscle. The FDMA passes dorsal to the deep transverse metatarsal ligament, which connects the plantar plates of the metatarsophalangeal (MTP) joints.

○ **Is there a classification system to describe the various positions of the FDMA?**

There are at least three different classification systems. Learning the classification systems is not necessary.

○ **Are the dorsal metatarsal and plantar metatarsal arterial systems connected?**

Yes: First, via the communicating vessels, which pass between the first and second metatarsals; secondly, the two systems converge at the first web space.

○ **Which digital artery of the toe is more important, the dorsal or plantar system?**

The plantar digital artery. The dorsal digital artery is rarely present.

○ **What venous system should be used to drain a great toe or second toe transfer?**

The intermediate level veins, which give rise to the greater saphenous vein.

○ **Which nerve supplies the first web space?**

The deep peroneal nerve.

○ **Which nerves are the most important for sensation of the transferred toe?**

The medial and lateral proper plantar digital nerves, which are terminal branches of the medial plantar nerve. The digital nerves are located plantar to the plantar digital arteries.

○ **Which tendon must be cut when dissecting the FDMA on the foot dorsum?**

Extensor hallucis brevis.

○ **In which types of congenital anomaly should a toe-to-hand transfer be considered?**

Constriction band syndrome, hands with no fingers but an adequate thumb, and thumb absence with a complex hand malformation. The latter two situations often have absent or anomalous recipient structures. A thorough work-up is mandatory. A well thought-out operative plan with alternative recipient vessels, nerves and tendons must be devised. Pollicization is the best procedure for isolated thumb aplasia/significant hypoplasia.

O   **In patients who may be future candidates for toe-to-hand transfer which structures should be preserved during the initial emergent treatment? Why?**

Skin: Toe transfers have a paucity of skin; Local flaps further injure and ultimately scar the hand making recipient site preparation more difficult; free flaps for skin coverage use all-important recipient vessels.
Joints: Intact proximal interphalangeal or metacarpophalangeal joints will enhance mobility and function following transfer; preservation of only the proximal articular surface of the metacarpophalangeal joint is better than saving no articular surface because a composite joint reconstruction is possible.
Bone: Adequate bony length allows restoration of the proper digital length with toe transfer, which improves appearance and function; the great toe should not be harvested proximal to the metatarsophalangeal joint, necessitating a staged reconstruction or second toe transfer if the thumb is excessively shortened.
Tendons: Maintaining flexor tendon length ensures preservation of flexor pulley system; the complex extensor mechanism should be saved as it is difficult to reconstruct; less donor site morbidity is incurred if tendons are preserved in the hand.
Vessels: Damage to recipient vessels either precludes transfer or necessitates riskier vein grafting.
Nerve: Preserving nerve length reduces donor site dissection; a more distal nerve repair during transfer will speed up sensory recovery.

O   **How can closure of wounds in potential toe-to-hand candidates be achieved?**

Pedicled distant flaps, which do not require sacrifice of local tissues or vessels.

O   **Should arteriography of the foot be performed prior to surgery?**

Preoperative arteriography is not required unless the donor foot has been injured. The vascular pedicle is dissected in a retrograde manner, thus it is not necessary to know the proximal course of the vessel.

O   **What type of secondary procedures might be necessary for patients who undergo toe-to-hand transfer?**

About 14% of patients require surgical revisions to improve function including: flexor tendon tenolysis (7%), arthrodesis (2%), web space deepening (2%), osteotomy for malunion (2%), or bone grafting for non-union. Pulp plasty improves the appearance of the toe transfer and may be indicated if the distal pulp is too bulky.

O   **How many motor units power the thumb?**

Nine: four extrinsic muscles and five intrinsic muscles.

O   **In which important way does the motion of the great toe metatarsophalangeal (MTP) joint differ from the thumb metacarpophalangeal (MCP) joint?**

The MTP range is one of hyperextension rather than flexion.

O   **What is the two point discrimination of the great toe in situ? Following transplantation and rehabilitation is the sensation in the transplanted toe better or worse than before transfer?**

The great toe in situ has an average static two-point discrimination (S2PD) of 10mm (2 X standard deviation = +/- 6mm). Following transfer sensation varies considerably. Mean S2PD of 6.5mm may be achieved in patients with optimal nerve coaptation and adequate sensory reeducation.

O   **What proportion of hand function does the thumb represent?**

Forty to fifty percent.

O   **What types of thumb to finger pinches are commonly discussed when analyzing prehensile function?**

Pulp-to-pulp, lateral (key) and chuck three-point (tripod) pinch. In addition the thumb assists the hand in power (cylinder) grasp. Hook grip requires only fingers. Without any digits present the hand may function as a bat.

○ **What are most common etiologies of a thumb absence/dysfunction that require reconstruction?**

Traumatic amputation, post-oncologic resection and certain types of congenital thumb anomalies.

○ **What is the best surgical procedure to treat an acutely amputated thumb?**

Replantation.

○ **If replantation is not possible, is primary toe-to-hand transfer possible?**

Yes. Advantages include decreased time in hospital and earlier return to work. There are no statistically significant differences in the rate of early post-operative complications between primary and secondary transfers. However, subjectively patients with primary reconstructions are less satisfied with the function and appearance of the reconstructed digit than patients who have lived for some time with the amputation.

○ **In assessing thumb amputations through the metacarpal, injury to which structures will most negatively influence the outcome of thumb reconstruction?**

Injury to the thenar muscles will dramatically affect thumb strength, stability and mobility.

○ **What are the elements of an ideal thumb reconstruction?**

There are three main components: Functional reconstruction: This requires adequate motor power/excursion, at least protective sensation, correct thumb length and position, stability, and absence of pain; Cosmetically acceptable, Minimal donor site morbidity.

○ **What is the minimum critical length of the thumb in an otherwise normal hand?**

The interphalangeal joint level. A reconstructed thumb may be made to this length if necessary or an amputation at this level may be tolerated.

○ **What factors determine the "correct" thumb length?**

A normal thumb reaches the middle of the proximal phalanx of the index finger when the thumb is adducted. The correct thumb length is determined by the thenar muscle function and the length and mobility of the remaining fingers. If the thumb will have minimal mobility slightly shorter is preferable. A shorter thumb may be tolerated if the fingers are normal or may be required in a metacarpal hand.

○ **What methods, other than toe-to-hand transfer, are available for thumb reconstruction?**

Pollicization of an injured digit, pollicization of an uninjured digit, osteoplastic thumb reconstruction, and distraction osteogenesis. Phalangization and the Gillies cocked-hat flap are rarely indicated. For soft tissue coverage of the distal tip local and regional flaps may be used. e.g. Moberg's palmar advancement flap and pedicled neurovascular island flaps.

○ **Is it necessary to use the ipsilateral great toe for thumb reconstruction? Why or why not?**

No. The left great toe is the first choice because the left foot is less important, especially for driving.

○ **How do the great toe and thumb differ in appearance?**

The widest diameter of the great toe is 60% bigger than the thumb. The great toe has a wider nail and larger bones.

❍   **Where on the thumb should the web space attach to avoid an arachnidactylous appearance?**

The web space should meet at the MCP joint of the thumb.

❍   **When might a second toe be considered for thumb reconstruction?**

Patient refuses/cannot tolerate first toe loss; Proximal metacarpal or transcarpometacarpal joint level injuries; when the second toe and thumb are similar in size; in children; Suboptimal reconstruction acceptable (age, non-dominant hand).

❍   **What are the advantages of the great toe over the second toe for thumb reconstruction?**

The great toe provides a broader, stronger, more stable reconstruction. The second toe is prone to sit in a flexed posture, has a small nail and two interphalangeal joints, which leads to less stability.

❍   **How can the flexed posture of the second toe be minimized?**

By releasing the extensor digitorum longus attachment from the metatarsophalangeal joint, suturing the extensor digitorum brevis to the extensor hood or interosseous tendon, tight extensor repair, pinning the interphalangeal joints in extension for 6 weeks and nighttime extension splinting for at least 1 year.

❍   **What are the main advantages of the second toe in thumb reconstruction?**

It may be harvested with a long segment of the second metatarsal, allowing for proximal thumb injury reconstructions. Donor site morbidity is less than that of the great toe.

❍   **What options are available for thumb reconstruction if the great toe is too big to give an acceptable aesthetic result?**

The great toe wrap-around, the trimmed great toe or the twisted two toe technique. The second toe generally gives a poorer aesthetic outcome.

❍   **What are the advantages of using the wrap-around great toe flap?**

Preservation of great toe skeleton/tendons; aesthetic thumb reconstruction; provision of glabrous skin, nail, pulp with fibrous septa and sensibility.

❍   **What are the disadvantages of the great toe wrap-around for total thumb reconstruction?**

At least 2 secondary donor sites are required: iliac crest for thumb skeleton and a skin graft and/or regional flap to cover the remaining great toe. The reconstructed thumb has no IP joint. There is a risk of bone resorption.

❍   **What are the advantages of the trimmed-toe transfer?**

The trimmed-toe provides a more aesthetic reconstruction than an entire great toe transplantation and preserves skin for donor site closure. However, there is a reduction in IP joint range of motion to around 18 degrees.

❍   **Do patients who undergo toe-to-hand transfer for thumb amputation do better than those who don't?**

Yes. Patients who undergo toe transfer have a statistically significant better hand function, aesthetics, and satisfaction than those who do not. The strength and dexterity of the hand with the toe transfer are comparable to the opposite normal hands.

❍   **What are possible donor site complications specific to the great toe transfer?**

Early: delayed wound healing, skin necrosis.

Late: Altered gait, changed weight bearing, pain, cold intolerance.

○ How can great toe donor site complications best be avoided?

Preservation of as much foot and web space skin as possible is important to allow direct closure without tension. The first metatarsal head should not be sacrificed and 1 cm of proximal phalanx should be preserved to maintain adequate of push-off.

○ If great toe is harvested proximal to the metatarsophalangeal joint how does gait change?

There is a small but statistically significant decrease in stride length.

○ List the flaps available for microvascular transfer from the forefoot for hand reconstruction.

Great toe, wrap-around great toe, trimmed great toe, pulp, hemi-pulp, onychocutaneous, first web-space, second toe, wrap-around second toe, vascularized second toe PIP joint, vascularized second toe MTP joint, combined second and third toe, combined third and fourth toe, third toe and twisted two toe technique.

○ List the unique physical characteristics of the fingertip that can only be replaced by tissue transplanted from a digit (toe or finger).

Glabrous skin, fibrous septa and the presence of a nail.

○ What is glabrous skin?

Glabrous skin, in distinction to hirsute skin, is thicker and hairless. Functionally important features of glabrous skin include friction ridges, increased mechanical strength, dense clustering of specialized sensory end organs and numerous sweat glands. Hair interferes with sensation and is therefore absent from glabrous skin.

○ Why are fibrous septa and nails important for manipulation?

Fibrous septa between the fat of the pulp prevent excessive shearing, but still allow the pulp to conform to the object being held. The nail provides dorsal support and counter pressure to the pulp.

○ What are indications for toe-to-hand transfer in a hand with only a single finger amputated?

To improve hand aesthetics and function and to treat painful finger tip/neuroma.

○ A patient has an index finger amputation at the middle of the proximal phalanx. Is she a good candidate for a second toe-to-index finger transfer?

No. At this level the reconstructed finger will be noticeably shorter than the rest of the intact fingers. In hands with single finger loss the best reconstructive outcome is obtained when the amputation level is from the middle of the middle phalanx to the base of the distal phalanx.

○ When using the second toe to reconstruct a distal finger, how is unnecessary bulkiness of reconstructed digit avoided?

Careful skeletonization of the vessels prevents bulky soft tissue marring the aesthetic result and precludes unsightly skin grafting. Removal of the thick plantar subcutaneous fat at the metatarsophalangeal joint level will not only improve the appearance, but will also allow greater range of motion for the transferred digit.

○ What are indications for toe-to-hand transfer in a mutilated hand?

To improve or provide pulp-to-pulp, chuck, lateral pinch and hook grip and therefore overall hand function.

O **What is a metacarpal hand?**

A hand that is unable to achieve any type of pinch or grip (no prehensile capacity) owing to amputation of all fingers. The thumb may or may not be preserved.

O **How should a metacarpal hand be reconstructed?**

The variety and complexity of the metacarpal hand injuries demands careful planning to ensure proper use of limited donor tissues and to correctly address the most important deficiencies. Classification of the metacarpal hand helps determine the most appropriate reconstructive method, which may include two second toe transfers, combined second and third toe transfer and great toe transfer.

O **Classify the metacarpal hand.**

Type I: Thumb preserved, all fingers amputated at or below the middle of the proximal phalanx. The level of finger amputation may be used to further subdivide patients into subtypes A, B or C.

Type I Metacarpal Hand

Subtype	Level of Finger Amputation	Recommendations
I A	Proximal to middle of proximal phalanx	2 second toes or combined $2^{nd}/3^{rd}$
I B	Through MCP joint (intact proximal articular surface)	Combined $2^{nd}/3^{rd}$ as composite joint transfer
I C	Proximal to MCP	Combined $2^{nd}/3^{rd}$

Type II metacarpal hands have all fingers amputated proximal to middle of proximal phalanx plus a thumb amputation. Subtypes A, B, C and D depend on the level of thumb amputation and status of two important structures: the thenar muscles and carpometacarpal (CMC) joint. Reconstruction of the fingers may be carried out concurrently or separate from the thumb reconstruction depending on the subtype.

Type II Metacarpal Hand

Subtype	Level of Thumb Amputation	Recommendations
II A	Distal to metacarpal neck	Great toe transfer
II B	Proximal to metacarpal neck, adequate thenar function	Preliminary procedure to lengthen thumb followed by great toe transfer or second toe transfer. Concurrent transfer of combined $2^{nd}/3^{rd}$ toe or two second toes.
II C	Inadequate thenar function	Two stage reconstruction. Opponensplasty
II D	CMC joint damage	Thumb reconstructed as an immobile post.

O **What is the vascular supply for a combined 2nd and 3rd toe transfer?**

The FDMA and/or a plantar digital metatarsal artery are taken as the vascular pedicle. There is no difference in early outcome between using one versus two arterial pedicles.

O **What are the advantages of providing a hand with two adjacent digits?**

This construct allows useful tripod (chuck) pinch, enhances lateral stability, provides a stronger hook grip and allows a wider span for grasping larger objects.

O **Is a combined $2^{nd}/3^{rd}$ toe transplant appropriate to reconstruct the fingers for a type I A metacarpal hand with a preserved web space? Why or why not?**

No, two second toes should be used when the amputation is distal to the web space in order to avoid a long palm-short finger appearance.

O **List the late donor site complications specific to combined $2^{nd}/3^{rd}$ toe transfer.**

Pain with ambulation and scissor deformity (migration of the 4th toe towards the great toe).

○ **What is the average range of motion obtained using a vascularized joint for finger arthroplasty?**

Approximately 32°.

○ **What are the indications for vascularized joint transfer?**

A painful joint with post-traumatic arthritis, instability and/or deformity. Patients must be highly motivated, young and have functioning flexor/extensor tendons.

○ **What advantages do vascularized joints have over other arthroplasty methods?**

Autologous tissue only; Growth potential in children; Allow reconstruction of compound defects involving joint, bone, skin, and tendon in a single procedure.

References

Bannister LH. Integumental system: skin and breasts. In Williams PL, Ed. Gray's Anatomy. 38th Edition. Toronto: Churchill-Livingstone, 1999: 375-424.

Berry MM, Standring SM, Bannister LH. Nervous system. In Williams PL, Ed. Gray's Anatomy. 38th Edition. Toronto: Churchill-Livingstone, 1999: 901-1398.

Cheng MH, Wei FC, Santamaria E, Cheng SL, Lin CH, Chen SH. Single versus double arterial anastomoses in combined second- and third-toe transplantation. Plast Reconstr Surg 1998; 108: 2408-12.

Chung KC, Wei FC. An outcome study of thumb reconstruction using microvascular toe transfer. J Hand Surg 2000; 25A: 651-8.

Eaton CJ, Lister GD. Toe transfer for congenital hand defects. Microsurgery 1991; 12: 186-195.

Foucher G, Binhammer P. Free vascularized toe transfer. In Foucher G, Ed. Reconstructive Surgery in Hand Mutilation. London: Mosby, 1997: 57-66.

Frykman GK, O'Brien BM, Morrison WA, MacLeod AM, Ciurleo A. J Hand Surg 1986; 11A: 9-17.

Gilbert A. Congenital absence of the thumb and digits. J Hand Surg 1989; 14 B: 6-17.

Gilbert A. Vascular anatomy of the first web space of the foot. In A Landi, Ed. Reconstruction of the thumb. London: Chapman and Hall, 1989 P. 199.

Gordon L. Toe-to-thumb transplantation. In Green DP, Hotchkiss RN, Pederson WC, Eds. Green's Operative Hand Surgery, Fourth Ed. Philadelphia: Churchill Livingstone. 1999: 1299-1326.

Kato H, Ogino T, Minami A, Usai M. Restoration of sensibility in fingers repaired with free sensory flaps from the toe. J Hand Surg 1989; 14A: 49-54.

Kleinman WB, Strickland JW. Thumb reconstruction. In Green DP, Hotchkiss RN, Pederson WC, Eds. Green's Operative Hand Surgery, Fourth Ed. Philadelphia: Churchill Livingstone. 1999: 2068-2170.

Leung PC. Sensory recovery in transplanted toes. Microsurgery 1989; 10: 242-244.

Leung PC. Thumb reconstruction using the second toe. In A Landi, Ed. Reconstruction of the thumb. London: Chapman and Hall, 1989 P 205.

Leung PC, Wong WL. The vessels of the first metatarsal web space. An operative and radiographic study. J Bone Joint Surg 1983; 65A: 235-9.

Lipton HA, May JW, Simon SR. Preoperative and postoperative gait analyses of patients undergoing great toe-to-thumb transfer. J Hand Surg 1987; 12A: 66-9.

Lister GD, Kalisman M, Tsai TM. Reconstruction of the hand with free microneurovascular toe-to-hand transfer: experience with 54 toe transfers. Plast Reconstr Surg 1983; 71: 372- 384.

Mathes SJ. Great toe (hallux) flap. In Mathes SJ, Nahai F, Eds. Reconstructive surgery: principles, anatomy, and technique. New York: Churchill Livingstone, 1997: 891-925.

May JW. Microvascular great toe to hand transfer for reconstruction of the amputated thumb. In McCarthy JG, May JW, Littler JW Eds. Plastic Surgery. Philadelphia: WB Saunders Co, 1990: 5183-5185.

May JW, Chait LA, Cohen BE, O'Brien BM. Free neurovascular flap from the first web of the foot in hand reconstruction. J Hand Surg 1977; 2: 387.

Morrison WA. The great toe wrap-around flap. In Serafin D, Ed. Atlas of microsurgical composite tissue transplantation. Philadelphia: WB Saunders Company. 1996:131-135.

Salmins S. In Williams PL, Ed. Gray's Anatomy. 38th Edition. Toronto: Churchill-Livingstone, 1999: 375-424.

Tsai TM, Wang WZ. Vascularized joint transfers. Hand Clinics 1992; 8: 525-536.

Wei FC. Tissue preservation in hand injury: the first step to toe-to-hand transplantation. Plast Reconstr Surg 1998; 102: 2497-2501.

Wei FC, Chen HC, Chuang CC, Chen SHT. Microsurgical thumb reconstruction with toe transfer: Selection of various techniques. Plast Reconstr Surg 1994; 93: 345-357.

Wei FC, Chen HC, Chuang CC, Noordhoff MS. Reconstruction of the thumb with a trimmed-toe transfer. Plast Reconstr Surg 1988; 82: 506-513.

Wei FC, Colony LH. Microsurgical reconstruction if opposable digits in mutilating hand injuries. Clin Plast Surg 1989; 16: 491.

Wei FC, Colony LH, Chen HC, Chuang CC, Noordhoff MS. Combined second and third toe transfer. Plast Reconstr Surg1989; 86: 651-661.

Wei FC, El-Gammal TA. Toe-to-hand transfer. Clin Plast Surg 1996; 23: 103-116.

Wei FC, El-Gammal TA, Lin CH, Chung CC, Chen HC, Chen SHT. Metacarpal hand: classification and guidelines for microsurgical reconstruction with toe transfers. Plast Reconstr Surg 1997; 99: 122-128.

Wei FC, Ma HS. Delayed sensory reeducation after toe-to-hand transfer. Microsurgery 1995; 16: 583-585.

Wei FC, Santamaria E. Toe-to-finger reconstruction. In Green DP, Hotchkiss RN, Pederson WC, Eds. Green's Operative Hand Surgery, Fourth Ed. Philadelphia: Churchill Livingstone. 1999:1327-1353.

Wei FC, Silverman RT, Hsu WM. Retrograde dissection of the vascular pedicle in toe harvest. Plast Reconstr Surg 1995; 96: 1211-4.

Wei FC, Yim KK. Pulp plasty after toe-to-hand transplantation. Plast Reconstr Surg 1995; 96: 661.

Woo, SH, Kim JS, Seul JH. Immediate toe-to-hand transfer in acute hand injuries: overall results, compared with results for elective cases. Plast Reconstr Surg 2004; 113: 882-892.

Yim KK, Wei FC. Secondary procedures to improve function after toe-to-hand transfers. Br J Plast Surg 1995; 48: 487-491.

Yim, KK, Wei, FC, Lin, CH. A comparison between primary and secondary toe-to-hand transplantation. Plast Reconstr Surg 2004; 114: 107-12.

NERVE INJURY/REPAIR

Jules Feledy, Jr MD and Michel Saint-Cyr, MD

I Anatomy of Peripheral Nerves

○   **What are the basic elements of the peripheral nerves?**

- internal epineurium
- external epineurium
- perineurium
- endoneurium

○   **What are the functions of the internal and external epineurium?**

The external epineurium surrounds the entire nerve and internal epineurium surrounds groups of fascicles.

○   **Which layer is an extension of the blood brain barrier?**

The perineurium. This layer has closely packed cells and surrounds individual fascicle which functions to block the spread of infection and to maintain a positive intrafascicular pressure.

○   **The layer which surrounds individual axons is termed?**

The endoneurium.

○   **What is a fascicular plexus?**

A region of interconnections between fascicles.

○   **How is the nerve potential propagated down the nerve?**

Depolarizing current achieving the threshold membrane potential leads to activation of voltage-gated sodium channels.

○   **What is a Node of Ranvier?**

A gap which represents a space between adjacent Schwann cells along the length of the axon.

○   **What is saltatory conduction?**

Propagation of the action potential via depolarization at the nodes of Ranvier (myelinated fibers 3-150m/s).

○   **What is the function of the neuromuscular junction?**

Transduce impulses across a synapse

○   **What is Wallerian degeneration?**

A process by which axoplasm and myelin are degraded and removed by phagocytosis

○   **What are key features of Wallerian degeneration?**

1. Granular disintegration of axoplasmic microtubules and neurofilaments
2. Disappearance of myelin sheath and axons distal to a nerve lesion
3. Loss of neural conductance within 48-96hrs
4. Axonometsis (Sunderland 2nd degree)

❍ **After laceration or injury to the nerve, Wallerian degeneration occurs in which segment?**

Distal segment

❍ **What are the Bands of Bungner?**

Collapsed columns of Schwann cells in the distal segment of a complete nerve injury

❍ **What is neurotrophism?**

The ability of appropriate distal receptors to enhance the maturation of nerve fibers, which includes the production of a gradient of diffusible substances that direct axonal growth during regeneration.

II Nerve Repair Classification and Assessment

❍ **How are nerve injuries classified (Sunderland based)?**

First-degree or Neuropraxia	Segmental demyelination
Second-degree or Axonotmesis	Axonal Injury
Third-degree combined with fibrosis of the endoneurium	Wallerian degeneration
Fourth-degree	Complete scar block
Fifth-degree or Neurotmesis	Transection
Sixth-degree	Combination of I-V injuries

❍ **How is fibrosis resulting from nerve injuries classified (Millesi)?**

Type I   Fibrosis of the epineurium
Type II   Interfascicular fibrosis
Type III Intrafascicular fibrosis

❍ **Which types of injuries can be expected to have complete recovery?**

Neuropraxia and Axonotmesis

❍ **Nerve fiber regeneration occurs at what rate?**

1 millimeter per day or 1 inch per month

❍ **What are clinical measurements of motor nerve injury?**

Weakness, loss of function, and atrophy

❍ **What are clinical measurements of sensory nerve injury?**

• Moving and static two-point discrimination for <u>innervation density</u> and number of fibers
• Semmes-Weinstein monofilaments and vibration instruments as <u>threshold tests</u> for performance levels

❍ **Describe and classify the six levels of motor recovery following motor nerve injury.**

- M0 no contraction
- M1 contraction in proximal muscles
- M2 contraction in distal muscles
- M3 contraction sufficient to resist gravity
- M4 contraction against strong resistance
- M5 return to full muscle strength

❍   **Describe and classify the six levels of sensory recovery following sensory nerve injury.**

S0 absence of sensibility
S1 deep pain sensibility
S2 superficial sensibility
S3 full recovery of pain and touch (moving 2PD > 15mm)
S3+ localization of stimulus (moving and static 2PD 7-15mm)
S4 complete recovery (2PD 3-6mm)

❍   **What does an "advancing Tinel's sign" after nerve injury signify?**

Effect of triggered electric-current like pain represents <u>outgrowing axon sprout ends</u>

❍   **What is the most sensitive test for eliciting nerve compression syndromes with demyelination?**

Nerve conduction velocity (NCV) tests

❍   **What is the most helpful test for eliciting a denervation with axonal loss?**

Electromyography (EMG)

❍   **What is the earliest that EMG studies will be helpful to evaluate a patient for a suspected peripheral nerve injury?**

Three weeks

❍   **Which imaging study is helpful in diagnosing injuries to peripheral nerves?**

Magnetic resonance imaging (MRI) neurograms

❍   **Which test is useful in helping to distinguish proximal and distal injuries?**

Somatosensory Evoked Potentials (SSEP)

III   Treatment of Nerve Injuries

❍   **What repair method is used when a nerve is partially transected and landmarks are preserved?**

Epineural repair

❍   **What repair method is generally used when a nerve injury includes a crushing component?**

Group fascicular repair

❍   **What repair method is generally used when there is a delayed repair requiring trimming of the nerve ends?**

Group fascicular repair

❍　**In an acute crush injury setting with evidence of transection and contusion of a peripheral nerve, what is the recommended treatment?**

Tagging the proximal and distal nerve endings followed by delayed repair after 3 weeks or until the wound permits

❍　**What is the advantage of early secondary nerve repair?**

Allows for terminated scar reaction along the nerve which the surgeon can estimate and graft

❍　**Have clinical studies demonstrated that fascicular repair is superior to epineural repair?**

No.

❍　**Nerve elongation in secondary nerve repairs can provide how much additional length**

Approximately 10%

❍　**Name six different types of nerve grafts.**

- Trunk graft
- Cable graft
- Pedicle nerve graft
- Interfascicular nerve graft
- Fascicular nerve graft
- Free vascularized nerve graft

❍　**What is the best way to treat segmental peripheral nerve injuries?**

Autogenous nerve grafts

❍　**Sural nerve grafts can be harvested up to how many centimeters?**

35-40 cm

❍　**Harvest of the sural nerve results in a sensory deficit in which region?**

Lateral aspect of dorsum of foot

❍　**Reverse vein autograft <u>conduits</u> can be used for defects less than how many centimeters in the forearm?**

Up to 3 cm

❍　**What is a non-suture method used in nerve coaptation?**

Fibrin glue

❍　**Collagen conduits can be used for defects less than how many centimeters in the forearm?**

2 cm

❍　**Synthetic grafts which incorporate combinations of synthetic hydrogels, biologic materials, extracellular matrix components, and neurotrophic factors are also termed?**

Axonal guidance channels

❍　**Failure of the nerve growth cone to reach its peripheral targets causes which conditions?**

Terminal neuroma or neuroma *in situ*

○ **The major treatment methods for treating neuromas include?**

- excision and repair
- embedding in muscle
- proximal ligation

○ **The overall success rate for burying neuromas is?**

Approximately 75%

○ **What is a nerve transfer?**

Transfer of a the proximal portion of an intact donor nerve to reinnervate the distal portion of a more important, injured nerve

IV   Peripheral Nerve Entrapment Syndromes

○ **What does the surgical treatment of entrapment syndromes consist of?**

Decompression and/or neurolysis

○ **What is the term given to compression of structures at the thoracic outlet?**

Thoracic Outlet Syndrome

○ **The interscalene triangle borders consist of which structures?**

- anterior scalene muscle anteriorly
- middle scalene muscle posteriorly
- medial surface of the first rib inferiorly

○ **The most common brachial plexus trunks involved in Thoracic Outlet Syndrome?**

C8 and T1

○ **Clinical maneuvers to diagnose Thoracic Outlet Syndrome include?**

- Adson or Scalene Test
- Costoclavicular or Military Test
- Hyperabduction Test
- Roos Test

○ **The supraclavicular approach for surgical treatment of Thoracic Outlet Syndrome endangers which nerve?**

The phrenic nerve

○ **The transaxillary approach for surgical treatment of Thoracic Outlet Syndrome endangers which nerve?**

The C8 or T1 nerve root

○ **Suprascapular nerve entrapment may cause pain, weakness, and even atrophy of which muscles?**

Supraspinatus and Infraspinatus

❍ **What is the most common anatomic site for suprascapular nerve entrapment?**

Suprascapular notch

❍ **The surgical treatment of suprascapular nerve entrapment consists of the release of which structure?**

Transverse scapular ligament

❍ **The two most common sites of ulnar nerve entrapment are located where?**

- Cubital Tunnel proximal to the elbow
- Guyon's Canal in the wrist

❍ **Inability to adduct the thumb without flexing the tip of the thumb is termed?**

Froment's Sign

❍ **Inability to adduct the little finger secondary to hypothenar and interossei atrophy is termed?**

Wartenberg's Sign

❍ **Hypothenar atrophy is secondary to compression or palsy of which nerve?**

Ulnar nerve

❍ **Surgical options for release of ulnar nerve compression at the elbow include?**

- simple decompression
- medial epicondylectomy
- anterior transposition (subcutaneous vs. intramuscular vs. submuscular)
- endoscopic decompression
- combinations of the above

❍ **As the ulnar nerve travels down the forearm, where is it positioned?**

Between the FDS and the FDP muscle bellies

❍ **The motor fascicular group of the ulnar nerve at the wrist is located in which position?**

Ulnar and dorsal.
Just remember that the motor branch of the ulnar nerve is the deep branch; so deep=more dorsal.

❍ **Fractures from which bone can impinge on the ulnar nerve at Guyon's Canal?**

Hamate via fracture of the hook segment (hamulus)

❍ **Laceration of the ulnar nerve in the distal forearm will result in the loss of which muscle groups?**

- interossei
- ulnar two lumbricals
- hypothenar muscles
- thumb adductor
- half of the thumb flexor brevis

❍ **Clawing of the hand is found with which types of ulnar nerve injuries?**

Low (distal) ulnar nerve injuries

❍ **Why does the hand claw with low ulnar nerve injuries?**

Unopposed FDP flexion of the IP joints and unopposed extension of the MP joints

❍ **What finding distinguishes a neuropathy of the ulnar nerve at the elbow from that at the wrist?**

Decreased sensation in the dorso-ulnar hand

❍ **What is the anatomic basis for the decreased sensation in the dorso-ulnar hand?**

The dorsal sensory branch of the ulnar nerve branches approximately 8 cm proximal to the pisiform. Thus, it is unaffected by compression at the wrist but its fascicles are still with the main ulnar nerve at the elbow.

❍ **What are sites of compression of the median nerve that cause pronator syndrome?**

- Ligament of Struthers
- Lacertus fibrosus (bicipital aponeurosis)
- pronator teres (musculofascial band or compression between two muscular heads)
- FDS proximal arch

❍ **What are the anatomic borders of the carpal tunnel?**

- carpal bones (floor)
- transverse carpal ligament (roof)
- scaphoid and trapezium radially
- pisiform and hook of the hamate ulnarly

❍ **The motor fascicular group of the median nerve at the wrist is located in which position?**

Radial and volar. Just remember that the recurrent motor (muscular) branch branches off radially toward the thenar muscle group.

❍ **Thenar atrophy is secondary to compression or palsy of which nerve?**

Median nerve

❍ **What is an important symptom to help distinguish the pronator syndrome from the carpal tunnel syndrome?**

Pain in the proximal palm

❍ **What is the anatomic basis for the above difference?**

The palmar cutaneous branch of the median nerve branches proximal to the wrist and is thus spared compression by the transverse carpal ligament.

❍ **A splint to minimize pressure within the carpal canal would be designed with how much wrist and finger extension/flexion?**

Wrist neutral and fingers in extension

❍ **A characteristic symptom of anterior interosseous syndrome is?**

Inability to form a circle by pinching the thumb and index finger (O sign)

○ **What is the anatomic basis for the above finding?**

The AIN provides motor innervation to the <u>FPL (thumb IP flexion)</u> and the <u>index and long FDP (index DIP flexion)</u>. You can't make an "O" without thumb IP and index DIP flexion. Incidentally, AIN also innervates the PQ.

○ **Does the anterior interosseous syndrome have any sensory component?**

No, motor only

○ **What is Gantzer's muscle?**

Accessory head of the FPL

○ **What is innervation through a Martin-Gruber anastomosis?**

Median to ulnar nerve in the <u>forearm</u>. Remember F.M.G. or **F**oreign **M**edical **G**raduate. (**F**orearm-**M**artin-**G**ruber).

○ **What is innervation through a Riche-Cannieu anastomosis?**

Median to ulnar nerve in the <u>hand</u>

○ **The radial nerve is derived from which cord of the brachial plexus?**

Posterior cord

○ **The most common site of compression of the radial nerve occurs at?**

The Arcade of Frohse, proximal fibrous edge of the supinator muscle. Remember the RAF or **R**oyal **A**ir **F**orce. (**R**adial Nerve-**A**rcade of **F**rohse).

○ **Other sites of compression of the radial nerve include?**

- Fibrous fascia over the radiocapitellar joint
- Vascular leash of Henry (radial recurrent artery) Remember RVH or **R**ight **V**entricular **H**ypertrophy. (**R**adial Nerve-**V**ascular leash of **H**enry)
- medial border of ECRB
- distal border of the supinator

○ **Pain and tenderness in the dorsal lateral forearm is most consistently associated with which compression syndrome?**

Radial tunnel syndrome

○ **What are symptoms commonly associated with posterior interosseous nerve syndrome?**

- pain in the upper extensor forearm
- dysesthesias in a superficial radial nerve distribution
- weakening of the extension of the fingers, thumb, or wrist

○ **Compression of the superficial radial nerve as it emerges from under the brachioradialis is termed?**

Wartenberg's Syndrome

○ **What structures pass through the tarsal tunnel?**

- tendons of the flexor hallucis longus muscle
- flexor digitorum longus muscle
- tibialis posterior muscle
- posterior tibial nerve
- posterior tibial artery

○ **Release of which structure is performed to decompress the tarsal tunnel?**

Flexor retinaculum (which is the roof of the tunnel).

○ **Erectile dysfunction following radical prostatectomy is considered to be largely neurogenic in origin; what is the origin of the fibers of the cavernous nerves?**

Parasympathetic fibers from S2-S4

○ **What is the location of the cavernous nerves in relation to the prostate?**

Within the cavernous nerve bundles along the posterolateral surface of the prostate, which corresponds anatomically to the peripheral zone, the most common site of prostate carcinogenesis

○ **What are common strategies to preserve erectile function after radical prostatectomy?**

Nerve-sparing radical prostatectomy
Cavernous nerve interposition grafting
Neurotrophic treatment

○ **What is the most common nerve graft used in cavernous nerve interposition grafting?**

Sural nerve

○ **What is the reported efficacy, or return of erectile function, for unilateral cavernous interposition nerve grafting? For bilateral cavernous interposition nerve grafting?**

Unilateral – approximately 50%
Bilateral – approximately 25%

○ **Spontaneous erectile activity following cavernous nerve regeneration has been observed how many months following surgery?**

5-8 months for mild tumescence
14-18 months for erectile activity

○ **What is the estimated probability of being able to have intercourse at 16 months?**

25%

References

Chang DW, Wood CG, Kroll SS, et al. Cavernous nerve reconstruction to preserve erectile function following non-nerve-sparing radical retropubic prostatectomy: a prospective study. Plast Reconstr Surg, 111: 1174-1181, 2003.

Mackinnon SE. Pathophysiology of nerve compression. Hand Clin. 18: 231-41, 2002.

Mackinnon SE, and Novak CB. Thoracic outlet syndrome. Curr Probl Surg. 39: 1070-145, 2002.

Penkert G, and Fansa H. Peripheral nerve lesions: nerve surgery and secondary reconstructive repair. 1st ed., Springer Verlag, Inc., NY, 2004.

Rummler LS, and Gupta R. Peripheral nerve repair: a review. Curr Opin Orthop, 15: 215-219, 2004.

Szabo, RM. Entrapment and compression neuropathies. In Green DP, Hotchkiss RN, Pederson WC (ed): Green's Operative Hand Surgery, 4th ed. Churchill Livingstone, NY, 1999.

HEAD AND NECK REGION

FACIAL TRAUMA

Ajaipal S. Kang, MD

○ **In a patient with panfacial fracture in a motor vehicle collision, what is the risk for cervical spine injury?**

The risk for cervical spine injury is closest to 10%.

FRONTAL SINUS

○ **What is the most important factor that determines the need for an urgent operation in a patient with a frontal sinus fracture?**

The integrity of the <u>posterior table</u>. A patient with a fracture of the <u>posterior table</u> should have urgent neurosurgical evaluation followed by an operation.

○ **During intra-operative evaluation of frontal sinus fracture, how do you check the adequacy of drainage?**

Intraoperative instillation of methylene blue into the sinus and its unobstructed flow into the nasal cavity indicates an intact and functional sinus.

○ **How would you treat a severely comminuted fracture of the posterior table?**

With cranialization of the frontal sinus, involving removal of the posterior wall. The intracranial contents (dura and brain) gradually expand to fill the open space. Also the mucosa is stripped, dural tears repaired and nasofrontal ducts plugged with fat, bone or a pericranial flap.

○ **Why is the mucosa stripped?**

To avoid the late complication of mucocele.

○ **Why are dural tears repaired?**

To avoid the complication of meningitis.

○ **Is there an alternative to plate and screw fixation in treatment of displaced anterior table of frontal sinus fracture?**

Yes, in case of thin bone fragments, cyanoacrylates (glues) such as butyl-2-cyanoacrylate provide comparable stability to plate and screw fixation.

○ **Name some advantages of glue fixation.**

Cyanoacrylates do not impede bone healing, need less operative time than plates and screws fixation, eliminate the need to contour plates and set within seconds.

○ **Name the common acute, subacute and chronic complications of frontal sinus fractures?**

<u>Acute</u>: Epistaxis, CSF leak, meningitis, and intracranial injury.
<u>Subacute</u>: Frontal sinusitis, mucocele, and meningitis.
<u>Chronic</u>: Osteomyelitis, mucocele, and intracranial or orbital abscesses.

ORBIT

○ **What are the bones of the orbit?**

1. Zygoma-most of the lateral wall and floor
2. Frontal-the roof and some of the lateral wall
3. Greater wing of the sphenoid-borders the superior and inferior orbital fissures
4. Lesser wing of the sphenoid
5. Maxilla-orbital floor (realize that the "roof" of the maxillary sinus is just on the otherside of the maxilla
6. Ethmoid-most of the medial wall
7. Lacrimal-part of the medial wall
8. Palatine-a tiny contribution from the palatine bone's orbital process.

○ **What bones border the lacrimal groove?**

The lacrimal bone posteriorly and maxilla anteriorly.

○ **What bone does Whitnall's tubercle lie on?**

The zygoma. Specifically, the frontal process of the zygoma about 5-10 mm from the lateral rim. The lateral canthal ligament attaches here.

○ **Where does the medial canthal ligament attach?**

The frontal process of the maxilla.

○ **What bone contains the optic canal?**

Lesser wing of the sphenoid.

○ **What bone does the superior oblique muscle originate on?**

The frontal bone. Specifically the trochlea.

○ **What bone does the inferior oblique muscle originate on?**

The maxilla.

○ **What are the common operative indications in case of an orbital blowout fracture?**

1. Orbital floor defect > 2 cm
2. Low vertical height of globe
3. Need to treat other fractures
4. Positive forced duction testing

○ **Discuss the transconjunctival approach to orbital floor fracture?**

Incision of capsulopalpebral fascia, entry into a plane between orbicularis oculi and orbital septum followed by periosteum incision along the infraorbital rim to expose the fracture.

○ **What is the direct pupillary response to light?**

The pupil <u>constricts in response to direct light</u> indicating intact function of the ipsilateral optic nerve and parasympathetics traveling along CN III.

❍   **What is the consensual response to light?**

The pupil <u>constricts when the contralateral pupil is illuminated</u> indicating intact function of the contralateral optic nerve (the one being illuminated) and the ipsilateral parasympathetic fibers in CN III (the one not being illuminated).

❍   **What is accommodation?**

Both pupils constrict when fixating on an object being moved towards them. Failure of a pupil to constrict indicates a problem on that sides optic nerve or parasympathetics in CN III.

❍   **What are the clinical findings in injury of ocular parasympathetic fibers during fracture reduction?**

Absence of direct and consensual responses to light and inability to constrict the pupil is noted. The parasympathetic fibers travel with the oculomotor nerve and can be injured during reduction of fractures.

❍   **What are the clinical findings in injury of optic nerve during fracture reduction?**

The most important finding is an <u>afferent pupillary defect</u>.

❍   **What is the afferent pupillary defect?**

Normally both pupils will alternately constrict and relax as a light is moved between them, with both pupils constricting as either one is illuminated and both pupils relaxing as the light moves between them.
If the <u>optic nerve</u> in a given eye is damaged, its consensual response will overcome its direct response and remain intact. Thus, the affected pupil constricts when the unaffected eye is illuminated (intact consensual response) but it <u>will paradoxically dilate when illuminated itself since it is being driven by the unaffected eye's (which is no longer being illuminated) consensual signal to dilate.</u>

❍   **What are the clinical findings in Marcus-Gunn pupil?**

The direct response to light is impaired but consensual response is preserved. Sound familiar? <u>It's just another name for an afferent pupillary defect.</u>

❍   **What is the mechanism of a carotid-cavernous fistula?**

Fractures of the orbital roof and middle cranial fossa allow a communication between the carotid artery and cavernous sinus. The result:
- Pulsating exophthalmos
- Associated bruit
- Blindness

ZYGOMA

❍   **Is OZMC fracture really a "tripod" fracture?**

No. This term is a misnomer as it's in fact a "tetrapod" since 4 processes are involved.

❍   **What are the four regions associated with OZMC fractures?**

1.   <u>Infraorbital rim</u> extending into floor medial to the zygomaticomaxillary suture often through the infraorbital foramen

2. <u>Lateral orbital wall</u> through the zygomaticofrontal suture extending inferiorly along the zygomaticosphenoid suture
3. <u>Zygomaticomaxillary buttress</u>-(look at a skull from the inferoposterior perspective)
4. <u>Zygomatic arch</u>-usually posterior to the zygomaticotemporal suture (a very thin, weak point along the arch)

❍ **Which anatomic landmark ensures accurate reduction of an OZMC fracture?**

<u>Lateral orbital wall</u> is the most important landmark.

❍ **What is the most common direction of displacement of OZMC fractures? How does this affect the palpebral fissure?**

Depressed and displaced laterally. Since the lateral canthus is attached to Whitnall's tubercle, the palpebral fissures pulled into a downward cant ("antimongoloid" slant).

❍ **What would be an indication for emergent ophthalmologic consultation in a patient with OZMC fracture?**

1. Blindness or blurred vision
2. Retrobulbar hematoma
3. Globe rupture
4. Eye pain
5. Hyphema, or blood within the anterior chamber

❍ **How can you prevent malar fat pad ptosis secondary to zygomatic fracture reduction?**

It can be prevented by performing <u>periosteal resuspension</u> of overlying soft tissue after reduction of the fracture.

❍ **What is the most common indication for zygomatic osteotomies?**

A post-panfacial fracture patient with persistent decreased malar projection is a candidate for this procedure.

❍ **For an isolated fracture of the zygomatic arch being treated with temporal (Gillies') approach, where should the instrument be passed for appropriate reduction?**

The incision is made in the temporal scalp and dissection proceeds through subcutaneous tissue, the superficial temporal fascia and deep temporal fascia. An elevating instrument is passed <u>between the deep temporal fascia and the temporalis muscle</u> and passed deep to the arch.

❍ **What about the "deep layer of the deep fascia" and the "superficial layer of the deep fascia"?**

It is critical to understand that <u>the deep temporal fascia doesn't divide into its deep and superficial layers until about 2 cm superior to the helical rim</u>. Cranial to that level, the only layers are the superficial temporal fascia (continuous with the SMAS) and the deep temporal fascia.

❍ **What is the most common cause of post-reduction persistent enophthalmos?**

Inadequate fracture reduction leading to <u>increased bony orbital volume</u> results in persistent enophthalmos.

❍ **What is the Superior Orbital Fissure Syndrome?**

It is a rare complication of high-velocity fractures extending into the superior orbital fissure.
- Eyelid ptosis
- Globe proptosis
- Ophthalmoplegia (paralysis of CN 3, 4, 6)
- Mydriasis (dilated pupil)

- Anesthesia in CN V1 distribution

○ **What is the anatomical basis for superior orbital fissure syndrome (SOFS)?**

- Eyelid ptosis-CN 3
- Globe proptosis-altered orbital volume or retrobulbar hemorrhage
- Ophthalmoplegia (paralysis of CN 3, 4, 6)
- Mydriasis (dilated pupil)-blocked parasympathetic outflow
- Anesthesia in CN V1 distribution-ophthalmic division CV 5

Anatomically, oculomotor (III), trochlear (IV), and abducens (VI) nerves, and the ophthalmic division of the trigeminal nerve (V1) pass through this fissure.

○ **What is Orbital Apex Syndrome?**

The findings are the same as in SOFS as well as <u>blindness secondary to optic nerve</u> involvement.

○ **Which fixation material causes the minimal scatter on a CT scan?**

<u>Lactasorb,</u> the nonmetallic copolymer of polylactic acid and L-glycolic acid causes the least scatter. <u>Among metals,</u> <u>titanium</u> causes the least scatter on CT scan.

○ **Which nerve injury results in cheek numbness following an orbital blowout fracture?**

Injury of infraorbital nerve, a branch of the maxillary division of the trigeminal nerve (V2).

○ **What is the typical presentation of patients with medial orbital wall fractures?**

- Enophthalmos
- Ipsilateral epistaxis
- Subcutaneous emphysema
- Periorbital ecchymosis

○ **What is the anatomic reason for subcutaneous emphysema?**

Fracture through the ethmoid's extremely thin *lamina papyracea* into the ethmoid air sinuses.

○ **What is the most common cause of posttraumatic enophthalmos?**

Increased bony orbital volume.

○ **What is the ideal location of subciliary incision for lowering the chances of post-operative ectropion?**

Incision into the first eyelid crease is recommended because it <u>preserves the innervation of pretarsal orbicularis oculi</u> and thus, maintains normal eyelid tone.

NASAL

○ **What are the most common types of facial fracture in children?**

Nasal fractures are most common type of facial fracture in children.
Mandibular fractures are the second most common type.

○ **What is the common sequela of an undiagnosed septal hematoma following nasal fracture?**

Undetected septal hematomas can cause pressure necrosis of the nasal mucosa and cartilage and lead to septal perforation.

❍   **How do you manage an acute septal hematoma?**

Following a nasal speculum examination, a #11 blade or a #16-18 needle and syringe can be used to drain the hematoma.

❍   **Outline the presentation and management of a patient with naso-orbito-ethmoid (NOE) fracture?**

- These patients have extensive comminution of the medial orbital walls, ethmoid sinus, frontal process of the maxilla and nasal bones.
- Classic findings include **telecanthus** and a **saddle nose deformity**.
- Management involves ORIF through a coronal approach.
- A **cantilever bone graft** may also be required to address the nasal deformity.
- **Transnasal canthopexy** and accurate reduction of the large fracture fragments containing the medial canthal tendons is key to managing the telecanthus.

❍   **What is the difference between telecanthus and hypertelorism?**

Hypertelorism is defined by the interorbital distance based on bony measurements between the two medial orbital walls. Typically congenital causes predominate.
Telecanthus is defined by the intercanthal distance and indicates displacement of the canthal bearing segments of the maxilla laterally. The relative positions of the orbits are normal.

❍   **How many types of naso-orbito-ethmoid fractures exist?**

Naso-orbito-ethmoid (NOE) fractures can be classified into three types based on the central segment that bears the medial canthal tendon.
- Type I is a simple fracture of central segment.
- Type II involves comminution of the central segment.
- Type III is avulsion of the attachment of the medial canthal tendon.

MAXILLA

❍   **What are the classic physical finding in a patient with a Le Fort I, II and III fractures?**

Le Fort I fracture-movement at the lower portion of the maxilla, but not at the nasal root (a maxillary rock).
Le Fort II patients have movement at the nasal root and a step deformity at the infraorbital rim. Bilateral circumorbital and subconjunctival ecchymosis are also typical.
In a Le Fort III fracture, the facial bone complex is disconnected from the cranium (a.k.a. craniofacial disjunction).

❍   **Which anatomic structure is most commonly affected in Le Fort I fractures?**

The pterygoid plate is most likely to be affected because it forms the most posterior aspect of the fracture.

❍   **So is the pterygoid plate fractured in LeFort I osteotomies during orthognathic surgery?**

No. In an elective osteotomy, a pterygomaxillary disjunction is performed to free the maxilla.

❍   **What is the most important principal in repair of LeFort I fracture?**

The most important principal is re-establishing the pretraumatic maxillomandibular occlusion. The fracture needs to be disimpacted before rigid fixation is applied.

MANDIBLE

○ **Which permanent tooth bud is at greatest risk of injury during rigid fixation in a child in mixed dentition?**

The canine is at greatest risk of injury.

○ **Which permanent teeth are the first to erupt in a child?**

The first molars generally erupt between ages 6 and 7 years.

○ **Name the site of mandibular fracture associated with future growth abnormalities in children.**

The fracture of <u>mandibular condyle, a primary growth center,</u> is associated with growth abnormalities.

○ **Is this a common place for children to fracture their mandibles?**

Extremely common. About 66% of mandibular fractures in children under 10 years old occur at the condyle, probably due to its thin cross-section.

○ **What is the most common facial fracture in children?**

<u>Nasal bone fractures</u> followed by mandible fractures.

○ **What are the most common sites of mandible fracture in adults?**

A.B.C. **A**ngle, **B**ody, **C**ondyle.

○ **What are indications for extracting teeth in a patient with a fracture?**

- A displaced or comminuted fracture of the mandible containing a tooth
- Fracture of the tooth itself or its root structure
- Periodontal disease of the supporting structures
- A functionless tooth without an opposing tooth
- Complete displacement of the tooth from its socket

○ **What nerve injury leads to lower lip numbness following mandibular fracture?**

Injury of <u>inferior alveolar nerve</u> from fractures of the mandibular body results in numbness of the lower lip.

○ **In cases of condylar neck fractures, what muscle is responsible for medial displacement of the proximal fragment?**

The lateral pterygoid muscle causes displacement of the proximal fracture fragment.

○ **What are the origins and insertions of muscles of mastication?**

<u>Temporalis:</u> Infratemporal fossa of the temporal bone and the coronoid process.
<u>Masseter:</u> Zygomatic arch and inferior lateral portion of the mandibular angle & body. <u>Medial pterygoid:</u> Pterygoid fossa and medial surface of the mandibular angle & ramus. <u>Lateral pterygoid:</u> Inferior head - lateral pterygoid plate and neck of condyle; Superior head - infratemporal crest and capsule and articular disk of TMJ.

○ **How do unilateral condylar fractures present? How do bilateral fractures present?**

Presentation for unilateral fracture includes malocclusion, pain, loss of posterior ramus height ipsilaterally, ipsilateral premature contact of the molars posteriorly, an ipsilateral upward cant and a <u>contralateral open bite</u>.

Bilateral condylar fractures present with <u>anterior open bite</u>, bilaterally decreased posterior facial height and pain.

○ **What are the common indications of open reduction of condylar fractures?**

- Displacement into the middle cranial fossa
- Inability of obtaining adequate dental occlusion by closed reduction
- Lateral extracapsular displacement of the condyle
- Invasion by a foreign body

○ **Outline the anatomy of the temporomandibular joint (TMJ).**

The <u>articular disk</u> separates the joint space into upper and lower spaces. At rest and during rotation, the mandibular condyle is located in lower joint space while during translation, the condyle moves into upper joint space.

○ **What is the maximal normal vertical incisal opening (interocclusal distance)?**

- 3.5 cm to 5 cm is maximal.
- The initial 1 cm to 2 cm of jaw opening involves <u>rotatory movements </u>(lower joint space).
- From 2 cm to 3 cm of jaw opening there is a combination of <u>rotation and translation</u>.
- The final 3 cm to 5 cm of jaw opening involves <u>translatory</u> movements only.

○ **What is the daily optimal distance of distraction osteogenesis of the mandible?**

A daily distraction rate of 1.0 mm has been shown to be optimal.

○ **What is the optimal management of coronoid fractures?**

An isolated non-displaced coronoid fracture is treated with short-term maxillomandibular fixation. Following removal of fixation, physical therapy is needed.

○ **How is the maxillomandibular relationship determined in an edentulous patient with displaced mandibular fractures?**

Custom-fabricated intraoral splints or the patient's own dentures can be rigidly fixed to the maxilla and mandible using wire or screws.

○ **In a patient with combined fractures of midface and mandible, what is the order of repair?**

The mandible is reduced first to <u>establish the posterior height of the face</u> followed by midface as long as the condylar head or high condylar neck is not fractured. If they are fractured, the mandible can't be used as a guide to posterior facial height and the midface should be treated first.

○ **When should external fixators be used for mandible fractures?**

External fixators are used in patients with comminuted mandible fractures or cases where medical instability precludes early ORIF.

○ **What is the anatomical site of mental foramen?**

The mental nerve exits the mental foramen below the second premolar, halfway down the mandible.

○ **What is the most common cause of posttraumatic opening click of the temporomandibular joint?**

The most common cause is subluxation of the articular disk.

○ **How do you handle acute infections following ORIF if hardware is stable?**

If hardware is stable, it is left in place and infection is treated with operative drainage and antibiotic therapy. If hardware is loose, appropriate management includes removal and replacement of the hardware with intermaxillary or external fixation.

References

Frontal Sinus

Dufresne CR, Manson PN. Pediatric facial trauma. In: McCarthy JG, ed. *Plastic Surgery*. Philadelphia, Pa: WB Saunders Co; 1990;2:1142-1187.

Rohrich RJ, Hollier LH. Management of frontal sinus fractures: changing concepts. Clin Plast Surg. 1992;19:219-232.

Wolfe SA, Johnson P. Frontal sinus injuries: primary care and management of late complications. Plast Reconstr Surg. 1988;82:781-791.

Gosain AK, Lyon VB. Use of tissue glue: current status. Perspectives in Plastic Surgery. 2001;15:129-145.

Orbit

Manson PN. Facial fractures. In: Aston SJ, Beasley RW, Thorne CH, eds. Grabb & Smith's Plastic Surgery. 5th ed. Philadelphia, Pa: Lippincott-Raven; 1997:383-412.

Manson PN, Iliff N. Management of blow out fractures of the orbital floor. Surg

Kelly KJ. Pediatric facial trauma. In: Achauer BM, Eriksson E, Guyuron B, et al, eds. Plastic Surgery: Indications, Operations, and Outcomes. Saint Louis, Mo: Mosby Ð Year Book, Inc; 2000;2:941-969.

Lettieri S. Facial trauma. In: Achauer BM, Erikson E, Guyuron B, et al, eds. Plastic Surgery: Indications, Operations, and Outcomes. Saint Louis, Mo: Mosby Ð Year Book, Inc; 2000;2:923-940.

Bite U, Jackson IT, Forbes GS, et al. Orbital volume measurements in enophthalmos using 3-D CT imaging. Plast Reconstr Surg. 1985;75:502..

Nasal/NOE

Pollock RA. Nasal trauma: pathomechanics and surgical management of acute injuries. Clin Plast Surg. 1992;19:133-147.

Markowitz BL, Manson PN, Sargent, L, et al. Management of the medial canthal tendon in nasoethmoid orbital fractures: the importance of the central fragment in classification and treatment. *Plast Reconstr Surg*. 1991;87:843-853.

Le Fort

Yaremchuk MJ. Fractures of the maxilla. In: Cohen, M, ed. *Mastery of Plastic and Reconstructive Surgery*. Boston, Mass: Little, Brown & Co; 1994;2:1156-1164.

Rohrich RJ, Shewmake KB. Evolving concepts of craniomaxillofacial fracture management. Clin Plast Surg. 1992;19:1-10.

Mandible

McGuirt WF, Salisbury PL III. Mandibular fractures: their effect on growth and dentition. Arch Otolaryngol Head Neck Surg. 1987;113:257.

Crawley WA, Sandel AJ. Fractures of the mandible. In: Ferraro JW, ed. Fundamentals of Maxillofacial Surgery. New York, NY: Springer-Verlag; 1997:192-202.

Zide BM. The temporomandibular joint. In: McCarthy JG, ed. *Plastic Surgery*. Philadelphia, Pa: WB Saunders Co; 1990;2:1475-1513.

FACIAL NERVE ANATOMY, PARALYSIS AND TREATMENT

Thomas A. Knipe, MD, and Rakesh K. Chandra, MD

ANATOMY AND EMBRYOLOGY

○ **What branchial arch does the facial nerve innervate?**

The second (hyoid) arch.

○ **What week of gestation do the muscles of facial expression develop?**

The sixth and seventh week.

○ **What cartilage is associated with the second branchial arch?**

Reichert's cartilage.

○ **Which muscles does the facial nerve innervate?**

Stapedius, stylohyoid, posterior belly of digastric and muscles of facial expression

○ **Through which foramen does the facial nerve exit the skull?**

Stylomastoid.

○ **What term is used to describe the network of anastomoses of the extratemporal facial nerve?**

The *pes anserinus.*

○ **What does *pes anserinus* mean?**

The foot of a goose.

○ **What landmarks are used to identify the nerve as it exits the skull?**

The tympanomastoid fissure: 6-8 mm inferior to the drop off of the fissure
The tragal pointer: 1cm anterior and 1cm inferior to the point.
Retrograde dissection of the posterior belly of the digastric muscle

○ **Where does the digastric muscle insert on the skull?**

The medial aspect of the mastoid portion of the temporal bone

○ **What are the extratemporal branches of the facial nerve?**

(Posterior auricular), Temporal, Zygomatic, Buccal, Marginal mandibular, Cervical.
Mnemonic: *To Zanzibar By MotorCar.*

❍   **What explains the fact that the parotid gland envelops the facial nerve within its substance while the marginal mandibular branch lies on the capsule of the submandibular gland?**

Unlike the submandibular gland, the capsule of the parotid gland develops after the facial nerve has coursed through it.

❍   **What important adjacent structures are developing at the same time as the facial nerve?**

The external, middle and inner ear.

❍   **What functional fiber types comprise the facial nerve?**

SVA: taste from anterior 2/3 of tongue via chorda tympani to the nucleus solitarius
SVE: Motor branches to muscles of facial expression, digastric, stapedius and stylohyoid from the motor nucleus
GSA: sensation from the conchal bowl and part of the external auditory canal
GVE: stimulation of lacrimal, submandibular, sublingual gland and minor salivary glands

❍   **What is the blood supply to the facial nerve.**

Stylomastoid artery branch of posterior auricular artery. Greater superficial petrosal artery from the middle meningeal artery.

❍   **What are the eighteen muscles of facial expression?**

Frontalis, Orbicularis oculi, Corrugator supercilii, Procerus, Zygomaticus major and minor, Levator labii superioris, Levator labii superioris alaeque nasi, Levator anguli oris, Nasalis, Buccinator, Depressor septi nasi, orbicularis oris, depressor anguli oris, depressor labii inferioris, Mentalis, Risorius, Platysma.

❍   **What is SMAS?**

Superficial musculoaponeurotic system. It is an inelastic fibrous tissue immediately below the skin and subcutaneous fat of the face which the facial muscles insert. It is contiguous with the platysma inferiorly and the superficial temporal fascia and the galea superiorly.

❍   **Where does the facial nerve course in the parotid region?**

Through the substance of the gland deep to the parotid fascia and SMAS.

❍   **Where do the nerve branches exit the parotid fascia to course superficially?**

At the anterior limit of the parotid gland continuing deep to the SMAS.

❍   **What is the most commonly injured branch of the facial nerve during rhytidectomy?**

The temporal branch at the zygomatic arch.

❍   **Where does the temporal branch cross the zygomatic arch?**

Halfway between the lateral canthus and the root of the auricular helix.

❍   **Between which fascial layers does the frontal nerve course as it crosses the arch?** The branch courses deep to

SMAS and immediately superficial to the superficial layer of deep temporal fascia.

❍   **What fascial layer does the marginal mandibular nerve lay deep to as it crosses the mandible?**

The nerve lies immediately below the superficial layer of the deep cervical fascia, deep to platysma.

FACIAL NERVE PATHOLOGY

○ **Why does a lesion proximal to the motor nucleus of VII produce paralysis of only the lower face, whereas a lesion below the motor nucleus produces complete facial paralysis?**

The lower face receives input from motor tract fibers that have crossed only once in the pons, while the upper face receives input from crossed and uncrossed fibers from the motor tract

○ **What is the House-Brackmann grading system?**

A standard system to evaluate the degree of facial nerve function from 1 (normal) to 6 (complete paralysis).

○ **What is the most common form of idiopathic facial paralysis?**

Bell's Palsy, 15-40 per 100,000.

○ **What percentage of Bell's palsy is recurrent?**

10-14%

○ **What is Bell's Palsy?**

A diagnosis of exclusion, it is idiopathic facial paralysis with sudden onset and spontaneous resolution.

○ **What percentage of Bell's Palsy presents with complete paralysis?**

66%.

○ **Over what time period do the majority of Bell's palsies resolve?**

4-6 months.

○ **What proportion of Bell's Palsy presenting with House Brackmann grade 6 resolve completely?**

70%. More than 90% presenting with incomplete paralysis resolve.

○ **What other characteristics do patients with Bell's palsy often present with?**

Viral prodrome, numbness of the ear, face, neck, dysgeusia, hyperacusis and decreased tearing.

○ **What is Bell's phenomena?**

Upward/outward rotation of the eye with attempted eye closure.

○ **What percentage of patients with Lyme disease develop facial paralysis?**

10%. Paralysis may be bilateral. All resolve with appropriate Lyme disease treatment.

○ **What is the most common cause of bilateral facial paralysis?**

Guillain-Barre.

○ **What is Melkersson-Rosenthal syndrome?**

Syndrome of unknown etiology characterized be recurrent facial nerve paralysis, woody facial edema and a deeply fissured tongue.

○   **What is neuropraxia?**

Compression of a nerve resulting in decreased transmission without disruption of axons

○   **What is axonotmesis?**

Disruption of axons resulting in wallerian degeneration distal to the lesion with preservation of the neural sheaths (complete recovery expected).

○   **What is neurotmesis?**

Disruption of axons and support cells leading to wallerian degeneration and uncertain return to function.

○   **What is synkinesis?**

Synkinesis is mass movement resulting from small groups of axons innervating separate facial muscles.

○   **At what rate does the facial nerve regenerate?**

3mm/day.

○   **What is Bogorad's syndrome?**

Nerves originally destined for the submandibular gland innervate the lacrimal gland leading to tearing during gustation. Also known as "Crocodile Tears."

○   **What is Frey's syndrome?**

Gustatory sweating secondary to autonomic branches to the parotid cross-innervating cheek sweat glands and blood vessels.

○   **What is the most common cause of facial paralysis in children?**

Bell's palsy.

○   **What is the most common cause of facial paralysis in neonates?**

Birth trauma.

○   **What is the most common cause of facial paralysis in adults?**

Blunt head trauma, including temporal bone fracture.

Facial Nerve Evaluation and Rehabilitation

○   **What is the significance of fibrillation potentials on EMG?**

Fibrillation potentials are spontaneous muscle action potentials which occur 2-3 weeks after injury and signify denervation of the muscle.

○   **What is the significance of polyphasic potentials on EMG?**

Polyphasic potentials are recorded from nearby nerve fibers and signify reinnervation of the muscle. They are the earliest sign of nerve regeneration.

❍   **What is ENoG?**

Electroneurography measures and compares the amplitude of summation potentials of the paralyzed face to the normal side.

❍   **When do you decompress the facial nerve in temporal bone fracture?**

When serial ENoG shows progression to degeneration of >90%. May be decompressed up to 3 or 4 weeks after injury.

❍   **When do you do decompress the nerve if there is voluntary activity on EMG?**

Do not decompress the nerve, its continuity is established.

❍   **What is the primary concern of facial paralysis?**

Ophthalmologic sequelae including exposure keratitis, corneal ulcer and potential blindness.

❍   **What non-surgical treatments exist for eye protection in facial paralysis?**

Hydrating drops, ointment, moisture chamber, lid taping at night, and physical therapy (using surface electromyography or mirror feedback).

❍   **What static surgical procedures are available for eye protection?**

Medial canthoplasty, sling procedure, lower lid shortening, tarsorrhaphy, gold weight placement.

❍   **Where is a gold weight placed?**

It is placed superficial to the upper tarsal plate and the levator aponeurosis with the inferior edge 2mm above the lash line.

❍   **What dynamic reanimation procedures may be accomplished?**

Temporalis transposition, free flap muscle transfer with microneuronal anastomosis

❍   **What is a static sling procedure?**

Suspension of the affected musculature with gore-tex, fascia lata, Alloderm

❍   **What procedures are used to restore neural input to the facial muscles?**

Neurorrhaphy, cable grafting, cross-face grafting, XII-VII crossover, XI-VII crossover, Jump grafts.

❍   **What nerve is used to provide cable graft of 10cm or less?**

Great auricular nerve.

❍   **What nerve is used for cable grafts requiring >10cm?**

Sural nerve, up to 35cm.

❍   **What is the technique of neurorrhaphy?**

Interrupted sutures of 9-0 nylon placed in the epineurium.

O **What is a XII-VII crossover with jump graft?**

The hypoglossal nerve is isolated and 1/3 to 1/2 of the nerve is incised. A greater auricular nerve graft is sutured to the proximal cut segment and anastomosed with the paralyzed facial nerve.

O **What is cross-facial nerve grafting?**

A nerve graft is anastamosed with contralateral buccal branches and tunneled to the opposite side of the face. The end is tagged and 9-12 months elapses while nerve fibers traverse the graft. The nerve is then anastamosed with branches of the involved facial nerve.

O **How long after paralysis may reinnervation techniques prove useful?**

After two to three years, progressive muscle atrophy precludes the use of these techniques.

O **Describe the two-stage technique of microvascular free tissue transfer.**

Sural nerve graft is tunneled from the anastomosis with contralateral buccal branches to the involved side of the face and tagged. 9-12 months later, free tissue transfer of gracilis muscle and neurovascular pedicle is performed and cross facial nerve is anastamosed with the pedicle.

O **What orientation is the sural nerve grafted?**

Reverse.

O **Describe the single stage technique.**

Free muscle transfer is performed with cross facial tunneling of the nerve pedicle to the contralateral buccal nerve branches.

O **What is the advantage of single stage repair?**

The axons need only traverse a single anastomotic line to reach the destination muscle.

O **What are common muscles used in single stage procedures?**

Gracilis, pectoralis minor, and serratus anterior.

References

Gantz BJ, Rubinstein JT, Gidley P, Woodworth GG. Surgical Management of Bell's Palsy. Laryngoscope. 1999;109:1177-88.

McCabe BF. Autoimmune Sensorineural Hearing Loss. Ann otol rhinol laryngol. 1979;88(5):585-89.

Papel ID, et al. Facial Plastic and Reconstructive Surgery. 2nd ed. New York:Thieme; 2002

Lee KJ. Essential Otolaryngology-Head and Neck Surgery. 8th ed. New York:McGraw-Hill; 2003

Bailey BJ. Head and Neck Surgery-Otolaryngology. 3rd ed. Philadelphia:Lippincott Williams and Wilkins; 2001

May M. The Facial Nerve. 1st ed. New York:Thieme; 1986

HEAD AND NECK EMBRYOLOGY

W. Stites Whatley, MD and Rakesh K. Chandra, MD

○ **Describe the anatomy of the branchial apparatus? (see Figure 1)**

The branchial apparatus consists of five paired mesodermal arches which are separated by invaginations of ectoderm and endoderm known respectively as clefts and pouches. Each arch has a cartilage bar, an artery, and a nerve. The derivatives of the cartilage of each arch form the facial skeleton and laryngeal framework, while the artery and nerve supply and innervate the derivatives of the arch. The ectoderm of the first cleft forms the major salivary glands, the mucosa of the oral cavity, and the lining of the anterior two-thirds of the tongue, while the ectoderm of the second, third and fourth arch fuse to form a common cervical sinus (of His), which normally degenerates. The endoderm of the branchial pouches form the middle ear, the glandular structures of the oropharynx, the parathyroid glands, and the thymus.

○ **What is the nerve of the first branchial arch?**

The trigeminal nerve.

○ **What is the artery of the first branchial arch?**

The artery of the first arch degenerates.

○ **What are the derivatives of the cartilage of the first arch?**

Meckel's cartilage is the cartilage of the first arch and its derivatives are the mandible, the malleus (except for the manubrium), and the incus (except for the long process).

○ **What are the muscular derivatives of the first branchial arch?**

The muscular derivatives are the muscles of mastication (temporalis, masseter, medial and lateral pterygoids), the tensor tympani, the mylohyoid, anterior belly of the digastric, and the tensor veli palatini.

○ **What is the nerve of the second branchial arch?**

The facial nerve.

○ **What is the artery of the second branchial arch?**

The stapedial artery, which degenerates.

○ **What are the derivatives of the cartilage of the second arch?**

Reichert's cartilage is the cartilage of the second arch and its derivatives are the manubrium of the malleus, the long process of the incus, the stapes suprastructure, the styloid process, the stylohyoid ligament, and the body and lesser cornu of the hyoid bone.

○ **What are the muscular derivatives of the second branchial arch?**

The muscular derivatives of the second arch are the muscles of facial expression, the platysma, stylohyoid, posterior belly of the diagastric, and the stapedius muscle.

○ **What is the nerve of the third branchial arch?**

311

The glossopharyngeal nerve.

O   **What is the artery of the third branchial arch?**

The internal carotid artery.

O   **What are the derivatives of the cartilage of the third arch?**

The body and greater cornu of the hyoid are the skeletal derivatives of the third arch.

O   **What are the muscular derivatives of the third branchial arch?**

The stylopharyngeus is the only muscle of the third arch.

O   **What is the nerve of the fourth branchial arch?**

The superior laryngeal nerve.

O   **What is the artery of the fourth branchial arch?**

The aortic arch is derived from the left arch, and the right subclavian artery is derived from the right arch.

O   **What are the derivatives of the cartilage of the fourth arch?**

The thyroid and cuneiform cartilage of the larynx.

O   **What are the mesodermal derivatives of the fourth branchial arch?**

The inferior pharyngeal constrictor, cricopharyngeus, and cricothyroid are the muscular derivatives of the fourth arch.

O   **What is derived from the fifth branchial arch?**

The fifth arch degenerates and has no derivatives in the human.

O   **What is the nerve of the sixth branchial arch?**

The recurrent laryngeal nerve.

O   **What is the artery of the sixth branchial arch?**

The pulmonary artery.

O   **What are the derivatives of the cartilage of the sixth arch?**

The skeletal derivatives are the cricoid, arytenoids, and corniculate cartilage.

O   **What are the muscular derivatives of the sixth branchial arch?**

The intrinsic muscles of the larynx.

O   **What are branchial cleft anomalies?**

Branchial cleft anomalies occur as cystic masses in the anterior triangle of the neck. The etiology of the masses is not known, but the most common theory is that they are the result of entrapped remnants of the cervical sinus of His. Branchial cleft anomalies may occur as cysts, sinuses (with a connection to the pharynx), or as fistulas (with a connection to the pharynx, and the skin). Branchial cleft anomalies are lined with squamous and respiratory epithelium.

❍   How do branchial cleft anomalies present?

Branchial cleft cysts typically present as fluctuant, nontender masses of the anterior cervical triangle. The may intermittently become infected during upper respiratory infections, and can present as a neck abscess. Branchial cleft sinuses and fistulas present with an opening along the anterior border of the sternocleidomastoid muscle. A mucoid discharge can often be expressed from the opening, and the opening may have increased or purulent drainage during an upper respiratory tract infection.

❍   Describe the classification of branchial cleft anomalies.

Branchial cleft anomalies are classified by anatomical location. They occur between the derivatives of two branchial arches, and are named for the arch whose structures they lie deep to.

❍   Describe the anatomical location of a first branchial cleft cyst.

There are two different types of branchial cleft cysts (type I and type II). A type I first branchial cleft cyst is a duplication of the external auditory canal, and exists as a fistulous tract lying in close association with the lower portion of the parotid gland. They often have tracts which terminate in the external auditory canal, or the middle ear. A type II first branchial cleft cyst is typically located in the anterior triangle of the neck just inferior to the angle of the mandible. The tract of a type II first branchial cleft cysts extends superiorly through the substance of the parotid gland, over the angle of the mandible to the bony cartilaginous junction of the external auditory canal. Type II cysts are intimately related to the facial nerve, putting it at risk for injury during excision.

❍   Describe the anatomical location of second branchial cleft cyst.

Second branchial cleft cysts are located deep to the structures of the second arch (the platysma), and superficial to the structures of the third arch (the internal carotid artery and the glossopharyngeal nerve). The tract of the second branchial cleft cyst ascends between the internal and external carotid arteries and opens into the pharynx at the tonsillar fossae.

❍   Describe the anatomical location of a third branchial cleft cyst.

Third branchial cleft cysts are located in the anterior triangle of the neck deep to the structures of the third arch, and superficial to the structures of the fourth arch. The tract of third branchial cleft cysts pass deep and posterior to the glossopharyngeal nerve and the internal carotid artery, crosses over the hypoglossal nerve and superior laryngeal nerves and enters the pharynx in the region of the thyrohyoid membrane, or piriform sinus.

❍   What are the embryologic components of the midface? (see Figure 2)

The maxillary prominence, the lateral nasal prominence, and the medial nasal prominence are paired embryologic structures which fuse in the midline along with the frontonasal prominence to form the nose and upper lip. These prominences are made of neural crest derived mesenchymal cells of the first branchial arch.

❍   Describe the embryogenesis of the nose and upper lip. (see Figure 2)

Nasal placodes invaginate to form nasal pits during the fifth week of development. Medial and lateral nasal prominences are created on either side of the nasal pits. During the next two weeks the maxillary prominences continue to grow in a medial direction and push the nasal prominences toward the midline. The medial nasal prominences fuse in the midline to form the tip of the nose, and the philtrum of the upper lip. The lateral nasal prominences form the ala of the nose, and fuse with the maxillary prominence which forms the cheeks and lateral portions of the upper lip. The frontonasal prominence which is located superiorly fuses with the medial and lateral nasal prominence and forms the remaining portion of the nasal dorsum.

❍   Describe the embryogenesis of the palate.

The primary palate is formed by the fusion of the medial nasal prominence. The primary palate is located anterior to the incisive foramen, and contains the four central incisors. Development of the secondary palate begins after development of the primary palate is complete. The secondary palate is formed from laterally based palatal shelves of the maxillary prominences. These shelves are initially directed obliquely downward on either side of the developing tongue. As the maxillary prominences move medially, and as the developing tongue descends, the palatal shelves achieve there correct orientation in a horizontal plane. The palatal shelves then fuse from anterior (incisive foramen) to posterior (uvula) and form the secondary palate.

O   **Describe the embryogenesis of the auricle.**

The external ear begins as six proliferations of mesenchymal tissue (known as Hillocks of His) located on either side of the dorsal end of the first branchial cleft. The first three hillocks are located on the first branchial arch and ultimately form the tragus (1), and the helix (2,3). Hillocks 4-6 are located on the second branchial arch and form the descending helix, antihelix (4,5), and the antitragus (6).

O   **Describe the embryogenesis of the tongue.**

The anterior two-thirds of the tongue is derived from components of the first pharyngeal arch, which include two paired lateral lingual swellings, and one medial swelling known as the tuberculum impar. The posterior one third of the tongue is formed by the second, third and fourth arch. The third arch component overgrows the second arch and the fourth arch component forms the most posterior portion of the tongue and the epiglottis.

O   **How does embryology explain tongue innervation?**

The embryologic origin and development of the tongue explain why the anterior two thirds is innervated by the lingual nerve (branch of trigeminal, nerve to first arch) and the posterior one third is innervated by the glossopharyngeal nerve (nerve to the third arch).

O   **How do thyroglossal duct cysts present?**

Thyroglossal duct cysts typically present as asymptomatic midline neck mass. They are located near the level of the hyoid bone, and elevate and descend with swallowing. Thyroglossal duct cysts are managed with excision of the cyst and the central portion of the hyoid bone (Sistrunk procedure).

Figure 1. Branchial arches

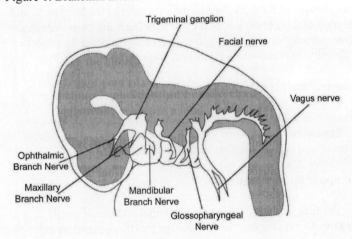

Figure 2. Seven week embryo

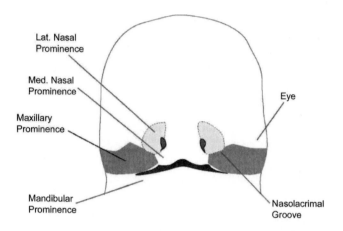

References

Chandler JR, Mitchell B. Branchial cleft cyst, sinuses, and fistulas. Otolaryngologic Clinics of North America 1981;14:175-186.

Friedman O, Wang TD, Miluzuk HA. Cleft Lip and Palate. In: Cummings CW, et al., eds. Otolaryngology-Head and Neck Surgery. 4th ed. Philadelphia: Elsevier Mosby, 2005: 4052-4085.

Goding, GS, Eisele, DW. Embryology of the Face,Head and Neck. In: Facial Plastic and Reconstructive Surgery. 2nd ed. New York: Thieme Medical Publishers, Inc., 2002:785-794.

Graney DO, Sie KCY. Developmental Anatomy. In: Cummings CW, et al., eds. Otolaryngology-Head and Neck Surgery. 4th ed. Philadelphia: Elsevier Mosby, 2005: 3938-3951.

Sadler, TW. Head and Neck. In: Langman's Medical Embryology. 7th ed. Baltimore: Williams & Wilkins, 1995:312-346.

Sadler, TW. Ear. In: Langman's Medical Embryology. 7th ed. Baltimore: Williams & Wilkins, 1995:347-357.

HEAD AND NECK CANCER

Gary Ross, MBChB, MRCS, MD

○ **A patient presents with a 3 cm biopsy proven SCC of the floor of mouth (midline) with invasion of the mandible on CT scan and no lymph node involvement or distant metastases. According to the TNM classification how would you stage this patient?**

T4N0M0

○ **Which surgical procedures are available for treating the mandible of the patient in question 1?**

Segmental mandibulectomy or marginal/rim resection depending on extent of disease. Marginal mandibulectomy can be used when the inner surface of the mandible is not involved.

○ **How would you treat the neck/s of the patient in question 1?**

The options are surgery +/- radiotherapy versus radiotherapy alone. Traditionally for midline T4 tumors, in-continuity bilateral neck dissections with postoperative radiotherapy to the both primary and bilateral necks.

○ **What are the advantages and disadvantages of an in-continuity neck dissection?**

It removes any lymphatic drainage pathways between the primary and levels I and II that lie in close proximity to the primary. Increased morbidity is the disadvantage especially fistula formation.

○ **How would you treat the surgical defect if a segmental mandibulectomy were required for tumor clearance?**

Free fibula flap for bone reconstruction taken with a cutaneous skin paddle to reconstruct the floor of mouth defect.

○ **How would you treat the surgical defect if a rim/marginal resection only were required for tumor clearance?**

A free radial forearm flap or anterolateral thigh flap for intraoral lining.

○ **A 50-year-old patient presents with a 2 cm non-pulsatile mass in the level III of the neck. What is your management plan?**

FNA biopsy and CT scan head and neck.

○ **If both CT and FNA are negative in the patient above what is your plan?**

Open biopsy with frozen sectioning and progression to neck dissection if diagnosis of SCC is obtained. Pan endoscopies of naso/oro/hypo- pharynx, larynx, esophagus, stomach. If all look normal multiple biopsies are performed including tonsils, base of tongue, nasopharynx and piriform fossa. Treatment of the primary depends on results of these biopsies.

○ **A patient presents with a 1cm biopsy proven tongue SCC and a palpable node in level II with no distant metastases. According to the TNM classification how would you stage this patient clinically?**

T1N1M0

○ **Following surgical excision pathological evaluation the tumor margins in the above patient were clear and the patient was staged as pT1N1M0. Would you perform radiotherapy to either the primary or the neck?**

No unless there is presence of extracapsular spread.

○ **What are the indications for postoperative radiotherapy to the neck?**

More than one neck node involved or evidence of extracapsular nodal disease.

○ **A patient requires segmental bony reconstruction of the mandible. This can be achieved by which methods?**

Reconstructive plate with no bone, reconstruction with non-vascularized bone, reconstruction with vascularized bone (free flap or pedicle flap)

○ **When would you use a reconstruction plate?**

For patients in whom no other reconstruction is possible, where good soft tissue exists, and/or when radiotherapy has not been performed or is not planned.

○ **What types of non-vascularized bone can be used?**

Free bone graft, freeze dried autoclaved or irradiated autogenous mandible, alloplastic materials.

○ **What types of vascularized bone on a pedicle flap exist?**

Clavicle on the sternocleidomastoid flap, rib on the pectoralis major muscle, scapula on the trapezius muscle.

○ **What types of vascularized bone as a free flap would you consider?**

Deep circumflex iliac artery flap, radial forearm flap, free fibula flap, free scapula flap

○ **Which free vascularized bone flap is most anatomically similar to a hemi-mandible?**

Deep circumflex iliac artery flap

○ **Which free vascularized bone flap could you place osteointegrated implants into?**

Fibula flap and deep circumflex iliac artery flap

○ **Which free vascularized bone flap provides the longest length of bone?**

Fibula flap

○ **A patient presents with a 2cm mass in the parotid gland. Is the mass likely to be benign or malignant?**

Benign

○ **What factors from the history in a patient with a parotid mass suggest malignancy?**

Pain, obstruction, facial nerve involvement, invasion of other structures, rapid progression

○ **What are the most common benign tumors of the parotid?**

Pleomorphic adenoma and adenolymphoma.

○ **What are the most common malignant tumors of the parotid?**

Mucoepidermoid, adenoid cystic carcinoma and malignant transformation of pleomorphic adenoma

○ **Which surgical methods are available to remove parotid tumors?**

Lumpectomy, Superficial parotidectomy, Total parotidectomy.

○ **What is Frey's syndrome?**

Gustatory sweating. Auriculotemporal secretomotor nerve fibers disrupted during surgery reinnervate sweat glands following parotid surgery. Subsequent eating induces sweating in the distribution of the auriculotemporal nerve.

○ **A patient has a biopsy proven T1 oropharyngeal SCC. Which types of surgical access are possible?**

Transorally or through pharyngotomy. Mandibulotomy/mandibular swings are used for larger tumors.

○ **Which regions of the oropharynx are accessible transorally?**

Tonsil, soft palate, superior pharyngeal wall.

○ **Which histological factors in the pathological report would influence your decision in performing postoperative radiotherapy to the primary?**

Close or positive margins, perineural or perivascular invasion, >5mm tumor depth, presence of a non-cohesive front, degree of differentiation, invasion of adjacent soft tissues, subglottic extension.

○ **A patient presents with a 3 weeks hoarseness of voice with a normal clinical examination. What is your management?**

CT scan, laryngoscopy/biopsy

○ **How are laryngeal tumors classified anatomically?**

Supraglottic, Glottic and Subglottic.

○ **What is the rate of nodal metastasis for a T1-2 glottic tumor?**

Less than 10% hence neck dissection rarely performed.

○ **What is the rate of nodal metastasis for a T1-2 supraglottic tumor?**

Approximately 50% hence bilateral neck dissections frequently performed.

○ **For advanced laryngeal tumors what are the treatment options?**

Surgical excision, radiotherapy, chemotherapy or a combination of all three. Organ preservation with chemoradiotherapy has shown comparable local control rates to traditional surgery.

○ **A patient presents with mandibular pain and trismus. He has previously had an excision of a T2N0M0 floor of mouth SCC with close margins and postoperative radiotherapy 1 year ago. What is your differential diagnosis?**

Osteoradionecrosis, recurrence/another primary. Dental related problems.

○ **Biopsy in the patient above suggests osteoradionecrosis. What is your initial management?**

Conservative – oral hygiene, antibiotics, analgesia

❍ **When would you consider surgery for osteoradionecrosis?**

Intractable pain, persistent bone exposure, fistulas, pathological fractures

❍ **Is there a role for hyperbaric oxygen in the management of osteoradionecrosis?**

Yes.

❍ **Frequently the involved mandible needs to be resected. How would you reconstruct the defect?**

With a free vascularized bone flap.

❍ **A patient presents with postnasal drip, pain around the upper first and second molar and cheek numbness on the left side. A CT scan shows a mass within the maxillary antrum and a biopsy confirms SCCa. Standard maxillectomy is planned. What access skin incision is traditionally used?**

Weber-Ferguson

❍ **Does a neck dissection need to be performed in the above patient?**

No. The risk of metastasis from maxillary tumors is rare.

❍ **How can the orbital floor be reconstructed?**

Usually with non-vascularized bone graft i.e. rib.

❍ **How is the maxillary defect reconstructed?**

Traditionally with an obturator and split skin graft. A split skin graft is usually placed within the cavity and the obturator used to contour the graft into the defect.

❍ **A patient presents with a 3 cm nodal mass in the posterior triangle following radiotherapy to a nasopharyngeal tumor 2 years previously. An FNA biopsy confirms SCCa. What type of neck dissection would you perform, comprehensive or selective?**

Traditionally a comprehensive neck dissection.

❍ **What is the difference between a selective and a comprehensive neck dissection?**

A selective neck dissection only removes the nodal levels most likely to harbor metastases. A comprehensive neck dissection removes lymph nodes from all levels.

❍ **What different types of comprehensive neck dissections do you know?**

Radical and modified radical neck dissections

❍ **How many types of modified radical neck dissection (MRND) are there?**

3

❍ **How do they differ?**

MRND Type 1 preserves only the accessory nerve, MRND Type 2 preserves both accessory and the internal jugular and MRND Type 3 preserves accessory, internal jugular and sternocleidomastoid.

○ **In a selective neck dissection which of the following structures are preserved: sternocleidomastoid, internal jugular vein or accessory nerve?**

All of them.

References

Haddadin KJ, Soutar DS, Oliver RJ et al. Improved survival for patients with clinically T1/T2, N0 tongue tumors undergoing a prophylactic neck dissection. Head Neck. 1999;21:517-525.

Leemans CR, Tiwari RM, Nauta JJP et al. Regional lymph node involvement and its significance in the development of distant metastases in head and neck carcinoma. Cancer 1993; 71:452-456.

Leemans CR, Tiwari R, van der Waal I et al. The efficacy of comprehensive neck dissection with or without postoperative radiotherapy in nodal metastases of squamous cell carcinoma of the upper respiratory and digestive tracts. Laryngoscope 1990;100:1194-8.

Pillsbury HC 3rd. Clark M. A rationale for therapy of the N0 neck. Laryngoscope 1997;107:1294-315.

Robbins KT. Classification of neck dissection: current concepts and future considerations. Otolaryngol.Clin.North Am. 1998;31:639-55.

Shah JP. Patterns of cervical lymph node metastasis from squamous carcinomas of the aerodigestive tract. Am J Surg 1990;160:405-409.

SALIVARY GLAND TUMORS

Alex Senchenkov, MD

○ **What are the histological features of salivary glands and how are they related to oncogenesis?**

The parenchyma of the salivary glands are formed from the acini that lead to the sequence of ducts. While origin of the salivary tumors is poorly understood, there is a correlation between the salivary neoplasms and the cells forming salivary units. This unit consists of acinus, intercalated, striated, and excretory ducts. **Table 1** (at the end of the chapter) illustrates the correlation between normal structure and tumor cells.

○ **Which salivary gland is the most common site for salivary tumors?**

Parotid gland harbors 70-85% of all salivary tumors

○ **What is the incidence of malignancy in different salivary glands?**

	Benign	Malignant
Parotid	80%	20%
Submandibular	50%	50%
Minor salivary	20%	80%

○ **Tumors of which salivary gland are most frequently malignant?**

Sublingual gland.
Starting with lowest to the highest chance of malignancy the sequence is as follows:
Parotid < submandibular < minor salivary < sublingual gland

○ **Overall, what salivary gland harbors the most of the malignant tumors?**

Parotid gland. Although about 80% of parotid tumors are benign, the remaining 20% are malignant, and since tumors in the parotid are much more frequent than in all other salivary glands combined, the majority of malignant salivary glands tumors occur in the parotid gland.

○ **What is the most common benign salivary neoplasm for all salivary glands?**

Pleomorphic adenoma is both most common benign parotid neoplasm and the most common benign salivary neoplasm overall, comprising about 60% of all salivary tumors and about 80% of benign tumors.

○ **The patient who was diagnosed with pleomorphic adenoma of the parotid (mixed parotid tumor) has another tumor in the same parotid gland. What is histology of the second primary parotid tumor most likely to be?**

Warthin's tumor

○ **Do any of the parotid tumors have propensity to be bilateral?**

Warthin's tumor

○ **A patient who has a symptomatic Warthin's tumor in the parotid gland is found to have an occult contralateral parotid tumor on the CT scan. What would you do about it?**

2% - 6% of Warthin's tumors are bilateral. The symptomatic side should be treated operatively, whereas you may observe an asymptomatic contralateral tumor. When it becomes symptomatic, you would remove it.

O **Why are oncocytomas frequently found on the Tc-99 scans and what do you do with them?**

Their origin is thought to correlate with striated ducts. This striation is related to the presence of large number of mitochondria. Tc-99 is preferentially picked up by tissues rich in mitochondria (gastric mucosa in the Meckel's diverticulum lights up on Tc-99 Meckel's scan). When oncocytoma is found on the scan and is not symptomatic, it may be observed initially.

O **What is the most common malignant tumor of the parotid gland?**

Mucoepidermoid carcinoma

O **What is the most common malignant tumor of the salivary gland outside the parotid?**

Adenoid cystic carcinoma is the most common submandibular, sublingual, and minor salivary gland malignancy

O **What is the most common malignant tumor of the salivary glands overall?**

Mucoepidermoid carcinoma. Low-grade variant is more common and is predominantly cystic, whereas high-grade tumors are solid with small amount of mucin.

O **How do salivary malignancies spread?**

Lymphatic, hematogenous, direct invasion of the surrounding structures, as well as perineurally

O **Which head and neck malignancies are notorious for perineural spread?**

Adenoid cystic carcinoma is a classic example. Malignant mixed tumor, melanoma, and squamous cell carcinoma also demonstrate perineural invasion.

O **What are peculiar features of adenoid cystic carcinomas?**

Lack a tumor capsule, directly invade surrounding tissues, and have a very high propensity for perineural invasion. Hematogenous route of spread common. Tumor frequently metastasizes to the lung, liver, and bone. Excellent five-year survival (75%), but lousy ten-year survival, and even worse twenty-year survival (13%); tends to recur late.

O **What are the important clinical features of acinic carcinoma?**

While the majority of the acinic carcinomas are curable, about 10% can manifest very aggressively and be tenacious; watch for recurrence.

O **What is an important consideration in planning the removal of malignant mixed tumors?**

Malignant mixed tumor (*or* carcinoma-ex-pleomorphic adenoma) is very locally destructive. Proper surgical control very often necessitates free flap reconstruction.

O **What is the most common parotid tumor of young children?**

Hemangioma

O **What are other common pediatric parotid tumors?**

Most common benign epithelial tumor is pleomorphic adenoma. Most common malignant tumor is mucoepidermoid carcinoma, similar to adults.

○ **Does the ratio 80:20 between benign and malignant parotid tumors apply for children?**

No. Pediatric parotid tumors are much more likely to be malignant. In fact, an older child with a parotid mass has 50% chance of harboring malignancy.

○ **What is the most common presentation of parotid tumors?**

Mass below the angle of the mandible, not in front of the ear

○ **Do you always feel parotid tumor on palpation?**

No. Sometimes the presentation is subtle. If the tumor is in the deep lobe, only diffuse enlargement of the gland can be appreciated, and you have to rely on imaging to demonstrate the tumor.

○ **What about the size of the tumor? If the tumor is large, is it more likely to be malignant?**

Not necessarily. You can have a large pleomorphic adenoma that has grown over past 20 years to be very large, but yet benign.

○ **So the patient presents to you with a parotid mass, when should you think about malignancy?**

Start with history and physical. Patient's age, history of head and neck radiation, history of previous malignancies and symptoms are important. Tumors in children and older individuals are more likely to be malignant. Pain and rapid growth are very suspicious for malignancy as are tumors that are adherent to surrounding structures on physical exam and have regional adenopathy. Facial nerve paralysis and eruption through the skin are rare even in advanced malignancy and are grave prognostic signs.

○ **A mass with facial nerve paralysis is a bad prognostic sign. What would be a benign condition that could have a similar presentation?**

Sarcoidosis is the most common cause for non-neoplastic parotid mass with facial nerve paralysis.

○ **What is importance of cystic parotid mass in an HIV patient?**

A benign lymphoepithelial cyst is a cystic degeneration of salivary gland inclusions within intercalated lymph nodes. The cyst is lined with lymphocytes. It is manifestation of progression to AIDS. Treatment is repeat aspiration and using a sclerosing agent.

○ **How can you tell whether it is malignant and how do you workup the parotid mass?**

After thorough history and physical, MRI is the best study; however, a good quality head and neck CT is acceptable. Evaluate locoregional extent of the disease (location of the tumor, tissue invasion, lymphadenopathy). If concerned about malignancy, a fine-needle aspiration (FNA) biopsy is the next important study. Threshold for FNA is low.

○ **How good is FNA for salivary tumors?**

It accurately diagnoses more than 95% of pleomorphic adenomas. It is very good in diagnosing malignancy, but rarely tells you the type.

○ **How do you perform FNA of a parotid mass?**

With a 25-gauge needle with or without ultrasound guidance. With each insertion of the needle directly into the mass and perform several passes back and forth with continuous aspiration. Then irrigate the syringe with saline and send it for cytopathology. The other alternative is to smear the aspirate for Diff-Quick stain, Papanicolaou, or hematoxylin-eosin stains.

❍   **What about core needle biopsy that we perform for breast masses? It gives us histological, not cytological diagnosis. Would it help to establish the type of parotid malignancy preoperatively?**

Core needle biopsy for breast masses is performed with 14 and 11-gauge needles. Its use is contraindicated for the parotid masses because of the danger of transsection of the facial nerve branch.

❍   **You have a young patient with a small mobile mass that is very superficial in the parotid lobe. You performed an FNA and it is a pleomorphic adenoma. You explained to her that although it is a benign tumor it needs to be removed. She is asking if you can do "minimally invasive surgery" and just take out the benign tumor.**

Enucleation or local excision of the adenoma is not an option. The minimal operation for the parotid tumor is a superficial parotidectomy. Partial parotid resection have high rate of complications and should not be done.

❍   **Some surgeons advocate not doing FNA, but just taking the patient with a parotid mass to the OR, performing superficial parotidectomy with frozen section and having that be the biopsy. Why is it important to know whether the tumor is malignant preoperatively?**

This approach is also valid. However, knowing preoperatively that the patient has a malignant parotid tumor will allow better planning of the operation. While treatment of benign tumors is straightforward, a malignancy may require radical parotidectomy with resection of the ramus of the mandible, neck dissection, facial nerve grafting, microvascular mandibular and soft tissue reconstruction and postoperative XRT. The patient and the family will have better understanding of what these all entail to make an informed consent.

❍   **How do you stage parotid malignancies?**

TNM Staging. T(primary tumor): T1: <2 cm, T2: 2 - 4 cm, T3: 4 – 6, T4: >6cm; a – no local extension, b – local extension
Stage I: T1a or T2a/N0;
Stage II: T1b, T2b, T3a/N0;
Stage III: T3b, T4a or any T (except T4b) with N1,
Stage IV: T4bN0 or Any T with N2-3 or M1

❍   **The patient presents to you pleural malignant effusion and multiple metastases in the lungs. He had a 1.5-cm high-grade mucoepidermoid carcinoma of the parotid removed 2.5 years ago. He did not have neck dissection at that time because the neck was clinically negative and distant workup did not show metastasis. What is his stage now?**

Stage 1(T1N0M0).
A cancer patient is staged only once on his initial treatment, and this stage remains unchanged. Stage is predictor of prognosis drawn from retrospective analysis of outcomes. You cannot "restage" or "downstage" the cancer patient.

❍   **What is the surgical treatment for parotid tumors?**

Benign tumor of the superficial lobe:	Superficial parotidectomy
Benign tumor of the deep lobe:	Total parotidectomy
Malignant parotid tumor:	Total parotidectomy *or* radical parotidectomy

❍   **What is the difference between total and radical parotidectomy?**

In total parotidectomy, the facial nerve is preserved. The operation starts with superficial parotidectomy, then the facial nerve is dissected free off the deep lobe and the deep lobe is removed. Release of stylomandibular ligament facilitates this step of the operation. In radical parotidectomy, the facial nerve is removed *en bloc* with both lobes of parotid.

❍   **How do you decide whether to perform total or radical parotidectomy?**

Direct invasion of the nerve is what determines the choice of the operation. If the patient's facial nerve is paralyzed preoperatively, radical parotidectomy is performed. If the nerve is not paralyzed, operation starts with superficial parotidectomy. If dissection plane between the tumor and the nerve branch cannot be established, that nerve or branch is resected with frozen section control of the nerve margin. If the main facial nerve trunk cannot be dissected free, radical parotidectomy is performed.

○ **You have mentioned superficial and deep lobes of the parotid. Could you define these terms?**

Division between the lobes of parotid is purely artificial. The parotid is one gland; however, during embryologic development facial nerve was trapped in the gland and the plane of the facial nerve branches defines the border between the lobes. Superficial lobe is much larger and encompasses approximately 80% - 90% of parotid parenchyma.

○ **The most critical part of the parotidectomy is finding of the facial nerve. How do you do that?**

1) **Tragal pointer** is the medial end of the tragal cartilage. The dissection is carried out in the subperichondrial plane to expose the tragal pointer. The facial nerve trunk is 1 cm deep and anteroinferior to the pointer. 2) The **Posterior belly of digastric muscle** is identified and followed superiorly to the digastric groove of the facial nerve. 3) **Tympanomastoid suture** is the most constant landmark that can be palpated. The facial nerve is 6-8 mm deep to the inferior end of the suture line. 4) As a last resort, alternative method is **retrograde dissection** of the branches of the facial nerve

○ **You have been called by your senior partner to give him a hand in the OR with a parotidectomy that he started three hours ago. He does not believe in preoperative FNA. The patient has a tumor of the superficial lobe of the parotid that was close to the nerve, but does not directly involve it. The pathologist is having a difficult time to determine the nature of the tumor on frozen section. How would you handle this situation?**

Some of the salivary malignancies are difficult to call on frozen section. In this case, sample any enlarged cervical nodes, and if they are not enlarged, sample normal-looking, cervical nodes below the posterior belly of digastric muscle and send them for frozen section. If tumor is present in the nodes, perform total parotidectomy with neck dissection. If there is no tumor present in the nodes, perform total parotidectomy if suspicious for malignancy. In the worst case, add postoperative radiation if the tumor is malignant on permanent section.

○ **When do you perform neck dissection for the parotid tumors?**

Neck dissection is never indicated based on histology of the primary tumor only. It is not recommended for high-grade tumors with N_0 neck. Neck dissection is performed in the presence of lymph node metastases.

○ **When is postoperative radiation therapy indicated?**

When microscopic disease might have been left behind, *e.g.* close margins, proximity of the tumor to the nerve, extensive soft tissue, skin, muscle, and bone invasion, extension into infratemporal fossa, malignant tumors of the deep lobe that cannot be excised with generous margins, tumors that exhibit perineural and vascular invasion, presence of lymph node metastasis.

○ **Is there any benign tumor that may benefit from postoperative radiation therapy?**

Recurrent pleomorphic adenoma

○ **When fast neutron radiation is indicated?**

Adenoid cystic carcinoma and recurrent acinic carcinoma

○ **You mentioned earlier that history of previous malignancies is important. Can you explain why?**

Parotid is a common site for metastases, both regional and distal.

❍ **Why is the parotid a common site of regional metastases?**

Because of the embryologic delay of formation of the parotid capsule, lymph nodes became incorporated into the parotid. These nodes serve as regional lymph nodes for the area of skin between line over temporozygomatic arch to labial attachment of the nose inferiorly, sagittal line from the base of the nose to the vertex medially, and imaginary line from the vertex to the temporozygomatic arch posteriorly. Additionally it drains the external auditory canal, part of external ear including tragus, helical root, and superior helix, orbital content, posterior oral cavity, part of the pharynx, and the parotid gland itself.

❍ **What is the most common metastatic tumor of the parotid?**

Malignant melanoma (40%) is the most common and squamous cell carcinoma is the next most common.

❍ **What hematogenous metastases are found in the parotid?**

For the reasons that are not understood, glandular tissue of parotid is favored by hematogenous metastases from breast, lung, kidney, and gastrointestinal carcinomas.

❍ **What is gustatory sweating?**

Gustatory sweating or Frey's syndrome occurs following parotidectomy or rhytidectomy. It is caused by dysfunction of the auriculotemporal nerve, a branch of the trigeminal nerve (V_3). The pathways of this nerve are disrupted during the operation, and they regenerate incorrectly. Cross innervation of parasympathetic nerves from IX occur with sweat glands of the skin flap. This results in parasympathetic innervation of sympathetic nerve receptors. Affected patients have facial sweating and flushing in response to gustatory stimulation.

❍ **How do you manage it?**

Injection of botulinum toxin (Botox) and operative placement of Alloderm, dermis, or fascia graft under the affected skin to prevent improper nerve regeneration.

❍ **What is the parapharyngeal space?**

It is an upside-down pyramid: superior border is skull base; inferior is lesser horn of the hyoid; medial is superior constrictor, tonsil, and eustachian tube; and lateral is ramus of the mandible. It is an important note that the lateral wall structures are rigid and the medial wall structures are pliable; tumors of the parapharyngeal space will present as a bulging tonsil.

❍ **What does the parapharyngeal space have to do with salivary tumors?**

Tumors of parapharyngeal space are frequently of salivary gland origin. They can be tumors extending from the deep lobe of the parotid or tumors of accessory salivary gland rest.

❍ **You have suspected that the patient has a parapharyngeal tumor, how do you work it up?**

Do not biopsy - some of the parapharyngeal tumors are highly vascular and orientation of the tumor and the carotid artery cannot be determined on physical exam. Workup is largely based on imaging - get a CT scan with contrast.

❍ **What in particular you look for on the CT scan?**

Axial cuts of the CT will show relation of the tumor to the styloid.
Prestyloid tumors are salivary in origin with the rare exception of connective tissue neoplasms
Poststyloid tumors are neurogenic (CN IX, X, XI, sympathetic chain), vascular (paragangliomas), or lymph node (metastases) in origin.

❍ **Overall, what is the most common tumor of the parapharyngeal space?**

Metastatic lesions are the most common. The most common primary tumor is pleomorphic adenoma (50%).

○   **What are the lymph nodes in the parapharyngeal space?**

Nodes of Rouviere drain the nasopharynx.

○   **What is Vernet syndrome?**

Enlargement of the nodes extending to the jugular foramen that causes compression of CN IX, X, XI and paralysis of their motor components.

○   **Does radical surgery for parotid tumors and radiation therapy significantly affect long-term survival?**

No. They do improve loco-regional control, but do not change long-term survival. Unfortunately, outcome of parotid malignancies is largely predetermined by the histology of the tumor.

Table 1. Histogenic scheme of salivary gland neoplasms

Normal structure	Cell of origin	Neoplasm
Excretory duct	Excretory duct reserve cells	Squamous cell Ca Mucoepidermoid Ca
Acinus	Intercalated duct reserve cells	Acinic cell carcinoma Mixed tumor Monomorphic adenoma Myoepithelioma
Intercalated duct		Adenoid cystic Ca
Myoepithelium		Adenocarcinoma
Striated duct		Oncocytic tumors

Regezi JA, Batsakis, JG. Histogenesis of salivary gland neoplasms. Otol Clin N Am 1977; 10:298

References

Batsakis JG. *Tumors of the head and neck: clinical and pathological considerations.* 2 ed. Baltimore: Williams Wilkins; 1979.

Close LG, Larson DL, Shah JP. *Essentials of head and neck oncology.* 1 ed. New York: Thieme Medical Publishers, Inc.; 1998.

Medina JE. Clinical Practice Guidelines for the Diagnosis and Management of Cancer of the Head and Neck. *American Head and Neck Society,* 2002.

Regezi JA, Batsakis JG. Histogenesis of salivary gland neoplasms. *Otol Clin N Am.* 1977;10:298.

Shah JP. *Head and neck surgery.* 2 ed. London: Mosby-Wolfe; 1996.

Spiro RH. Salivary neoplasms: overview of a 35-year experience with 2,807 patients. *Head Neck Surg.* 1986;8(3):177-184.

Woods JE. Parotidectomy versus limited resection for benign parotid masses. *Am J Surg.* 1985;149(6):749-750.

INTEGUMENT

BENIGN SKIN LESIONS

Ned Snyder IV, MD

○ **What is a nevus?**

Latin for spot or blemish. Describes a cutaneous hamartoma or benign proliferation of cells. Usually refers to a melanocytic nevus.

○ **Are there types of melanocytic nevi?**

Yes. Classified by histology (junctional, compound, or intradermal). Can also be classified by appearance or acquired vs. congenital.

○ **T/F: Melanocytes develop from neural crest cells.**

True

○ **During fetal development neural crest cells migrate to what eventual location?**

Epidermal side of the dermal/epidermal junction.

○ **What is a blue nevus?**

A deep dermal accumulation of melanocytic cells. Its deep dermal location gives a blue, gray, or black appearance.

○ **Can blue nevi become malignant?**

Yes, rarely.

○ **What is a Spitz nevus?**

A melanocytic nevus that occurs most commonly in children.

○ **Where does a Spitz nevus appear?**

Usually presents as a small pink nodule on the face or lower extremities. Histologically composed of pleomorphic and cytologically atypical cells, sometimes confused for a melanoma.

○ **Is the risk of malignancy within a congenital melanocytic nevus (CMN) related to size?**

Yes.

○ **When is the risk of malignant transformation of a CMN greatest in childhood?**

Usually before age 9.

○ **What is a Becker's nevus?**

Area of hyperpigmentation and hypertrichosis, most commonly found on the upper back, shoulder, or chest in males. Usually presents at puberty.

○ **What is the recommended treatment for an atypical nevus?**

Excision with 2 mm margins.

O **What is a nevus of Ota?**

It is a blue to gray hyperpigmentation of the skin, mucosa, or conjunctiva in the distribution of the trigeminal nerve.

O **What is a nevus of Ito?**

Similar in appearance to a nevus of Ota but found on the neck or shoulder.

O **What is the recommended treatment for melanoma in-situ?**

Excision with 5 mm margins.

O **What is a Mongolian spot?**

Congenital hyperpigmented spot found in the sacrococcygeal region. Usually disappears in the first 3-5 years of life.

O **What is a nevus spilus?**

An irregularly shaped light brown macule with darkly pigmented macules or papules scattered randomly within the lesion.

O **What is labial lentigo?**

Hyperpigmented macule that develops on the lip, usually in young women

O **What is the most common vascular neoplasm of childhood?**

Hemangioma

O **What is a hemangioma?**

It is a benign tumor of vascular endothelium. Presents at age 4-8 weeks.

O **What is the natural history of a hemangioma?**

The lesion proliferates for the first 6 months to a year then goes through involution (regression). Classically, 50% completely regress by age 5.

O **What is the most common complication of hemagiomas?**

Ulceration

O **What are complications after regression of a hemangioma?**

Hypopigmentation, telangiectasia, excess skin, fibrofatty deposits, and scarring after ulceration.

O **What is a port-wine stain?**

A capillary malformation present at birth that grows proportionate to the patient and has normal endothelial turnover.

O **What laser is used to treat a port-wine stain? Why?**

Pulsed dye. Wavelength (585nm) specific for absorption of oxyhemoglobin with an extremely short duration (400 ms). The short duration limits heating of adjacent tissues.

O   **When a facial port-wine stain is seen with leptomeningeal angiomatosis, what is it called?**

Sturge-Weber syndrome.

O   **Where does the port-wine stain occur most commonly in Sturge-Weber Syndrome?**

The cutaneous areas innervated by CN V1 and V2.

O   **Regular ophthalmologic exams are important for which patients with port-wine stains?**

All patients with V1 facial distribution.

O   **What are blue-black hyperkeratotic vascular papules?**

Angiokeratomas.

O   **Who gets cherry angiomas?**

Middle-aged and elderly patients

O   **What occurs in the extremity as a painful, purple nodule? (Hint: sometimes seen in the fingertip)**

Glomus tumor.

O   **T/F: A condition with inherited multiple glomus tumors is transmitted in an autosomal dominant fashion.**

True.

O   **What syndrome has telangiectasias on the face, lips, tongue, ears, hands, feet, GI, GU, pulmonary, CNS, and liver?**

Osler-Weber-Rendu syndrome.

O   **What are the common causes of facial telangiectasias?**

Chronic UV light, rosacea, connective tissue disease, abuse of potent topical steroids, and radiation.

O   **What is a solitary, firm, hyperkeratotic, sometimes pedunculated papule frequently found on the digits overlying an IP joint, but can be found anywhere on the hands or feet?**

Acquired digital fibrokeratoma.

O   **What is a lesion that is skin colored or red found on the lateral or dorsal surface of a digit on an infant or young child?**

Infantile digital fibromatosis.

O   **T/F: Seborrheic keratoses are pre-malignant lesions.**

False.

O   **What is the ideal treatment of a keratoacanthoma?**

Complete excision when the lesion is first recognized

❍ **Cutaneous horns are related to what premalignant skin lesion?**

Actinic keratoses.

❍ **Name the acceptable treatment modalities for actinic keratoses.**

Excision, curettage, cryosurgery, dermabrasion, chemical peels, topical 5-FU, and laser ablation.

❍ **What is the natural history of Bowen's disease?**

10% will develop into invasive squamous cell carcinoma.

❍ **What is an eczematous condition of the nipple and areola with or without an underlying mass?**

Paget's disease.

❍ **What is a firm nodule or papule often found on the extremities?**

Dermatofibroma.

References

Grevelink SV, Mulliken JB. Vascular Anomalies and Tumors of Skin and Subcutaneous Tissues. In: Freedberg IM, Eisen AZ, Wolff K, et al., eds. Fitzpatrick's Dermatology in General Medicine. Sixth Edition. New York, McGraw-Hill, 2003:1002-1019.

Grichnik JM, Rhodes AR, Sober AJ. Benign Hyperplasias and Neoplasias of Melanocytes. In: Freedberg IM, Eisen AZ, Wolff K, et al., eds. Fitzpatrick's Dermatology in General Medicine. Sixth Edition. New York, McGraw-Hill, 2003:881-905.

Tsao H and Sober AJ. Atypical Melanocytic Nevi. In: Freedberg IM, Eisen AZ, Wolff K, et al., eds. Fitzpatrick's Dermatology in General Medicine. Sixth Edition. New York, McGraw-Hill, 2003:906-916.

Netscher D, Spira M, Cohen V. Benign and Premalignant Skin Conditions. In: Achauer BM, Eriksson E, Guyuron B, et al. eds. Plastic Surgery Indications, Operations, and Outcomes. First Ed. St. Louis, Mosby, 2000:293-314.

Kint A, Baran R, De Keyser H: Acquired (digital) fibrokeratomas. J Am Acad Dermatol 12:816-821, 1985.

Morelli JG, Tan OT, Yohn JJ, et al. Management of ulcerated hemangiomas in infancy. Arch Pediatr Adol Med 1994;148:1104-1108.

Walsh P. Benign melanocytic tumors. In: Fitzpatrick JE and Aeling JL. Dermatology Secrets. First ed. Philadelphia, Hanley & Belfus, Inc, 1996: 269-274.

Morelli JG. Vascular neoplasms. In: Fitzpatrick JE and Aeling JL. Dermatology Secrets. First ed. Philadelphia, Hanley & Belfus, Inc, 1996: 275-277.

Giandoni MB. Fibrous tumors of the skin. In: Fitzpatrick JE and Aeling JL. Dermatology Secrets. First ed. Philadelphia, Hanley & Belfus, Inc, 1996:278-283.

PEDIATRICS

CRANIOFACIAL SYNDROMES

Mark W. Kiehn, MD and Christopher Forrest, MD, MSc, FRCSC, FACS

❍ **What process involves the premature fusion of the sutures between cranial bones?**

Craniosynostosis

❍ **What type of synostosis is commonly associated with anterior plagiocephaly?**

Unicoronal synostosis

❍ **What type of synostosis is associated with turribrachycephaly?**

Bicoronal synostosis

❍ **Synostosis of which suture is associated with scaphocephaly?**

Sagittal suture

❍ **Synostosis of which suture is associated with the Harlequin deformity?**

Coronal suture

❍ **Synostosis of which suture is associated with trigonocephaly?**

Metopic suture

❍ **Which suture is the most commonly affected by craniosynostosis?**

Sagittal suture

❍ **Are the majority of craniosynostosis cases syndromic or non-syndromic?**

Non-syndromic

❍ **What is the incidence of sporadic synostosis?**

0.04% to 0.1%

❍ **What is Virchow's Law?**

Growth restriction occurs perpendicular to a synostotic suture. Compensatory overgrowth can occur at other unaffected sutures, typically parallel to the affected suture.

❍ **What is the incidence of elevated intracranial pressure with single suture synostosis?**

13%

❍ **What is the incidence of elevated intracranial pressure with multiple suture synostoses?**

42%

O **What functional ocular problem has an increased incidence in patients with coronal synostosis?**

Strabismus

O **What is the typical age for surgical intervention for synostosis?**

3 to 12 months

O **What is the primary stimulus for cranial growth?**

Brain growth

O **Does microcephaly require surgical intervention to prevent increased intracranial pressure?**

No. It is not caused by growth restriction.

O **What are the causes of posterior plagiocephaly?**

Lambdoidal synostosis and positioning (molding)

O **Of the causes of posterior plagiocephaly, which is more common?**

Positional plagiocephaly

O **What factors contribute to non-synostotic posterior plagiocephaly?**

Supine positioning and torticollis

O **What features distinguish positional from synostotic posterior plagiocephaly?**

Positional
    Head Shape – parallelogram shaped
    Ear position – more anterior on side of flattening

Synostotic
    Head Shape – trapezoid shaped
    Ear position – more posterior on affected side

O **What head shape results from fusion of all sutures except the metopic and squamosal sutures?**

Kleeblattschadel (clover leaf skull)

O **What receptor complexes have been linked to syndromic craniosynostosis?**

Transforming growth factor-Beta (TGF- B) and fibroblast growth factor receptor (FGFR), TWIST, MSX2

O **What syndrome is characterized by nasomaxillary hypoplasia, absent anterior nasal spine, short columella, and poor nasal projection?**

Binder Syndrome

O **What syndrome involves hypoplasia of the mandible, maxilla, and zygomas, downward slanting palpebral fissures, lower eyelid colobomas, absence of eyelashes, and auricular anomalies?**

Treacher Collins syndrome

❍ **What are the 3 findings required for the diagnosis of Pierre-Robin Sequence?**

Micrognathia, glossoptosis, and respiratory obstruction

❍ **Is cleft palate required for the diagnosis of Pierre-Robin Sequence?**

No

❍ **What is the first line treatment for the respiratory distress associated with Pierre-Robin sequence?**

Prone positioning

❍ **What syndrome involves an acquired progressive atrophy of skin, fat, muscle and bone, typically in a hemifacial distribution?**

Parry-Romberg disease

❍ **Which cranial nerve's function can be affected by hemifacial microsomia?**

Facial nerve (Cranial nerve VII)

❍ **What syndrome involves mandibular hypoplasia, epibulbar dermoids, microtia and vertebral anomalies?**

Goldenhar Syndrome (Oculoauriculovertebral dysplasia)

❍ **What autosomal dominant syndrome involves craniosynostosis, a low hairline, midface hypoplasia, and brachydactyly?**

Saethre-Chotzen syndrome

❍ **What autosomal dominant syndrome involves craniosynostosis, exorbitism, and midface retrusion, but not extremity anomalies?**

Crouzon syndrome

❍ **What autosomal dominant syndrome involves turribrachycephaly due to bicoronal synostosis, midface hypoplasia, symmetric complex or complicated syndactyly, and acne?**

Apert's syndrome

❍ **What syndrome is associated with craniosynostosis, broad thumbs and great toes, and syndactyly?**

Pfeiffer syndrome

❍ **What autosomal recessive disorder involves hypoplasia of the zygomas, orbits, maxilla, mandible and soft palate, auricular anomalies, and preaxial aplasia or hypoplasia of the upper extremity?**

Nager syndrome

❍ **What autosomal recessive syndrome involves pits of the lower lip and cleft lip and palate?**

van der Woude Syndrome

❍ **What autosomal recessive syndrome involves craniosynostosis, brachydactyly, mental retardation?**

Carpenter syndrome

❍   **What Pierre-Robin like syndrome is autosomal dominant, and also involves cleft palate, myopia, retinal detachment, and progressive blindness?**

Stickler Syndrome-(remember a <u>stick</u> in your eye causes blindness)

❍   **What syndrome involves submucous cleft palate and velopharyngeal insufficiency, in addition to a characteristic facies featuring a broad flat nose, poor malar projection, epicanthal folds, vertical maxillary excess, retrognathia, cardiac anomalies, and learning disabilities?**

Velocardiofacial syndrome (Shprintzen Syndrome)

❍   **What chromosomal abnormality is associated with velocardiofacial syndrome?**

Chromosome q 22 deletion

❍   **Patients with velocardiofacial syndrome who require surgical treatment for velopharyngeal insufficiency should be evaluated for what anatomic variation?**

Medial positioning of the internal carotid arteries

❍   **Which of the atypical clefts (Tessier classification) is the most common?**

Number seven

❍   **Which of the atypical clefts (Tessier classification) is associated with macrostomia?**

Number seven

References

Bartlett SP, Mackay GJ. Craniosynostosis syndromes. In: Aston SJ, Beasley RW, Thorne CH, eds. Grabb & Smith's Plastic Surgery. 5th ed. Philadelphia, Pa: Lippincott-Raven; 1997:295.

Huang MH, Gruss JS, Clarren SK, et al. The differential diagnosis of posterior plagiocephaly: true lambdoid synostosis versus positional molding. Plast Reconstr Surg. 1996; 98:765.

Kawamoto HK Jr. Rare craniofacial clefts. In: McCarthy JG, ed. Plastic Surgery. Philadelphia, Pa: WB Saunders Co; 1990;4:2945.

McCarthy JG, Epstein FJ, Wood-Smith D. Craniosynostosis. In: McCarthy JG, ed. Plastic Surgery. Philadelphia, Pa: WB Saunders Co; 1990;4:3054.

Mulliken JB, Vander Woude DL, Hansen M, et al. Analysis of posterior plagiocephaly: deformational versus synostotic. Plast Reconstr Surg. 1999; 103: 371.

Munro IR, Jay PP, Randall P, et al. Craniofacial syndromes. In: McCarthy JG, ed. Plastic Surgery. Philadelphia, Pa: WB Saunders Co; 1990;4:3106.

Robin NH: Molecular genetic advances in understanding craniosynostosis. Plast Reconstr Surg. 1999; 103: 1060-1070.

Ruff GL. Progressive hemifacial atrophy: Romberg's disease. In: McCarthy JG, ed. Plastic Surgery. Philadelphia, Pa: WB Saunders Co; 1990;5:3135-3143.

Tessier P. Anatomical classification of facial, craniofacial and latero-facial clefts. J Maxillofac Surg. 1969;4:69.

CRANIOSYNOSTOSIS

Wellington J. Davis III, MD

○ **What is the incidence of craniosynostosis?**

1 in 2000 births.

○ **T/F: Facial sutures fuse before cranial sutures.**

False.

○ **When do the facial sutures fuse?**

Facial sutures (except for the midpalatal suture) fuse in the seventh decade. Suture-Time of fusion: frontonasal-68yrs, frontozygomatic-72yrs.

○ **When do the cranial sutures fuse?**

Cranial sutures fuse earlier than the facial sutures.

Suture-Time of fusion: metopic-2yrs (may persist throughout life in 10%), sagittal-22yrs, coronal-24yrs, lamboid-26yrs, palatal 30-35yrs.

○ **What is the pattern of cranial suture fusion?**

Front to back, lateral to medial.

○ **What is the function of cranial and facial sutures?**

Cranial- bone overlap during birth, principle site of skull expansion, and shock-absorbing function in childhood.
Facial- shock-absorbing function related to mastication.

○ **What is Moss's functional matrix theory?**

Cranial bones enlarge as a result of growth and expansion of the underlying brain.

○ **What role may osteoblast-derived growth factors have in craniosynostosis?**

In-vitro studies of craniosynostotic bone cells reveal a longer population doubling time, which suggests that suppression of osteoblastic-derived growth factors (IGF-I, IGF-II, TGF-b1, PDGF, and bFGF) may be a factor.

○ **What is the genetic abnormality of Crouzon, Apert and Jackson Weiss Syndromes?**

Chromosome 10, mutation of fibroblast growth factor receptor 2 gene.

○ **What is the genetic abnormality of Pfeiffer syndrome?**

Chromosomes 8 and 10, mutation of the fibroblast growth factor receptor 1 or 2 gene.

○   **Which form of suture synostosis has an increased frequency of mutation in the genetic loci for fibroblast growth factor receptor 3 (FGFR-3)?**

Coronal.

○   **What is the genetic transmission of Saethre Chotzen, Crouzon, Apert and Pfeiffer Syndromes?**

Autosomal dominant.

○   **What is the genetic transmission of Carpenter and Baller Gerhold Syndromes?**

Autosomal recessive.

○   **What is the cause of contralateral frontal bone bossing and bilateral temporal bulges in coronal suture craniosynostosis?**

Bone growth occurs at the perimeter sutures with increased bone deposition directed away from the abnormally fused bone plate.

○   **T/F: Virchow (1851) noted that skull growth is inhibited parallel to the synostosed suture.**

False (inhibited perpendicular, compensatory expansion parallel).

○   **What are the three types of forehead plagiocephaly (asymmetry of the head)?**

Synostotic plagiocephaly, compensational plagiocephaly, deformational plagiocephaly.

○   **What is the incidence of synostotic forehead plagiocephaly?**

1 in 10,000 live births.

○   **T/F: 79% of synostotic forehead plagiocephaly occurs in females.** True.

○   **What are the distinguishing features of synostotic forehead plagiocephaly?**

- Forehead flat on affected side
- Eyebrow elevated on affected side
- Ear on affected side rotated anterior-superiorly
- Face C-shaped with nose and chin deviated to opposite side
- Forehead prominence opposite side
- Ipsilateral cheek forward

○   **What is the cause of head tilting in uncorrected unilateral synostosis?**

Strabismus secondary to paresis of the ipsilateral superior oblique muscle.

○   **What are the radiographic features of synostotic forehead plagiocephaly?**

- Radiographs- perisutural sclerosis, absence of coronal suture, harlequin mask appearance of orbit.
- 3D CT scan- fused suture, extent of skull and facial deformity.

○   **What percentage of patients with synostotic forehead plagiocephaly have torticollis?**

14%, usually contralateral side.

○ **What is the cause of compensational plagiocephaly?**

Premature fusion of the contralateral lamboid suture. Uncommon condition, fused suture revealed on radiographs. Clinical distinguishing factor from deformational plagiocephaly, no improvement on follow up.

○ **What is the cause of deformational plagiocephaly?**

Compressive forces in utero, by birth trauma and postnatally.

○ **What is the incidence of deformational forehead plagiocephaly?**

1 in 300 live births.

○ **What are the distinguishing features of deformational plagiocephaly?**

- Superior orbital rim lower on the affected side
- Eyebrow down;
- Ear rotated posterior-inferiorly on the flattened side;
- Malar eminence flattened ipsilaterally;
- Nose and chin rotated to affected side.
- Deformity not as severe as in synostosis

○ **What are the radiographic findings?**

Patent sutures.

○ **T/F: Torticollis is most commonly ipsilateral in deformational forehead plagiocephaly.**

True.

○ **T/F: Unlike synostotic forehead plagiocephaly, 76% of patients are male in deformational forehead plagiocephaly.**

False.

○ **T/F: On follow-up examination physical findings in deformational plagiocephaly do not improve.**

False.

○ **What is the cause of brachycephaly?**

Bilateral coronal suture craniosynostosis.

○ **What are the clinical features of brachycephaly?**

Reduced anterior-posterior distance, increased bitemporal distance.

○ **What is the normal ratio of anterior-posterior to bitemporal distance? What is the ratio in brachycephaly?**

3:2, 1:1.

○   **What are the radiographic findings of brachycephaly?**

- X-ray- bilateral fused coronal sutures and harlequin mask appearance.
- CT scan- fused sutures, abnormal shape of frontal bone.
- 3-D CT scan receding supraorbital borders, compensatory bulging of upper forehead.

○   **What is the cause of trigonocephaly?**

Metopic suture craniosynostosis.

○   **What are the clinical features of trigonocephaly?**

Triangular forehead with bilateral recession of lateral supraorbital borders and hypotelorism.

○   **What are the radiographic findings of trigonocephaly?**

- X-ray- hypotelorism.
- CT scan- triangular shaped forehead.
- 3-D CT scan- altered shape of forehead.

○   **Which form of synostosis is most frequently associated with abnormalities of the corpus callosum and increased incidence of developmental delay?**

Metopic synostosis, trigonocephaly.

○   **What is the cause of scaphocephaly?**

Sagittal suture craniosynostosis.

○   **T/F: Scaphocephaly is the most common form of craniosynostosis, more than 50% of cases.**

True.

○   **What are the clinical features of scaphocephaly?**

Dolichocephalic (scaphocephalic) cranial shape with biparietal narrowing and often frontal and/or occipital bossing. Palpable midline ridge.

○   **What percentage of patients also have lamboid synostosis?**

5-10%.

Clinical findings- foreshortening of skull in occipital region with prominent frontal bossing.

○   **What is the incidence of lamboid suture craniosynostosis?**

1-5% of all craniosynostosis cases. Much less common than deformational posterior plagiocephaly.

○   **What are the clinical features of lamboid craniosynostosis?**

Flatness on one or both sides of the posterior skull, posterior rotation of ipsilateral ear, compensatory flatness on contralateral frontal area- brachycephaly.

○ **What are the radiographic findings?**

Extensive sclerosis along the suture line difficult to distinguish from the mild sclerosis of deformational plagiocephaly.

○ **What is Kleeblattschadel (cloverleaf skull)?**

It is the most severe form of craniosynostosis, fusion of the coronal, lamboid and metopic sutures. Anterior sagittal and squamosal sutures open.

○ **What are the clinical features of Kleeblattschadel?**

- Bulging of frontal and temporal bones
- Markedly receding supraorbital borders
- Severe exorbitism
- Skull circumference significantly reduced
- Hydrocephalus usually present

○ **What are some of the congenital anomalies which may be associated with Kleeblattschadel?**

- Choanal atresia
- High arched palate
- Cleft palate

○ **What are the ocular complications seen in Kleeblattschadel?**

Because of retraction of the eyelids behind the globe, corneal opacity and perforations may occur if surgery is delayed.

○ **Which craniosynostosis syndrome is commonly associated with Kleeblattschadel?**

Pfeiffer syndrome.

○ **What is cranioscoliosis?**

Curvature of the midline of the craniofacial skeleton without fusion of sutures or torticollis or neck deformities. Diagnosis of exclusion.

○ **What are the features of Saethre Chotzen Syndrome (Craniocephalosyndactyly)?**

- bilateral coronal synostosis
- brachycephaly
- ptosis
- maxillary hypoplasia
- low hair line
- prominent ear crus along concha
- strabismus
- cleft or high arched palate
- syndactyly
- brachydactyly or clinodactyly

- vertebral anomalies
- normal intelligence

○ **What are the features of Crouzon Syndrome (Craniofacial Dysostosis)?** Bilateral coronal synostosis,

- oxycephaly (high, wide forehead, bulging anterior fontanelle)
- cranial base synostosis, hypertelorism
- exophthalmos
- maxillary hypoplasia
- parrot beak nose
- micrognathia
- no hand or feet abnormality

○ **What are the features of Apert Syndrome (Acrocephalosyndactyly)?**

- Skull- bilateral coronal synostosis, brachycephaly
- Maxillary hypoplasia- high arched palate, cleft palate or submucosal cleft palate, crowding dental arch, anterior open bite
- Orbit- hypertelorism, exorbitism, oculomotor paralysis, ptosis, down-slanting palpebral fissure
- Hands- syndactyly all fingers (mitten hands), short humerus
- Feet- syndactyly all toes
- Coarse skin and acne
- Enlarged ear lobes
- Mental retardation: variable

○ **What are the features of Carpenter Syndrome (Group of Acrocephalosyndactyly)?**

- craniosynostosis single or multiple sutures
- deafness
- mental retardation
- brachydactyly (hands and feet)
- syndactyly (hands and feet)
- polydactyly (hands, preaxial)

○ **What is the incidence of Crouzon and Apert Syndromes?**

1 in 60,000 and 16 per million births.

○ **What are the clinical features of Pfeiffer Syndrome?**

- craniosynostosis
- wide thumbs and great toes
- brachydactyly
- partial syndactyly
- maxillary hypoplasia
- intelligence usually normal

○ **What is Jackson-Weiss Syndrome?**

- craniosynostosis
- hypertelorism
- midface hypoplasia
- broad great toes

- syndactyly toes (occasionally fingers)
- medial deviation tarsal-metatarsal coalescence

❍   **What is Baller-Gerhold Syndrome?**

- craniosynostosis
- radial aplasia
- anal anomalies
- urologic defects
- cardiac deformity
- CNS abnormalities
- vertebral defects

❍   **What is the timing of surgery in Kleeblattschadel, sagittal synostosis, coronal synostosis?**

First few days of life (urgent decompression), 2 months of age, 6 months of age.

❍   **What is the risk of increased intracranial pressure and adverse effect on mental development in synostosis of one suture?**

7% chance, risk increases with multiple sutures.

❍   **T/F: Cosmetic appearance is the primary factor for operative intervention in craniosynostosis?**

False.

❍   **What are the goals of therapy in craniosynostosis?**

- Release the synostosis and provide adequate skull volume for brain development.
- Create an aesthetically normal forehead and skull shape.

❍   **What are the nonoperative interventions for skull deformity without evidence of craniosynostosis?**

- Sternomastoid stretching exercises for torticollis.
- At feeding times baby encouraged to turn head toward breast or bottle.
- Orthotic cranioplasty- helmet to mold skull as it grows.

❍   **At what age is orthotic cranioplasty effective and what is the time course of therapy?**

 Molding can be begun after age 6 months, not effective after 18 months of age. Helmet is worn 23 hours a day for 2-4 months. Inadequate response may require surgical intervention.

❍   **What is the surgical management of unilateral coronal suture synostosis?** Unilateral (mild deformity) or bilateral (severe deformity) fronto-orbital advancement.

❍   **What is the determining factor in the surgical management of bilateral coronal suture synostosis?**

Presence of concomitant brachycephaly.

❍   **What is the surgical management of bilateral coronal suture synostosis?**

Bilateral fronto-orbital advancement in patients without brachycephaly. Total calvarial reconstruction with barrel staving of occipital bones in patients with brachycephaly.

❍ **What is the surgical management of metopic synostosis?**

Removal of supraorbital bar, corticotomy and correction of midline angle to 150 degrees with bone graft or miniplates. Correction of coronal synostosis. Examination of metopic suture and release. Hypotelorism corrects with growth.

❍ **What is the primary determinant in the choice of operation for patients with sagittal synostosis?**

Patient age followed by previous intervention. Procedures are most effective and less extensive in younger patients less than 6 months. Ideal age 2-4 months. More extensive procedures are needed age 6-9 months. Children older than 1 year even more extensive procedures are needed and morbidity increases significantly due to increased blood loss.

❍ **What are the surgical interventions for Sagittal Synostosis?**

The "pi" or "t" craniectomy techniques (or modifications thereof) which utilize strip craniectomies with partial wedge osteotomies. In selected cases with more severe deformity (frontal and occipital bossing) anterior and posterior parietal wedges or barrel-stave osteotomies to facilitate biparietal expansion. Total calvarial reconstruction may be used in children older than 1 year or reops, may require bone replacement.

❍ **What is the major risk of surgical management of sagittal synostosis?**

Sagittal sinus injury with blood loss or venous infarction.

❍ **What is the disadvantage of simple suture removal?**

Immediate correction of cranial shape is not achieved, many patients have residual deformity secondary to suture reclosure before adequate cranial remodeling.

❍ **What is the advantage of early operation in sagittal synostosis?**

High potential for new bone growth, quicker operative options with less blood loss, continued brain growth for skull expansion, increased skull flexibility for easier remodeling.

❍ **How long does it take for bone defects to fill in?**

Approximately 6 months.

❍ **What is the rate of reoperation, what are the outcomes?**

Less than 5% reoperation. >90% excellent cosmetic results, the remaining good cosmetic results.

❍ **What is the surgical management of lamboidal synostosis?**

Under age 6 months excision of lamboid suture. Over age 6 months posterior skull remodeling with occipital bandeau, barrel staving of bone below the bandeau and bending with Tessier bone bender. Alternate method: spiral osteotomy.

❍ **What is the preoperative management of Kleeblattschadel?**

- Management of more serious medical problems
- Airway management
- Eye protection- artificial tears, ophthalmic ointment
- R/O cervical spine and craniovertebral anomalies
- Radiologic work-up 3-D CT scans

○ **What is the indication for emergent management?**

- Management of hydrocephalus
- VP shunt may be indicated at the same time or at a subsequent procedure

○ **What is the operative management of Kleeblattschadel?**

Anterior calvariectomy with fronto-orbital advancement. Bone removal from constricting band of coronal, frontosphenoid, frontoethmoid and lamboid sutures.

○ **Will further intervention be needed?**

In severe cases a second-stage posterior calvarial release is necessary at 1-2 months of age. A second anterior surgical release often required at 6-12 months. A third correction of anterior and/or posterior skull deformities again before age 4.

○ **What is the surgical management of cranioscoliosis?**

Fronto-orbital advancement on the receding side and expansion of the flattened parietal area with interdigitating cuts in the parietotemporal area.

○ **What are some of the potential operative and early postop complications of craniosynostosis cases?**

- death
- anesthetic complications
- excessive blood loss
- sagittal sinus tear with venous infarction
- cerebral edema
- increased ICP
- dural leak
- subdural hematoma
- periorbital injury
- nerve injury (frontal branch VII, supraorbital nerve)
- loss of vision
- corneal abrasion
- CSF leak
- infection
- skin necrosis
- SIADH

○ **What are some of the late postop complications of craniosynostosis operations?**

- alopecia
- hypertrophic scarring
- palpable hardware
- forehead defects and irregularities
- deficient frontal bone advancement

- temporal depression
- pseudomeningoceles
- metal plates
- orbital deformities
- asymmetry
- recurrence
- bone graft Resorption
- increased ICP
- patient dissatisfaction

References

Losken HW, Pollack IF. Craniosynostosis. In: Bentz, ML, ed. Pediatric Plastic Surgery. 1st ed. Stamford: Appleton & Lange, 1998: 129-157.

Delashaw JB, et al. Cranial vault growth in craniosynostosis. J. Neurosurg 70: 159-165, 1989.

Bruneteau RJ, Mulliken JB. Frontal plagiocephaly: Synostotic, compensational, or deformational. Plast Reconstr Surg 89: 21-31, 1992.

Anderson FM, Geiger L. Craniosynostosis: A Survey of 204 cases. J. Neurosurg 22: 229-240, 1965.

David DJ, Poswillo D, Simpson DA. The Craniosynostosis; Causes, Natural History and Management. New York: Springer-Verlag, 1982.

Hinton DR, Becker LE, Muakkessa KF, Hoffman HJ. Lamboid synostosis. Part 1. The lamboid suture: Normal development and pathology of "synostosis." J. Neurosurg 61: 333-339, 1984.

Watters EC, Hiles DA, Johnson BL. Cloverleaf skull syndrome. Am J Ophthalmol 76: 716-720, 1973.

Fearon JA, Munro IR. Cranioscoliosis. Plast Reconstructive Surg 92: 202-208, 1993.

Cassileth LB, Bartlett SP, Glat PM, et al. Clinical characteristics of patients with unicoronal synostosis and mutations of fibroblast growth factor receptor 3: a preliminary report. Plast Reconstr Surg. 2001;108:1849-1854.

Sidoti EJ Jr, Marsh JL, Marty-Grames L, et al. Long-term studies of metopic synostosis: frequency of cognitive impairment and behavioral disturbances. Plast Reconstr Surg. 1996;97:276-281.

Zampino G, DiRocco C, Butera G, et al. Opitz C trigonocephaly syndrome and midline brain anomalies. Amer J Med Genet. 1997;73:484-488.

Gosain AK, Steele MA, McCarthy JG, et al. A prospective study of the relationship between strabismus and head posture in patients with frontal plagiocephaly. Plast Reconstr Surg. 1996;97:881-891.

CLEFT LIP/PALATE

Reuben A. Bueno, Jr., MD

○ **What facial elements fuse to form the face?**

Frontonasal
2 lateral maxillary segments
2 mandibular segments

○ **Failure of fusion of what components results in the cleft lip deformity?**

Medial nasal prominence to the maxillary nasal prominence

○ **Failure of fusion of what components results in primary cleft palate?**

Lateral palatine processes and median palatine process

○ **Failure of fusion of what components results in secondary cleft palate?**

Lateral palatine processes to each other and with the nasal septum

○ **What structures arise from the frontonasal prominence?**

Lateral nasal prominence
Medial nasal prominence
Median palatine process
Nasal placodes

○ **What methods are used to narrow a wide unilateral cleft lip prior to definitive repair?**

Presurgical orthodontics and lip adhesion

○ **What structures meet at the incisive foramen?**

The lateral maxillary bones meet the midline premaxilla

○ **What is the significance of the incisive foramen?**

It separates the primary and secondary palates, just behind the central incisors.

○ **Clefts of the primary palate involve what structures?**

Alveolus, lip, and nasal tip cartilages

○ **Clefts of the secondary palate involve what structures?**

Hard palate, soft palate, and uvula

○ **When is alveolar bone grafting usually done?**

During the time of <u>mixed dentition</u> (ages 6-12 years) prior to eruption of permanent dentition

❍ **What is the most common cleft combination?**

Unilateral cleft lip and palate

❍ **What is the anatomical failure in a cleft palate?**

Failure of the palatal shelves to assume a horizontal orientation and fuse in the midline

❍ **What is more common: right or left side cleft palate?**

Left sided clefts are more common. 6 left: 3 right: 1 bilateral

❍ **Why is the left more commonly cleft?**

Possibly because the right palatal shelf assumes its fully horizontal position before the left, leaving the left susceptible to developmental insults for a greater period of time.

❍ **The eruption of what tooth is most likely to be impaired in a unilateral cleft lip and palate deformity?**

Canine on the cleft side

❍ **What is the usual age for cleft lip repair?**

Between 3-6 months of age

❍ **What is the estimated incidence of clefting by race?**

Asian: 3/1000
Caucasian: 1/1000
Black: 0.5/1000

❍ **If a parent gives birth to a child with cleft lip and palate, what is the estimated risk of a future child having a cleft lip and palate deformity?**

- 3% if one sibling has the deformity
- 3-4% if one parent has the deformity
- 15-17% if one sibling and one parent has the deformity

❍ **What are the features of a submucosal cleft palate?**

Bifid uvula
palpable notch at posterior edge of hard palate
zona pellucida

❍ **What is a zona pellucida?**

A thin area where the levator muscle fibers have failed to fuse in the midline

❍ **What is the significance of a submucosal cleft palate?**

It may lead to VPI

❍ **What are considered the most important muscles for velopharyngeal closure?**

The levator veli palatini muscles

○   **What is the action of the levator veli palatini muscles?**

These muscles pull the middle third of the soft palate superiorly and posteriorly to produce contact with the posterior pharyngeal wall, thereby separating the nasopharynx from the oropharynx.

○   **What palatal muscles are innervated by the vagus nerve?**

Levator veli palatini
Pharyngeal constrictors
Musculus uvulae
Palatoglossus
Palatopharyngeus

○   **The hamulus serves as a pulley for what muscle?**

Tensor veli palatini

○   **Is the tensor veli palatini involved in normal velopharyngeal closure?**

No

○   **What is the primary indication to repair a cleft palate?**

To provide more normal speech

○   **At what age is a cleft palate usually repaired?**

Between 8-12 months

○   **Describe the von Langenbeck palatoplasty.**

Incisions are made along the cleft margin and laterally. Mucoperiosteal flaps are raised. Abnormal muscle attachments are taken down. Midline closure involves three layers: nasal layer, muscle layer, and oral layer.

○   **Describe the Veau-Wardill-Kilner palatoplasty.**

V-Y advancement of mucoperiosteal flaps allows palatal lengthening. Bare areas laterally heal in secondarily. As with the von Langenbeck, abnormal muscular attachments are taken down, and the nasal, muscle, and oral layers are closed separately.

○   **What is the blood supply of the mucoperiosteal flaps in the von Langenbeck and Veau-Wardill-Kilner repairs?**

The greater palatine artery coming through the greater palatine foramen.

○   **Describe the Furlow palatoplasty.**

Double opposing Z-plasty allows closure of the cleft palate and reorientation of the muscle. For the oral layer, oral mucosa-muscle flap is raised on one side, and an oral mucosa flap is raised on the opposite side. For the nasal layer, a nasal layer flap is raised on one side with a muscle-nasal layer flap on the opposite side. Flaps containing muscle must always be posteriorly based to preserve muscle blood supply.

○   **What is the problem in VPI (velopharyngeal incompetence)?**

The soft palate does not reach the posterior pharyngeal wall during speech leading to hypernasal speech.

❍ **How is VPI evaluated?**

A speech pathologist is involved in evaluation. Assessment of palatal motion can be made by videofluoroscopy or nasoendoscopy. Pressure flow or objective nasal resonance can also be measured.

❍ **What are the surgical options for VPI?**

With minor VPI, speech therapy may improve speech and prevent the need for any surgery. Surgical options include a Furlow palatoplasty, pharyngeal flap or sphincteroplasty.

❍ **Describe sphincter pharyngoplasty.**

Palatopharyngeal (palatopharyngeus muscle) myomucosal flaps with intact neurovascular supply are elevated from the posterior tonsillar pillar and inset into the posterior wall of the nasopharynx where it joins the palate to create a dynamic velopharyngeal sphincter.

❍ **What anatomical anomaly must be evaluated prior to a pharyngoplasty?**

In patients with **velocardiofacial syndrome** who demonstrate VPI, the position of the carotid arteries must be evaluated, usually by MR angiography. **The carotid arteries may be ectopic** and in a more superficial and medially displaced position in the posterior pharyngeal wall.

❍ **What is a major complication of surgery to correct VPI?**

Obstructive sleep apnea

❍ **What percentage of cleft palate repair patients develop VPI?**

Approximately 20% of patients who undergo cleft palate repair develop VPI requiring surgical intervention

Syndromes

❍ **What are the features of Pierre Robin Sequence?**

Retrognathia
Glossoptosis
Respiratory distress
U-shaped cleft palate

❍ **What are the characteristics of velocardiofacial syndrome?**

Cleft palate
Cardiac abnormalities
Abnormal facial features

❍ **What are the abnormal facial features associated with velocardiofacial syndrome?**

Broad, prominent nose
Malar flattening
Epicanthal folds
Retrognathia
Vertical maxillary excess

❍ **What chromosomal abnormality is associated with velocardiofacial syndrome?**

Deletion on the long arm of chromosome 22q

○ **What diagnostic test is used for velocardiofacial syndrome?**

Fluorescent in situ hybridization (FISH) analysis

○ **What is Van der Woude's syndrome?**

An autosomal dominant disorder characterized by cleft lip and palate and <u>lip pits</u>

References

David DJ, Bagnall AD: Velopharyngeal incompetence. In McCarthy JG (ed): *Plastic Surgery*. Philadelphia, W.B. Saunders, 1990, pp 2903-21.

Johnson MC, Bronsky PT, Millicorsky G: Embryogenesis of cleft lip and palate. In McCarthy JG (ed): *Plastic Surgery*. Philadelphia, W.B. Saunders, 1990, pp 2451-95.

Millard DR Jr. *Cleft craft: The evolution of its surgery*. Boston, Little, Brown & Co., 1976.

Randall P, LaRosa D: Cleft palate. In McCarthy JG (ed): *Plastic Surgery*. Philadelphia, W.B. Saunders, 1990, pp 2723-52.

VELOPHARYNGEAL INCOMPETENCE/INSUFFICIENCY

Jugpal S. Arneja, MD and Arun K. Gosain, MD

○ **Describe what is meant by velopharyngeal incompetence (VPI)?**

a) the velopharyngeal structures cannot produce full closure of the port
b) the velopharyngeal system is structurally inadequate for production of good speech
c) the structure of the velopharyngeal system or its neuromotor control is inadequate for production for good speech
d) an individual's speech is perceived as showing characteristics associated with disorders of the velopharyngeal system

○ **What synonyms have been used to describe VPI?**

Velopharyngeal incompetence, inadequacy, deficiency, or insufficiency

○ **What are the symptoms & signs of VPI?**

Speech - Hypernasality, Compensatory misarticulations, Airflow escape, Facial grimacing
Reflux - Oro-nasal regurgitation (fluids >>solids)
Hearing Loss (conductive) - Eustachian tube dysfunction

○ **What is the incidence of VPI post cleft palate repair?**

The incidence varies between 7-25% post-palate repair

○ **What are the etiologies of VPI?**

a) idiopathic insufficiency of palatal musculature
b) congenital palatal insufficiency
c) submucous cleft palate
d) post cleft palate repair (most common)
e) post pharyngeal flap or pharyngoplasty
f) post adenoidectomy
g) enlarged tonsils
h) post midface advancement
i) neurogenic causes
j) lack of velopharyngeal sphincter movement for speech
k) functional or hysterical hypernasality

○ **What anatomically makes up the velopharygeal space?**

Velum (anterior border); posterior pharyngeal wall (posterior border); right lateral pharyngeal wall (lateral border); left lateral pharyngeal wall (lateral border)

○ **What muscles contribute to closure of the velopharynx?**

Levator veli palatini, superior pharyngeal constrictor, palatopharyngeus, tensor tympani, musculus uvulae

○ **Discuss functions during opening and closing of the velopharynx.**

Opening of the velopharynx - facilitates breathing and normal speech production of nasal articulations
Closure of the velopharynx - allows normal speech production of oral consonants and prevents oro-nasal reflux

○ How does the velopharynx close?

The velum moves posteriorly and superiorly; the posterior pharyngeal wall moves anteriorly; the lateral pharyngeal walls move medially; the tonsils and adenoids may augment or interfere with the function of the walls during velopharyngeal closure

○ Who contributes to the evaluation of VPI?

An interdisciplinary team consisting of :
a) Plastic Surgeon
b) Speech/Language Pathologist
c) Otolaryngologist
d) Audiologist
e) Radiologist
e) Geneticist

○ How should VPI be evaluated?

Indirect Methods: Perceptual Speech Assessment, Pressure-Flow Measurements, TONAR (The Oral Nasal Acoustic Ratio)

Direct Methods: Nasopharyngeal Endoscopy, Multiview Videofluoroscopy

○ What does the speech pathologist evaluate?

Perceptually (auditory and visual input), the patient's speech is evaluated by a trained speech pathologist establishing the diagnosis of VPI.
Speech criteria evaluated include:
     i.   Articulation (+/- errors)
     ii.   Facial grimace
     iii.   Nasal emission
     iv.   Quality (laryngeal resonance)
     v.   Quality (nasal resonance)

○ At what age should a perceptual speech assessment be performed

An initial evaluation should be performed at 3 years of age

○ What are the closure patterns seen with nasopharyngeal endoscopy?

4 types of closure patterns found on nasopharyngeal endoscopy:
Coronal (most common, 55%), circular (20%), circular with Passavant ridge (15-20%), sagittal (10-15%)

○ What modality has been recently studied that might have efficacy in the evaluation of VPI?

Magnetic Resonance Imaging (MRI)

○ What non-surgical treatments are available for VPI?

Speech therapy, palatal lift, palatal prosthesis, velopharyngeal obturator

○ What surgical treatments are available for VPI?

Palatal lengthening (Furlow palatoplasty or V-Y pushback palatoplasty), posterior wall augmentation (alloplastic or autogenous materials), sphincter pharyngoplasty, pharyngeal flap

❍ **What materials are available for posterior wall augmentation?**

Alloplastic: Teflon, Silastic, Silicone gel, Proplast

Autogenous: autologous cartilage, autologous fascia

❍ **Is posterior wall augmentation used in practice today?**

Most centers have abandoned posterior wall augmentation because of unpredictable results

❍ **What is a sphincter pharyngoplasty?**

A surgical procedure designed to tighten the central orifice and occlude the lateral aspects of the velopharyngeal sphincter

❍ **What muscle forms the basis for a successful sphincter pharyngoplasty? How is it done?**

Palatopharyngeus; Two (right and left) myomucosal (palatopharyngeus) flaps are elevated from the posterior tonsillar pillars and are sutured to each other and to the posterior pharyngeal wall

❍ **When should a sphincter pharyngoplasty be performed?**

There is no consensus in the literature, but historically sphincter pharyngoplasties have been performed for documented cases of sufficient palatal length and mobility, with poor lateral wall motion

❍ **What are the complications of a sphincter pharyngoplasty?**

Sleep apnea, snoring, airway obstruction.

❍ **What is a pharyngeal flap?**

The creation of a midline subtotal obstruction of the oral and nasal cavities with two small lateral openings (ports) which remain patent during respiration and nasal consonant production and closed during oral consonant production.

❍ **How is a pharyngeal flap done?**

A myomucosal flap is elevated from the posterior pharyngeal wall and is attached to the soft palate creating an incomplete midline obstruction; the donor site can be closed primarily or allowed to heal secondarily.

❍ **Should a superiorly or inferiorly based pharyngeal flap be performed?**

Superiorly based flaps are most frequently used as inferiorly based flaps can tether the flap in an inferior direction, opposite to the necessary direction for correct velopharyngeal closure

❍ **When should a pharyngeal flap be performed**

Again, there are no clear indications, but historically pharyngeal flaps are performed when there is sufficient lateral wall motion with a short or adynamic central palate

❍ **What are the complications of a pharyngeal flap?**

Sleep apnea, snoring, airway obstruction

○   **What is Velocardiofacial (VCF) Syndrome? What is the concern to a surgeon treating patients with VPI?**

An autosomal dominant condition associated with deletions on the long arm of chromosome 22.
Major clinical findings include cleft palate, congenital heart anomalies, cognitive impairment and abnormal facies; of concern to the VPI surgeon, patients with VCF may have medially displaced carotid arteries which make injury to the carotids a possibility during pharyngeal surgery.

○   **What test is essential prior to surgical correction of velopharyngeal incompetence in patients with VCF?**

Magnetic Resonance Angiography (MRA)

○   **What is the recommended surgical treatment for VPI in VCF patients?**

A high, wide pharyngeal flap

○   **What is a submucous cleft palate (SMCP)?**

A SMCP is classically defined as patients having a bifid uvula, a zona pellucida (palatal muscle diastasis), and a bony notch of the hard palate

○   **What is the incidence of VPI in patients with a SMCP?**

1 in 9 (11%)

○   **What should the treatment be of a SMCP?**

SMCP should be initially evaluated by perceptual speech evaluation; surgery should only be performed for documented cases of VPI following a thorough speech evaluation.

References

Bicknell S, McFadden LR, Curran JB. Frequency of pharyngoplasty after primary repair of cleft palate. J Can Dent Assoc 2002; 68:688-692.

Conley SF, Gosain AK, Marks SM et al. Identification and assessment of velopharyngeal inadequacy. Am J Otolaryngol 1997; 18:38-46.

Croft CB, Shprintzen RJ, Rakoff SJ. Patterns of velopharyngeal valving in normal and cleft palate subjects: a multiview videofluoroscopic and nasendoscopic study. Laryngoscope 1981; 91:265-271.

David DJ, Bagnall AD. Velopharyngeal incompetence. In: McCarthy JG, ed. Plastic Surgery. 1st ed. Philadelphia, PA: WB Saunders Co., 1990:2903-2921.

Denny AD, Marks SM, Oliff-Carneol S. Correction of velopharyngeal insufficiency by pharyngeal augmentation using autologous cartilage: a preliminary report. Cleft Palate Craniofac J 1993; 30:46-54.

Folkins JW. Velopharyngeal nomenclature: incompetence, inadequacy, insufficiency, and dysfunction. Cleft Palate Craniofac J 1988; 25:413-416.

Gosain AK, Conley SF, Marks S, et al. Submucous cleft palate: diagnostic methods and outcomes of surgical treatment. Plast Reconstr Surg 1996; 97:1497-1509.

Marsh JL. The evaluation and management of velopharyngeal dysfunction. Clin Plastic Surg 2004; 31:261-269.

Marsh JL. Management of velopharyngeal dysfunction: differential diagnosis for differential management. J Craniofac Surg 2003; 14:621-628.

Mitnick RJ, Bello JA, Golding-Kushner KJ, et al. The use of magnetic resonance angiography prior to pharyngeal flap surgery in patients with velocardiofacial syndrome. Plast Reconstr Surg 1996; 97:908-919.

Schendel SA, Lorenz HP, Dagenais D, et al. A single surgeon's experience with the Delaire palatoplasty. Plast Reconstr Surg 1999; 104:1993-1997.

Sirois M, Caouette-Laberge L, Spier S, et al. Sleep apnea following a pharyngeal flap: a feared complication. Plast Reconstr Surg 1994; 93:943-947.

Sloan, GM. Posterior pharyngeal flap and sphincter pharyngoplasty: the state of the art. Cleft Palate Craniofac J 2000; 37:112-122.

Tatum SA 3rd, Chang J, Havkin N, et al. Pharyngeal flap and the internal carotid in velocardiofacial syndrome. Arch Facial Plast Surg 2002; 4:73-80.

Vedung S. Pharyngeal flaps after one- and two-stage repair of the cleft palate: a 25-year review of 520 patients. Cleft Palate Craniofac J 1995; 32:206-215.

Witt PD. Velopharyngeal insufficiency. In: Achauer B, ed. Plastic Surgery: Indications, Operations, and Outcomes. 1st ed. St. Louis, MO: CV Mosby Co., 2000:819-833.

Witt PD, D'Antonio LL. Velopharyngeal insufficiency and secondary palatal management. Clin Plast Surg 1993; 20:707-721.

Witt PD, Marsh JL, Muntz HR et al. Acute obstructive sleep apnea as a complication of sphincter pharyngoplasty. Cleft Palate Craniofac J 1996; 33:183-189.

PHARYNGOPLASTY/ PHARYNGEAL FLAPS

Steven L. Henry, MD

○ **Name the six primary muscles of the velopharyngeal mechanism.**

Levator veli palatini, tensor veli palatini, musculus uvulae, palatoglossus, palatopharyngeus, superior constrictor.

○ **Which of these muscles is innervated by V3?**

Tensor veli palatini.

○ **What is the primary function of tensor veli palatini?**

Opening of the eustachian tube.

○ **In what direction(s) does the soft palate move to close the velopharyngeal portal?**

Posteriorly and superiorly.

○ **What muscle is primarily responsible for this movement?**

Levator veli palatini.

○ **What muscle is primarily responsible for medial movement of the lateral pharyngeal walls during closure of the velopharyngeal portal?**

Levator veli palatini.

○ **Name the four patterns of velopharyngeal closure.**

Coronal, sagittal, sphincteric, sphincteric with Passavant's ridge.

○ **What is Passavant's ridge?**

Transversely oriented ridge on the posterior pharyngeal wall, due to bulging of the uppermost fibers of superior constrictor

○ **Where does Passavant's ridge usually lie relative to the level of velopharyngeal closure?**

Approximately 1 cm inferior.

○ **Which arteries supply the soft palate?**

Lesser palatine artery, ascending palatine branch of facial artery, palatine branches of ascending pharyngeal artery.

○ **What is the difference between velopharyngeal incompetence and velopharyngeal insufficiency?**

Incompetence refers to neuromuscular deficit, as in myasthenia gravis, cerebral palsy, stroke, head injury, or upper/lower motor neuron lesions. Insufficiency refers to an anatomic defect, as in cleft palate, congenitally short palate/large pharynx, or after ablative surgery.

○   **What is rhinolalia aperta?**

Hypernasal speech due to inadequate closure of the velopharyngeal portal.

○   **Besides hypernasality, what other category of speech disturbance is associated with VPI?**

Misarticulations.

○   **What is a fricative?**

Consonant sound produced by the constriction of the air stream to create friction, as in f, v, s, z, th, or sh.

○   **What distinguishes the different fricatives?**

Position of the articulators (e.g., the tongue articulates with the teeth for th, and with the alveolar ridge for s or z).

○   **What is a pharyngeal fricative?**

Fricative produced by articulation of the tongue against the posterior pharyngeal wall.

○   **Name an example of a pharyngeal fricative in normal English speech.**

There is none. A pharyngeal fricative is used by patients with VPI as a substitute for a normal oral fricative.

○   **What is a stop plosive?**

Consonant sound produced by the sudden release of intraoral pressure, as in p, b, t, d, k, or g.

○   **What is a glottal stop?**

Plosive sound made by suddenly releasing the laryngeal valve. It is a common misarticulation by patients with VPI. The only example in normal English is "uh," as in "uh huh" or "uh uh."

○   **What is a posterior nasal fricative?**

Nasal snort (attempt to close posterior nasal aperture).

○   **What is an anterior nasal fricative?**

Nasal grimacing (attempt to close anterior nasal aperture).

○   **What is a diphthong?**

Single syllable with two vowel sounds (e.g., cow, toy, about). Diphthongs require significant velar elevation and mobility, and are thus difficult for patients with VPI.

○   **Besides VPI, what are other common reasons for misarticulation in the pediatric plastic surgery population?**

Mental retardation, abnormal dentition (e.g., V-shaped maxillary dentition in Apert's syndrome), malocclusion, hearing deficit.

○ **Describe the cul-de-sac test.**

Ask the patient to repeat a word like "bat" or "boot" twice, the second time with the patient's nose pinched. If the resonance is different, the oral and nasal cavities are coupled (i.e., there is inadequate velopharyngeal closure).

○ **What is pressure-flow instrumentation?**

Objective assessment of nasal airflow and differential oral-nasal air pressure.

○ **What are the two most common imaging modalities for the assessment of VPI?**

Videofluoroscopy and nasal endoscopy.

○ **What is the advantage of videofluoroscopy?**

Ability to define the level of velopharyngeal closure in the sagittal plane (i.e., with respect to Passavant's ridge).

○ **What is the advantage of nasal endoscopy?**

Ability to visualize the entire velopharyngeal mechanism during speech.

○ **What are the indications for a palatal obturator?**

Extremely wide cleft with little or no velar movement (in whom surgery would be expected to have a poor outcome), neuromuscular deficit, poor surgical candidate, surgical failure.

○ **What is the orientation of the levator fibers within the normal soft palate and in the cleft palate?**

Transverse in the normal palate; longitudinal in the cleft palate.

○ **What is an intravelar veloplasty?**

Redirection of the aberrantly oriented levator muscles to the transverse plane, permitting functional mobility of the soft palate.

○ **What is the incidence of VPI after standard palatoplasty and intravelar veloplasty?**

About 20%.

○ **What common palatoplasty technique has the lowest incidence of post-operative VPI?**

Furlow double opposing Z-plasty.

○ **What is pharyngeal augmentation?**

Placement of a substance in the retropharyngeal space in an attempt to create a ridge against which the soft palate can more easily close. Reported substances include bone, cartilage, fascia, mucosa, and fat.

○ **The retropharyngeal space lies between what two fascial planes?**

Buccopharyngeal fascia and prevertebral fascia.

○ **Who first reported the posterior pharyngeal flap (PPF)?**

Schoenborn, in 1876.

❍   **What layers are included in the PPF?**

Mucosa, muscle (superior constrictor), buccopharyngeal fascia.

❍   **What important vascular structure lies 1-1.5 cm lateral to the posterior pharyngeal wall?**

Internal carotid artery.

❍   **The internal carotid artery is often medially displaced in what common craniofacial syndrome?**

Velocardiofacial syndrome.

❍   **What are the advantages of a superiorly based PPF compared to an inferiorly based PPF?**

The superiorly based flap can be made longer. In theory, it may provide suspension (rather than inferior tethering) of soft palate, and hence better facilitate velopharyngeal closure. Friable adenoid tissue must often be dissected and sutured in the inferiorly based flap; this is avoided in the superiorly based flap.

❍   **Follow up studies have shown that superiorly and inferiorly based PPFs heal at the same level and orientation. How is this possible?**

Contracture of the donor site pulls the superiorly based flap downward, and the inferiorly based flap upward.

❍   **What can be done to prevent contracture and rolling of a PPF?**

Lining the raw surface with mucosal flaps from the hard or soft palate.

❍   **What potentially deleterious maneuver must often be done to provide lining for the raw (inferior) surface of a superiorly based PPF?**

The soft palate often must be incised, transversely or in the midline, to provide access to the nasal surface of the palate. This is a disadvantage of the superiorly based PPF compared to the inferiorly based PPF.

❍   **What is the Millard island push-back flap?**

Island flap of hard palate mucosa based on the greater palatine artery, used for palatal lengthening and/or lining of a PPF.

❍   **T/F: the superiorly based PPF has been shown to result in better outcomes than the inferiorly based PPF.**

False. Large reviews by Skoog in 1965, Hamlen in 1970, and Whitaker in 1972 found no difference in outcomes between the two flaps.

❍   **When is PPF surgery usually performed?**

At the time of diagnosis of VPI, usually between the ages of 2 and 6 years.

❍   **What is a primary PPF?**

PPF performed at the time of cleft palate repair.

❍   **What are the theoretic advantages of the primary PPF?**

Obviates the development of bad speech habits, reduces the need for speech therapy, avoids a second surgery, improves exposure of the posterior pharyngeal wall, enables the surgeon to work with unscarred mucosa, provides additional tissue for the palate repair.

○ **What are the most serious complications of PPF surgery?**

Hemorrhage and sleep apnea.

○ **What are the risk factors for post-operative sleep apnea?**

Age < 5 years, microretrognathia, upper respiratory tract infection, history of perinatal respiratory dysfunction.

○ **What are the most common complications of PPF surgery?**

Persistent hypernasality, hyponasality, dehiscence.

○ **What is a sphincter pharyngoplasty (SP)?**

Wrapping of superiorly based lateral pharyngeal flaps along posterior pharyngeal wall to create a dynamic ridge.

○ **What muscle is included in the lateral pharyngeal flaps?**

Palatopharyngeus.

○ **What is the difference between the Hynes and Orticochea pharyngoplasties?**

Hynes: the palatopharyngeal flaps are inset within a transverse incision in the posterior pharyngeal wall.

Orticochea: the palatopharyngeal flaps are inset under an inferiorly-based mucosal flap from the posterior pharyngeal wall. Jackson modified the Orticochea procedure by insetting the flaps under a superiorly-based mucosal flap.

○ **At what level should the palatopharyngeal flaps be inset?**

At the level of velopharyngeal closure, as determined by videofluoroscopy. Usually this means insetting the flaps as high as possible, above Passavant's ridge and above the level of the arch of the atlas.

○ **In what fraction of SPs does the transferred palatopharyngeus muscle retain significant contractility?**

Approximately 1/3.

○ **What are the advantages and disadvantages of the SP compared to the PPF?**

SP has a lower rate of nasal obstruction and sleep apnea, but a higher rate of persistent hypernasality. It is also thought to be easier to perform, with no need to divide the soft palate.

○ **For each of the following velopharyngeal closure patterns, what treatment is most appropriate?**

Coronal pattern, with little lateral wall movement:	SP
Sagittal pattern, with good lateral movement but poor velar movement:	PPF
Sphincteric pattern, with small gap:	SP
Sphincteric pattern, with large gap:	PPF
No closure (poor velar and lateral movement):	PPF or obturator

References

Armour A, Fischbach S, Klaiman P, et al. Does velopharyngeal closure pattern affect the success of pharyngeal flap pharyngoplasty? Plast Reconstr Surg 2005; 115(1):45-52.

Millard DR. Cleft Craft: The Evolution of Its Surgery, Vol. III: Alveolar & Palatal Deformities. Boston: Little, Brown & Co., 1980.

Sadove MA, et al. Velopharyngeal insufficiency. In: Bentz ML, ed. Pediatric Plastic Surgery. Stamford: Appleton & Lange, 1998.

Serafin D, Riski JE. The velopharyngeal port: anatomy, physiology, and the management of incompetence. In: Serafin D, Georgiade NG, eds. St. Louis: Mosby, 1984.

Stal S, et al. Pharyngeal flap. In: Evans GRD, ed. Operative Plastic Surgery. New York: McGraw-Hill, 2000.

Witt PD. Velopharyngeal insufficiency. In: Vander Kolk CA, ed. Plastic Surgery: Indications, Operations, & Outcomes, Vol. II: Craniomaxillofacial, Cleft, & Pediatric Surgery. St. Louis: Mosby, 2000:819-834.

Ysunza A, et al. Velopharyngeal surgery: a prospective randomized study of pharyngeal flaps & sphincter pharyngoplasties. Plast Reconstr Surg 2002; 110(6):1401-1407.

DISTRACTION OSTEOGENESIS

Wellington J. Davis III, MD

○ **When was the field of craniofacial surgery established?**

In 1967 after publication of Paul Tessier's work in the paper "Osteotomies totales de face, Syndrome de Crouzon, Syndrome D'Apert, Oxycephalies, Scaphocephalies, Turricephalies".

○ **What are the main insights over the past 25 years which have helped to overcome the limitations in craniofacial surgery?**

Understanding of the pathologic anatomy through better imaging (3-D CT Scan), extensive bone grafting of bony defects, rigid fixation of osteotomized segments, most recently the evolving applications of distraction osteogenesis.

○ **What is distraction osteogenesis?**

A concept of fixation that actively mobilizes osteotomy segments and promotes osteogenesis. Also know as callostasis (stretching of callus, as in a fracture).

○ **What are the advantages of distraction osteogenesis?**

Reduced risk of infection seen in nonvascularized bone grafts, eliminated need for a donor site hence no donor site morbidity or limitations, simple design, more predictable bone survival, potential for three dimensional changes, reduced operative blood loss, reduced number of subsequent procedures, possibility of repeated applications, avoids in situ metal plates and screws or MMF, early closure of tracheostomy in cases of micrognathia, ability to be used in irradiated bone, well tolerated, no known evidence of growth retardation, possibility of better aesthetic results.

○ **T/F: Distraction osteogenesis has a higher rate of morbidity and greater need for secondary midface procedures compared to bone grafting.**

False.

○ **What are the disadvantages of distraction osteogenesis?**

Hypertrophic scarring at pin site (most common disadvantage), pin tract infection (osteomyelitis not reported to date), pin extrusion or migration, facial nerve injury, sensory deficits of inferior alveolar nerve, intolerance or noncompliance (uncommon), dentigerous cyst formation, ankylosis, tooth bud injury in patients less than 1 year.

○ **How is new bone formed during distraction osteogenesis?**

Intramembranous ossification.

○ **What are the zones of distraction osteogenesis which result in mature bone formation?**

Zone of fibrous tissue (zone I)- The fibrous interzone (FIZ) is composed of highly organized, longitudinally oriented, parallel strands of collagen with spindle-shaped fibroblasts and undifferentiated mesenchymal precursor cells through the matrix. Central region of the distraction gap.

Zone of extending bone formation (zone II)- the primary mineralization front (PMF) found on both edges of the FIZ composed of fibroblasts and undifferentiated mesenchymal precursor cells in direct continuity with osteoblasts on the surface of bone spicules (Osteoblasts longitudinally oriented and parallel to direction of distraction). Spindle-shaped fibroblastic cells transform into bone-forming cells. Increased levels of alkaline phosphatase, pyruvic acid and lactic acid. Also known as the transitional zone.

Zone of bone remodeling (zone III)- Advancing fields of bone resorption and apposition, increased number of osteoclasts.

Zone of mature bone (zone IV)- early compact cortical bone located adjacent to mature bone in unexpanded areas. Bone spicules thicker, less longitudinal orientation.

❍   **When are chondrocytes present during distraction osteogenesis?**

When there is excessive motion, fibrocartilage nonunion occurs.

❍   **T/F: The blood supply in the distraction zone is decreased compared to the normal side.**

False.

❍   **How long does it take the bone in the distraction zone to achieve 90% of normal bony structure?**

Usually within 8 months.

❍   **What are the clinical phases of distraction osteogenesis?**

Latency phase: 5-7 days post corticotomy or osteotomy, initial fracture healing bridges the cut bony surfaces before initiating distraction.

Distraction phase: 3-5 week period of active stretching of the fibrous interzone at 1 mm/day.

Mineralization phase: The period of consolidation, a 7-9 week period post-distraction when the PMF advances from each end toward the center, bridging the FIZ with bone.

❍   **T/F: Failure of distraction osteogenesis has not been reported clinically in the craniofacial skeleton.**

True.

❍   **Although failure of distraction osteogenesis has not been recorded in the craniofacial skeleton, what are some of the factors Aronson has suggested could contribute to failure?**

Ischemic fibrogenesis - inadequate local blood supply fibrous tissue formation without bone formation, cystic degeneration - caused by blockage of venous outflow, distraction gap fills with cystic cavity, fibrocartilage nonunion - caused by unstable fixation, cartilage fills distraction gap, buckling of regenerate bone - fixation device destabilized or removed prematurely.

❍   **At what age are bones potentially too soft to allow distraction?**

Before age 18 months distraction is used with caution. Distraction is primarily used in the mandible between 18 months to 22 years of age.

❍   **What is the only indication for distraction in patients younger than 2 years of age?**

Tongue-based airway compromise secondary to mandibular hypoplasia. Pulling the mandible forward pulls the tongue forward relieving the obstruction.

❍ **T/F: Children younger than 2 years with hypoplasia or aplasia of the mandible without airway compromise should not undergo distraction osteogenesis of the mandible because of the risk for permanent dental injury.**

True.

❍ **In which grades of mandibular hypoplasia is distraction osteogenesis indicated?**

Grade I, IIA and IIB. In grade III elongation is not possible because the ramus is absent.

❍ **T/F: Distraction can be accomplished regardless of soft tissue deficiency since the soft tissues are simultaneously expanded with bone distraction.**

True.

❍ **What is included in the clinical assessment of patients for mandibular distraction?**

Anthropometric measurements, facial nerve function, dental occlusion, dental cast impressions, preop photos (full face, profile, 3/4, basal views, biting tongue blade for occlusal slant), cephalometric radiographs (Lateral, AP), Panorex and or 3D CT scans- most accurate measure of mandible size and deficiency.

❍ **T/F: Bone grafting is preferred over distraction osteogenesis for advancements of more than 10mm because a more stable result that is less prone to relapse can be attained.**

False.

❍ **Why is distraction less prone to relapse than bone grafting in advancements larger than 10mm?**

There is a more gradual stretching of the soft tissues which makes relapse less likely.

❍ **What are the principles of distraction?**

Preserve periosteum if possible; place osteotomy and pin sites with adequate bone stock away from tooth buds; corticotomy preferred to osteotomy (to avoid inferior alveolar nerve injury)

❍ **What are the surgical approaches to the mandible?**

Extraoral approach (Modified Risdon) or internal approach.

❍ **What is the primary advantage of an external distraction device vs. an internal distraction device?**

It can be removed in the office avoiding a second operative procedure.

❍ **What is the protocol for mandibular distraction after device placement?**

Begin distraction on fifth to seventh postop day by rotating the screw 0.25mm four times a day (better tolerated than 0.5mm twice a day) or 1mm of distraction a day. Distraction completed in 3-5 weeks, slight overcorrection useful to prevent postop relapse. Pins and device left in place 8-9 weeks longer or until radiographic evidence of new bone bridging seen.

❍   **When should the distraction device be removed?**

Only when new bone has a radiodensity equivalent to the host bone surfaces and a macrostructure resembling host bone with equivalent cross-sectional area and formation of cortex and medullary canal.

❍   **How is the posterior open bite achieved during distraction maintained?**

Biteblock or similar orthodontic appliance until maxillary growth and tooth eruption fill the gap.

❍   **What are the complications of mandibular distraction?**

Injury to the inferior alveolar nerve (direct injury or slow traction when distraction distance is significant), pin tract infection, loosening of pins, relapse after device removal, injury to tooth buds, ankylosis of TMJ, failure of distraction (not reported).

❍   **T/F: Osteomyelitis of the mandible during distraction has not been reported.**

True.

❍   **What patient population may benefit most from the clinical application of distraction osteogenesis of the midface?**

Cleft palate patients with maxillary hypoplasia. Maxillary advancement may cause speech problems, distraction may limit velopharyngeal compromise.

❍   **What patient population may benefit from orbital expansion by distraction in the future?**

Patients with anophthalmos, congenital absence of ocular tissue. It is predicted to result in fewer surgical procedures, better fit of orbital prosthesis, improved cosmetic outcome.

❍   **What are the indications for palatal distraction?**

Anatomic or relative maxillary deficiency, nasal stenosis when conchae are compressed against the septum, all types of class III occlusion, mature cleft patient, anteroposterior maxillary deficiency, selected arch length problems.

References

Singhal, VK, Losken HW, Patterson G. Craniofacial Distraction. In: Benz, ML, ed. Pediatric Plastic Surgery. 1st ed. Stamford: Appleton & Lange, 1998: 341-357.

Ilizarov GA. The tension-stress effect on the genesis and growth of tissues: I. The influence of stability of fixation and soft-tissue preservation. Clin Orthop 238:249-281, 1989.

Ilizarov GA. The tension-stress effect on the genesis and growth of tissues: II. The influence of rate and frequency of distraction. Clin Orthop 239:263-285, 1989.

Karp IS, McCarthy JG, Schreiber JS, Sissons HA, Throne CH. Membranous bone lengthening: A serial histological study. Ann Plast Surg 29: 2-7, 1992.

Aronson J. Experimental and clinical experience with distraction osteogenesis. Cleft Palate-Craniofac J 31:473-482, 1994.

Gantous A, Phillips JH, Catton P, Holmberg D. Distraction osteogenesis in the irradiated canine mandible. Plast Reconstr Surg 93: 164-168, 1994.

McCarthy JG, Schrieber J, Karp N, Throne CH, Grayson BH. Lengthening the human mandible by gradual distraction. Plast Reconstr Surg 89: 1-8, 1992.

Haas AJ. Long-term post treatment evaluation of rapid palatal expansion. Angle Orthod 50:189-217, 1980.

Cruz MJ, Kerschner JE, Beste DJ, et al. Pierre Robin sequence: secondary respiratory difficulties and intrinsic feeding abnormalities. Laryngoscope. 1999; 109: 1632-1636.

Gosain AK. Distraction osteogenesis of the craniofacial skeleton. Plast Reconstr Surg. 2001; 107: 278-280.

McCarthy JG, Stelnicki EJ, Mehrara BJ, et al. Distraction osteogenesis of the craniofacial skeleton. Plast Reconstr Surg. 2001; 107: 1812-1827.

Glat PM, McCarthy JG. Distraction of the mandible: experimental studies. In: McCarthy JG, ed. Distraction of the Craniofacial Skeleton. New York, NY: Springer-Verlag; 1999: 67-79.

Cohen SR, Holmes RE, Machado L. Midface distraction. In: Samchukov ML, Cope JB, Cherkashin AM, eds. Craniofacial Distraction Osteogenesis. Saint Louis, Mo: Mosby-Year Book, Inc; 2001: 520-530.

ORTHOGNATHIC SURGERY

Mark W. Kiehn, MD, and Christopher Forrest, MD

○ **What are cranial base planes that are commonly used when evaluating lateral cephalograms?**

Sella-Nasion plane and Frankfort horizontal plane

○ **What is the Frankfort Horizontal Plane?**

Line from the superior edge of the external auditory meatus (Porion) to the inferior orbital rim (Orbitale).

○ **What angle describes the position of the anterior extent of the maxilla relative to the cranial base?**

Sella-Nasion-PointA (SNA)

○ **What angle describes the position of the anterior extent of the mandible relative to the cranial base?**

Sella-Nasion-PointB (SNB)

○ **What classification scheme describes occlusion by molar relationships?**

Angle Classification

○ **What is Angle I relation?**

Normo-occlusion. Mesial-buccal cusp of first maxillary molar seated in buccal groove of first mandibular molar.

○ **What is Angle II relation?**

Mesial-buccal cusp of first maxillary molar anterior to buccal groove of first mandibular molar placing the mandible relatively posterior to the maxilla.

○ **What is Angle III relation?**

Mesial-buccal cusp of first maxillary molar anterior to buccal groove of first mandibular molar placing the mandible relatively anterior to the maxilla.

○ **What term describes the <u>horizontal relation</u> of the maxillary incisors to the mandibular incisors in centric occlusion?**

Overjet

○ **What term describes the <u>vertical relation</u> of the maxillary incisors to the mandibular incisors in centric occlusion?**

Overbite

○ **Which tooth has the longest root?**

Canine

○ **What cranial nerve branch provides sensation to the maxillary teeth?**

Infraorbital nerve from CN V

❍   **What is the major arterial supply for the palate?**

Greater palantine artery

❍   **What is the blood supply to the mobilized segment in a Le Forte I osteotomy if the greater palantine arteries are divided?**

*   Ascending palatine branch of the facial artery
*   Anterior branch of the ascending pharyngeal artery

❍   **What operation is indicated for maxillary retrusion in association with persistent oronasal fistulas and alveolar bone gaps in a patient with bilateral cleft lip and palate?**

3 piece Le Forte I osteotomy

❍   **What procedure is indicated for a patient with severe (20mm) maxillary retrusion and normal mandibular position?**

Le Forte I osteotomy with distraction osteogenesis

❍   **At what point in development is orthognathic surgery generally performed?**

Skeletal maturity (females 16-18 years, males 18-20 years)

❍   **What subcranial operation is generally indicated for the orbitomaxillary deformity associated with craniofacial dysostosis syndromes (Crouzon's, Pfeiffer's, etc)?**

Le Forte III osteotomy

❍   **What condition involves Angle class II malocclusion, full incisal show at rest, excessive gingival show with smiling, and labiomental (mentalis) strain to achieve lip closure?**

Vertical maxillary excess (Long face syndrome)

❍   **What surgical procedure is generally required for vertical maxillary excess?**

Le Forte I with impaction, with or without mandibular osteotomy and genioplasty

❍   **What clinical condition can be exacerbated by Le Forte I osteotomy and maxillary advancement in the cleft palate patient?**

Velopharyngeal insufficiency-VPI

❍   **What is the most common cause of temporomandibular joint ankylosis?**

Trauma

❍   **When is alveolar bone grafting performed for clefts involving the alveolus?**

Prior to eruption of the canine teeth (9 to 12 years of age)

❍   **What is the optimal amount of upper central incisor show at rest?**

Males = 2 to 3 mm, females = 4 to 6 mm

❍   **What is the probable cause of an anterior open bite upon release of intermaxillary fixation following bilateral sagittal split osteotomy of the mandible?**

Inadequate seating of the condyles within the glenoid fossae at the time of fixation of the mandibular osteotomy

❍   **A patient with increased SNB angle and normal SNA angle has what deformity?**

Mandibular prognathism

❍   **What points define the Frankfort horizontal line?**

Porion (tragion) and orbitale

❍   **Upon performing a sagittal split osteotomy (BSSO) of the mandible, within which segment are the mandibular nerve and associated vasculature are found?**

The distal segment

❍   **What are the advantages of a bilateral sagittal split osteotomy (BSSO) versus other types of osteotomy for the mandible?**

Greater bone contact, easier to achieve rigid fixation, and less need for bone grafting

❍   **Patients with cleft lip and palate that require orthognathic surgery generally have what pattern of malocclusion?**

Class III due to maxillary hypoplasia/retrusion

❍   **What is the indication for multiple part Le Forte I osteotomy?**

Alveolar clefting and dental gaps in a patient with facial skeletal-dental imbalance

❍   **What operation is indicated for a patient with an excessively long lower face and microgenia?**

Jumping genioplasty

❍   **What operation is indicated for a patient with a prominent chin and long lower face?**

Reduction genioplasty

❍   **What operation is indicated for a patient with microgenia and an acceptable lower facial height?**

Sliding or implant genioplasty

❍   **What is the primary blood supply to the genioplasty segment?**

Posterior muscle attachments

❍   **In patients with hemifacial microsomia, what is the factor that most determines the ability to lengthen the mandible with distraction osteogenesis?**

Extent of the condylar development

❍   **At what rate is distraction osteogenesis of the mandible performed?**

1 mm per day

References

Bessette RW, Jacobs JS. TMJ dysfunction. In: Aston SJ, Beasley RW, Thorne CH, eds. Grabb & Smith's Plastic Surgery. 5th ed. Philadelphia, Pa: Lippincott-Raven; 1997:335-347.

Gosain AK. Distraction osteogenesis of the craniofacial skeleton. Plast Reconstr Surg. 2001;107:278-280.

McCarthy JG, Ruff GL, Zide BM. A surgical system for the correction of bony chin deformity. Clin Plast Surg. 1991; 18:139-152.

Polley JW, Figueroa AA. Rigid external distraction: its application in cleft maxillary deformities. Plast Reconstr Surg. 1998; 102:1360.

Posnick JC, Goldstein JA. Surgical management of temporomandibular joint ankylosis in the pediatric population. Plast Reconstr Surg. 1993;91:791-798.

Schendel SA. Vertical maxillary deformities. In: Ferraro JW, ed. Fundamentals of Maxillofacial Surgery. New York, NY: Springer-Verlag; 1997:284-286.

Shprintzen RJ. Velocardiofacial syndrome. Otolaryngol Clin North Am. 2000; 33:1217-1240.

Siebert JW, Angrigiani C, McCarthy JG, et al. Blood supply of the Le Fort I maxillary segment: an anatomic study. Plast Reconstr Surg. 1997;100:843.

Zide BM. The temporomandibular joint. In: McCarthy JG, ed. Plastic Surgery. Philadelphia, Pa: WB Saunders Co; 1990;2:1475-1513.

Zide B, Grayson B, McCarthy JG. Cephalometric analysis: part I. Plast Reconstr Surg. 1981;68:816.

Zide B, Grayson B, McCarthy JG. Cephalometric analysis for upper and lower midface surgery: part II. Plast Reconstr Surg. 1981;68:961.

CONGENITAL EAR DEFORMITIES

Reuben A. Bueno, Jr., MD

❍ **What embryologic structures give rise to the tragus, helical crus, and superior helix?**

The three anterior hillocks of the first branchial arch

❍ **What embryologic structures give rise to the helix, scapha, concha, antihelix, antitragus, and lobule?**

The three posterior hillocks of the second branchial arch

❍ **What embryologic structure gives rise to the external auditory meatus?**

The first branchial groove

❍ **What is the normal size of the ear?**

5.5-6.5 cm for the normal adult ear height and 3-4.5 cm for the normal adult width

❍ **Describe normal ear growth?**

85% of ear development occurs by 3 years of age with full development achieved between 6-15 years of age

❍ **What is the normal position of the ear?**

1. One ear length posterior to the lateral orbital rim
2. Lateral protrusion of the helix from the scalp between 1.5-2.0 cm
3. Mean inclination from vertical of 20 degrees posteriorly

❍ **The helical root arises from what external ear structure?**

The concha, dividing it into the concha cavum and concha cymba.

❍ **The superior crus of the antihelix is bordered by what structures?**

The scapha and the triangular fossa

❍ **The inferior crus of the antihelix is bordered by what structures?**

The triangular fossa and the concha cymba

❍ **What is the triangular fossa?**

The concave area between the superior crus and the inferior crus

❍ **Describe the arterial blood supply to the ear.**

1. Superficial temporal artery supplies the lateral surface
2. Posterior auricular artery supplies the posterior surface of the ear, lobule, and retroauricular skin
3. Occipital artery may contribute to the posterior ear blood supply.

❍ **Describe the venous drainage of the ear.**

Anterior ear is drained by the superficial temporal and retromandibular veins. Posterior ear is drained by posterior auricular veins draining into the external jugular vein.

O   **What nerve supplies sensation to the lower half of the lateral ear, including the lobule, antihelix, scapha, postauricular sulcus, helix, concha, and the lower part of the cranial surface of the ear?**

Great auricular nerve from C2 and C3

O   **What nerve supplies sensation to the superolateral surface and the anterior and superior surfaces of the external auditory canal?**

Auriculotemporal nerve from the mandibular branch of the trigeminal nerve

O   **What nerve supplies sensation to the superior ear?**

Lesser occipital nerve

O   **What nerve supplies sensation to the concha and posterior auditory canal?**

Arnold's nerve from the vagus nerve

O   **Microtia is seen in what syndromes?**

1. Hemifacial microsomia, or first and second branchial arch syndrome
2. Goldenhar's
3. Treacher Collins

O   **What vascular event is the proposed mechanism for microtia?**

Obliteration of the stapedial artery

O   **For the microtia patient, at what age is it usually recommended for the child to undergo total ear reconstruction?**

Usually by age 6 or 7 prior to starting school

O   **How many stages are usually required for total ear reconstruction?**

Between 2 and 3 depending on the particular technique

O   **What is usually involved in the first stage?**

Creation of a subcutaneous pocket and insertion of a cartilage framework

O   **What is usually involved in the second and third stages?**

Lobule rotation, tragal reconstruction, and elevation of the helical rim

O   **Which ribs are usually harvested for the cartilage framework?**

Ribs 6 through 9

O   **Adequate soft tissue coverage of the framework can be achieved with what local flap?**

The temporoparietal fascial flap based on the superficial temporal artery with split thickness skin graft

○ **In microtia patients, what must be present for middle ear reconstruction?**

Wide pneumatization of the middle ear

○ **What are the characteristics of a prominent ear deformity?**

1. Loss of antihelical fold
2. Conchal hypertrophy
3. Conchoscaphal angle > 90 degrees.
Surgical treatment should address each of these factors independently depending on severity.

○ **What is the role of ear taping and splinting in the management of the prominent ear deformity?**

In the neonatal period up to a maximum of 6 months of age, molding the ear with taping and splinting may improve ear appearance and prevent the need for surgical correction

○ **Why is this limited to the first 3-6 months of life?**

Circulating maternal estrogen increases hyaluronic acid in cartilage rendering it more deformable. This probably facilitates passage through the birth canal during delivery but can be exploited to reshape deformities of the ear.

○ **What methods have been described to weaken the anterior surface of the cartilage?**

Scoring with a scalpel, abrasion with a otobrader or rasp, and incision of the cartilage

○ **What is the effect of conchomastoid sutures?**

Reduction of conchal projection. Conchal reduction can also be achieved by direct excision through an anterior or posterior incision.

○ **What is the effect of Mustardè sutures?**

Permanent conchoscaphal sutures are placed to recreate the antihelical fold

○ **Anterior scoring in otoplasty is more likely to be associated with what complication?**

Sharp antihelical fold deformity

○ **Concha-mastoid sutures are more commonly associated with what complication?**

Meatus distortion

○ **What is the most common complication following otoplasty surgery?**

Recurrent deformity with 8-24% undergoing revision otoplasty

○ **What is telephone ear?**

Prominent upper and lower thirds of the ear relative to the middle third as a result of inadequate correction of the lower third of the ear

○ **What is the percentage of patients who present with residual deformity after correction of prominent ears?**

10-25%

❍   **What is cryptotia and how is it treated?**

"Hidden ear" deformity is characterized by the absence of the superior auriculocephalic sulcus and can be corrected with helical release and skin grafting or z-plasty

❍   **What is lop ear?**

Lop ear is characterized by protrusion of the ear and folding of the superior helix

❍   **What is Stahl's ear?**

Stahl's ear is characterized by a 3rd crus, flattened antihelix, and malformation of the scaphoid fossa

References

Allison GR. Anatomy of the auricle. *Clin Plast Surg.* 17:209-12, 1990.

Brent B. The acquired auricular deformity: a systematic approach to its analysis and reconstruction. *Plast Reconstr Surg.* 59:475-85, 1977.

Brent B. Microtia repair with rib cartilage grafts: a review of personal experience with 1000 cases. *Clin Plast Surg.* 29:257-71, 2003.

Eriksson E, Vogt PM. Ear reconstruction. *Clin Plast Surg.* 19:637-43, 1992.

CONGENITAL NEVI/TISSUE EXPANSION

Stephen Colbert, MD, Matthew J. Concannon, MD, and Charles L. Puckett, MD

O **Does "congenital" imply "hereditary"?**

No

O **What is a nevus?**

A congenital mark or pigmented area on the skin; synonymous with "birthmark." Some state that all nevi are not congenital; in general, nevi are divided into two classifications, congenital and acquired

O **What is a giant nevus?**

Greater than 20 cm in largest diameter; greater than 2% body surface area; or, a size that cannot be excised in a single procedure

O **What is the incidence of congenital nevi?**

1-2%

O **What is the incidence of giant nevi?**

For lesions greater than or equal to 9.9 cm, approximately 1 in 20,000

O **Nevi result from a proliferation of what cells?**

Melanocytes

O **In what layer(s) of the skin do nevi occur?**

Dermis and epidermis

O **For what cancer are nevi generally considered a risk factor?**

Malignant melanoma

O **What is the risk of melanoma in one who has a giant congenital nevus?**

5-7% by the age of 60 is the most often reported range; however, reported incidence in the literature ranges from 0% to 42%

O **What is an acquired nevus?**

The more common "mole" the occurrence of which begins in childhood, increases rapidly in adolescence and young adulthood

O **How are nevi classified by location and histologic pattern?**

Compound, intradermal, and junctional.

○   **What is a compound nevus?**

A nevus with fully formed nests of cells in the epidermis and newly forming cells in the dermis

○   **What is an intradermal nevus?**

A nevus with nests of cells located exclusively within the dermis; clinically indistinguishable from a compound nevus

○   **Define a junctional nevus.**

A nevus with nests of cells confined to the dermoepidermal junction; usually presenting as a small discrete flat or slightly raised macule

○   **How are congenital nevi classified by size?**

Small <1.5 cm, medium 1.5 – 20 cm, large >20 cm

○   **How are small congenital nevi managed medically?**

Baseline photography and regular follow-up

○   **What features of small nevi warrant biopsy?**

Asymmetry, border irregularity, color variegation, and diameter larger than 6 mm represent the traditional ABCDs of melanoma; in addition, any nevi that has changed appearance

○   **At what location(s) are congenital nevi associated with leptomeningeal melanoma?**

Congenital nevi of the head, neck and trunk, particularly over the spine

○   **What is a nevus of Ota?**

Pigmented nevus in the distribution of the ophthalmic (V1) and maxillary (V2) division of the trigeminal nerve; seen in early infancy, approximately 50% congenital

○   **What demographic segment are nevi of Ota seen in?**

Early adolescence, most common in females and Asian populations; usually unilateral, may affect mucosa, associated with development of glaucoma and rare malignant degeneration

○   **What is the recommended treatment of small and large congenital nevi?**

Giant nevi should be removed surgically as soon as possible, as there is risk of melanoma even in the first 3-5 years of life; surgical excision remains the most acceptable method;

○   **How are small and medium congenital nevi treated?**

Remains controversial with recommendations ranging from excision of all congenital nevi as soon as tolerated by the patient to lifetime observation of small and medium congenital nevi with excision only for specific changes

TISSUE EXPANSION

❍ **What is the main advantage of using tissue expansion in reconstruction?**

Replacing missing or pathologic tissue with normal-appearing like tissue

❍ **What are other advantages?**

Expanded tissue is typically sensate and well vascularized, and final donor defects are minimized

❍ **In what type of situations should tissue expanders be avoided?**

Immediate traumatic or infected fields, open wounds, proximity to malignant tumor, non-expandable or high risk tissue such as a skin graft or irradiated tissue

❍ **What are the common disadvantages of tissue expansion?**

Requires two operations, creates an aesthetic deformity during expansion, and may cause transient discomfort during expansion

❍ **What is "creep"?**

Viscoelastic deformation occurring immediately with expansion

❍ **Besides creep, what factors increase dimensions of expanded tissue in the short-term?**

Loss of interstitial fluid by pressure, and recruitment of adjacent mobile tissues

❍ **Does stretch of tissue have any effect on cellular proliferation?**

Yes, tension has been shown to induce DNA synthesis and cellular mitosis

❍ **Does expansion affect blood flow in expanding tissue?**

Yes, blood flow increases in expanding tissue; in addition, the placement of an expander functions as a delay for the overlying flap

❍ **What happens to the epidermis during expansion?**

The epidermis thickens

❍ **What happens to the dermis during expansion?**

The dermis thins

❍ **What are the risks to fat, muscle, and nerves during expansion?**

Compression could cause atrophy of all of these tissues; in addition, compression of sensory nerves may lead to paresthesias or discomfort

❍ **What tissues are particularly amenable to expansion?**

The scalp and breast; in general, the farther from these tissues, the less successful expansion becomes

❍ **What may happen if an expander is placed beneath an incision?**

Dehiscence and expander exposure

○   **How should exposure of a tissue expander be treated?**

In general, exposure of an expander is best treated by removal, pocket drainage, and expander replacement at a later date; in select situations, removal, sterilization, and immediate replacement may be appropriate; in other select situations, some may consider completion of expansion in the setting of exposure appropriate.

○   **Does tissue expansion require placement of an expandable implant?**

No, techniques such as presuturing, external expanders, and lacing devices allow tissue expansion and ultimate wound closure without placement of internal expanders

○   **Is placement of incisions for expander insertion important?**

Yes, one of the most critical factors affecting outcome is the placement of the final scar, which is usually affected by placement of the initial incision; in addition, placement of the incision in tissue that is to be expanded may lead to a widened scar or even dehiscence and expander exposure

○   **What technical error committed during expander placement will likely lead to expansion failure?**

Inadequate development of the pocket where the expander will be placed

○   **What complications are associated with tissue expanders?**

Seroma formation, transient alopecia during scalp expansion, contour deformities such as dog-ears post-operatively, widened scars, hematoma, infection, expander exposure, expander extrusion, and tissue necrosis

○   **What is the benefit of a textured surface on a tissue expander?**

Relative immobility due to tissue adherence, maintenance of proper expander orientation, increased capsular compliance and reduction in capsular contracture

References

Dorland's Illustrated Medical Dictionary, 28th ed. Philadelphia: W.B. Saunders Co., 1994.

Fitzpatrick TB, Johnson RA, Wolff K, and Suurmond D. Color Atlas and Synopsis of Clinical Dermatology: Common and Serious Diseases, 4th ed. New York: McGraw-Hill, 2001.

Gosain AK, Santoro TD, Larson DL, and Gingrass RP. Giant congenital nevi: a 20-year experience and an algorithm for their management. Plas Reconstr Surg 2001; 108(3):622-631.

Sahin S, Levin L, Kopf AW, Rao BK, Triola M, Koenig K, Huang C, Bart R. Risk of melanoma in medium-sized congenital melanocytic nevi: a follow-up study. J Am Acad Dermatol. 1998; 39(3):428-33.

Tannous ZS, Mihm MC Jr, Sober AJ, Duncan LM. Congenital melanocytic nevi: clinical and histopathologic features, risk of melanoma, and clinical management.
J Am Acad Dermatol. 2005; 52(2):197-203.

Zaal LH, Mooi WJ, Sillevis Smitt JH, van der Horst CM. Classification of congenital melanocytic naevi and malignant transformation: a review of the literature.
Br J Plast Surg. 2004; 57(8):707-19.

Watt AJ, Kotsis SV, and Chung KC. Risk of melanoma arising in large congenital malanocytic nevi: a systematic review. Plas Reconstr Surg 2004; 113(7):1968-1974.

Tissue Expansion

Concannon MJ, and Puckett CL. Wound coverage using modified tissue expansion. Plas Reconstr Surg 1998; 102(2):377-384.

De Filippo RE, and Atala A. Stretch and growth: the molecular and physiologic influences of tissue expansion. Plas Reconstr Surg 2002; 109(7):2450-2462.

Hammond DC, Perry LC, Maxwell GP, and Fisher J. Morphologic analysis of tissue-expander shape using a biomechanical model. Plas Reconstr Surg 1993; 92(2):255-259.

Manders EK. Reconstruction using soft tissue expansion. In: Cohen M, ed. Mastery of Plastic and Reconstructive Surgery. Boston: Little, Brown and Co., 1994:201-213.

CONGENITAL BREAST

Wellington J. Davis III, MD

O   **What organ system should always be included in the initial preoperative evaluation of patients with gynecomastia?**

Genitalia may reveal an underlying cause such as testicular tumors, nonpalpable and/or undescended testes. These findings should prompt genetic and/or endocrine evaluation prior to surgery.

O   **Where are accessory mammary structures found most frequently in patients with polymastia?**

The axilla followed by the inframammary region.

O   **What is the primary feature of Poland syndrome?**

Unilateral aplasia or hypoplasia of the pectoralis major muscle (absence of sternal head) and breast hypoplasia.

O   **What is the incidence of Poland syndrome?**

1 in 20,000-30,000. Most cases are sporadic and 75% occur on the right side. Some reports of familial cases. M:F ratio 3:1.

O   **What is the suggested primary defect in Poland syndrome?**

Subclavian artery disruption sequence resulting in diminished blood supply to affected limb yielding partial loss of tissue in the affected regions.

O   **What are the other associated deformities of Poland syndrome?**

Absence of ribs 2 to 4, hypoplasia of the muscles of the shoulder girdle including the latissimus dorsi, brachysyndactyly, shortening of forearm bones, deficiency of subcutaneous fat, absence of axillary hair, aplasia or hypoplasia of nipple-areolar complex.

O   **What pharmaceutical agents are linked to the development of gynecomastia?**

Cimetidine, digitalis, minocycline, spironolactone, anabolic steroids, haloperidol, opiates, marijuana, phenothiazines, tricyclic antidepressants, progestins, amphetamines, isoniazid, methyldopa, minocycline, estrogens, diazepam, reserpine, theophylline

O   **What are the three components of the tuberous breast deformity?**

Herniation of breast tissue into nipple-areola complex with cylindrical projection accompanied by a relatively large areola; deficiency of lower pole in vertical and horizontal axes; hypoplasia.

O   **What is the surgical management of the tuberous breast deformity?**

In most cases augmentation with a periareolar mastopexy. In severe breast ptosis augmentation with wise-pattern mastopexy. In severely deficient skin envelope, two-stage reconstruction with tissue expansion.

O   **What is the treatment of choice in juvenile breast hypertrophy?**

Reduction mammoplasty. High recurrence rates may require further surgery.

❍ **Which areas are commonly affected in ectopic polymastia?**

Ectopic polymastia- breast tissue in areas outside the milk line. Reported in midline, face, ear, neck, back, buttock, posterior or dorsal thigh, scalp, shoulder, epigastrium.

❍ **What is the difference between amastia, amazia, and athelia?**

Amastia- congenital absence of the breast (nipple-areola complex and glandular tissue). Amazia- absence of glandular tissue only. Athelia- absence of nipple alone.

❍ **How is gynecomastia classified?**

There are three grades. Grade I: small enlargement, no skin excess; Grade IIA: moderate enlargement, no skin excess; Grade IIB moderate enlargement with extra skin; Grade III: marked enlargement with extra skin.

❍ **What is the modification of gynecomastia classification for surgical planning?**

Simplify to the three grades. Grade I: localized button of tissue localized to areola. Chest not fatty, no skin excess. Simple excision. Grade II: diffuse gynecomastia on fatty chest, indistinct tissue edges. Suction lipectomy adjunct to excision. Grade III: Diffuse gynecomastia with excessive skin, require skin excision outside areola and/or nipple repositioning.

❍ **What are the options for surgical management of gynecomastia?**

Suction lipectomy only, glandular resection through periareolar incision +/- suction lipectomy, skin and glandular resection, concentric circle resection, pedicled relocation of nipple with skin resection, breast amputation with free nipple grafting. Wise-pattern mastopexy should NOT be performed in gynecomastia.

❍ **What is the incidence of gynecomastia in males at puberty?**

75%. 75% of those 75% disappear within several years. 30-55% of men.

❍ **What is the typical time length until spontaneous resolution of gynecomastia in adolescent boys?**

16 to 18 months. Best to wait as long as two years prior to intervention. If psychosocial disturbance may intervene earlier.

❍ **What percentage of males with gynecomastia present at puberty have residual gynecomastia at age 17?**

7.7%.

❍ **In which medical condition is gynecomastia associated with an increased incidence of breast cancer?**

Klinefelter's syndrome (at least 20 times general population), breast biopsy indicated.

❍ **What is the most common complication after correction of gynecomastia?**

Hematoma.

❍ **What is the management of gynecomastia in the neonate?**

Requires no therapy, typically resolves in several weeks.

❍ **What is the management of breast enlargement before puberty?**

Rare condition, requires search for chromosomal abnormalities, drug and endocrine workups.

❍ **What are the common causes of gynecomastia?**

Increase in estrogens, decrease in androgens or deficit in androgen receptors.

❍ **What are the multiple disease states in which gynecomastia can be seen?**

Primary testicular failure (Klinefelter's, XXY syndrome), secondary testicular failure (orchitis, mumps), endocrine disorders (hyper- or hypothyroidism, adrenocorticohyperplasia), liver disease (most common alcoholic cirrhosis), tumors (lung cancer, testicular cancer, adrenal tumors, pituitary tumors, colon or prostate cancer), congenital syndromes, debilitated disease states (eg. severe burn).

❍ **What are the incidence and most common location for polythelia (supernumerary nipple)?**

5% and inframammary region (commonly misdiagnosed as nevi).

❍ **What study is a useful adjunct in the preoperative workup of patients with Poland syndrome?**

High resolution CT scan to confirm status of latissimus dorsi and define associated skeletal anomalies.

❍ **What are the three aspects of chest wall reconstruction in Poland syndrome?**

Stabilization of chest wall; creation of a soft tissue "fill"; breast reconstruction.

❍ **What is the surgical management of the breast deformity in male patient's with Poland syndrome?**

Latissimus dorsi neuromuscular island flap reconstruction. As early as 5-6 years of age.

❍ **What is the surgical management of the breast deformity in the female patient with Poland's syndrome?**

At age 12-13 temporary expander for symmetry during breast development, exchange for permanent implant at the end of breast development. Latissimus dorsi used in cases of inadequate subcutaneous tissue. In adults patients pedicled TRAM flap may be used, not used in adolescent patients or those considering childbirth.

❍ **What are the options for skeletal chest wall deformity reconstruction in patients with Poland syndrome?**

No contraindication to single stage repair. Customized silicone prosthesis placed subcutaneously or beneath latissimus dorsi muscle flap OR split rib grafts; if soft tissue lacking cover grafts with prosthetic patch or latissimus dorsi muscle flap (preferred) which serves as base for mammary prosthesis. Some cases may require contralateral mastopexy.

❍ **What are the causes of unilateral hypoplasia?**

Congenital condition or acquired secondary to iatrogenic injury to breast bud.

❍ **What is the surgical management of unilateral hypoplasia?**

Delay reconstruction until 13 years if possible. At age 13 temporary expander for symmetry during breast development, exchange for permanent implant at the end of development. Submusculofascial position preferred. Nipple-areola reconstruction at completion of expansion.

❍ **What is the other anatomic consideration at the time of implant placement in the hypoplastic breast?**

Breast constriction with a shortened and high inframammary fold. Must be addressed at time of implant placement.

❍ **What number of patients with syndactyly of the hand have Poland syndrome?**

10%.

References

Neuman JF. Evaluation and treatment of gynecomastia. Am Fam Physician. 1997; 55:1835-1844, 1849-1850.

Wood RJ, Bostwick J. Congenital Breast Deformities. In: Benz, ML, ed. Pediatric Plastic Surgery. 1st ed. Stamford: Appleton & Lange, 1998: 739-746.

Tuerk M. Medications that cause gynecomastia. Plast Reconstr Surg. 1993; 92: 1411.

Bostwick J. Plastic and Reconstructive Surgery of the Breast. St. Louis. Quality medical Publishing, 1990: 478.

May N, Vasconez LO, Jurkiewicz MJ. Treatment of macromastia in the actively enlarging breast. Plast Reconstr Surg. 1977; 59: 575.

Georgiade NG, Georgiade GS, Riefkohl R. Esthetic breast surgery. In: McCarthy JG, ed. Plastic Surgery. Philadelphia, Pa: WB Saunders Co; 1990; 6: 3839-3840.

Skandalakis JE, Gray SW, Ricketts R, et al. The anterior body wall. In: Skandalakis JE, Gray SW, eds. Embryology for Surgeons: the Embryologic Basis for the Treatment of Congenital Anomalies. 2nd ed. Baltimore: Williams & Wilkins; 1994: 559-563.

Hoehn JG, Georgiade GS. Congenital and developmental deformities of the breast and breast asymmetries. In: Georgiade GS, Riefkohl R, Levin LS, eds. Plastic, Maxillofacial and Reconstructive Surgery. 3rd ed. Baltimore: Williams & Wilkins; 1997: 715-729.

Mc Kinney P. Gynecomastia. In: Aston SJ, Beasley RW, Thorne CHM, eds. Grabb and Smith's Plastic Surgery. 5th ed. Philadelphia-New York: Lippincott-Raven; 1997: 753-757.

Simon BE, Hoffman S, Kahn S. Classification and surgical correction of gynecomastia. Plast Reconstr Surg. 1973; 51: 48-52.

Riefkohl R, Zavitsanos GP, Courtiss EH. Gynecomastia. In: Georgiade GS, Riefkohl R, Levin LS, eds. Textbook of Plastic, Maxillofacial and Reconstructive Surgery. Baltimore: Williams and Wilkins; 1997: 820-828.

Albanese CT, Rowe MI. Congenital Thoracic Deformities. In: Benz, ML, ed. Pediatric Plastic Surgery. 1st ed. Stamford: Appleton & Lange, 1998: 730-733.

Jones KL. Smith's Recognizable Patterns of Human Malformation. 5th ed. Philadelphia: WB Saunders, 1997: 302-303.

CONGENITAL HAND

Abdulaziz Jarman, MB.BS, FRCSC

○ **How many stages of human embryonic development have been described by Streeter?**

23 Horizons or stages

○ **At what age does the limb bud develop and differentiate?**

Between the third and eighth postovulatory weeks.

○ **What is the limb bud called and at what age does it develop?**

Wolf's crest and it is well defined at day 30 embryonic life.

○ **What are the three critical regions of the limb bud that signal or control its outgrowth and pattern of development?**

1. Apical ectodermal ridge (AER).
2. Dorsal ectoderm.
3. Zone of polarizing activity (ZPA).

○ **What does the dorsal ectoderm control**

It controls the palmar to dorsal differentiation.

○ **At what day of development are the fingers finally separated?**

By the day 52 or 53.

○ **What does the apical ectodermal ridge control?**

It induces the underlying mesoderm to differentiate. It also responsible for morphogens that maintain the apical ectodermal ridge.

○ **What does the zone of polarizing activity control?**

It controls anteroposterior develpment.

○ **What is currently the most widely used classification for congenital differences of the hand?**

The current classification was proposed by Swanson and revised by the congenital anomalies committee of the International Federation of Societies for Surgery of the Hand (IFSSH).

○ **List the types of the classification?**

1. Failure of formation of parts (arrested development).
2. Failure of differentiation / separation of parts.
3. Duplication.
4. Overgrowth.
5. Undergrowth.
6. Congenital constriction band syndrome.

7.   Generalized skeletal abnormalities.

O   **Where does longitudinal radial deficiency fit into this classification?**

Under failure of separation of parts.

O   **What are the types of radial club deformity?**

Type 1: short distal radius.
Type 2: hypoplastic radius.
Type 3: partial absence of the radius.
Type 4: absent radius.

O   **Name five syndromes associated with radial club hand?**

1.   Fanconi's anemia.
2.   TAR syndrome.
3.   Holt-Oram syndrome.
4.   VATER association.
5.   Treacher –Collin's syndrome.

O   **List the key features of Holt-Oram Syndrome?**

Most common "heart-hand" syndrome
Autosomal Dominant
Carpal abnormalities
Atrial or ventricular septal defects (**Hol**t-**Hol**es)
Thumb abnormalities-hypoplasia or triphalangeal
Possible radial dysplasia (O**r.a.**m-**R**adius **A**nomalies)
No hematologic abnormalities

O   **List the key features of Fanconi's Anemia?**

Autosomal Recessive
Seen with radial border abnormalities that are more severe distally (e.g. thumb hypoplasia or aplasia)
<u>Progressive</u> aplastic anemia
Does NOT present at birth but around 6 years of age
If early diagnosis, treatment with bone marrow transplant possible

O   **How is Fanconi's Anemia diagnosed?**

The chromosome challenge test.
Early diagnosis and a high index of suspicion critical since late treatment much less effective

O   **Describe TAR Syndrome?**

Thrombocytopenia-presents by 4 months (contrast with Fanconi's at 6-8 years)
Anemia limited to platelets
Much better prognosis than Fanconi's
Radius-bilateral absence or hypoplasia
Thumbs may be hypoplastic, but are always present

O   **Why would hematologic and musculoskeletal anomalies be linked like this?**

The radii, platelet producing megakaryocytes and the heart all develop around 6-8 weeks gestation.

O   **List the key features in VATER or VACTERL Association?**

V-vertebral anomalies (hypoplasia often resulting in later scoliosis)
A-anal atresia or imperforate anus
C-cardiac anomalies (VSD/ASD)
TE-tracheoesophageal fistulae
R-renal and/or radial anomalies
L-limb anomalies (typically thumb hypoplasia
The point of surgery is to improve the child's ability to reach their hand to their mouth or head. Without the ability to flex the elbow, the radial deviation of the hand at the wrist is often critical in allowing them to reach their hand to their mouth and head.

○   **Name four contraindication in considering surgery for radial club hand?**

1.   Children with life threatening conditions.
2.   Older children with adequate function.
3.   Bilateral affliction with stiff elbow.
4.   Type 1 and mild type 2 cases.

○   **Why is a stiff elbow a contraindication to treatment of radial club hand (typically ulnar centralization)?**

The point of surgery is to improve the child's ability to reach their hand to their mouth or head. Without the ability to flex the elbow, the radial deviation of the hand at the wrist is often critical in allowing them to reach their hand to their mouth and head.

○   **What are the main characteristics of a typical cleft hand?**

•   V-shaped
•   Autosomal dominant inheritance
•   No finger nubbins
•   Syndactyly
•   One to all four limbs can be affected

○   **What are the main characteristics of an _atypical_ cleft hand?**

•   U- shaped
•   Sporadic
•   Finger nubbins exist
•   Usually one limb is affected(no feet)

○   **What is the most common congenital anomaly of the hand?**

Duplication.

○   **What is the incidence?**

Varies between 3.8-12.0/1000 live births.

○   **Which side of the hand is most commonly involved in duplication or polydactyly?**

In Asian and Caucasian populations preaxial (thumb) duplication is most common while in African Americans and Native Americans post-axial (ulnar) duplication is more common.

○   **What does syndactyly means?**

"Syn" means together and "dactylos" means digits; both are Greek.

○   **What is the name of the process of the finger separation in embryological life?**

It is called Apoptosis or programmed cell death.

O   **What is the prevalence of syndactyly?**

1 in 2000 birth.

O   **What are the types of syndactyly**

Simple (no bony or cartilaginous involvement)
- Complex (bony and cartilaginous involvement)
- Complicated
- Complete or incomplete.

O   **What is complete and incomplete syndactyly?**

In complete syndactyly the webbing between the digits extends to the tips of the fingers, while in incomplete syndactyly there is more proximal termination.

O   **What is complicated syndactyly?**

Refers to abnormally duplicated skeletal parts within the interdigital space.

O   **What is the most common pattern?**

Bilateral simple incomplete syndactyly of the long and ring finger (the third web space).

O   **What is the most important web space in the hand?**

The thumb – index web space (First web space).

O   **Name five syndromes associated with syndactyly?**

- Trisomy 21
- Apert's syndrome
- Carpenter's syndrome
- Holt-Oram syndrome
- Pfeiffer's syndrome.

O   **What is the most common web involved in the hand?**

The long-ring web space (third web space).

O   **What is the most common web involved in the foot**

Second toe- third toe web space (Second web space).

O   **What is the most important investigation for syndactyly?**

X-ray; to distinguish simple from complex syndactyly.

O   **What is the timing in syndactyly surgery?**

A- Surgery before 4-6 months of age is recommended for complex syndactyly involving the border ring-small web space or other web space when continued growth is expected to cause tethering and abnormal growth.
B- Otherwise usually it is performed at 12-18 months.

○ **Name 3 flaps commonly used for release of the first web space?**

1. Single Z-plasty (75% expansion).
2. Four flap Z-plasty (164% expansion).
3. Butterfly flap (Jumping man flap).

○ **What is a malformation?**

It is a sequence of poor formation of tissue within the fetus that initiates the chain of defects that can range from mild to severe e.g. VATER.

○ **What is deformation?**

It involves abnormal external or structural forces that cause secondary distortion or deformation e.g. constriction ring syndrome.

○ **What is disruption?**

The normal fetus or embryo is subjected to tissue breakdown or injury which may be vascular, infection, mechanical or metabolic in origin e.g. Thalidomide ingestion.

○ **What are the genetics of the constriction ring syndrome (CRS)?**

There is no positive inheritance in CRS.

○ **What is the incidence of CRS?**

Less than 10%.

○ **What is the cause of constriction ring syndrome?**

It is related to an *in utero* deformation where strands of the inner layer of the chorionic sac detach and wrap around part of the fetus.

○ **How deep can the ring band be?**

It can be superficial or deep extending into periosteum and can be completely or partially around the circumference of the part.

○ **What associated anomalies can be found with CRS?**

Most cases happen with normal pregnancies, but oligohydramnios and prematurity have been noted.

○ **How do you clinically classify congenital hand duplication?**

Preaxial (radial), central and postaxial (ulnar) duplications.

○ **What classification describes thumb duplication?**

Wassel classification.

○ **How many types are in Wassel classification?**

There are seven types

○ **How can I remember the classification?**

<u>Odds (I, III, V, VII) are clefts</u> into the bones resulting in bifid distal phalanx, proximal phalanx, metacarpal; <u>evens (II, IV, VI) represent complete separation</u> of a given bone resulting in duplicated distal phalanx, proximal phalanx, metacarpal.

❍ **What is the most common type?**

Wassel type 4 is the most common.

❍ **Describe type 4?**

Duplicated proximal phalanx. A broad thumb metacarpal articulates with two proximal phalanges sitting side by side.

❍ **What is Wassel type 7?**

A triphalangeal thumb or delta phalanx. Many consider this a separate entity.

❍ **What are the basic principles of thumb duplication correction?**

1. Using the best parts to create the best thumb.
2. Preserve the ulnar collateral ligament.
3. Reattach all thenar intrinsics.
4. Release first web space.
5. Preserve as much mobility as possible.

❍ **Will the reconstructed thumb be normal?**

No, usually weaker and smaller with less range of motion.

❍ **What are the genetics and incidence of the central polydactyly?**

- Usually bilateral
- Often result of an autosomal dominant trait
- Less than 10% of all duplications.

❍ **What is the classification of central polydactyly?**

Stelling's classification.

❍ **What are the types of Stelling's classification?**

1. Type 1: soft tissue mass not adherent to existing skeleton.
2. Type 2: supernumerary part with normal bone component attached to an enlarged metacarpal or phalanx.
   a. Hands are not attached to adjacent digits.
   b. Central synopolydactyly (syndactylized to adjacent digits).
3. Type 3: complete duplication of central digit including metacarpal. (rare).

❍ **What are the types of postaxial duplication of the fifth finger?**

1. Type1: soft tissue nubbin with a skin bridge.
2. Type 2: type 1 with skeletal connection.
3. Type 3: complete duplication of the entire ray.

❍ **What is the most common type of postaxial duplication?**

Type 1 is the most common.

○   **What is the other name for ulnar dimelia?**

Mirror hand.

○   **Describe the mirror hand?**

An upper limb with two ulnae, no radius, seven to eight fingers and no thumb. The wrist and elbow appear thick and arm appears short.

○   **What does symphalangism mean?**

Greek Sym = together and phlyx means bone and it refers to fused phalanges.

○   **What is the deformity of symphalangism according to congenital hand classification?**

It is failure of differentiation.

○   **What is the most important clinical sign in symphalangism?**

Lack of flexion crease.

○   **What are the classification of symphalangism?**

3 types by Flatt and Wood:
•   Type 1: true symphalangism
•   Type 2: symbrachydactyly
•   Type 3: syndromic symphalangism

○   **What is the full name of the sporadic form of the arthrogryposis?**

It is Arthrogryposis multiplex congenital.

○   **What is the characteristic pattern of this disease?**

It is paralysis and joint contracture that affect all joints in all limbs.

○   **Define the position of each part of the upper limb in arthrogryposis?**

1. Shoulder: thin, adducted and internally rotated.
2. Elbow: extended.
3. Forearm: semiflexed and pronated.
4. Wrist: flexed and ulnarly deviated.
5. Thumb: flexed and adducted.
6. Digits: flexed at the MP joint and ulnarly deviated.

○   **What are the three elements of windblown hand?**

1. Flexion and adduction of the thumb.
2. Narrowing of the first web space.
3. Ulnar deviation of the fingers at the MP joint.

○   **What is camptodactyly?**

General term to congenital flexion deformity of the digits in an anteroposterior plane (just think of a camping tent).

○   **What is the most commonly affected digit?**

The fifth finger.

○ **Mention four main anatomic problems in camptodactyly?**

1. Abnormal extrinsic muscles.
2. Abnormal distal insertion of the intrinsics.
3. Tight joint capsule.
4. Joint contracture with tight collateral ligaments.

○ **What are the x-ray findings of camptodactyly?**

- Narrowing of the joint space.
- Indentation within the surface of the middle phalanx
- Flattening of both the palmar and dorsal surfaces of the condyles of the proximal phalanx.
- Widened base of the middle phalanx.

○ **What is clinodactyly?**

It refers to a digit that is deviated (or in<u>clin</u>ed)in a radio-ulnar or medio-lateral direction.

○ **Where is the most common site for a simple clinodactyly?**

Middle phalanx of the small finger.

○ **Mention conditions that should be considered in macrodactyly?**

1. Neurofibromatosis.
2. Nerve-territory-oriented lipofibromatosis not associated with neurofibromatosis.
3. Multiple hereditary exostosis.
4. Proteus syndrome with hyperostotic lesions and overgrowth of phalanges.
5. Vascular malformation.
6. Hemihypertrophy of the limb

○ **What is the classification for thumb hypoplasia?**

Blauth's classification

○ **What are the types of Blauth's classification?**

Type 1: Minor generalized hypoplasia.
Type 2: Absence or hypoplastic intrinsic thenar muscles with narrow first web and ulnar collateral ligament insufficiency.
Type 3: as in type 2 with extrinsic muscles and tendons abnormality with skeletal deficiency:
      a: stable carpometacarpal joint.
      b: unstable carpometacarpal joint.
Type 4: *Pouce flottant* or floating thumb.
Type 5: Absence of the thumb.
Realize this is a <u>progressive description</u> of hypoplasia extending from minor undergrowth with all structures present extending through MCP instability (Type 2) to CMC instability (3A) to total absence of the thumb.

○ **Which types are treated with pollicization?**

Type 3B and type 4&5

○ **What is the key decision point distinguishing a thumb that is reconstructible versus one that should be ablated followed by pollicization?**

The presence of a stable CMC joint; thus 3B and worse get pollicized.

○ **What is the role of toe-to-thumb transfer for thumb hypoplasia?**

Results are very poor relative to pollicization.

○ **What is Poland syndrome?**

Described by Alfred Poland in 1849 and it may include:
Absence of the sternal head of the pectoralis major muscle: This is the one consistent feature of Poland's syndrome.
Hypoplastic hand.
Brachysyndactyly (short, webbed fingers).
Absence of ribs 2 to 4.
Hypoplasia of the breast and nipple areola complex.
Hypoplasia of the shoulder muscles including the latissimus dorsi muscle.
Short forearm bones.
Deficiency of subcutaneous fat.
Absence of axillary hair.

○ **What is the incidence of Poland's syndrome and which side and sex is most affected?**

It occurs in 1 in 30,000 live births, most commonly in the right side and exists in a male: female ratio of 3:1.

○ **How is the chest deformity corrected in Poland syndrome patients?**

Nothing is usually done in childhood. In adolescence correction of the chest deformities can be addressed with a latissimus dorsi muscle flap (with or without the use of custom made silicone implants in boys) or (breast implants with or without the use of tissue expanders in girls).

References

Ezaki M, Kay S, Light T, et al. Congenital Hand Deformities. In: Green PG HR, Pederson WC, ed. *Green's Operative Hand Surgery.* Vol One. New York: Churchill Livingstone; 1999:325-551.

Moore K. *The Developing Human.* Philadelphia: WB Saunders; 1988.

Upton J, Childers B. Congenital Anomalies. In: J W, ed. *Plastic Surgery Secrets.* Philadelphia: Hanley & Belfus; 1999:545-554.

Upton J. Congenital anomalies of the hand and forearm. In: McCarthy JG MJ, Littler JW, ed. *Plastic Surgery.* Vol vol.8. Philadelphia: WB Saunders; 1990:5213-5398.

Summerbell D. The zone of polarizing activity. Evidence for a role in normal chick limb morphogenesis. *J Embryol Exp Morph.* 1979;50:217-233.

Swanson A, Swanson G, Tada K. A Classification for congenital limb malformation. *J Hand Surgery.* 1983;8:693-702.

Cox H, Viljoin D, Versfeld G, et al. Radial ray defects and associated anomalies. *clin genet.* 1989;35:322-330.

Flatt A. *The care of congenital hand anomalies.* 2nd ed. St. Louis: Quality Medical publishing; 1994.

Tada K, Kurisaki E, Yonenobu K, et al. central polydactyly a review of 12 cases and their surgical treatment. *J Hand surgery.* 1982;7A:460-465.

Yang S, Jackson L, Green D, et al. A rare variant of mirror hand: a case report. *J Hand surgery.* 1996;21A:1048-1051.

Hall J, Green G, Powers E. Arthrogryposis- clinical and genetic heterogenicity. Paper presented at: Fifth International Conference on Birth Defects; August 1997, 1997; Montreal.

Kozin SH. Congenital Anomalies. In: Trumble TE, ed. *Hans Surgery Update 3, Hand, Elbow, & Shoulder.* Rosemont: American Society for Surgery of the Hand; 2003:599-624.

Kleinman WB, Strickland JW. Thumb Reconstruction. In: Green DP, Hotchkiss RN, Pederson WC, eds. *Green's Operative Hand Surgery.* Vol Two. New York: Churchill Livingstone; 1999:2068-2170.

Wood RJ, Bostwick J. Congenital Breast Deformities. In: Bentz ML, ed. *Pediatric Plastic surgery.* First ed. Pittsburgh: McGraw-Hill Professional; 1998:739-746.

HEMANGIOMAS

Jayant Agarwal, MD, Cori Agarwal, MD and Alvin Cohn, MD

O **Who proposed the biologic classification scheme for vascular anomalies?**

Mulliken and Glowacki in 1982.

O **What is the most common tumor of infancy?**

Hemangioma.

O **What is the incidence of hemangiomas in infants?**

1-2% of neonates and 12% by the age of one year.

O **Who has an increased incidence of hemangioma?**

Premature infants with a birth weight of less than 1000 grams (23% incidence vs. 1-2%).

O **What is the male:female ratio of hemangioma frequency?**

1:3.

O **Where do most hemangiomas occur?**

Head and neck 60%.
Trunk 25%.
Extremities 15%.

O **Do most hemangiomas present as multiples or singularly?**

Singularly.

O **What percent of patients have multiple hemangiomas?**

20%.

O **Which patients are at increased risk for harboring visceral hemangiomas?**

Infants with multiple cutaneous hemangiomas (hemangiomatosis).

O **Is this a serious diagnosis?**

Absolutely. Patients must be evaluated for:
1) hepatomegaly
2) congestive heart failure
3) anemia
Even with treatment this condition is fatal in up to 30% of patients.

O **Do hemangiomas usually present at birth?**

No; however, there is an entity known as congenital hemangioma that proliferates in utero.

O   **What is the usual presentation of a hemangioma?**

A "herald spot" (a blanched area or a telangectasia surrounded by a pale halo).

O   **How long is the proliferative phase?**

From presentation to 6-20 months.

O   **What phase occurs after proliferation?**

Involution.

O   **What are some characteristics of involution?**

Decrease in cellularity and tumor size, fibrofatty replacement, and development
of lobular architecture.

O   **Can proliferation and involution be seen simultaneously within a given lesion?**

Yes.

O   **T/F: Most hemangiomas resolve spontaneously.**

True.

O   **At what age does complete involution occur?**

50-65% by 5 years, 70% by 7 years, and 90% by 9 years. After 10 years of age there is rarely further regression.

O   **What cell type is abundant in hemangiomas?**

Mast cell.

O   **How are mast cells thought to affect hemangiomas?**

It is thought that they influence angiogenesis by stimulating capillary endothelium, although the precise mechanism
is not known.

O   **T/F: Hemangiomas result from a derangement in angiogenesis characterized by increased endothelial
cell turnover.**

True.

O   **What is the hallmark ultrastructural feature of hemangiomas?**

Multilaminated basement membranes.

O   **What percent of hemangiomas are complicated by bleeding and ulceration?**

About 10%.

O   **What is Kasabach-Merritt Syndrome?**

Profound thrombocytopenia with petechiae, ecchymoses, intralesional hemorrhage, or internal bleeding as a result of
a localized intravascular coagulopathy, not DIC.

○ **Which tumors are associated with this syndrome?**

Kaposiform hemangioendotheliomas and tufted angiomas.

○ **Are systemic antibiotics indicated in the treatment of hemangiomas?**

Only if there is evidence of cellulitis.

○ **What should you be concerned about if a child has a lumbar hemangioma?**

Possibility of spina bifida occulta. Evaluate with ultrasound or MRI.

○ **Why are periorbital hemangiomas concerning?**

They can block the visual field resulting in deprivation amblyopia.

○ **What are the possible complications of total visual obstruction for one week or more in an infant?**

Strabismus, amblyopia, optic atrophy.

○ **What is the outcome of untreated subglottic hemangioma?**

40-70% of affected patients die from respiratory compromise.

○ **How do subglottic hemangiomas typically present?**

They present with stridor at 6-8weeks of age and are associated with cervicofacial hemangiomas in 50% of affected infants.

○ **What complication can result with carbon dioxide laser treatment of circumferential subglottic hemangiomas?**

Subglottic stenosis.

○ **What complication can be seen with diffuse neonatal hemangiomatosis or large visceral hemangiomas?**

Congestive heart failure.

○ **What is the most common parotid tumor of childhood?**

Hemangioma.

○ **What complication can occur with parotid hemangioma?**

Obstruction of the external auditory meatus resulting in a conductive hearing loss and possible speech impairment.

○ **Is skeletal overgrowth a common feature of hemangiomas?**

No. Hypertrophy, erosion, or deformation of skeletal structures occur in about 1% of cases.

○ **Which hemangiomas require aggressive treatment?**

Large lesions or lesions which have the potential to cause functional impairment or psychosocial trauma.

○ **When is surgical excision recommended?**

Surgical excision is recommended for any tumors unresponsive to pharmacologic therapy, that are ulcerated, that obstruct both ears, or that obstruct the visual axis or airway.

O **What is the mainstay of treatment for hemangiomas?**

Systemic corticosteroids.

O **What is the usual systemic dose?**

Oral prednisone 2-3 mg/kg body weight for 2-3 weeks followed by a slow taper.

O **When are IV steroids indicated?**

These are usually not indicated other than in cases of life threatening Kasabach-Merritt syndrome.

O **What are some of the side effects of steroid use?**

Cushingoid facies, irritability, gastric upset, infection, and growth retardation.

O **Intralesional steroids have been used for eyelid and perioral hemangiomas. How is it given?**

Single dose of triamcinolone (40-80 mg) and/or betamethasone (6-12 mg) administered under general anesthesia.

O **What are some of the complications of intralesional injection?**

Blindness, ulceration, and eyelid necrosis.

O **What are the mechanisms of alpha-interferon?**

1. inhibiting endothelial cell, fibroblast, and smooth muscle cell proliferation
2. inhibiting growth factor release
3. inhibiting collagen synthesis

O **When are interferons used in the treatment of hemangiomas?**

1. For the treatment of hemangiomas that are life threatening
2. Those that require rapid involution (e.g. to protect the visual axis)
3. Those that have failed intensive steroid therapy.

O **What is the usual regimen for interferon use?**

Subcutaneous injection of 1 to 3 million units/m^2/day of either interferon-alpha-2a or interferon-alpha-2b. Some lesions may require treatment for up to 3 years and regression is seen in as many as 84% with complete resolution in almost 42%.

O **What are some of the side effects of interferon use?**

Flu-like symptoms, neutropenia, liver enzyme abnormalities, and spastic diplegia.

O **What types of lasers have been used in the management of hemangiomas?**

Carbon dioxide, flashlamp-pumped pulsed-dye, neodymium: yttrium-aluminum-garnet, potassium-titanyl-phosphate, and argon lasers.

O **What is the mechanism by which these lasers work in the treatment of hemangiomas?**

Selective photocoagulation (or selective photothermolysis) acting on oxyhemoglobin.

❍   **What lesions do lasers work best for?**

Superficial or flat lesions. Most lasers are unable to penetrate deeper than about 1.5 mm.

❍   **What other treatment modalities exist for hemangiomas?**

Embolization, chemotherapy, radiation, and cryotherapy.

❍   **What is Parkes-Weber Syndrome?**

1.   Arteriovenous malformations (or AV fistulas)
2.   Cutaneous capillary malformations
3.   Skeletal or soft-tissue hypertrophy (typically of the lower extremity)

❍   **What is Klippel-Trenaunay-Weber Syndrome?**

1.   Extremity hypertrophy (can include skin, muscle and/or bone with the lower limb affected 95% of the time)
2.   Cutaneous capillary malformation (port-wine stain) of the extremity
3.   Venous and lymphatic malformations
4.   Upper extremity involvement in 10% of patients with or without concomitant lower limb involvement
5.   No AVM present as in Parkes-Weber

❍   **What is Sturge-Weber Syndrome?**

1.   Vascular malformations (classically port-wine stain) of the face (V1-V2 particularly)
2.   Glaucoma (in the eye ipsilateral to the facial lesion)
3.   Vascular malformations of the choroid plexus and meninges
4.   Possible seizures depending on intracranial involvement

❍   **What is Maffucci Syndrome?**

1.   Multiple enchondromas (80% occurring in the hand)
2.   Hemangiomas although venous malformations also occur
3.   25% of patients have degeneration of enchondromas into chondrosarcomas
4.   6 cases of hemangioma degeneration into angiosarcoma have been reported

❍   **What is Rendu-Osler-Weber disease?**

1.   Autosomal dominant disorder (strong family history is typical)
2.   Telangiectasias (red spots)
3.   Multiple mucosal, visceral, cutaneous AVMs
4.   A.K.A. hereditary hemorrhagic telangiectasia

References

Mulliken JB. Classification of vascular birthmarks. In: Mulliken JB and Young AE (eds.). Vascular Birthmarks: Hemangiomas and Malformations. Philadelphia: Saunders, 1988.

Mulliken JB and Glowacki J. Hemangiomas and vascular malformations in infants and children: A classification based on endothelial characteristics. Plast Reconstr Surg 1982; 69:412-422.

Gampper TJ and Morgan RF. Vascular anomalies. Plast Reconstr Surg 2002; 110:572.

Boon LM, Enjolras O, and Mulliken JB. Congenital hemangioma: Evidence of accelerated involution. J Pediatr 1996; 128:329-335.

Drolet BA, Esterly NB, and Frieden IJ. Hemangiomas in children. N Eng. J Med 1999; 341: 173-181.

Enjolras O. Classification and management of the various superficial anomalies: Hemangiomas and vascular malformations. J Dermatol 1997; 24:701-710.

Enjolras O and Mulliken JB. The current management of vascular birthmarks. Pediatr Dermatol 1993; 10:311.

Sarkar M, Mulliken JB, Kozakewich HP et al. Thrombocytopenic coagulopathy (Kasabach-Merritt phenomenon) is associated with kaposiform hemangioendothelioma and not with common infantile hemangioma. Plast Reconstr Surg 1997; 100:1377-1386.

Kushner BJ. Intralesional corticosteroid injection for infantile adnexal hemangioma. Am J Ophthalmol 1982; 93:496-506.

Healy GB, Fearon B, French R et al. Treatment of subglottic hemangioma with the carbon dioxide laser. Laryngoscope. 1980; 90:809-813.

Ezekowitz RA, Mulliken JB, and Folkman J. Interferon alfa-2a therapy for life-threatening hemangiomas in infancy. N Engl J Med 1992; 326:1456-1463.

Lasser AE and Stein AF. Steroid treatment of hemangiomas in children. Arch Dermatol 1973; 108:565-567.

Geller JD, Topper SF, and Hashimoto K. Diffuse neonatal hemangiomatosis: A new constellation of findings. J Am Acad Dermatol 1991; 24:816-818.

Barlow CF, Priebe CJ, Mulliken JB et al. Spastic diplegia as a complication of interferon alfa-2a treatment of hemangiomas of infancy. J Pediatr 1998; 132:527-530.

Garden JM and Bakus AD. Clinical efficacy of the pulsed dye laser in the treatment of vascular lesions. J Dermatol Surg Oncol 1993; 19:321-326.

VASCULAR ANOMALIES

Ananth S. Murthy, MD

❍ **Are all strawberries hemangiomas?**

No, and not all hemangiomas are strawberries.

❍ **What is the ISSVA classification of vascular anomalies?**

Classification into vascular tumors and vascular malformations:

Tumors	Malformations
Hemangioma 　　Infantile 　　Congenital Hemangioendotheliomas Angiosarcoma Other	Slow-Flow 　　Capillary (CM) 　　Lymphatic (LM) 　　Venous (VM) Fast-Flow 　　Arterial (AM) Combined

❍ **What is the overall incidence of hemangiomas?**

4-10%; 23% in low-birth-weight (<1200g) infants.

❍ **What is the prevalence of hemangiomas in the head and neck?**

60%.

❍ **Is there a sex predilection of infantile hemangiomas?**

Yes; female preponderance 3:1.

❍ **How often do multiple hemangiomas occur?**

Incidence 20%.

❍ **When is there an increased likelihood of visceral involvement of hemangiomas?**

If >5 cutaneous hemangiomas, CT scan of liver should be obtained to R/O visceral involvement (hemangiomatosis).

❍ **What are the three phases in the life cycle of an infantile hemangioma?**

Proliferative, involuting, involuted.

❍ **How long does the proliferative phase of an infantile hemangioma last?**

From 0-1 year of age.

○ **What are the histopathologic changes in the involuting phase?**

Downregulation of angiogenesis, endothelial apoptosis and accumulation of mast cells.

○ **At what age is apoptosis at its highest rate in an involuting hemangioma?**

48 months.

○ **What percent of hemangiomas involute by age 5? By age 7?**

50% by age 5; 70% by age 7.

○ **Describe the MRI features of an infantile hemangioma?**

T1-parenchymous tissue with intermediate intensity; T2-moderate hyperintensity; flow voids; homogenous enhancement with gadolinium.

○ **What is the difference between congenital and infantile hemangioma?**

Congenital hemangioma is fully grown at birth or a "fetal" hemangioma.

○ **What are the two types of congenital hemangiomas?**

RICH (rapidly involuting congenital hemangioma) and NICH (non-involuting congenital hemangioma).

○ **What is the treatment of a congenital hemangioma?**

Observation. Corticosteroids are not indicated.

○ **What are some other infantile vascular tumors?**

Hemangioendotheliomas, tufted angioma, hemangiopericytoma, fibrosarcoma.

○ **What is the lesion in a 5-year-old child presenting with fruit-like cutaneous vascular tumor with episodic bleeding?**

Pyogenic granuloma.

○ **What is the treatment of pyogenic granuloma?**

Curettage, shave excision, laser or full-thickness excision.

○ **You are asked to see a patient in the NICU with an innocuous hemangioma on the cheek on the OR schedule for repair of a congenitally split-sternum. What is your concern?**

Hemangiomas (plaque-like) can be associated eye abnormalities, persistent intracranial arterial, great vessel abnormalities, posterior cranial fossa malformations, split sternum: PHACES syndrome. Order an MRI of the brain, an echocardiogram, and an ophthalmology consult.

○ **What does a lumbosacral hemangioma portend?**

Spinal dysraphism.

○ **What specific vascular tumors are associated with Kasabach-Merritt phenomenon (KMP)?**

Kasabach-Merritt phenomenon is caused by Kaposiform hemangioendothelioma and tufted angioma.

○ **Can KMP be caused by hemangioma (infantile or congenital)?**

No, neither causes KMP.

○ **What are the findings of KMP?**

Severe thrombocytopenia (<10,000/mm^3), fibrinogen level low, D-dimers increased, and PT/PTT **minimally** elevated or not at all.

○ **Do you transfuse platelets for KMP-associated thrombocytopenia?**

No. Since it is a localized intravascular coagulopathy, transfusion will cause more consumption of platelets. Treatment of the lesion will also treat the thrombocytopenia. Nevertheless, platelets can be transfused when spontaneous bleeding is encountered, or in anticipation of a surgical procedure. Heparin should be avoided.

○ **Platelets drop further (<10,000), in spite corticosteroid therapy. Now what?**

Interferon therapy (50% effective).

○ **What is the mortality rate of KMP?**

20-30%.

○ **What complications can a periorbital hemangioma cause?**

Periorbital hemangiomas can cause amblyopia, strabismus, proptosis, and astigmatism.

○ **What is the dosage of corticosteroids for treatment of infantile hemangioma?**

Oral steroid dose: Prednisone 2-3 mg/kg/day.

○ **Can hemangiomas be injected?**

Yes, for small hemangiomas (1-2 cm diam.) intralesional Triamcinolone (3-5 mg/kg) can be injected.

○ **What is the overall response rate for corticosteroids?**

85%.

○ **What are the complications encountered with corticosteroid therapy?**

Serious complications include: diminished gain of weight and height, infection, hypertension, myopathy, bone resorption.

○ **A 5 month old baby in the NICU has a very large cervicofacial hemangioma refractory to corticosteroid therapy. What is the next step?**

Recombinant interferon (IFN) alpha, 2a or 2b—second line treatment of life-endangering hemangioma/hemangioendothelioma. There is no documented synergy with corticosteroids; therefore, they may be discontinued prior to starting IFN Rx.

○ **What is the dose of IFN?**

2-3 million U/m2 SQ qD—response rate 90% (even if failed steroids).

○ **What is the most feared complication of IFN Rx?**

Spastic diplegia (incidence 5%), is reversible with discontinuation.

O   **How effective is laser in the treatment of hemangiomas?**

Laser is effective on telangiectasias that persist in involuting/involuted hemangiomas.

O   **Which live-vaccines are tolerated while on corticosteroids?**

None (polio, MMR, varicella vaccines should be withheld).

O   **What are the indications for resection?**

Proliferative phase—obstruction of airway or vision, painful or recalcitrant ulceration, and persistent localized bleeding.
Involuting phase—if excision is deemed inevitable, then prior to school age.
Involuted phase—resection of excess, stretched skin and contouring.

O   **The common name of *nevus flammeus neonatorum*?**

"Stork bite" or "angel kiss" (present in 50% of newborns).

O   **What common vascular anomaly can occur along with CM?**

Pyogenic granuloma.

O   **What other underlying anomalies can a CM signal?**

Scalp-midline: encephalocele.
Cervical/lumbosacral spine: spinal AVM (*Cobb's syndrome*).
Parkes Weber syndrome (CAVM).

O   **Capillary malformation covers dermatomes V1 and V2—what is it?**

Sturge-Weber syndrome (SWS).

O   **What is the concern with *Sturge-Weber syndrome*?**

Diagnose extension via MRI into: leptomeninges and choroid.

O   **What are the ocular findings associated with SWS?**

Funduscopic exam and tonometry: choroidal VM—retinal detachment, glaucoma and blindness.

O   **What type of laser can be used for treatment of CM?**

Tunable flashlamp pulsed dye laser (585 nm wavelength)—makes no difference after 1 year; 70% have obvious lightening of CM.

O   **What can be accomplished with surgical treatment of CM?**

Soft-tissue and skeletal hypertrophy can be improved.
Fibrovascular nodules can be excised.
Contour resection for labial hypertrophy and macrochilia.

O   **What is the order of frequency of LM?**

1. Cervicofacial, 2. Axilla/Chest/Mediastinum, 3. Retroperitoneum, 4. Buttock, 5. Anogenital area.

❍ **What are the 2 major types of LM?**

Macrocystic LM=soft; microcystic LM=firm/hard (19th century names: cystic hygroma and lymphangioma, respectively).

❍ **What is a well recognized side-effect of LM?**

Overgrowth of skeletal and soft tissues.

❍ **LMs are associated with what conditions?**

Aneuploidy (45XO-Turners), Trisomy 13, 18, and 21, Noonan and Roberts syndromes.

❍ **What is the best test to assess LM?**

MRI.

❍ **What are MRI findings of LM?**

Gadolinium show "rim enhancement."
LMs are hyperintense on T2-weighted images.

❍ **What is the radiographic differential diagnosis for such a lesion?**

Infantile fibrosarcoma, teratoma.

❍ **Sudden enlargement of LM is usually indicative of what?**

Intralesional bleeding/cellulitis.

❍ **What is the overall incidence of infection with LM?**

17%.

❍ **Describe the duration of ABX therapy for cellulitis in LM.**

ABX Rx for 6-8 weeks.

❍ **What is the first-line treatment for macrocystic LM?**

Sclerotherapy (ineffective against microcystic LM).

❍ **What are some of the options of sclerotherapy?**

Absolute ethanol, sodium tetradecyl sulfate, doxycycline, and OK-432

❍ **What is OK-432?**

OK-432: killed protein derived from Group A *Strep pyogenes*.

❍ **How do you treat dermal LM?**

Dermal LM or *lymphangioma circumscriptum* (tiny lymphatic vesicles with occasional intravesicular bleeding leading to dark-red dome shaped nodules) can be treated with excision.

○ **When does a lymphangioma start to involute?**

Trick question! Lymphangioma or cystic hygroma are quaint terms for LMs: LMs do not involute.

○ **What is the recurrence rate after resection?**

40% after incomplete excision; 17% after macroscopically complete excision.

○ **What are some problems with intra-osseus VMs?**

Structural weakening of the bone (predisposing to fractures) and hemarthrosis (if involves the joint).

○ **You are examining a patient with multiple cutaneous VMs—what's the next step?**

Multiple cutaneous VMs should raise suspicion of familial VMs: get a family history.

○ **What are examples of familial VMs?**

Glomuvenous malformations "glomangioma" (*glomulin* mutation), cutaneous-mucosal malformation (*TIE2* mutation), and cerebral-"cavernous" VM (*KRIT1* mutation).

○ **What are the MRI findings of VM?**

Hyperintense on T2 (similar to LM); enhancement of contents in T1 (unlike LM).

○ **Can you encounter coagulopathy with VMs?**

Localized intravascular coagulopathy (LIC) can be encountered due to stagnant flow in large VMs (very different from KMP).

○ **What is the primary modality of treatment of VM?**

Sclerotherapy. Indications: near critical nerves (no alcohol for sclero), multiple thrombi, VM involving palm/digits.

○ **What are the complications of sclerotherapy?**

Blistering, full-thickness cutaneous necrosis, damage to local nerves. Usually requires several sessions (VMs can re-canalize).

○ **When do you plan resection of VMs?**

Resection planned several (4) weeks after sclerotherapy. Unlike KMP, heparin may be used for preoperative control of LIC.

○ **Adjuvant therapy for VMs?**

Elastic garments are important, low dose ASA minimizes painful phlebothrombosis.

○ **What is the Schobinger staging system of AVMs?**

I (quiescence)-pink, warm.
II (expansion)-enlargement, pulsation and thrill.
III (destruction)-ulceration, bleeding or persistent pain.
IV –high output cardiac failure.

○ **What is the best diagnostic modality for AVMs?**

MRI. Angiography is not indicated unless intervention is planned.

○   **What are the treatment modalities of AVM?**

Embolization (*no* indication of ligation of feeding vessel since it results in rapid recruitment of flow and denies access for future embolization).
Resection within 24-72 hrs after embolization (observation of type of bleeding from margins of resection is most accurate to assess adequacy of removal).

○   **What are two examples of inheritable arterial malformations?**

1. Parkes Weber syndrome, or CM-AVM with a *RASA1* mutation is familial.
2. Osler-Weber-Rendu, or hereditary hemorrhagic telangiectasia (HHT).

○   **What is HHT?**

Autosomal dominant disorder, characterized by visceral, cutaneous and mucosal AVMs. There are three types of mutations along the TGFβ signaling pathway, HHT1 (endoglin receptor mutation), HHT2 (activin receptor mutation), and HHT3 (with intestinal polyposis, gene mutation not localized).

○   **Are intracerebral AVMs more common than extracerebral AVMs?**

Yes, by 20 fold.

○   **Geographic capillary malformation with lymphatic/venous malformation?**

Klippel-Trenaunay (CLVM) (look for associated limb hypertrophy).

○   **What is the association of lymphedema from lymphatic hypoplasia in KTS?**

>50% of patients

○   **What are the limb risks secondary to lymphedema?**

Cellulitis, thrombophlebitis, and thromboembolism.

○   **What is *Parkes Weber* syndrome?**

High flow combined capillary-AVM (look for *RASA1* mutation if familial).

○   **What is Bannayan-Riley-Ruvalcaba/Cowden syndrome?**

Overgrowth syndrome associated with vascular malformation, macrocephaly, macrosomia, pigmented macules of the penis, hamartomas of the GI tract, malignancy of the thyroid and breast, lipomas and trichilemmomas (*PTEN* mutation in 60-80% of cases).

○   **What is Maffucci syndrome?**

Hemangioendotheliomas of the extremity associated with enchondromas. 20-30% will progress to chondrosarcomas.

○   **What is Proteus syndrome?**

Complex and variable disorder characterized by overgrowth of limbs, epidermal nevi, vascular malformations, and cranial hyperostosis.

❍   **Describe the findings of blue rubber bleb syndrome.**

Intestinal and multiple palmar and plantar VMs.

This chapter was possible only after being awakened to the field of vascular anomalies by my mentor, Dr. John B. Mulliken.

References

Mulliken JB, Young AE. Vascular Birthmarks: Hemangiomas and Malformations. Philadelphia: Saunders; 1988

Holmdahl K. Cutaneous hemangiomas in premature and mature infants. Acta Paediatr Scand 44:370-9, 1955.

Amir J, Metzker A et al. Strawberry hemangioma in preterm infants. *Pediatr Dermatol* 3:331, 1986.

Bowers RE, Graham EA, Tomlinson KM. The natural history of the strawberry nevus. *Arch Dermatol* 82:667, 1960.

Martinez-Perez D, Fein NA, Boon LM, Mulliken JB. Not all hemangiomas look like strawberries: uncommon presentations of the most common tumor of infancy. *Pediatr Dermatol* 12:1-6, 1995.

Takahashi K, Mulliken JB, Kozakewich HPW, et al. Cellular markers that distinguish the phases of hemangioma during infancy and childhood. *J Clin Invest* 93:2357-64, 1994.

Razon MJ, Kraling BM, Mulliken JB, Bischoff J. Increased apoptosis coincides with onset of involution in infantile hemangioma. *Microcirculation* 5:189-95, 1998.

Mulliken JB, Enjolras O. Congenital hemangiomas and infantile hemangioma: missing links. *J Am Acad Derm* 50(6):875-82, 2004.

Patrice SJ, Wiss K, Mulliken JB. Pyogenic granuloma (lobular capillary hemangioma): a clinicopathologic study of 178 cases. *Pediatr Dermatol* 8:267-76, 1991.

Frieden IJ, Reese V, Cohen D. PHACE syndrome: the association of posterior fossa brain malformations, hemangiomas, arterial anomalies, coarctation of the aorta and cardia defects and eye abnormalities. *Arch Dermatol* 132:307-11, 1996.

Sarkar M, Mulliken JB, Kozakewich HP, Robertson RL, Burrows PE. Thrombocytopenic coagulopathy (Kasabach-Merritt phenomenon) is associated with kaposiform hemangioendothelioma and not with common infantile hemangioma. *Plast Reconstr Surg* 100:1377-86, 1997.

Boon LM, MacDonald DM, Mulliken JB. Complications of systemic corticosteroid therapy for problematic hemangiomas. *Plast Reconstr Surg* 104:1616-23, 1999.

Ezekowitz RAB, Mulliken JB, Folkman J. Interferon alfa-2a therapy for life-threatening hemangiomas of infancy. *N Engl J Med* 326:1456, 1992.

Mulliken JB, Boon LM, Takahashi K, et al. Pharmacologic therapy for endangering hemangiomas. *Curr Opin Dermatol* 2:109-13, 1995.

Tan OT, Sherwood K, Gilchrest BA. Treatment of children with port-wine stains using the flashlamp pumped tunable dye laser. *N Engl J Med* 320:416-21, 1989.

Boyd JB, Mulliken JB, Kaban LB, Upton J III, Murray JE. Skeletal changes associated with vascular malformations. *Plast Reconstr Surg* 74:789, 1984.

Vikkula M, Boon LM, Mulliken JB, Osen BR. Molecular basis of vascular anomalies. *Trends Cardiovasc Med* 8:281-92, 1998.

Guttmacher AE, Marchuk DA, White RI Jr. Hereditary hemorrhagic telangiectasia. *N Engl J Med* 333:918-24, 1995.

Vikkula M, Boon LM, Carraway KL III, et al. Vascular dysmorphogenesis caused by an activating mutation in the receptor tyrosine kinase TIE2. *Cell* 87:1181-90, 1996.

Laberge-le Couteulx S, Jung HH, Labauge P, et al. Truncating mutations in CCM1, encoding KRIT1, cause hereditary cavernous angiomas. *Nat Genet* 23:189-93, 1999.

Boon LM, Mulliken JB, Enjolras O, Vikkula M. Glomuvenous malformation (glomangioma) and venous malformation: distinct clinicopathologic and genetic causes. *Arch Dermatol* 140(8): 971-6, 2004.

Enjolras O, Riche MC, Merland JJ. Facial port-wine stains and Sturge-Weber syndrome. *Pediatrics* 76:48-51, 1985.

Padwa BL, Hayward PG, Ferraro NF, Mulliken JB. Cervicofacial lymphatic malformation: clinical course, surgical intervention, and pathogenesis of skeletal hypertrophy. *Plast Reconstr Surg* 95:951-60, 1995.

Alqahtani A, Nguyen LT, Flageole H, et al. 25 years' experience with lympangiomas in children. *J Pediatr Surg* 34:1164-8, 1999.

Oranje AP. Blue rubber bleb nevus syndrome. *Pediatr Dermatol* 3:304-10, 1986.

Berenguer B, Burrows PE, Zurakowski D, Mulliken JB. Sclerotherapy of craniofacial venous malformation: complications and results. *Plast Reconstr Surg* 104:1-11, 1999.

Kohout MP, Hansen M, Pribaz JJ, Mulliken JB. Arteriovenous malformations of the head and neck: natural history and management. *Plast Reconstr Surg* 102:643-54, 1998.

Eerola I, Boon LM, Mulliken JB, et al. Capillary malformation-arteriovenous malformation, a new clinical and genetic disorder caused by RASA1 mutations. *Am J Hum Genet* 73(6):1240-9, 2003.

Jacob AG, Driscoll DJ, Shaughness WJ, et al. Klippel-Trenaunay syndrome: spectrum and management. *Mayo Clin Proc* 73:28-36, 1998.

Marsh DJ, Kum JB, Lunetta KL, et al. PTEN mutation spectrum and genotype-phenotype correlations in Bannayan-Riley-Ruvalcaba syndrome suggest a single entity with Cowden syndrome. *Hum Mol Genet* 8:1461-72, 1999.

Mulliken JB, Fishman SF, Burrows PE. Vascular Anomalies. *Curr Probl Surg* 37(8):517-84, 2000.

Marler JJ, Mulliken JB. Current management of hemangiomas and vascular malformations. *Clin Plast Surg* 32(1):99-116, 2005.

RECONSTRUCTION

WOUND HEALING/KELOIDS

Ali Al-Attar, MD, Ph.D.

PRINCIPLES

○ **What are the steps involved in wound healing?**

1. Inflammation-1-2 days
2. Proliferation-3-30 days (depends on bacterial load)
3. Remodeling/differentiation-up to 1 year

○ **What are the cell types primarily responsible for each of these stages?**

1. Inflammation-PMN's, macrophages
2. Proliferation-macrophages, fibroblasts
3. Remodeling-myofibroblasts (wound contraction), epithelial cells (re-epithelialization)

○ **What are the steps involved in epithelialization across a wound?**

Mobilization, migration, mitosis, and differentiation of epithelial cells. The loss and reestablishment of **contact inhibition** initiate and terminate the process.

○ **What is the key cell involved in wound remodeling?**

Macrophage. The macrophage is probably the most critical cell in wound healing in general—it initiates the growth factor cascade that results in fibroblast proliferation and thus collagen production.

○ **Which cells are responsible for wound contracture?**

Myofibroblasts—fibroblasts that contain myofibrils permitting contractile activity similar to muscle.

○ **What provides tensile strength to a healing wound?**

Collagen.

○ **Which cells produce collagen in the healing wound, and when does production peak?**

Fibroblasts produce collagen; maximal net collagen production occurs at about one to two weeks.

○ **When is a scar fully matured, and how much tensile strength does it achieve?**

A scar matures in one year, at which point it has gained approximately 80-90% of its initial tensile strength. The most rapid increase in tensile strength occurs between ten to thirty days, secondary to **collagen cross-linking**.

○ **What are the different types of collagen?**

There are many types of collagen (over ten). Critical to wound healing are:
Type I: most common; in skin, bone, and tendon/ligament
Type II: hyaline cartilage
Type III: vessel walls; intestine; skin

423

Type IV: basement membrane
Type V: fetal and placental tissue

O   **What is the ratio of type I to type III collagen in normal skin and scars?**

Normal skin: 4:1 (i.e., predominantly type I collagen)
Immature scar: 2:1
Hypertrophic scar: 2:1
Keloid: 3:1 (varies)
Fetal skin: predominantly type III collagen

O   **Which conditions adversely affect key steps in collagen synthesis?**

1.   Vitamin C deficiency-inhibits hydroxylation of proline and lysine (required for collagen cross-linking).
2.   Colchicine-inhibits secretion of tropocollagen from the cell.
3.   Copper deficiency and penicillamine-prevent lysine oxidation (which is necessary for intra- and intermolecular bonding).

O   **What are the detrimental effects of corticosteroids on wound healing?**

Corticosteroids inhibit macrophages, resulting in poor fibroblast stimulation and wound contraction.

O   **What strategy can overcome the effects of steroids?**

Vitamin A (25,000 IU by mouth daily for three to five days, alternatively 200,000 IU topically three times a day).

O   **How long should you wait before revising a scar?**

One year to allow scar remodeling to complete.

O   **What factors impair wound healing?**

1.   Foreign bodies and infection
2.   Radiated tissue-decreases blood supply
3.   Inadequate blood supply-any cause
4.   Local trauma
5.   Systemic factors (steroid use, obesity, edema, smoking, co-morbidities)

O   **What are the escalating strategies that can be used to close a defect (the "reconstructive ladder")?**

Secondary intent
Primary intent
Skin graft
Local tissue rearrangement
Transposition flap
Free tissue transfer

KELOIDS

O   **What is the difference between keloids and hypertrophic scars?**

1.   Keloids extend beyond the margin of the initial scar, whereas hypertrophic scars do not.
2.   Keloids have an increased ratio of types I/III collagen unlike hypertrophic scars.
3.   More significant cellular and biochemical abnormalities are found in keloids.

○ **What are the principles of keloid and hypertrophic scar management?**

1. Excision plus adjuvant therapy (intradermal steroids, silicone gel, radiation therapy)
2. Meticulous tissue handling and closure with intradermal sutures
3. Pressure earrings/garments

○ **What are the contraindications to radiation therapy for keloids?**

1. Pediatric patients
2. Pregnant women
3. Tissue with underlying visceral structures

Despite the theoretical risk of neoplastic transformation, less than ten cases of cancer due to radiation therapy for keloids have been reported.

○ **What is the mechanism of intralesional steroid (triamcinolone acetonide) therapy for keloids?**

1. Inhibits fibroblast proliferation and collagen production
2. Stimulates collagenase production
3. Normalizes collagen ultrastructural organization that is disrupted in keloid nodules

○ **What is the optimal treatment for earlobe keloids?**

Surgical excision with or without steroid injection, followed by wearing of pressure earrings.

○ **Can a partial-thickness burn scar be left to heal by secondary intention?**

Generally, partial-thickness burn scars can be given up to three weeks to close by secondary intent. If not closed by three weeks, they need to be grafted to avoid hypertrophic scar formation.

○ **Where does scarless wound healing occur?**

Wound healing occurs without scar in the early mammalian fetus (including human). Levels of hyaluronic acid are significantly higher in fetal skin and appears to correlate with scarless wound healing.

○ **What is the Fitzpatrick classification of skin types?**

   --based on density of melanin pigment
Type I: White or freckled skin (always burns)
Type II: White skin (usually burns)
Type III: White to olive skin (equally burns and tans)
Type IV: Brown skin (tans easily, rarely burns)
Type V: Dark brown skin (very rarely burns)
Type VI: Black skin (never burns)

○ **What is the staging of sacral wounds?**

Stage 1: Skin intact; non-blanching erythema
Stage 2: Partial-thickness skin loss, abrasions and blisters included (so into epidermis or dermis)
Stage 3: Full-thickness skin loss with extension into subcutaneous tissue/muscle
Stage 4: Full-thickness skin loss with extension into bone, joint, tendon

○ **What are the principles of sacral wound management?**

1. Remove pressure
2. Maintain hygiene in region (diverting colostomy if needed)
3. Optimize medical issues

4.   Serial wound debridements
5.   Dressing changes (wet-to-dry; enzymatic therapy if necrotic tissue or dilute acetic acid if infected, especially with pseudomonas)
6.   Repair with excision and choice of flap once above factors addressed

❍   **In the evaluation of a pressure ulcer, what is the imaging modality of choice for diagnosis of osteomyelitis?**

MRI is the current imaging modality of choice
Bone biopsy is the gold-standard to confirm osteomyelitis

❍   **Where can pressure ulcers occur?**

Anywhere bony prominences exist.
1.   Ischial tuberosity
2.   Trochanter
3.   Sacrum
4.   Calcaneus
5.   Occiput
6.   Scapula

❍   **During wound therapy with leeches, which bacteria grow in the leech gut?**

Aeromonas hydrophila. Ciprofloxacin, Bactrim or tetracycline can be used for prophylaxis.

❍   **What is the antibacterial mechanism of Acticoat?**

Acticoat contains silver ions that are directly bactericidal. Acticoat needs to be moistened with distilled water prior to application (ions in normal saline will negate the antibacterial effect of Acticoat). Acticoat is efficacious against Pseudomonas, MRSA, VRE and some species of yeast.

❍   **What are the clinical indications for Regranex gel (becaplermin, PDGF)?**

Regranex is indicated for lower extremity ulcers:
    --of diabetic neuropathy
    --that extend into the subcutaneous tissue
    --that have a good vascular supply
    --that are not infected.
Regranex is not FDA-approved for use in ischemic, infected, or superficial wounds, or those that are being closed primarily.

❍   **Which biologic dressings contain cultured cells?**

1.   Trancyte-a dermal substitute that is composed of cultured neonatal dermal fibroblasts seeded on a silicone/collagen matrix, covered with a nylon sheet.
2.   Dermagraf-contains neonatal fibroblasts on a sheet of Dexon (polyglycolic acid) or Vicryl.
3.   Epicyte- a matrix of cultured autologous keratinocytes (i.e., from the same patient).
4.   Apligraf-contains both neonatal keratinocytes and fibroblasts; these cells are seeded onto a collagen matrix.

❍   **Which other biologic dressings contain dermal matrix?**

1.   Biobrane-a nylon sheet covering a silicone layer containing dermal collagen.
2.   Integra-a silicone sheet coated with collagen and glycosaminoglycan obtained from bone tendon cartilage.
3.   Alloderm-cadaveric acellular dermis that has been de-epithelialized.

❍   **Which wounds are best treated with alginates?**

Highly exudative wounds. Calcium alginate gels are made from seaweed and are hydrophilic, so they can absorb significant amounts of fluid. Alginates prevent tissue maceration, trap bacteria, and can be rinsed off.

TISSUE EXPANSION

O   **What are the effects of tissue expansion on flap properties?**

1.   Increased tissue surface area, collagen and ground substance content
2.   Increased vascularity (similar to flap delay)
3.   Decreased tensile strength and elasticity (since thinner dermis)
4.   Markedly increased sensitivity to epinephrine-induced necrosis

Tissue expansion results in a <u>net gain of tissue</u> that is due to both stretching of existing tissue as well as de novo tissue generation.

O   **What are the histologic changes seen following tissue expansion?**

a.   Subcutaneous fat atrophies.
b.   Dermis becomes thinner.
c.   Epidermis becomes thicker, particularly the **stratum spinosum** (increased mitotic activity).
d.   Rete ridges become flatter.

O   **What are the tissue zones that result from tissue expansion?**

Tissue expansion results in formation of a capsule surrounding the expander, which is essentially a foreign body reaction. These zones are, from inside to outside:
         Zone A: Inner zone, cellular (predominantly macrophages)
         Zone B: Central zone, fibrous, with fibroblasts and myofibroblasts
         Zone C: Transitional zone, with loose collagen
         Zone D: Vascular zone

O   **What is mechanical creep?**

1.   A response to constant mechanical force
2.   Collagen realigns and results in a change in tissue elasticity
3.   Interstitial fluid and ground substance are displaced
4.   Depends on viscoelastic properties of skin

O   **What is stress-relaxation?**

Less force is needed to keep tissue stretched to a given length the longer it is held at that length.

O   **Which tissue expansion protocol results in maximal tissue recruitment?**

Cyclic loading: repeated cycles of stretching followed by relaxation.

O   **How can extra tissue be recruited intraoperatively?**

Approximately 15-20% tissue expansion can be gained with a brief one to two hour session (acute tissue expansion). Clinical studies suggest acute tissue expansion provides tissue of comparable quality to that expanded over a much longer time frame (weeks).

O   **What are the concerns with lower extremity tissue expansion, especially below the knee?**

1.   Extensive tissue expansion can cause sural nerve neuropraxia.

2. The region below the knee has relatively limited lymphatic outflow (compared with the trunk); and a tissue expander is at increased risk for cellulitis.
3. Tissue expansion in the lower extremity is particularly problematic in the pediatric population.

❍ **What effect does tissue expansion have on hair growth?**

Tissue expansion, such as in the scalp, decreases the telogen, or growth arrest, phase.

❍ **How does irradiated tissue differ from normal during tissue expansion?**

Irradiated tissue does not undergo the histologic changes that are seen with normal tissue during tissue expansion. Previous irradiation decreases the net tissue gain from expansion by about 25%.

❍ **What is the mechanism of vacuum-assisted closure (VAC)?**

Continuous or intermittent negative pressure is applied to the wound bed increasing collagen production by fibroblasts and fibroblast mitotic activity. The actual mechanism is believed to involve structural re-alignment of fibroblast cells that triggers collagen production and mitosis.

❍ **How does a split thickness skin graft initially receive nutrition?**

<u>Plasma imbibition</u> for the first 48 hours until an adequate vascular supply is established.
<u>Inosculation</u>-connection of recipient and donor vessels in the graft and recipient bed
<u>Neovascularization</u>-sprouting of new blood vessels

❍ **What are the steps in adherence of a skin graft?**

Phase 1: <u>fibrin</u> phase (first 72 hours).
Phase 2: fibrovascular phase (after 72 hours)—vascular ingrowth and anastomosis

❍ **What are the causes of skin graft failure?**

1. Hematoma
2. Seroma
3. Infection
4. Shearing forces disrupting skin graft adherence and thus nutrition

❍ **What bacterial load is required to cause clinical infection in a split thickness skin graft?**

10^5 bacteria per cm^3 of tissue

❍ **Which flap type offers the greatest resistance to bacterial infection?**

Musculocutaneous flaps bring in a large proportionate blood supply that best wards off bacterial infection.

❍ **What histologic layer mediates skin graft contraction?**

<u>Elastin within the dermis</u>-thicker skin grafts mean more dermis which means more elastin which means more primary or immediate contraction.
Conversely elastin inhibits delayed (secondary) graft contraction so those grafts without dermis, such as cultured epithelial cells, demonstrate the most delayed contraction.

❍ **What is the maximal dose of lidocaine that can be used for local anesthesia?**

Plain lidocaine: 4 mg/kg
Lidocaine with epinephrine: 7 mg/kg

Tumescent technique: up to 35 mg/kg has been suggested to be safe

❍ How long do sutures retain tensile strength?

Catgut—one week or less.
Vicryl, Dexon—four weeks.
PDS—six weeks.

❍ Which animals can potentially transmit rabies?

Carnivores: dog, cat, raccoon, bat, fox, skunk, coyote. Incidence of rabies from cats is increasing. Exposure alone without a bite can transmit rabies and is an indication for prophylaxis (entering a cave harboring rabid bats).
    Rodents do not carry rabies.

❍ How is a rabies exposure managed?

1. Wash the wound in virucidal agent (dilute Betadine).
2. Rabies immune globulin: give single dose of 20 IU/kg around the wound.
3. Rabies vaccine (human diploid cell vaccine): give five 1cc doses over a 28-day period (days 0, 3, 7, 14, 28); intramuscular injection in the deltoid.
--Give both rabies immune globulin and vaccine to all patients, except for patients with a documented antibody titer, who do not need immune globulin.

❍ Which wounds are "tetanus prone"?

1. Wounds that are contaminated
2. Contain devitalized tissue
3. Are open greater than 6 hours
4. Are deeper than 1 centimeter

❍ What tetanus measures are required for a wound in a "fully immunized" patient?

A fully immunized patient is one who has received complete tetanus toxoid immunization (three to five doses) with a booster within five years of the current injury. If the wound is "tetanus prone", give tetanus toxoid (0.5 ml of adsorbed toxoid intramuscularly). If the wound is not "tetanus prone", do nothing.

❍ What tetanus measures are required for a wound in a patient of unknown or inadequate immunization status?

These patients need to receive tetanus toxoid for all wounds. In addition, if the patient has received less than two injections of immunization, also give immune globulin (250 Units of human tetanus immune globulin).

❍ Which cytokines are produced by macrophages?

IL-1, IL-6, IL-8, IL-10, TNFa, IFNg.

❍ What isomers mediate the pro-fibrotic phenotype of TGF-b?

TGF-b has three isomers. TGF-b1 and TGF-b2 are pro-fibrotic.
TGF-b3 is anti-fibrotic.
Various fibrotic diseases (such as keloids) might result from aberrant ratios of TGF-b isomers (i.e., increased TGF-b1 and TGF-b2 and decreased TGF-b3).

❍ What are the biologic effects of FGF?

• Fibroblast and epithelial proliferation

- Collagen production
- Potent angiogenic factor

○   What is the role of FGF in wound healing?

- FGF-1 and FGF-2 (acidic and basic FGF) are the major proteins in this family and drive rapid proliferation of fibroblasts, epithelial cells and endothelial cells.
- FGF-7 (keratinocyte growth factor) is a major epidermal growth factor, and is involved in dermal-epidermal signaling.
- The sequence of events in wound healing is largely mediated by orchestration of intra- and extra-cellular regulation of FGF proteins in a defined pattern.

References

Argenta LC, Morykwas MJ: Vacuum-assisted closure: a new method for wound control and treatment: clinical experience. *Ann Plast Surg* 1997;38:563-577.

Fitzpatrick TB: The validity and practicality of sun reactive skin types I-VI. *Arch Dermatol* 1988; 124:869-871.

Goldman R: Growth factors and chronic wound healing: past, present, and future. *Adv Skin Wound Care* 2004;17:24-35.

Liu W, Wang DR, Cao YL: TGF-beta: a fibrotic factor in wound scarring and a potential target for anti-scarring gene therapy. *Curr Gene Ther* 2004; 4:123-136.

Morkywas MJ, Argenta LC, Shelton-Brown EI, McGuirt W: Vacuum-assisted closure: a new method for wound control and treatment: animal studies and basic foundation. *Ann Plast Surg* 1997;38:553-562.

Pandya AN, Vadodaria S, Coleman DJ: Tissue expansion in the limbs: a comparative analysis of limb and non-limb sites. *Br J Plast Surg* 2002;55:302-306.

Powers CJ, McLeskey SW, Wellstein A: Fibroblast growth factors, their receptors and signaling. *Endocr Relat Cancer* 2000;7:165-197.

Ratner D: Skin grafting. *Semin Cutan Med Surg* 2003;22:295-305.

Rumalla VK, Borah GL: Cytokines, growth factors, and plastic surgery. *Plast Reconstr Surg* 2001;108:719-733.

Saxena V, Hwang CW, Huang S, Eichbaum Q, Ingber D, Orgill DP: Vacuum-assisted closure: microdeformations of wounds and cell proliferation. *Plast Reconstr Surg* 2004;114:1086-1096.

Zeng YJ, Xu CQ, Yang J, Sun GC, Xu XH: Biomechanical comparison between conventional and rapid expansion of skin. *Br J Plast Surg* 2003;56:660-666.

PRINCIPLES OF SKIN GRAFTING

Douglas M. Sammer, MD

○ **What are the two main types of skin graft?**

Split-thickness and full-thickness.

○ **Which parts of skin are included in skin grafts?**

The epidermis and part (STSG) or all (FTSG) of the dermis.

○ **What structures are included with the dermis in both split-thickness and full-thickness skin grafts?**

Adnexal structures including sebaceous glands, hair follicles, sweat glands, and capillaries.

○ **How thick is a "thin" split-thickness skin graft?**

0.005 to 0.012 inch.

○ **How thick is an "intermediate" split-thickness skin graft?**

0.012 to 0.018 inch.

○ **How thick is a "thick" split-thickness skin graft?**

0.018 to 0.028 inch.

○ **What are the advantages of meshing a partial-thickness skin graft?**

Expansion of graft surface area up to six times, better contouring, decreased seroma or hematoma formation beneath the graft.

○ **How does the mesher ratio affect the graft surface area?**

A mesher expansion ratio of 1:1.5 (most commonly used) increases surface area by 50%, a ratio of 1:2 increases surface area by 100%, etc.

○ **What are the disadvantages of meshing?**

Waffled appearance, increased graft contraction (may be an advantage in some situations).

○ **Where should meshing be avoided?**

On the face, hand, or forearm (cosmetically sensitive areas), and over joints, where contracture becomes a problem.

○ **What is the postoperative bolster made of?**

Xeroform, cotton balls or batting moistened in saline/mineral oil, secured with tie-over sutures or a stapled-on foam dressing.

○ **How long should the bolster stay on postoperatively?**

Five to seven days. Two to three days if the recipient site is contaminated.

❍ **What are typical donor sites for split-thickness skin grafts?**

Anterior or lateral thigh in adults, buttock in children (for concealment of scar). The abdomen, back, chest, and scalp are often used if other donor sites are limited.

❍ **What is an appropriate donor-site dressing?**

Xeroform gauze dried with a hair-dryer or heat lamp is the traditional dressing. An occlusive semipermeable dressing such as Opsite or Tegaderm may be used.

❍ **What is the advantage of Tegaderm or Opsite for the donor-site dressing?**

Faster healing and pain reduction.

❍ **Do the dermis and epidermis regenerate in split-thickness donor sites?**

The donor site epidermis regenerates from the periphery and from adnexal structures, but the dermis does not regenerate. The donor site can be reharvested after it is well healed, if the underlying dermis is thick enough.

❍ **How long does a split-thickness donor site take to heal?**

A thin STSG donor site will heal within one week, whereas thicker STSG donor sites will take 2-3 weeks to heal.

❍ **What are the advantages of full-thickness skin grafts?**

Better color, thickness, and texture match with recipient site, decreased contraction.

❍ **What are the disadvantages of full-thickness skin grafts?**

Donor site must be closed primarily, limited donor sites, more difficult take compared to split-thickness skin grafts.

❍ **What are typical full-thickness skin graft donor sites?**

Supraclavicular, preauricular, postauricular, volar forearm, inguinal region.

❍ **Why should a FTSG be defatted after harvesting?**

Full-thickness skin grafts should be aggressively defatted to improve imbibition and take.

❍ **What is a composite graft?**

A graft that includes fat, muscle, or cartilage in addition to skin.

❍ **What is the maximum size of a composite graft?**

Variable, but composite grafts that contain cartilage will not take if greater than 1 to 1.5 cm in diameter.

❍ **What is the difference between an isograft / autograft, an allograft / homograft, and a xenograft / heterograft?**

Autograft or isograft: from same person, or an identical twin.
Allograft or homograft: from same species.
Xenograft or heterograft: from different species.

○ **What is the purpose of allograft or xenograft?**

Used for temporary coverage of wounds until they are suitable for autografting. Cadaver allograft or more rarely porcine xenografts can be used. Cadaveric allografts do take initially, but are rejected after ten days. Xenografts are more quickly rejected.

○ **What is the difference between primary and secondary skin graft contraction?**

Primary contraction is the immediate shrinkage of a skin graft after harvesting which is due to dermal elastin. Secondary contraction is the contracture that occurs with healing, and is due to myofibroblast activity.

○ **Do split-thickness or full-thickness skin grafts contract more?**

Primary contraction is greater with thicker skin grafts, whereas secondary contraction is greater with thinner skin grafts.

○ **How does graft thickness affect the ability of the graft to sweat?**

Thicker grafts contain more dermis, and therefore more sweat glands, and will have a greater potential to sweat.

○ **How does graft thickness affect the ability of the graft to grow hair?**

More hair follicles are harvested with thicker grafts, and these will have greater hair growth.

○ **How does graft thickness affect the ability of the graft to develop sensation?**

Thicker grafts contain more neurilemmal sheaths, allowing greater ingrowth of nerve fibers, and greater potential for sensation over time. Thin grafts have less potential for sensation, but may develop sensation more quickly.

○ **What type of sensation develops first in a healing skin graft?**

Pain returns first, then light touch, then hot/cold sensation.

○ **What are the phases of skin graft take?**

Imbibition, inosculation, and revascularization.

○ **What is imbibition?**

The first phase of take, involving the uptake of nutrients from serum in the wound bed by capillary action, lasting 48-72 hours.

○ **What is inosculation?**

The second phase of take, involving donor and recipient capillary alignment.

○ **What is revascularization?**

The third phase of take, revascularization occurs through the aligned capillaries, complete at 7 days.

○ **How does revascularization occur?**

Controversial: new recipient site vessels may grow into the graft along the path of graft vessels, new ingrowth may occur randomly, recipient and donor vessels may anastomose, or a combination of the above.

○ **To what type of tissue will a skin graft not take?**

Exposed bone, cartilage, or tendon (unless there is overlying periosteum, perichondrium, or paratenon).

○ **What are the most common causes of failure of skin graft take?**

Hematoma or seroma, poorly debrided or poorly vascularized wound, shearing of the graft, and infection. The most common is hematoma or seroma beneath the graft.

○ **What level of bacterial load in the recipient site precludes skin graft take?**

Skin grafts will not take in wounds with bacterial loads of 10^5 per gram or greater.

○ **What are the two phases of graft adherence?**

The first phase is due to fibrin deposition between the graft and the wound bed, lasting 72 hours. The second phase involves ingrowth of vessels into the graft and production of fibrous tissue.

○ **Once a skin graft is well healed, how should it be taken care of?**

Hand-lotion or cream should be used to prevent dessication. Skin grafts have decreased sweat and sebaceous glands. Sweat glands do not function until innervated. Sebaceous gland function is also delayed, although innervation is not required for function.

References

Chang E. Grafts. In: Brown DL, Borschel GH, eds. Michigan Manual of Plastic Surgery. Philadelphia: Lippincott Williams&Wilkins, 2004:16-21.

Place MJ, Herber SC, Hardesty RA. Basic techniques and principles in plastic surgery. In: Aston SJ, Beasley RW, Thorne CHM, eds. Grabb and Smith's Plastic Surgery. 5th ed. Philadelphia: Lippincott-Raven, 1997:13-26.

Preuss S, Breuing KH, Eriksson E. Plastic surgery techniques. In: Achauer BM, Eriksson E, eds. Plastic Surgery Indications, Operations, and Outcomes. St. Louis: Mosby, 2000:147-162.

Vasconez HC. Skin grafts. In: Cohen M, ed. Mastery of Plastic and Reconstructive Surgery. Boston: Little, Brown and Company, 1994:45-55.

Wolf SE, Herndon DN. Burns and radiation injuries. In: Mattox, Feliciano, Moore, eds. Trauma. 4th ed. New York: McGraw-Hill, 2000:1137-1152.

SKIN GRAFTING

Samuel J. Lin, MD and John B. Hijjawi, MD

○ **After the age of 35, what happens to the histology of skin?**

Gradual thinning of dermis, decreased skin elasticity, progressive loss of sebaceous gland content

○ **What percentage of the skin is dermis?**

95%

○ **Where are sebaceous glands located?**

In the dermis

○ **What are advantages of split thickness skin grafts over full thickness skin grafts?**

The best "take," and can be used under unfavorable wound conditions

○ **What are disadvantages of STSGs?**

They shrink considerably, pigment abnormally, and are susceptible to trauma.

○ **What are advantages of FTSGs?**

They do not contract upon grafting, resist trauma, and generally look more natural after healing

○ **How long does plasmic imbibition last for?**

24-48 hours

○ **How long does it take before neovascularization of a skin graft?**

5-6th day

○ **What is secondary revascularization of a skin graft?**

Occurs when vascular connections in the bed and the graft are delayed; granulation tissue accumulates under the graft

○ **What are methods of adherence in skin grafting techniques?**

Absorbable staples, fibrin glue, bolsters, VAC, lyofoam

○ **What is the clinical appearance of healing grafts?**

As described by Medawar, the graft is first white but then becomes pink over the next few days after application to the recipient site

○ **How much do FTSGs and STSGs contract primarily?**

FTSG – 40%, STSG 10-20%

○   **When will a skin graft become innervated?**

Between 5 weeks and 5 months; normal sensation may be complete at 12-24 months

○   **What happens to the pigment of skin grafts taken from the abdomen, buttocks, and thigh?**

Over time these skin grafts darken; grafts from the palm lighten

○   **What is the best treatment for hyperpigmented grafts?**

Dermabrasion only when graft innervation has occurred

○   **What are alternative methods of skin graft expansion?**

Pinch grafting, relay transplantation, meshing

○   **What is relay transplantation?**

Cutting a skin graft into strips (approx. 5 mm wide and 10 mm apart) and placing them in the bed for a short period of time (7 days) followed by removing and transplanting the skin to a adjacent area for epithelial growth to occur

○   **What is the Meek technique of graft expansion?**

Use of a special dermatome to achieve 1:9 mesh ratios

○   **Can excessive pressure on a skin graft cause graft failure?**

Yes, pressures exceeding 30 mmHg

○   **What nutritional supplements can be given for increasing skin graft success?**

Zinc and vitamin C

○   **What is Millard's crane principle?**

Utilizing a local or regional flap to cover an exposed area of interest temporarily in order to prepare a wound bed for future skin grafting; the flap is summarily lifted off and the graft applied to the wound.

References

Kelton PL. Skin grafts and skin substitutes. In <u>Selected Readings in Plastic Surgery</u>. Dallas, TX: Selected Readings in Plastic Surgery. Vol. 9, No. 1, 1999.

Millard DR: The crane principle for the transport of subcutaneous tissue. PRS 43:451, 1969.

FLAPS

Scott L. Hansen, MD

○ **What is a flap?**

Tissue that is either transferred or transplanted with intact circulation

○ **How are muscle flaps classified by Mathes and Nahai?**

Type I: Single vascular pedicle
Type II: Dominant vascular pedicle(s) and minor vascular pedicle(s)
Type III: Two dominant pedicles
Type IV: Segmental vascular pedicles
Type V: Dominant vascular pedicle and secondary segmental vascular pedicles

○ **What is the mnemonic for remembering one muscle of each type?**

Type I: Ten (Tensor Fascia Lata)
Type II: Graceful (gracilis)
Type III: Glutei (gluteus maximus)
Type IV: Sat (sartorius)
Type V: on Latrines (latissimus dorsi)

○ **What is the vascular supply of the sartorius muscle?**

Superficial femoral artery and vein, segmental

○ **What type of ultrasonography will most reliably image and locate vascular perforators preoperatively?**

Duplex ultrasonography

○ **What is most likely to improve the survival of the distal portion of a random pattern cutaneous flap?**

Surgical delay prior to flap elevation

○ **What is the vascular supply of the gastrocnemius muscle?**

Sural vessels

○ **The lateral arm flap is supplied by what artery?**

Posterior radial collateral artery

○ **The arterial pedicle to the radial forearm flap arises between what two muscles?**

Brachioradialis and flexor carpi radialis

○ **What are the indications of leech therapy?**

Venous congestion

○ **What method of flap monitoring is most reliable?**

Clinical observation

○ **What flap receives its motor innervation from the obturator nerve?**

Gracilis

○ **What is the dominant vascular supply of the gracilis flap?**

Ascending branch of the medial circumflex femoral artery

○ **The rectus femoris receives its blood supply from what source?**

Lateral circumflex femoral artery

○ **What organism is associated with medicinal leeches?**

Aeromonas hydrophila (gram negative rod)

○ **What artery provides the primary blood supply to a cutaneous groin flap?**

Superficial circumflex iliac artery

○ **The gluteal thigh flap is supplied by what vessel?**

Inferior gluteal artery

○ **The periosteal perforators of the peroneal artery will be found bordering what aspect of the fibula.**

Posteromedial

○ **The parascapular flap is based on what vessel?**

Circumflex scapular artery

○ **What space does this vessel traverse?**

Triangular space

○ **Which muscles comprise the borders of the triangular space?**

Triceps, teres major and teres minor

○ **Which nerve provides sensation to the lateral arm flap?**

Posterior brachial cutaneous nerve (C5-6)

○ **The venous outflow of the reverse radial forearm flap depends on what vessel?**

Radial venae comitantes

○ **The fibular flap is based on what vessel?**

Peroneal vessels

○ **The fibula and radial forearm osteocutaneous flap can provide up to what length of bone?**

25cm and 10cm, respectively

○   **What is the dominant vascular supply to the vastus lateralis muscle?**

Descending branch of the lateral femoral circumflex artery

○   **The gracilis muscle is immediately posterior to what muscle?**

Adductor longus muscle

○   **What is the *pes anserinus*?**

The confluence of the sartorius, gracilis and semitendinosus at the medial knee, in that order from superficial to deep. This is important when harvesting full length gracilis for free functional muscle transfer.

○   **Name the three subtypes of fasciocutaneous flaps according to Cormack-Lamberty.**

Type A: Multiple perforators
Type B: Solitary perforator
Type C: Segmental perforator

○   **Name the three subtypes of fasciocutaneous flaps according to Nahai-Mathes.**

Type A: Direct cutaneous perforator
Type B: Septocutaneous perforator
Type C: Musculocutaneous perforator

○   **Describe a flaps arc of rotation.**

The range of reach of the flap when transposed at its point of rotation (usually the vascular pedicle)

○   **What is the vascular supply of the temporoparietal fascia flap?**

Superficial temporal artery and vein

○   **The saphenous artery originates from what artery?**

Genicular

○   **What is the secondary vascular supply of the gracilis flap?**

Superficial femoral artery and vein (provides segmental vessels)

○   **The paramedian forehead flap is based on what vessel?**

Supratrochlear

○   **What is the source of free radicals in the ischemic flap?**

Xanthine oxidase

○   **What is the blood supply of the deltopectoral flap?**

First, second and third perforating branches of the internal mammary artery

○   **The posterior thigh flap involves transfer of what three muscles?**

Biceps femoris, semimembranosus, and semitendinosus muscles

❍ **What are the main functions of the gluteus maximus muscle?**

Extension of the hip joint and adductor of the thigh

❍ **The deep inferior epigastric artery arises from what artery?**

External iliac

❍ **What is the dominant pedicle to the latissimus dorsi muscle?**

Thoracodorsal

❍ **Where does the gluteus maximus muscle insert?**

Greater trochanter of the femur

❍ **What is the blood supply to the trapezius flap?**

Transverse cervical artery

❍ **What is an angiosome?**

Composite area of tissue supplied by the same source artery

❍ **Which gastrocnemius muscle has a longer reach?**

Medial head

❍ **What structure is at risk when transposing a lateral gastrocnemius flap?**

Peroneal nerve at the fibular head where it is subcutaneous

❍ **What is the blood supply to the soleus muscle?**

Popliteal

❍ **The radial forearm neurosensory flap is innervated by what nerve(s)?**

Lateral and medial antebrachial cutaneous nerves

❍ **The great toe flap is based on what vessel?**

First dorsal metatarsal artery and venae comitantes

❍ **What is the blood supply of the external oblique?**

Lateral cutaneous branches of the inferior eight posterior intercostal arteries

❍ **What are the muscles that define the boundaries of the quadrilateral space?**

Long head of the triceps, humerus, teres major and teres minor

❍ **What structures traverse the quadrilateral space?**

Posterior circumflex humeral vessels and axillary nerve

○ **What are the two dominant pedicles of the omental flap?**

The right and left gastroepiploic artery and vein

○ **Can the anterolateral thigh flap be neurotized?**

Yes, from the lateral femoral cutaneous nerve

○ **What is the origin and insertion of the gracilis muscle?**

The pubic symphysis and the medial tibial condyle

○ **The forehead flap is based on what vessel?**

Superficial temporal artery and vein

○ **The paramedian forehead flap is based on what vessel?**

Supratrochlear artery and vein

References

Mathes SJ, Nahai F: Reconstructive surgery: principles, anatomy & technique. Quality Medical Publishing, 1997.

Mathes SJ, Nahai F: Classification of the vascular anatomy of muscles: experimental   and clinical correlation. Plast Reconstr Surg 1981, 67, 177.

Tolhurst DE, Haeseker B, Zeeman RJ: The development of the fasciocutaneous flap and its clinical applications. Plast Reconstr Surg 1983; 71, 597.

Cormack GC, Lamberty BG: A classification of fascio-cutaneous flaps according to their patterns of vascularization. Br J Plast Surg 1984; 37, 80.

Taylor GI, Palmer JH: The vascular territories (angiosomes) of the body: experimental study and clinical applications. Br J Plast Surg 1987; 40, 113.

Mathes SJ, Nahai F: Clinical Atlas of Muscle and Musculocutaneous Flaps. St. Louis, MO, C. V. Mosby Company, 1979.

Burget GC, Menick FJ: Aesthetic Reconstruction of the Nose. S. Louis, MO. Mosby, 1994.

MICROSURGERY

Matthew M. Hanasono, MD

○ **What is the average tissue survival rate for a microvascular free flap?**

95% or better.

○ **What is the salvage rate for microvascular free flaps that require reexploration for flap ischemia?**

About 50%.

○ **What is the maximum warm ischemia time tolerated by muscle flaps?**

Less than 2 hours.

○ **What is the maximum warm ischemia time tolerated by bone flaps?**

Less than 3 hours.

○ **What is the maximum warm ischemia time tolerated by skin and fasciocutaneous flaps?**

About 4-6 hours.

○ **What is the warm ischemia time tolerated by jejunal flaps?**

Under 2 hours.

○ **How can the maximum tolerated ischemia time be increased?**

Cooling of tissues: up to 12 hours of ischemia tolerated for fasciocutaneous tissues, 8 hours for muscle, and 24 hours for bone.

○ **Which results higher flap survival rates, end-to-end or end-to-side anastomoses?**

Most studies demonstrate similar patencies.

○ **Which type of arteriotomy, slit or circular/oval, is more successful?**

Most studies demonstrate similar patencies.

○ **Under what circumstances might an end-to-side anastomosis be advantageous?**

Vessel size discrepancy (larger donor vessel), only one artery available and needed for distal organ/tissue perfusion, limited exposure/availability of similar size donor vessels.

○ **What anastomotic angles are thought to be the most desirable and result in the greatest amount of blood flow to the recipient vessel in an end-to-side anastomosis?**

Based on technical factors and blood flow rates, angles of 45 to 90° result in greater arterial flow than obtuse angles up to 135°.

❍ **What methods relieve vasospasm?**

Topical anesthetics (e.g., lidocaine), topical papaverine, dilation, adventitial stripping, sympathetic nerve block (e.g., epidural anesthesia for lower extremity reconstruction).

❍ **What is the reason for adventitial stripping?**

To relieve vasospasm and to prevent loose adventitia from being caught in the vessel lumen, a potential trigger for thrombosis.

❍ **Which method of adventitial stripping is preferred, blunt or sharp?**

Sharp adventitial stripping is associated with less vessel trauma resulting less vasospasm and improved blood flow to the flap.

❍ **What are the characteristics of a viable flap?**

Warmth, color, softness, capillary refill, and detectable pulse (e.g., Doppler).

❍ **What are signs of inadequate arterial flow?**

Pale, cool flap with slow (>2 sec) capillary refill.

❍ **What are signs of inadequate venous flow?**

Dark, congested flap with fast (<1 sec) capillary refill.

❍ **What are the most reliable methods of free flap monitoring?**

Clinical observation, Doppler ultrasound flowmetry, pulse oximetry, quantitative fluorometry, surface temperature probing.

❍ **How long before a pseudointima forms at the anastomotic site?**

About 5 days.

❍ **How long before a new intima forms at the anastomotic site?**

About 1-2 weeks.

❍ **Which has superior patency rates, coupled or hand-sewn anastomoses?**

They are similar when used appropriately.

❍ **Under what circumstances can microvascular coupling anastomotic devices generally be used?**

Coupling devices are usually used for minimally discrepant, soft, pliable venous microvascular anastomoses.

❍ **What is the maximum closing pressure of vascular clips that should be used in order to minimize damage to vessels?**

30 g/mm^2.

❍ **What are some key points when performing an anastomosis for preventing exposure of subendothelium and thereby inducing platelet aggregation?**

Use small needles, avoid repeated needle punctures, equal placement of sutures, avoid tying sutures too loose or too tight, avoid use of too many sutures, which can cause endothelial slough.

❍   **How does heparin prevent coagulation?**

Primarily by increasing the action of antithrombin-3, which inactivates thrombin. It also decreases platelet adhesion and inhibits the conversion of fibrinogen to fibrin.

❍   **How does aspirin function to prevent platelet aggregation?**

Aspirin blocks the endothelial cyclooxygenase pathway with subsequent blockage of thromboxane A2 preventing vasoconstriction and thrombus formation.

❍   **How does Dextran work to prevent clotting?**

Dextran is a volume expander that prevents platelet adhesion by increasing the negative electric charge and an inactivator of von Willebrand factor, a major contributor to platelet aggregation and adhesion to vessel wall collagen.

❍   **What are some possible complications associated with the use of low molecular weight dextran?**

Bleeding, pulmonary edema, and allergic reaction including anaphylaxis

❍   **What is the mechanism of the no-reflow phenomenon?**

Ischemia results in cellular swelling in the vascular endothelium with subsequent intravascular platelet aggregation and leakage of intravascular fluid into the interstitial space.

❍   **What pharmacologic agents can be used to rescue some free flaps in which anastomotic revision fails to restore flap perfusion or is associated with recurrent thrombosis?**

Thrombolytic agents such as streptokinase, urokinase, tissue plasminogen activator.

❍   **What is the mechanism of thrombosis in microvascular anastomosis?**

Exposure of subendothelial collagen-containing surfaces to which platelets adhere eventually leading to fibrin deposition, vasospasm, stenosis and thrombosis, causing loss of blood flow.

❍   **Why is bipolar electocautery preferable to monopolar electrocautery in the control of bleeding from or around a recipient or donor blood vessel used in microvascular free tissue transfer?**

Bipolar cautery damages tissue, including endothelium and media, over a much more limited distance (approximately 1-2 mm) compared to unipolar cautery.

❍   **Why is the number of sutures placed in an anastomosis critical?**

Too few sutures results in excessive bleeding and thrombus formation; too many results in increased damage to the endothelium and thrombus formation.

❍   **Which anastomotic technique demonstrates greater success rates, interrupted suture placement or continuous sutures?**

In experienced hands, similar success rates are observed.

❍   **Does smoking tobacco increase free flap failure rate?**

Most retrospective studies demonstrate similar (non-digital) flap survival and thrombosis rates between smokers and nonsmokers, although smokers have a higher incidence of healing complications at the flap interface and at the donor-site wound.

O   **What happens to vein grafts when they are used to bridge intraarterial gaps?**

There is ingrowth of smooth muscle cells and creation of a neo-intima that results in significant thickening of the vein wall. Also, graft length decreases by 26 to 30 percent when used as an intraarterial or intravenous graft.

O   **In addition to excellent vascular and neural anastomoses what other factor determines the success of functional free skeletal muscle transfer?**

Reestablishment of the correct resting tension since very small decreases in resting tension can markedly reduce the power and amplitude of muscle contraction.

O   **Name some commonly used donor sites for free osseous and osseocutaneous flaps.**

Rib, fibula, iliac crest, second metatarsal, radius, calvarium, scapula.

O   **In what ways are vascularized bone transfers superior to nonvascularized bone grafts?**

Vascularized bone grafts demonstrate earlier incorporation, bone hypertrophy, mechanical strength to failure, osseous mass retention, and resistance to local infection.

O   **What techniques can be used to prolong ischemia time in limb replantation?**

Cooling and AV shunting.

O   **What are the major contraindications to replantation?**

Concomitant life-threatening injury, multiple segmental injuries to the amputated part, severe crushing or avulsion of the tissues, extreme contamination, inhibiting systemic illness (small vessel disease, diabetes mellitus, etc.), prior surgery or trauma to the amputated part precluding replantation.

O   **How do leeches function to relieve venous congestion?**

By secreting hirudin, a selective thrombin inhibitor that is injected into the hosts tissue as they feed on host blood.

O   **What pathogenic bacterium do leeches commonly transmit?**

Aeromonas hydrophila.

O   **What antibiotics should be used in the prophylaxis or treatment of bacterial infections associated with the use of leeches?**

Ciprofloxacin, tetracycline, trimethoprim-sulfamethoxazole, or second- and third-generation cephalosporins.

O   **Does the order of anastomosis and microvascular clamp removal affect the survival of free flaps?**

There are no significant differences in flap survival based on order of anastomosis or microvascular clamp removal seen in an animal model, although early, transient venous congestion does develop if the artery is anastomosed first and the clamp on the artery is removed prior to venous anastomosis and clamp removal.

O   **Can loupe magnification be safely used for microvascular anastomoses?**

High power loupes have been used for anastomosing vessels greater than 1 mm in diameter with success rates comparable to those achieved using a microscope.

O **Can microvascular surgery be successfully performed in children?**

A success rate of 93% has been observed in children under age 15.

References

Shaw WW. Microvascular free flaps: The first decade. Clin Plast Surg 1983;10:3-20.

Lineaweaver WC, Buncke HI. Complications of free flap transfers. Hand Clin N Am 1986;2:347-351.

Godina M. Preferential use of end-to-side arterial anastomoses in free flap transfers. Plast Reconstr Surg 1979;64:673-682.

Zhang L, Moskovitz M, Piscatelli S, Longaker MT, Siebert JW. Hemodynamic study of different angled end-to-side anastomoses. Microsurgery 1995;16:114-117.

Zhang F, Pang Y, Buntic R et al. Effect of sequence, timing of vascular anastomosis, and clamp removal on survival of microsurgical flaps. J Reconstr Microsurg 2002;18:697-702.

Jones NF. Intraoperative and postoperative monitoring of microsurgical free tissue transfers. Clin Plast Surg. 1992;19:783-797.

Khouri RK, Shaw WW. Monitoring of free flaps with surface-temperature recordings: is it reliable? Plast Reconstr Surg 1992;89:495-499.

Ahn CY, Shaw WW, Berns S, Markowitz BL. Clinical experience with the 3M microvascular coupling anastomotic device in 100 free-tissue transfers. Plast Reconstr Surg 1994;93:1481-1484.

Wieslander JB. Endothelialization following end-to-end and end-in-end (sleeve) microarterial anastomoses: A scanning electron microscopic study. Scand J Plastic Reconstr Surg 1984;18:193-199.

Lohman R, Siemionow M, Lister G. Advantages of sharp adventitial dissection for microvascular anastomoses. Ann Plast Surg 1998;40:577-585.

Acland RD. Microvascular anastomosis: A device for holding stay sutures and a new vascular clamp. Surgery 1974;75:185-187.

Johnson PC, Barker JH. Thrombosis and antithrombotic therapy in microvascular surgery. Clin Plast Surg 1992;19:799-807.

Goldberg JA, Pederson WC, Barwick WJ. Salvage of free tissue transfers using Thrombolytic agents. J Reconstr Microsurg. 1989;55:351-356.

Seuter F. Inhibition of platelet aggregation by acetylsalicylic acid and other inhibitors. Haemostasis 1976;5:85-95.

Weinstein PR, Mehdorn HM, Szabo Z: Microsurgical anastomosis: Vessel injury, regeneration, and repair. In: Serafin D, Buncke HJ Jr, Microsurgical Composite Tissue Transplantation. St Louis, CV Mosby, 1979, Ch9, 111-144.

Rhee RY, Donayre CE, Ouriel K, Neschis DG, Shortell CK. Low dose heparin therapy: In vitro verification of antithromonbotic effect. J Vasc Surg 1991;14:628-634.

Rosenberg RD. Actions and interaction of antithrombin and heparin. N Engl J Med 1975;292:146-151.

Hood JM, Lubahn JD. Bipolar coagulation at different energy levels: effect on patency. Microsurgery 1994;15:594-597.

Cordeiro PG, Santamaria E. Experience with the continuous suture microvascular anastomosis in 200 consecutive free flaps. Ann Plast Surg 1998;40;1-6.

Chang LD, Buncke G, Slezak S, Buncke HJ. Cigarette smoking, plastic surgery, and microsurgery. J Reconstr Microsurgery 1996;12: 467-474.

Reus WF 3rd, Colen LB, Straker DJ. Tobacco smoking and complications in elective microsurgery. Plast Reconstr Surg 1992;89:490-494.

Frey M, Gruber H, Freilinger G. The importance of the correct resting tension in muscle transplantation. Experimental and clinical aspects. Plast Reconstr Surg 1983;71:510-518.

Mitchell GM, Zeeman R, Rodegers IW, Pribaz JJ, O'Brien BM. The long-term-fate of microvenous autografts. Plast Reconstr Surg 1988:82:473-479.

Weiland AJ. Bone grafts: A radiologic, histologic, and biomechanical model comparing autografts, allografts, and free vascularized bone grafts. Plast Reconstr Surg 1984;74:368-379.

Nunley A, Koman LA, Urbaniak JR. Arterial shunting as an adjunct to major limb revascularization. Ann Surg 1981;193:271-273.

Wilson CS, Albert BS, Buncke HJ, Gordon L. Replantation of the upper extremity. Clin Plast Surg 1983;10:85-101.

Valauri FA. The use of medicinal leeches in microsurgery. Blood Coagul Fibrinolysis 1991;2:185-187.

Braga A, Lineaweaver WC, Whitney TM, Follansbee S, Buncke HJ. Sensitivities of Aeromonas hydrophila cultured from medicinal leeches to oral antibiotics. J Reconstr Microsurg 1990;56:135-137.

Shenaq SM, Klebuc MJ, Vargo D. Free-tissue transfer with the aid of loupe magnification: Experience with 251 procedures. Plast Reconstr Surg 1995;95:261-269.

Devaraj VS, Kay SP, Batchelor AG, Yates A. Microvascular surgery in children. Br J Plast Surg 1991;44:276-280.

PERFORATOR FLAPS

Ming-Huei Cheng, MD, and Betul Gozel Ulusal, MD

❍ **What is the definition of a "cutaneous perforator vessel"?**

Any vessel that perforates the outer layer of the deep fascia to supply the overlying subcutaneous fat and the skin.

❍ **Where do cutaneous perforator vessels derive from?**

They derive from "source" or "segmental" vessels that usually course parallel to the bony skeleton.

❍ **How are the cutaneous vessels defined according to their course?**

They are defined as septocutaneous and myocutaneous vessels. Septocutaneous vessels course either between the tendons or muscles following the intermuscular septa. Myocutaneous perforators penetrates the muscle to follow the intramuscular septa.

❍ **What is the arterial source of a perforator flap?**

Either septocutaneous or musculocutaneous vessels.

❍ **What is an angiosome?**

The angiosomes of the body are distinct vascular territories that are composed of muscle and the overlying skin and the adipose tissue. The angiosomes define the anatomical borders from which tissues are available for composite transfer.

❍ **What is the anatomical basis for perforator based skin flap design and harvest?**

The size, length, direction, and connections of the cutaneous perforators provide basis of flap design. At least one adjacent anatomical cutaneous vascular territory can be captured with safety when based on a particular perforator.

❍ **What is the contribution of Taylor and Daniel to the evolution of the perforator flap surgery?**

These authors were the first who attempted to harvest skin flaps on the septocutaneous and myocutaneous perforators that they had identified during their vascular anatomy studies on cadavers.

❍ **What is a true perforator flap?**

A "true" perforator flap relies on perforator vessels from a given source vessel that must first penetrate a muscle before piercing the deep fascia to reach the skin.

❍ **What are the advantages of the perforator flaps?**

1) Less donor site morbidity 2) muscle sparing 3) versatility in design to include as little or as much tissue as required and 4) improved postoperative recovery of the patient.

❍ **What is the definition of a reliable perforator vessel?**

The reliable perforator is defined as a perforator that sprouts from the carrier muscle with a "visible" pulsation. A reliable perforator is believed to have the ability to expand its perfusion over its territory after the perforator flap elevation.

○   **How are the perforator vessels identified?**

Currently, the most practical, simple, safe, speedy and inexpensive method is use of handheld doppler ultrasound probe. Other techniques include magnetic resonance imaging, thermography, and color-flow duplex scanning.

○   **How are the axial artery and perforators discriminated with the doppler probe?**

The axial artery has a unidirectional pulsating course whereas there is no evident pulsating sound around the perforator.

○   **What is the most common consequence when a tiny perforator is selected?**

Marginal flap necrosis beyond the territory of the perforator.

○   **What are the requirements for an acceptable perforator flap donor site?**

a) Predictable and consistent blood supply b) at least one large perforator (diameter >= 0.5 mm) c) sufficient pedicle length for the procedure and d) primary closure of the donor site with the absence of excessive wound tension.

○   **What are the most commonly used perforator flaps?**

Anterolateral thigh perforator flap, deep inferior epigastric perforator flap, superior gluteal artery perforator flap, inferior gluteal artery perforator flap, thoracodorsal perforator flap, tensor fascia lata perforator flap, medial plantar perforator flap, and deep circumflex iliac perforator flap.

○   **What is a free style free flap?**

An anatomic region with the appropriate texture, color, and pliability is selected, and using a Doppler probe, the skin vessels in that region are mapped. Mapped perforators are dissected towards source vessels to provide adequate vessel length and size.

○   **What is the main advantage of free style free flap?**

The advantage of this concept is that it allows the surgeon an extra sense of freedom and variability when approaching a flap harvest and when choosing the recipient site.

○   **What are the most common causes of the perforator thrombosis?**

Stretching, twisting, drying and compression of the perforator.

○   **What are the strategies to reexplore a thrombosed perforator flap?**

a) Explore early b) open the vessels and squeeze the flap to evacuate the thrombi c) do not inject any solution from the cut end since this maneuver may cause migration and plugging of thrombi into the small perforator and kill the flap d) Relieve the tension from the flap f) use PGE-1 if available.

○   **What are the principles in "thinning" of a perforator flap?**

a) preserve the fat and the fascia within a circle of 1 cm diameter around the perforator b) use loupes or microscope to perform the procedure c) perform thinning when there is circulation in the flap, either before division of pedicle or after restoration of blood circulation.

○   **What is "supermicrosurgery" technique?**

Supermicrosurgery technique involves division of the perforator flap pedicle above the deep fascia and anastomosing small vessels that are less than 1mm (0.5-0.7 mm).

O   **What are the advantages in applying supermicrosurgery technique in perforator flap surgery?**

The donor site morbidity is reduced since the fascia remains intact and the muscle is not dissected.

O   **What are the disadvantages to apply supermicrosurgery technique in perforator flap surgery?**

The primary disadvantage is the short and small pedicle rendering the inset and the anastomosis difficult.

O   **List the perforator flaps and their accompanying nerves that can be harvested as a sensate flap.**

Thoracodorsal perforator flap - lateral branch of the intercostal nerve
Medial plantar artery perforator flap - medial plantar nerve
Anterolateral thigh flap - lateral musculocutaneous nerve
Deep inferior epigastric perforator flap - sensory branch of the intercostal nerve
Superior gluteal artery perforator flap - superior and middle cluneal nerve

O   **Who first described anterolateral thigh perforator flap?**

Song et al. described it as a septocutaneous perforator flap in 1984.

O   **What is the source artery of the ALT perforator flap?**

Septocutaneous or musculocutaneous perforators derived from the lateral circumflex femoral system.

O   **What is the landmark for the perforators in the thigh region?**

A line is drawn from anterior superior iliac spine to the lateral border of the patella and the perforators are usually located in a circle 3 cm around the midpoint of this line.

O   **What is the ratio of septocutaneous vessels / myocutaneous perforators in the anterolateral thigh perforator flap?**

In different series, only 12% - 33% of the patients were reported to have septocutaneous vessels while 67% - 88% have myocutaneous perforators.

O   **What can be the maximum dimensions of an anterolateral thigh perforator flap?**

The maximum dimension of the nonthinned anterolateral thigh flap can be up to 25 × 18 cm.

O   **What can be the range of the pedicle length of an anterolateral thigh perforator flap?**

8-20 cm

O   **What are the advantages of thinning anterolateral thigh perforator flaps?**

a) Uniformly thin and pliable flaps become available especially for reconstruction of oral cavity, neck, hand and fingers, axilla, forearm and anterior tibial area b) avoids secondary defatting procedures c) improved sensory recovery d) early range of motion training when used in hands and fingers.

O   **What is the upper width limit of the anterolateral thigh flap that can be usually closed primarily?**

Although the laxity is important for this issue, generally up to 8 cm defect can be closed primarily.

O   **What are the variations in the anatomy of the anterolateral thigh flap?**

Variations occur in 2% of the cases. a) absence of any perforator to the skin b) small perforator c) perforator pedicle that contains an artery but no vein d) artery not going with the vein side by side.

O   **What is the technical management when anatomical variations are encountered during elevation of anterolateral thigh flap?**

a) try to dissect a perforator from the transverse branch in the upper thigh b) use an anteromedial thigh flap c) shift to the opposite thigh.

O   **What are the main application areas of the anterolateral thigh flap?**

Head and neck reconstruction, esophagus reconstruction, chest emphyema with bronchocutaenous fistula, abdominal wall reconstruction, upper and lower extremity reconstruction.

O   **How is the decision made if an anterolateral thigh perforator flap should be used pedicled or as a free flap in abdominal wall reconstruction?**

This depends on the location of the defect and length of the pedicle. The flap is raised first without division of the pedicle. If simple transposition is enough, microvascular anastomosis can be saved. If not, the recipient vessels should be explored.

O   **What are the advantages of using ALT flap in head and neck reconstruction?**

a) Long pedicle (12.01 ± 1.50 cm) with sufficient diameter (2.0 to 2.5 mm) b) pliable and wide flap c) allows for two team approach d) feasibility to design as either a single skin paddle for one-layer defect reconstruction or double-skin paddles for through-and-through defects e) Moderate flap thickness f) possibility for thinning g) possibility to harvest as a chimeric flap or composite flap along with the neighboring tissues h) potentially sensate by including the lateral femoral cutaneous nerve i) inconspicuous scar over the donor thigh.

O   **What are the contraindications of the anterolateral thigh flap?**

The absolute contraindications are severe atherosclerosis, previous injury or incision in the thigh region and infection in the recipient site (myocutaneous flap is preferred) and a relative contraindication is obesity.

O   **Describe the thigh flaps according to their source artery.**

Anterolateral thigh flap - descending branch of the lateral femoral circumflex artery (LFCA)
Medial thigh flap - a branch from the LFCA or descending branch of LFCA
Proximal 2/3 of lateral thigh skin - transverse branch of the LFCA
Skin at medial thigh - medial femoral circumflex artery
Skin at posterolateral thigh - third or fourth perforator from the deep femoral artery
Inferior gluteal thigh flap - inferior gluteal artery
Posterior popliteal thigh flap - a branch of the popliteal artery

O   **Compare the tensor fascia lata perforator flap and anterolateral thigh flap.**

The most remarkable difference is the anatomy of the vessels. The descending branch of the lateral femoral circumflex artery which supplies the anterolateral thigh flap runs longitudinally in the intermuscular septum between the rectus femoris and vastus lateralis muscle whereas the transverse or ascending branch of the TFL flap runs laterally. Tensor fascia lata flap has a shorter and a narrower diameter, the skin is thicker but the scar is hidden better when compared to the anterolateral thigh flap.

O   **Which perforator flaps are available for breast reconstruction?**

Deep inferior epigastric perforator (DIEP) flap, thoracodorsal artery perforator (TAP) flap, gluteal artery perforator flap, anterolateral thigh perforator flap.

○ **What is the blood supply of DIEP flap?**

Indirect perforating vessels originating from the deep inferior epigastric artery.

○ **What are the advantages of DIEP flap over TRAM flap?**

The rectus abdominis muscle and fascia is preserved in DIEP flap and therefore is associated with less donor site morbidity and shorter recovery period.

○ **What are the contraindications for the DIEP flap?**

Abdominal scar, previous abdominal operations, caeserean delivery, obesity

○ **What are the most significant risk factors of fat necrosis in the DIEP flap?**

Radiotherapy and smoking.

○ **What are risk factors for flap failure in DIEP flap?**

Tobacco use, small sized perforator, venous congestion in zone 3 and 4.

○ **What are the indications for bilateral breast reconstruction with DIEP flap?**

a) bilateral prophylactic mastectomy b) therapeutic and contralateral prophylactic mastectomy c) after explantation of bilateral implant failures.

○ **Which vein is considered as a "lifeboat" and spared during the harvest of DIEP flap?**

The superficial inferior epigastric vein.

○ **What are alternative perforator flaps for breast reconstruction if abdominal tissue is not available?**

Anterolateral thigh perforator flap, thoracodorsal perforator flap and superior gluteal artery flap.

○ **What is the main indication of the pedicled superior gluteal artery perforator (SGAP) flap?**

Since the SGAP flap has a thick subcutaneous layer and as a pedicled flap, it is an excellent tool to cover large sacral midline defects and gluteal defects and successfuly fills the dead space.

○ **What are the disadvantages of the traditional gluteus maximus myocutaneous flap?**

The exposure of the donor vessels is difficult, the vascular pedicle is short, the flap dissection is challenging and may result in injury to the adjacent sciatic nerve. In addition, partial resection of the gluteus maximus muscle can eventually result in weakness of muscle function in abduction and extension of the thigh.

○ **What are the advantages of SGAP flap over gluteus maximus flap?**

In SGAP flap, the anatomical and functional integrity of the muscle is preserved therefore exposure of any nerves or bony eminences is avoided, postoperative pain is decreased and hospitalization period is shortened. In addition, it provides a better intraoperative exposure and a longer vascular pedicle, the scar is well hidden and contour deformities are minimized.

○ **What are the preferred recipient vessels in breast reconstruction with SGAP flap?**

The axillary vessels should not be used for SGAP breast reconstruction. Pedicle length is often insufficient. The preferred recipient vessels are either the perforators of the internal mammary vessels at the second or third intercostal space or the internal mammary vessels themselves at the third or fourth intercostal junction.

O   **Who first described the use of SGAP flap in breast reconstruction?**

In 1995, Allen and Tucker first reported the use of the SGAP flap in breast reconstruction.

O   **What are the indications of SGAP flap in breast reconstruction?**

SGAP flap can be used for total and partial breast reconstruction and is indicated in patients who have an asthenic body habitus or excessive abdominal scarring.

O   **Who first described the thoracodorsal artery perforator flap?**

Angrigiani et al. in 1995.

O   **What are the various compositions of the thoracodorsal artery perforator flap?**

Dermoadiposal flap, a composite or chimeric pattern including bone or regional muscle flap or a flow-through pattern flap.

O   **What are the advantages of the thoracodorsal artery perforator flap over scapular and parascapular flaps?**

Thoracodorsal artery perforator flap has a longer pedicle, can have variable compositions and a thinner dermis and subcutaneous tissue.

O   **What are the application areas of the thoracodorsal perforator flap?**

Because the thoracodorsal perforator flap is a large and thin flap without hair, it can be used effectively for resurfacing the skin and soft tissue defect over the hand or thumb, pretibia, and foot, as well as defects after release of burn scar contracture, resection of malignant skin lesions or radiation ulcers.

O   **What are the advantages the thoracodorsal perforator flap?**

Large flap size, well-hidden donor scar, long pedicle and variable composition.

O   **What are the and disadvantages of the thoracodorsal perforator flap?**

Unreliable anatomy and the extended operation time.

O   **Describe the anatomic location of the deep circumflex iliac perforator (DCIP) artery.**

The perforator is usually 1 cm to 2 cm above the iliac crest and 5 cm posterior to the anterior superior iliac crest.

O   **How is the skin paddle designed?**

The skin paddle is designed over the perforator as its central long axis along the upper border of the anterior part of the iliac crest.

O   **What are the advantages of deep circumflex iliac perforator (DCIP) flap over standard iliac crest osseocutaneous flap?**

a) easier contouring b) eliminates the need for secondary debulking procedure c) minimal sacrifice of the abdominal muscles and reduced the donor site morbidity.

○ **Describe the anatomic location of the medial plantar perforator vessels.**

The medial plantar system emerges through the septum between the abductor hallucis muscle and the flexor digitorum brevis and sends several perforators through this intermuscular septum into the medial plantar skin.

○ **What are the main application areas of medial perforator flap?**

This flap provides thick, glabrous skin and is especially suitable for the repair of a finger pulp, flexor surfaces of the digits, palm or foot plantar defects.

○ **Propose a perforator-based free flap for one stage repair of an ischemic finger with pulp defect.**

Medial plantar perforator free flap.

○ **What are the advantages of the medial plantar perforator flap?**

a) minimum donor site morbidity c) possibility of primary defatting d) availability of two venous drainage systems (concomitant and cutaneous venous systems) e) good color and texture match with the finger skin f) concealed location of the donor site g) ease in elevation.

○ **What is a chimeric flap?**

A chimeric flap has separate components with separate vascular supplies that are attached to a common source vessel.

○ **What is a perforator based chimeric flap?**

Skin paddles can be elevated based on at least two perforators from different vascular systems and separated into two skin paddles with at least one cutaneous perforator per each.

○ **What are the advantages of using a chimeric flap?**

Easy three dimensional insetting, acceptable aesthetic appearance, reduced donor-site morbidity, design with the least effort and operation time, one pair of recipient vessels.

○ **What are the disadvantages of using a chimeric flap?**

The disadvantages are the variations of perforators, the requirement of a learning curve, easy twisting of perforators and / or pedicle and sometimes the need for a second venous drainage or shifting to double flaps.

○ **Which flaps are available to harvest chimeric flaps?**

Anterolateral thigh and thoracodorsal perforator flaps.

○ **Propose a flap for one stage reconstruction of wide and through and through cheek defect involving the commissure.**

Anterolateral thigh chimeric flap.

References

Ahn CY, Narayanan K, Shaw WW. In vivo anatomic study of cutaneous perforators in free flaps using magnetic resonance imaging. J Reconstr Microsurg. 1994; 10: 157–163.

Allen RJ, Treece P. Deep inferior epigastric perforator flap for breast reconstruction. Ann Plast Surg. 1994; 32:32-8.

Allen RJ, Tucker Jr.C. Superior gluteal artery perforator free flap for breast reconstruction. Plast Reconstr Surg. 1995; 95:1207-12.

Angrigiani C, Grili D, Siebert J. Latissimus dorsi musculocutaneous flap without muscle. Plast Reconstr Surg 1995; 96:1608-14.

Blondeel PhN. The sensate free superior gluteal artery perforator flap: a valuable alternative in autogenous breast reconstruction. Br J Plast Surg. 1999; 52:185-93.

Blondeel P, Landuyt VK, Hamdi M, et al. Soft tissue reconstruction with the superior gluteal artery perforator flap. Clin Plastic Surg. 2003; 30: 371-382.

Blondeel PN. One hundred free DIEP flap breast reconstructions: a personal experience. Br J Plast Surg. 1999; 52(2):104-11.

Callegari PR, Taylor GI, Caddy CM, et al. An anatomic review of the delay phenomenon: I experiment studies. Plast Reconstr Surg. 1992; 89:397-407.

Chijiwa T, Arai K, Miyazaki N, et al. Making of a facial perforator map by thermography. Ann Plast Surg. 2000; 44: 596–600.

Celik N, Wei FC. Technical tips in perforator flap harvest. Clin Plastic Surg. 2003; 30: 469-472.

Celik N, Wei FC, Lin CH, et al. Technique and strategy in anterolateral thigh perforator flap surgery, based on an analysis of 15 complete and partial failures in 439 cases. Plast Reconstr Surg. 1998; 101: 72-84.

Chen HC, Tang YB. Anterolateral thigh flap: an ideal soft tissue flap. Clin Plastic Surg. 2003; 30: 383-401.

Geddes CR, Morris SF, Neligan PC. Perforator flaps: evolution, classification, and applications. Ann Plast Surg. 2003; 50:90-9. Review.

Gedebou TM, Wei FC, Lin CH. Clinical experience of 1284 free anterolateral thigh flaps. Handchir Mikrochir Plast Chir. 2002; 34:239-44.

Gill PS, Hunt JP, Guerra AB, et al. A 10-year retrospective review of 758 DIEP flaps for breast reconstruction. Plast Reconstr Surg. 2004;113:1153-60.

Guerra AB, Metzinger SE, Lund KM, et al.The thoracodorsal artery perforator flap: clinical experience and anatomic study with emphasis on harvest techniques. Plast Reconstr Surg. 2004; 114:32-41.

Guerra AB, Metzinger SE, Bidros RS, et al. Bilateral breast reconstruction with the deep inferior epigastric perforator (DIEP) flap: an experience with 280 flaps. Ann Plast Surg. 2004; 52: 246-52.

Guerra AB, Soueid N, Metzinger SE, et al. Simultaneous bilateral breast reconstruction with superior gluteal artery perforator (SGAP) flaps.Ann Plast Surg. 2004; 53:305-10.

Hallock GG. Doppler sonography and color duplex imaging for planning a perforator flap. Clin Plastic Surg. 2003; 30: 347-357.

Hallock GG. Simultaneous transposition of anterior thigh muscle and fascia flaps:an introduction to the chimera flap principle. Ann Plast Surg. 1991; 27:126-31.

Hamdi M, Blondeel P, Van Landuyt K, et al. Bilateral autogenous breast reconstruction using perforator free flaps: a single center's experience. Plast Reconstr Surg. 2004;114:83-9.

Huang WC, Chen HC, Wei FC, et al. Chimeric flap in clinical use. Clin Plastic Surg. 2003; 30: 457-467.

Inoue T, Kobayashi M, Harashina T. Finger pulp reconstruction with a free sensory medial plantar flap. Br J Plast Reconstr Surg. 1988; 41:657-9.

Ishida LH, Busnardo FF, Montag E, et al. Thoracodorsal artery perforator flap and scapular flap: comparative anatomic study (abstract). Plastic Surgical Forum of the 69th annual scientific meeting of the American Society of Plastic Surgeons. Los Angeles: 2000. p. 48-9.

JT Kim. Latissimus dorsi perforator flap. Clin Plast Surg. 2003; 30: 403-431.

Kaplan JL, Allen RJ, Guerra A, et al. Anterolateral thigh flap for breast reconstruction: review of the literature and case reports. J Reconstr Microsurg. 2003; 19:63-8.

Kimata Y. Deep circumflex iliac perforator flap. Clin Plast Surg 2003; 30: 433-438.

Kimata Y, Uchiyama K, Ebihara S et al. Versatility of the free anterolateral thigh flap for reconstruction of head and neck defects. Arch Otolaryngol Head Neck Surg. 1997; 123:1325-31.

Kimura N, Satoh K, Hasumi T, et al. Clinical application of the free thin Anterolateral thigh flap in 31 consecutive patients. Plast Reconstr Surg. 2001;108:1197-1208.

Kimura N, Satoh K, Hosaka Y. Tensor fascia latae perforator flap. Clin Plastic Surg. 2003; 30: 439-446.

Koshima I, Nanba Y, Tustsui T, et al. Medial perforator flaps with microsurgery. Clin Plastic Surg. 2003; 30: 447-455.

Koshima I, Sashio H, Kawada S, et al. Flow-through thin latissimus dorsi perforator flap for repair of soft tissue defects in the legs. Plast Reconstr Surg. 1999;103: 1483-90.

Koshima I, Fukuda H, Yamamoto H, et al. Free anterolateral thigh flaps for   reconstruction of head and neck defects. Plast. Reconstr. Surg. 1993; 92: 421-8.

Koshima I, Moriguchi T, Soeda S, et al. Gluteal perforator-bases flap for repair of sacral pressure sores. Plast Reconstr Surg 1993; 91(4):678-83.

Kroll SS, Sharma S, Koutz C, et al. Postoperative morphine requirements of free TRAM and DIEP flaps. Plast Reconstr Surg. 2001; 107:338-41.

Kroll SS, Schusterman MA, Reece GP, et al. Abdominal wall strength, bulging, and hernia after TRAM flap breast reconstruction. Plast Reconstr Surg 1995; 96: 616-9.

Lee HB, Tark KC, Rah DK, et al. Pulp reconstruction of fingers with very small senate medial plantar free flap. Plast Reconstr Surg. 1998; 101:999-1005.

Morris SF, Taylor GI. Predicting the survival of experimental skin flaps based on a knowledge of the vascular architecture. Plast Reconstr Surg. 1993; 92:1352-71.

Rand RP, Cramer MM, Strandness Jr DE. Color-flow duplex scanning in the preoperative assessment of TRAM flap perforators: a report of 32 consecutive patients.
Plast Reconstr Surg. 1994; 93: 453–459.

Rowsell AR, Eisenberg N, Davies DM, et al. The anatomy of the thoracodorsal artery within the latissimus dorsi muscle. Br J Plast Surg 1986; 39: 206-9.

Safak T, Klebuc MJA, Mavili E, et al. A new design of the iliac crest microsurgical free flap without including the "obligatory" muscle cuff. Plast Reconstr Surg. 1997; 64:595-604.

Shieh SJ, Chiu HY, Yu JC. Free anterolateral thigh flap for reconstruction of head and neck defects following cancer ablation. Plast Reconstr Surg. 2000; 105:2349-57

Song YG. Chen GZ, Song YL. The free thigh flap: a new flap concept based on the septocutaneous artery. Br J Plast Surg. 1984: 37: 149-59.

Taylor GI, Palmer JH. The vascular territories (angiosomes) of the body: experimental study and clinical applications. Br J Plast Surg. 1987; 40:113-41.

Taylor GI, Daniel RK. The anatomy of several free flap donor sites. Plast Reconstr Surg. 2002; 55:83-5.

Taylor IG. The angiosomes of the body and their supply to perforator flaps. Clin Plastic Surg 2003; 30: 331-342.

Taylor IG, Townsend P, Corlett R. Superiority of deep circumflex iliac vessels as the supply for free groin flaps: clinical work. Plast Reconstr Surg. 1997; 100: 1703-9.

Verpaele AM, Blondeel PN, Van Landuyt K, et al. The superior gluteal artery perforator flap: an additional tool in the treatment of pressure sores. Br J Plast Surg. 1999; 52:385-91.

Wei FC, Jain V, Celik N, et al. Have we found an ideal soft tissue flap? An Experience with 672 anterolateral thigh flaps. Plast Reconstr Surg. 2002; 109: 2219-26.

Wei FC, Jain V, Suominen S, et al.Confusion among perforator flaps: what is a true perforator flap? Plast Reconstr Surg. 2001; 107: 874–876.

Wei FC, Mardini S. Free-style free flaps. Plast Reconstr Surg. 2004;114: 910-6.

Zetterman E, Salmi A, Suominen S, et al. Effect of cooling and warming on thermographic imaging of the perforating vessels of the abdomen. Eur J Plast Surg 1999; 22: 58–61.

BURN CARE

Nicole L. Nemeth, MD

○ **What is the first step in management of a burn victim?**

Primary Survey—maintain airway patency, breathing, circulation
Secondary Survey—identify associated life-threatening injuries and remove burned clothing and jewelry

○ **What are the ABA criteria for transfer to a specialized burn center?**

1. Partial thickness burns involving greater than 10% total body surface area (TBSA)
2. Burns that involve the face, hands, feet, genitalia, perineum or major joints
3. Third degree burns in any age group
4. Electrical burns, including lightening injury
5. Chemical burns
6. Inhalation injury
7. Burn injury in patients with preexisting medical disorders that could complicate management
8. Any patients with traumatic injury in which the burn injury poses the greatest risk of morbidity or mortality
9. Any burned children if the hospital initially receiving the patient does not have qualified personnel or equipment for children
10. Any patient with burns that require special social, emotional, or long-term rehabilitative intervention

○ **What methods are used to estimate burn size?**

Lund and Brower chart—most accurate, accounts for body proportions by age group

Wallace's 'Rule of Nines'—head and neck (9%), anterior torso, (18%), posterior torso (18%), each upper extremity (9%), each lower extremity (18%), perineum (1%).

'Patient's Palm' method—the patient's palm is roughly equivalent to 1% of the TBSA

○ **When should fluid resuscitation begin in a burn victim?**

Fluid resuscitation should begin immediately. Resuscitation for burns > 20% TBSA in an adult is based on the Parkland formula.

○ **What is the Parkland formula?**

4cc X weight (kg) X %TBSA = Total volume of Lactated Ringer's (LR) to be given over the first 24 hours.

○ **At what rate should fluid resuscitation begin for a 70 kg man with a 40% TBSA second- and third-degree flame burn, now 3 hours post-injury?**

4cc X 70kg X 40% = 11200cc of LR over first 24 hours

½ of volume is given over the first 8 hours; the remainder is given over the next 16 hours

11200 ÷ 2 = 5600cc needed within the first 8 hours

5600 ÷ 5 = **1120cc/hr**

❍ **How are the resuscitation requirements determined for children?**

Based on body surface area;

Galveston Shriner's Burns Institute formula: $5000cc/m^2$/BSA burn + $2000cc/m^2$/ Total BSA = total LR for 1st 24 hours

❍ **What is the single best monitor of fluid resuscitation?**

Urine output (0.5cc/kg/hr for adults; 1.0cc/kg/hr for children)

❍ **By what percent does inhalation injury increase fluid resuscitation requirements?**

40 – 75% (~2cc/kg/%TBSA)

❍ **What is the fluid regimen for patients with myoglobinuria or hemoglobinuria?**

Discontinue Lactated Ringer's and begin Normal saline with sodium bicarbonate

❍ **What osmotic diuretic may be added to assist in clearing the urine of these pigments?**

Mannitol

❍ **Which burn patients should receive tetanus immunization?**

>10% TBSA burn injury should receive 0.5cc of tetanus toxoid; if unknown immunization history or >10 years since last booster, add 250 units of immunoglobulin

❍ **What are the depth classifications of burn injury?**

1st Degree—involves epidermis only

2nd Degree—involves partial thickness of dermis

3rd Degree—involves full thickness of dermis and all adnexal structures

4th Degree—involves underlying muscle, bone, or tendon

❍ **In what order do different sensory modalities return in a healed burn wound?**

Pain (first), light touch, temperature, vibration (last)

❍ **What are the 3 histologic zones of burn injury?**

Zone of necrosis—area of tissue necrosis due to destruction from burn injury

Zone of ischemia—surrounds zones of necrosis; can convert to zone of necrosis due to inadequate tissue perfusion

Zone of hyperemia—surrounds zone of ischemia; usually reversible injury

❍ **When should escharotomies be performed?**

For deep, circumferential extremity burns with decreased or absent pulses or deep burns involving the torso that impair ventilation

❍ **How should escharotomy incisions be planned?**

Release of eschar should occur immediately at the bedside using a Bovie electrocautery

Midaxial incisions release eschar of extremities

Axial incisions along the flanks that connect across the midline release the chest / torso

Unilateral midaxial incisions on the digits on the radial surface of the small finger and thumb; escharotomy incisions on the index, long, and ring finger generally should be placed on the ulnar surface

❍ **What is the cardiovascular response to a burn injury?**

Cardiac output (C.O.) initially decreases and systemic vascular resistance (SVR) increases

After the first 24 to 48 hours, the heart rate and CO increase and SVR decreases

❍ **How are red blood cells affected by burn injury?**

Their $T_{1/2}$ is shortened

❍ **What are some causes of early renal insufficiency in burned patients?**

Hypovolemia, vasoconstriction due to catecholamine release, myoglobinuria, nephrotoxic medications

❍ **Which muscle relaxant should be avoided in burned patients?**

Succinylcholine—causes marked hyperkalemia

❍ **What is the immunologic response to thermal injury?**

Decreased levels of lymphocytes, macrophages, immunoglobulins, and lysosomal enzymes

❍ **What is the hypermetabolic response?**

After an early "ebb" phase, a more prolonged period of protein catabolism, lipolysis, tachycardia, increased urinary output, increased oxygen consumption, nitrogen loss, and elevated body temperature ensues

❍ **What are the hormonal manifestations of the hypermetabolic response?**

Increased levels of cortisol, catecholamines, and glucagons; there is an overall increase in the blood glucose level

❍ **What are signs and symptoms of inhalation injury?**

Facial burns, singed nasal hairs, carbonaceous sputum, hypoxemia with or without an elevated carbon monoxide level, hoarseness, stridor

❍ **What is an accurate and practical test for diagnosing an inhalation injury?**

Fiberoptic bronchoscopy

O   **How may parenchymal thermal lung injury be detected?**

^{133}Xenon lung scan

O   **What is the T$_{1/2}$ of carbon monoxide at room air and on 100% oxygen?**

~ 4 hours on room air, ~45 minutes on 100% oxygen (at sea level)

O   **What is the initial treatment of suspected inhalation injury?**

100% oxygen via face mask or nasal cannula

O   **What is a low-voltage versus a high-voltage electrical exposure?**

Low-voltage— < 1000 Volts, mostly cutaneous manifestations of burn injury

High-voltage— > 1000 Volts, extent of injury usually involves deeper structures (based on resistance of different tissues to passage of current)

O   **How does a lightning injury differ from a high-voltage electrical accident?**

Lightning injuries result in a "flashover" and do not tend to cause devastating internal thermal injuries

O   **What is the most common cause of death in a lightning victim?**

Cardiopulmonary arrest

O   **Which tissue has the greatest amount of resistance and therefore produces the most heat?**

Bone

O   **Which tissues have the least resistance to electrical current?**

Nerves, blood vessels, muscle

O   **What are emergent management considerations for electrical injury?**

Evaluate for associated injuries, including cervical spine or extremity fractures, pneumothorax, neurologic changes, cardiac arrhythmias

Escharotomy or fasciotomy alone or in combination (for compartment syndrome) and nerve decompression (ex: release of Carpal tunnel, Guyon's canal) may also be warranted emergently

O   **What are long-term management considerations for a patient with an electrical injury?**

Debridement of all non-viable tissue, especially muscle; involved extremities may require amputation

Cataracts may present with a slow and progressive onset years after the injury

O   **What are the first steps in management of a chemical burn?**

Disrobe patient, early irrigation of affected area with copious amounts of plain water, identify offending agent, identify and treat systemic toxicity

○ **Why should a chemical burn NOT be treated with a neutralizing agent?**

The heat generated can induce a thermal injury

○ **Which causes a deeper burn: acids or alkalis?**

Alkalis

○ **What are some commonly encountered alkali agents?**

Lime, Bleach, Sodium hydroxide, Potassium hydroxide (usually agents found in household cleaning products)

○ **What are the mechanisms by which alkali chemicals induce tissue injury?**

1) Fat saponification
2) Water extraction from cells
3) Formation of hydroxide ion-containing alkaline proteinates, leading to deeper tissue penetration

○ **What are examples of some commonly encountered acidic agents?**

Acetic acid, Hydrochloric acid, Hydrofluoric acid, Trichloroacetic acid

○ **By what mechanisms do acid chemicals induce tissue injury?**

Hydrolysis of proteins, generation of heat in contact with skin

○ **How does hydrofluoric acid differ in its mechanism of injury?**

Free fluoride ions complex with bivalent cations (Ca^{++}, Mg^{++}), forming insoluble salts, and depleting the available Ca^{++} and Mg^{++} in circulation

○ **What can be applied topically to chelate fluoride ions and reduce pain?**

2.5% Calcium gluconate in a water-soluble gel

○ **If pain relief is refractory to topical calcium gluconate, what is the next step in management?**

Subcutaneous injection of 10% calcium gluconate

○ **How are phosphorous and phosphoric acid similar to hydrofluoric acid?**

They bind calcium ions

○ **What can be applied topically to impede oxidation and burn injury from phosphorous compounds?**

0.5% copper sulfate solution—upon contact, copper sulfate forms a black film which delineates the area of phosphorus injury

○ **What is the basic tenet of surgical treatment for burn wounds?**

Wounds that will not heal within two weeks should be excised and skin grafted

○   **Which wounds tend to require excision and autografting?**

Deep partial-thickness and full thickness burn wounds

○   **What is the 'overlay' grafting method?**

The use of widely expanded (4:1 meshed) split-thickness autograft with a meshed, unexpanded homograft overlay (used for patients with large burns and minimal donor sites)

○   **What is the most common side effect of silver sulfadiazine (Silvadene)?**

Transient leukopenia

○   **What is the most common side effect of mafenide (Sulfamylon)?**

Carbonic anhydrase inhibition / hyperchloremic metabolic acidosis

○   **What are the side effects of Silver nitrate solution?**

Electrolyte leaching, methemoglobinemia, silver discoloration of tissues

○   **What is Acticoat?**

Antimicrobial silver-coated barrier dressing

○   **What is Biobrane?**

Knitted nylon mesh bonded to a thin silicone membrane with a porcine collagen matrix

○   **How do TransCyte compare to Biobrane?**

Both are temporary skin replacement products—TransCyte has a polymer membrane with newborn human fibroblasts cultured onto a porcine collagen nylon mesh

○   **What is Integra?**

Bilaminate membrane—outer silicone layer and inner dermal layer made up of bovine Type I collagen that is cross-linked with shark glycosaminoglycans and chondroitin-6-sulfate

○   **What are some advantages and disadvantages of using Integra for wound closure or contracture release?**

The disadvantages are the need for a 2ⁿᵈ surgery to remove the outer silicone layer, the risk of collecting fluid under the Integra and infection

The advantage is the creation of a "neodermis" and the ability to take a very thin (~0.005 inch) split-thickness skin graft

○   **When should the outer silicone layer be removed?**

~ 21 days

○ **How does Alloderm differ from Allograft?**

Alloderm is chemically treated cadaver skin which incorporates as a neodermis and can also be grafted with a much thinner skin graft

Allograft is cadaveric homograft

○ **What is CEA?**

Cultured epithelial autograft—keratinocytes cultured in a laboratory setting over 3 to 4 weeks from a single punch biopsy of patient's normal skin

Utilized for near total 100% TBSA burns that require excision and grafting

○ **How is a skin graft perfused within the first 24 – 48 hours?**

By plasmatic imbibition; the graft becomes vascularized by inosculation over a period of 3 to 4 days

○ **In what order do skin grafts undergo increasing amounts of primary contraction?**

Full-thickness, thick split-thickness, thin split-thickness, meshed split-thickness

○ **What quality of the skin graft determines the degree of primary contraction?**

Elastin present in increasing amounts with the thickness of the dermal component provides a greater potential for primary contraction

○ **What is an important aspect of burn rehabilitation / reconstruction that begins during the acute phase of the injury?**

Early range of motion, mobilization, and proper positioning / splinting

○ **How should burned areas be splinted?**

Neck in slight extension, shoulder abducted, elbow in full extension, hand in intrinsic plus position, hips in extension / abduction, knees in full extension, and foot in neutral position / 90° of dorsiflexion

References

Hansen, SL, Voigt DW, Wiebelhaus, P et al. Using skin replacement products to treat burns and wounds. Adv Skin Wound Care 2001; 14(1): 37-46.

Herndon D,ed. Total Burn Care. 2nd ed. London: W.B. Saunders Company Ltdl, 2002.

Nguyen TT, Gilpin DA, Meyer NA et al. Current treatment of severly burned patients. Ann Surg 1996; 223(1): 14-25.

Press B. Thermal, Electrical, and Chemical Injuriesl In: Aston SJ, Beasley RW, Thorne C, eds. Grabb and Smith's Plastic Surgery. 5th ed. Philadelphia: Lippincott-Raven, 1997: 161-189.

Sheridan RL. Burns. Crit Care Med 2002; 30(11 Suppl): S500-S514.

INJECTABLE SOFT TISSUE FILLERS

Viki Fripp, MD and Mia Talmor, MD

❍ **What are the categories of injectable fillers available today?**

Temporary injectable fillers	– Collagen, Restylane, Hylaform
Injectable Micro Implants	– Artecoll, Silicone
Injectable Bio-catalyst	– Isolagen
Synthetic Lip implants	– Gore-Tex
Cadaver-derived Bio-implants	– Alloderm, Cymetra, Fascian
Autologous Options	– Fat Grafting

❍ **Where are injectable fillers used most?**

Injected collagen and fat are primarily used to improve the appearance of the skin's texture. They can help fill out deep facial wrinkles, creases and furrows, "sunken" cheeks, skin depressions and some types of scars. They can also be used to add a fuller, more sensuous look to the lips.

❍ **What are the forms of collagen?**

Zyderm I, Zyderm II and Zyplast.

Zyderm I and II are sterilized fibrillar bovine collagen, 95% type I and 5% type III. Zyplast results from cross-linking the collagen with glutaraldehyde to give it a longer lifespan. These products differ primarily in rates of resorption. Zyderm I and II require overcorrection to 1.5 or 2 times the initial depth of the defiency is recommended, because absorption of the saline carrier leaves 30% of the injected volume.

❍ **Is overcorrection advocated for Zyplast?**

Zyplast retains the injected volume and overcorrection is not advocated.

❍ **Where is collagen injected?**

Within the dermis to minimize contour irregularities.

❍ **What is the major concern with the use of injectable collagens?**

The potential allergic reaction.

❍ **Why is skin testing necessary for collagen?**

Circulating antibodies to bovine collagen can induce an allergic response. The peptide end regions are thought to be the most antigenic sites on the molecule. Skin testing is therefore, required: collagen is injected into the volar forearm, and the skin is observed at 48 hours and again at 4 weeks (very important).

❍ **What are the indications of injectable collagen?**

Zyderm I - It is useful for superficial dermal defects in thin skin, such as fine periorbital and perioral wrinkles.
Zyderm II (concentration of 65mg/cc) – used for defects in thicker skin, such as glabellar lines, nasolabial lines,

transverse forehead lines or acne scarring. Zyplast is recommended for glabellar folds, nasolabial folds, and postrhinoplasty defects in the deep dermis.

○   **What are the contraindications of injectable collagen?**

Contraindications include autoimmune disease, viral pock marks, "ice-pick" acne scars or indurated scars and hypersensitivity reactions to skin testing.

○   **How often should collagen be given?**

Reinjection for maintenance is required every 6 months to 2 years.

○   **What is Restylane?**

Restylane is a based on a non-animal hyaluronic acid.   It is a clear get that is injected into the lips as well as wrinkles, to provide a desired augmentation. Once injected it works together with the body's own hyaluronic acid and lasts longer than bovine-derived collagen. It is injected into the mid dermis and does not need overcorrection. Additionally, no pre-test is necessary.

○   **What is Hylaform?**

Hylaform is a viscoelastic gel made of avian hyaluronic acid. Hyaluronan is chemically, physically and biologically identical in the tissue of all species. No allergic reaction to the material; however, allergies to poultry may be an issue. Hylaform lasts from 3 to 6 months.

○   **Which filler is permanent?**

Artecoll. Polymethylmethylmethacrylate microspheres suspended in 3.5% denatured bovine collagen, mixed with 0.3% Lidocaine. It is injected into the dermis. The bovine collagen within the Artecoll mixture resorbs within 2 to 3 months and the microspheres are then encapsulated by the body's own collagen within 2 to 4 months creating added tissue augmentation. Allergy testing is required secondary to the collagen carrier.

○   **What is Silicone?**

Not FDA approved for cosmetic use. The injection of silicone oil triggers a foreign body response. The body forms collagen layers around the silicone and eventually augmentation is gained in the form of fibrous tissue. This augmentation is permanent as Silicone is difficult to remove.

○   **What is Isolagen?**

Not FDA approved. It is derived by from cultured human fibroblasts. When injected into the body it encourages tissue growth for an undetermined amount of timed. No allergy testing necessary because the body accepts the fibroblast. It is reported to be indefinite although the collagen is susceptible to natural aging.

○   **What is Gore-Tex?**

Gore-Tex is expanded polytetrafluoroethylene (ePTFE). Used in medical implants throughout the body. Extremely strong and is not likely to tear or disintegrate. Can be palpable when not placed correctly. The ends must be trimmed the correct length or inflammation can occur where the ends meet the suture areas. It is permanent, yet reversible. Allergy testing is not necessary.

○   **Which agent requires that the donor be tested for AIDS, Hepatitis B, C, HIV types 1 and 2 and syphilis?**

Alloderm. Unlike Gore-Tex, which can be removed, Alloderm cannot be removed. Great for lip augmentation because the native tissue attaches to the allograft scaffold. It is injected into the submucosa at the border of the wet and dry vermillion.

○   **What product is rehydrated with Lidocaine before injection?**

Cymetra. It is composed of micronized acellular human cadaveric dermis. It is rehydrated with Lidocaine and Epinephine and saline if desired. No allergy test is required because it is human tissue and metabolically compatible with the patient's body. Its use is contraindicated in patients with autoimmune connective tissue disease and in infected or nonvascular surgical sites. It lasts 3 –9 months.

○   **What is Fascian?**

Fascian is an injectable form of preparation of human fascia, especially fascia lata, collected from human cadaveric donors. It is used for pitted acne scars, volume enhancers for the nasolabial fold, and lip augmentation. Some degree of absorption is expected so overcorrection is performed. Trace amounts of polymyxin B sulfate, bacitracin and/or gentamicin may be present. Recipients who may be allergic to these antibiotics should be managed accordingly.

○   **What are the pros and cons of fat injections?**

Fat is non-antigenic and can be harvested from thighs and abdomen. The cons of fat injections are the fast resorption rate. Overcorrection is required for fat injections as only 30% to 50% remains on average after 1 year. Can last anywhere form 6 months to several years.

References

Aston S, Beasley R, Thorne, C. In: Aston S, ed. Grabb and Smith's Plastic Surgery. 5th ed. Philadelphia: Lippinocott-Raven; 1999: 45.

Weinzweig J. In: Weinzweig J, ed. Plastic Surgery Secrets. 1st ed. Philadelphia: Hanley and Belfus; 1999: 25.

Cheng JT, Perkins SW, Hamilton MM. Collagen and injectable fillers. Otolaryngol Clin North Am 2002; 35 (1): 73-85.

Jordan DR. Soft-tissue fillers for wrinkles, folds and volume augmentation. Can J Ophthalmol 2003; 38(4): 285-8.

Cohen SR, Holmes RE. Artecoll: a long-lasting injectable wrinkle filler material: Report of a controlled, randomized, multicenter clinical trial of 251 subjects. Plast Reconstr Surg 2004; 114(4): 964-79.

EYELID RECONSTRUCTION AND BLEPHAROPLASTY TECHNIQUES

Viki Fripp, MD and Mia Talmor, MD

○ **What are the analogous structures in the upper and lower eyelid?**

The levator aponeurosis is specific to the upper eyelid and is analogous to the capsulopalpebral fascia of the lower lid.

○ **What is the most commonly injured muscle in upper lid blepharoplasty?**

The superior oblique

○ **What is the difference between blepharochalasis and dermatochalasis?**

Blepharochalasis is characterized by intermittent swelling of the eyelid with redundancy of the lid. No associated pain or erythema and it primarily affects young women. Dermatochalasis is age related eyelid wrinkling.

○ **What structure is often mistaken for fat in the upper eyelid?**

The upper lid has three compartments: the nasal fat compartment, medial fat compartment and the lacrimal gland compartment. During fat resection the lacrimal gland may be mistaken for fat.

○ **How are retrobulbar hematomas diagnosed?**

Patients with retrobulbar hematomas typically complain of steady, severe, lancinating pain in the globe and orbit. Other characteristic symptoms include firmness and tenderness of the globe and early discharge from the eye.

○ **How are retrobulbar hematomas diagnosed and treated?**

Immediate release of the sutures, operative exploration, intravenous corticosteroids and acetazolamide to decrease swelling. Consider ophthalmology.

○ **What are the differences between the Asian eyelid and the Occidental eyelid?**

Presence of epicanthal folds, lack of supratarsal folds and puffy upper lids. The supratarsal fold, which is formed by dermal attachments of the levator aponeurosis, is lacking in the Asian eyelid.

○ **What is the relation of the preaponeurotic fat in the Asian eyelid?**

The preaponeurotic fat may extend lower secondary to a lower insertion of the orbital septum to the levator aponeurosis.

○ **What are the goals of Asian eyelid surgery?**

The double eyelid surgery focuses on establishing a visible lid fold. Incisions are made within the lid at the desired level of fold creation, excess fat is removed and fixation sutures are placed.

○ **How are the degrees of upper lid ptosis characterized?**

Repair is based on the degree of ptosis and levator function. Minimal (1-2mm), moderate (3-4mm), or severe (>4mm).

○   **What are the degrees of levator function?**

Levator function is expressed as the distance between excursion of upper lid margin from full downgaze to full upgaze without brow movement. Excellent (>10mm), good (8-10mm), fair (5-7mm), or poor (1-4mm).

○   **What are the surgical options for minimal upper lid ptosis repair with good levator function?**

For minimal ptosis, Müeller's muscle conjunctival resection or the Fasanella Servat procedure is proposed.

○   **What are options for moderate ptosis with fair levator function?**

Shortening of the levator palpebrae or levator muscle advancement are proposed.

○   **What is the treatment for severe ptosis with poor levator function?**

For severe ptosis with a levator function <5mm, a brow/frontalis suspension is indicated.

○   **What is the Fasanella Servat procedure?**

The procedure involves the excision of conjunctiva, Müeller's muscle toward the fornix, and accessory lacrimal glands.

○   **What is the success rate of the Fasanella Servat procedure?**

Approximately 70%

○   **What are guidelines of resection in the Fasanella Servat procedure?**

Resection is carried out according to the following algorithm: 1mm ptosis: 4 mm resection; 1.5 mm ptosis: 6 mm resection; and 3 mm ptosis: 11-12 mm resection.

○   **When should the Fasanella Servat procedure be avoided?**

Patients with significant corneal disease or filtering blebs. Some believe there is promotion of a poor lid crease and partial removal of the tarsal plate that causes secondary problems.

○   **What is the indication for lower lid arcus marginalis release?**

Arcus marginalis release is warranted when lower lid bags and/or infraorbital skeletonization is encountered.

○   **How does the inferior margin of the bony orbit change with time?**

In the youthful face, the inferior margin of the bony orbit is concealed entirely by overlying soft tissue. With age, this tissue progressively atrophies and sags, creating a prominent ridge along the infraorbital rim.

○   **What is accomplished with arcus marginalis release?**

With the arcus marginalis release procedure the orbital fat is advanced to reconstruct the soft tissue of the lower lid.

○   **How does this differ from traditional blepharoplasty?**

Directly opposite to traditional blepharoplasty in which orbital fat is resected in an attempt to eliminate bags, which may accentuate the ridge by creating a depression above the infraorbital rim.

❍ **How is lower lid ectropion acutely treated?**

Application of Steri-Strips obliquely and with tension at the lateral canthus can be done at the time of surgery. This provides the lower lid with superolateral support that mitigates against development of ectropion.

❍ **How is persistent ectropion treated?**

Release of all scar tissue, skin grafting of the internal or external lid lamella to make up for deficits or canthoplasty. A portion of the deformity usually persists.

❍ **When is the lower lid subciliary approach used?**

When there exists excessive amounts of skin in the lower lid. If any doubt exists regarding the presence of excess skin, a subciliary skin incision may be done at a later date. A transcutaneous subciliary incision also is indicated when combined with a skin-muscle flap for exposure in orbital fat translocation and as access for midface correction.

❍ **What is the general approach of the lower lid transconjunctival approach?**

Incisions placed within the lower conjunctival sac, and going through the lower lid retractors to obtain access to the lower eyelid fat.

❍ **What are the benefits of the lower lid transconjunctival approach?**

Useful when only fat removal or orbital septum tightening is desired; no visible external scar.

❍ **What are the drawbacks of the lower lid transconjunctival approach?**

Potential ectropion-producing scarring (though less than the skin approach), difficulty identifying the correct tissue planes, hematoma (greater chance with this approach), inability to excise lower eyelid skin (lid-tightening ability), and injury to the inferior oblique muscle.

❍ **Which lid is more dynamic – the upper or the lower?**

The lower lid is more dynamic than the upper lid and its function as a corneal protection is essential.

❍ **Describe the options for horizontal defects up to 25% in lower lid reconstruction.**

Direct approximation is possible.

❍ **What are options for 25-60% defects?**

Selective cantholysis and medial transposition of the lid with or without a local skin flap or Tenzel semicircular rotation flap.

❍ **What are options for 75-100% defects?**

Hugh's tarsoconjunctival flap or a Mustarde cheek flap with composite grafting for lid support and lining.

❍ **What eyelid defects are best suited for the Hugh's tarsoconjunctival flap?**

The Hugh's flap is a well-accepted example of a lid-sharing technique, best suited for defects that have a vertical dimension of 4-5mm.

❍ **What is the principle of the Hugh's lid-sharing procedure?**

Staged advancement flap using the posterior lamella of the upper lid to reconstruct lower lid; flap includes conjunctiva, tarsus, levator aponeurosis, and Müeller's muscle. Approximately 4-5 mm of inferior upper lid tarsus preserved for upper lid support and lid margin stability. After the flap is advanced and inset a full-thickness skin graft is secured onto the flap. Flap division at 6-8 weeks.

❍ **Describe the principle behind performing a canthoplasty.**

Designed to reposition and firmly reinforce the lower eyelid by dividing and permanently repositioning the lateral canthal tendon.

❍ **Describe a canthopexy.**

Refers to a much simpler and less invasive procedure designed to stabilize the eyelid by placement of a single suture; effect usually minimal.

❍ **When is a canthopexy performed?**

To maintain eyelid position during blepharoplasty, offer a more almond-shaped eye, improve the weakness in lower lid canthal tendons and allow for eyelid skin excision and tightening of the lower eyelid.

❍ **What is the primary goal of both canthopexy and canthoplasty?**

Strengthening of the tissues at the outer corner of the eyelid; helps to prevent ectropion and may also create a slight upward pull that can soften wrinkles and improve handling of tears.

❍ **What is the midface approach in blepharoplasty?**

Transblepharoplasty malar fat pad lifting is carried out through a skin-muscle flap approach, which is dissected down the orbital rim where the arcus marginalis is released. The periosteum is left intact on the orbital rim and the plane that is naturally entered is a subcutaneous plane just anterior to the muscles of facial expression.

❍ **What advantages are there in midface rejuvenation with lower blepharoplasty?**

Advantages of this approach are that midface rejuvenation can be accomplished in association with lower lid blepharoplasty with less dissection than more aggressive sub-periosteal techniques.

References

Jelks G, Jelks E. Blepharoplasty. In: Peck GC, ed. Complications and Problems in Plastic Surgery. 5th ed. New York, NY: Gower Medical Publishing; 1992:18- 19.

Aston S, Beasley R, Thorne, C. In: Aston S, ed. Grabb and Smith's Plastic Surgery. 5th ed. Philadelphia: Lippinocott-Raven; 1999: 609-20.

Weinzweig J. In: Weinzweig J, ed. Plastic Surgery Secrets. 1st ed. Philadelphia: Hanley and Belfus; 1999: 200-7, 276-286.

Finsterer J. Ptosis: Causes, Presentation, and Management. Aesthetic Plast Surg 2003; 27:1-24.

Jacobs S. Prophylactic lateral canthopexy in lower blepharoplasties. Arch Facial Plast Surg 2003; 5: 1-13.

Shin YH, Hwang K. Cosmetic lateral canthoplasty. Aesthetic Plast Surg 2004; 28: 1-9.

Glatt, HJ. Transconjunctival flap supplementation: an approach to the reconstruction of large lower eyelid defects. Plast Reconstr Surg 1997; 13: 90-7.

Eser Y, Potochy J, Spira M. A differential approach to the midface lift: an anatomic and clinical study. ASPS meeting Nov 3, 2002.

NASAL RECONSTRUCTION

Clark F. Schierle, MD, PhD

❍ **What is the first recorded documentation of nasal reconstruction?**

The *Sushruta Samhita*, an ayurvedic treatise authored by the healer Sushruta around 600 B.C.E., describes the reconstruction of nasal amputation for adultery using a forehead flap traced using a leaf as a template.

❍ **What are the first Western accounts of nasal reconstruction?**

Branca is believed to have rediscovered Arabic translations of Sushruta's original texts. Tagliacozzi described the use of a pedicled arm flap in his 1597 treatise *De Curtorem Chirurgia per Insitionem*, widely regarded as the first modern text of plastic surgery.

❍ **What are the aesthetic subunits of the nose?**

The alae, the columella, the soft triangles, the tip, the sidewalls, and the dorsum.

❍ **What are the two general contour classes into which the subunits fall?**

Convex and flat.

❍ **What is the ideal reconstructive element for each class?**

Convexities are best replaced by flaps which contract spherically, flat areas are best replaced by full thickness skin grafts which contract in a linear fashion.

❍ **What is the basic tenet of the subunit theory?**

If a defect encompasses more that 50% of a given subunit, a better aesthetic result will be achieve by complete excision and replacement of the subunit with suitable tissue.

❍ **What is the rationale for this theory?**

Incisional scars will fall in natural anatomic grooves and shadows and produce less noticeable light reflexes.

❍ **What are the differences in skin quality between the different nasal subunits?**

The skin of the dorsum and sidewalls tends to be thin and smooth, while the skin of the tip and alae is denser and more sebaceous.

❍ **What are the three principles that guide reconstruction of any full thickness nasal defect?**

A satisfactory reconstruction must provide a suitable nasal **lining**, adequate structural **framework**, and aesthetically appropriate skin **cover**.

❍ **What are potential donor sites for full thickness skin grafting of nasal defects?**

Preauricular, postauricular and supraclavicular skin provide the best color and quality match for nasal skin.

❍ **What are common donor sites for reconstructing the cartilaginous framework of the nose?**

The nasal septum, auricular conchal cartilage and rib cartilage.

○   **When may a superficial nasal defect be closed by a local flap?**

Defects of less than 1.5 cm can generally be filled through the rotation of the relatively mobile and pliable skin of the nasal sidewall.

○   **What are options for reconstruction of larger defects?**

A nasolabial or forehead flap.

○   **What is the ideal donor for reconstruction of an isolated alar defect?**

A nasolabial flap

○   **What is the blood supply of the nasolabial flap?**

Tributaries of the facial artery and its angular branch which perforate the levator labii muscle near the ala and radiate across the cheek.

○   **What is the ideal donor tissue for larger defects of the nasal tip and alae?**

A forehead flap

○   **Why?**

The dense, sebaceous skin of the forehead provides the ideal replacement for nasal tip and alar skin.

○   **What is the blood supply of the forehead flap?**

The supraorbital and supratrochlear arteries primarily, with contribution from the rich anastomotic arcade comprised of the infratrochlear, dorsal nasal, and angular arteries.

○   **Does tissue expansion play a role?**

Generally no. Tissue expansion potentially thins the otherwise ideally dense skin of the forehead and compromises its blood supply.

○   **What is the approach for an adequately sized forehead flap that leaves too large a forehead defect for primary closure?**

The donor site defect can be easily treated. Most contract adequately with time and heal by secondary intention or can be easily camouflaged with a skin graft. Do not compromise the reconstruction of the recipient site for the sake of the donor site. You will be left with two defects to fill.

○   **When must framework be supplied?**

Anytime the inherent cartilaginous architecture of the nose is compromised.

○   **The alar wings do not normally contain cartilage, why must they be supported by cartilage when reconstructed?**

To resist the centripetal contractile forces of a healing tissue flap.

○   **What are the principles guiding selection of adequate nasal lining?**

Adequate vascular supply, sufficient pliability to conform to a concave contour, appropriate thinness to avoid airway obstruction.

❍ **What are options for nasal lining?**

Redundant skin folded over from the coverage flap, skin graft, mucoperichondrial flaps from the septum, rotational or advancement flaps from residual vestibular lining, facial artery musculo-mucosal (FAMM) flaps, or free flaps from the radial forearm and anterolateral thigh.

❍ **What is the role of free microvascular tissue transfer in nasal reconstruction?**

Recent work has made use of thin pliable free flaps for reconstruction of the nasal lining. Although quite bulky, the robust vascular supply of the free flap results in negligible contraction of the tissue, which can be carefully thinned in subsequent procedures.

❍ **What is generally the upper limit of defect size when using a bilobed flap?**

1.5 cm

❍ **Besides suture package, what other material may be used as a template?**

Aquaplast molding material

LIP RECONSTRUCTION

Russell R. Reid, MD, PhD

○ **What is the function of the lips?**

Establishment of oral competence, modulation of the spoken word, facial expression, as well as a role in social importance (relationships).

○ **What is cheiloscopy?**

Using an individual's lips which have a unique topographic, just like a fingerprint pattern, for identification.

○ **What are the critical and unique anatomic landmarks of the lip?**

Philtral columns, philtral groove, Cupid's bow and tubercle for the upper lip; the vermilion (white roll or mucocutaneous junction) and oral commissures are found on both upper and lower lips and bilaterally, respectively

○ **When do the lips begin to develop embryologically?**

At 4-5 weeks of gestation.

○ **What are the important processes that occur during embryologic development of the lips?**

The two medial nasal prominences fuse with the maxillary prominences to form the upper lip. The mandibular prominence contributes to lower lip development. Failure of neural crest cell migration (as early as day 22) results in variable clefting of the upper lip.

○ **Discuss the perioral subunit principle of the lips.**

Burget and Menick described the lateral subunit, bordered by the philtral column, nasal sill, alar base and nasolabial fold, as well as the medial subunit, which represents one-half of the philtrum.

○ **What is the subunit principle?**

When the majority of a subunit has been lost, replacement of the entire subunit with like tissue yields the most superior aesthetic reconstruction.

○ **What is the blood supply to the lip?**

The external carotid system via the facial artery, inferior/superior labial artery,

○ **What muscle planes does the facial artery travel within?**

Deep to the platysma, risorius, and zygomaticus major and minor muscles and superficial to the buccinator and levator anguli oris

○ **Where does the inferior labial artery branch from the facial artery?**

2.6 cm lateral and 1.5 cm inferior to the oral commissure

○ **What does the facial artery continue as in the midface?**

It ascends as the angular artery, forming branches to the nasal ala and anastomosing with the dorsal nasal artery. The facial and labial arteries communicate with the subdermal plexus through a dense population of musculocutaneous perforators.

O   **Where does lymphatic drainage occur from the lips?**

Submental, submandibular, periparotid nodes. Submandibular and parotid nodes secondarily drain into ipsilateral jugulodigastric nodes.

O   **How are the lips innervated (motor-wise)?**

Motor innervation to the lips is via the facial nerve, whose buccal and marginal mandibular branches supply the perioral musculature on their undersurface.

O   **What muscles of facial expression are innervated on their superficial surface?**

The buccinator, levator anguli oris, and mentalis

O   **What is the sensory innervation of the lips? What innervates the upper lip?**

Maxillary and mandibular divisions of the fifth cranial nerve. The infraorbital nerve, which is a terminal branch of the maxillary nerve, innervates the upper lip. The lower lip and chin receive sensory innervation from branches of the mandibular nerve.

O   **Where does the inferior alveolar nerve travel?**

The inferior alveolar nerve, a branch of the mandibular nerve, travels through the body of the mandible to exit from the mental foramen.

O   **What landmarks are used for an infraorbital nerve block?**

The nerve exits the infraorbital foramen 4-7 mm below the inferior orbital rim on a vertical line that descends from the medal limbus of the iris.

O   **What does the infraorbital nerve supply?**

It runs beneath the levator labii superioris and superficial to the levator anguli oris to supply the lateral nasal sidewall, ala, columella, medial cheek, and upper lip.

O   **What landmarks are used to find the mental foramen?**

It is located below the apex of the second mandibular bicuspid with 6-10 mm of lateral variability.

O   **What territory does the mental nerve supply?**

The lower lip skin down to the labiomental fold and, occasionally, down the chin as well. The nerve is located in the submucosa as it exits the foramen and frequently is visible in this location.

O   **What are the goals of lip reconstruction?**

Complete skin cover and oral lining, re-establishment of the vermilion, maintenance of an adequate stomal diameter, maintenance of sensation, and to restore normal oral sphincter function (competence).

O   **What are the limits of primary closure of the lower lip in terms of tissue loss? What about the upper lip?**

Up to one third of lower lip loss may be tolerated with primary closure techniques, before microstomia and oral incompetence become a concern. Up to 25% tissue loss of the upper lip allows for reasonable primary closure.

O   **What is the difference between primary closure of the upper lip as opposed to the lower lip?**

The unique anatomic landmarks of the upper lip (Cupid's bow, philtral columns) make the upper lip less flexible than its lower counterpart for primary closure.

O   **How is primary closure performed?**

Precise layered closure should be suture specific. Fast-absorbing material (4-0 or 5-0 chromic gut) in the buccal mucosa (which heals rapidly). The orbicularis oris is commonly repaired with large bites of a long-absorbing (vicryl or PDS) suture or permanent suture (clear nylon). Interrupted, buried sutures of fine vicryl (5-0) may be used for dermal approximation, followed by a running or interrupted monofilament suture (e.g., 6-0 nylon) in the skin.

O   **How does one treat vermilion lesions?**

The vermilion should be handled with care. Discrepancies of 1mm can be detected at a conversational distance. Lesions near the vermilion border must be excised with a vertical ellipse.

O   **What technique may be used when incising across the vermilion?**

When crossing the vermilion with an incision, one should cross this critical junction at a 90-degree angle. The fine anatomic borders of the uninvolved, marginal vermilion should be tattoed with dye prior to local infiltration.

O   **Where are the majority of malignancies of the lip – the upper or lower?**

95% of lip cancers involve the lower lip (more sun-exposed component)

O   **What histologic type are most lip malignancies?**

90% of all lip cancers are SCC. Other, more rare, subtypes (sebaceous carcinoma, adenoid cystic carcinoma, acinic cell carcinoma, Merkel cell carcinoma), may also occur.

O   **What margins should one take when excising lip malignancies?**

In one prospective study, (72 consecutive patients with primary Stage I/II SCC of the lower lip), full-thickness excision with 3mm margins yielded a 89.9% tumor-free specimen rate with a 2.8% recurrence rate after a 5-year median follow-up. 3-5mm margins appear to be sufficient in most series.

O   **What techniques may be used when excising a SCC from the lower lip?**

A flared W-plasty, single barrel, or double barrel incision (in contrast to conventional V-excisions) aid in wider margins and avoidance of crossing the labiomental fold.

O   **What general principles apply in lip reconstruction?**

A wide variety of flaps are available for reconstitution of the upper and lower lips. Two main strategies are available: rotation-advancement of remaining uninvolved lip peripheral to the defect and lip-switch flaps.

O   **What is the reconstructive technique of lip-switching?**

The concept is based on the dual blood supply to the lips from the facial artery and using tissue from one lip to reconstruct the other lip.

O   **What is an Abbé flap based upon and what is it used for?**

More commonly from the lower lip, it is based upon the coronal branch of the inferior labial artery, and is used to close a paramedian or philtral defect.

○ **How is an Abbé flap designed?**

Designed so that it measures one-half the width of the upper lip defect. A secondary division of the pedicle is performed at 3 weeks post-elevation.

○ **How does the Estander flap differ from the Abbé flap?**

The Estlander's derivation of the Abbé flap involves a triangular designed flap, based on the superior labial artery. It provides coverage for lateral lower lip defects involving the commissure.

○ **What is the Gillies fan flap used for?**

As a rotational advancement flap, the Gillies fan flap donates upper lip and cheek tissue to close large central lower lip tissue losses (>50%). Several modifications of this original concept have been established. McGregor (1983) initially described a rectangular-shaped musculocutaneous flap similar to Gillies, but with a more narrow base and thus without the distortion at the oral commissure present in its predecessor. Typically, the width of the flap is the same as the vertical defect height and the length of the flap is equivalent to the width of the defect in addition to the width of the flap.

○ **What is unique about the Karapandzic flap?**

Originally described in 1974, this is an innervated orbicularis oris (composite) flap. Used to repair midline upper and lower lip defects, this flap is elevated by semicircular incisions camouflaged within the nasolabial folds, and mobilized based on neurovascular pedicles consisting of trigeminal and facial motor and sensory supply. This flap provides a functionally competent oral sphincter. Other innervated composite flaps incorporate levator anguli oris or depressor anguli oris for muscle units. Each of these flaps can restore up to 50% defects unilaterally and may be raised bilaterally to restore total lip defects.

○ **When local or regional flaps are not available, what is the next step in lip reconstruction?**

Free flap options are available for total lip reconstitution, but are plagued by bulky reconstruction, the failure to restore a competent oral sphincter, and aesthetic limitations.

○ **For each flap (Abbé, Bernard-Burow, Estlander, Gillies, Karapandzic) describe the advantages and disadvantages.**

Abbé flap: Ideal for central defects of the upper lip (philtral). Color match and rapid reinnervation are well described. Pedicled flap configuration (requiring secondary division), minor secondary vermilion discrepancies, and upper lip asymmetries are all negative characteristics.

Modified Bernard-Burow flap: Postoperative scars are camouflaged with natural creases along alar base and sill. Displacement of philtral columns and distortion of nasolabial fold contribute to disfavor of this flap.

Estlander flap: Optimal for reconstruction of lateral lower commissural defects. Adverse effect of microstomia and ablation of the natural fold of the oral commissure are potential outcomes.

Gillies fan flap: Designed for large lower lip defects (>50%), it has a generous arc of rotation. Similar to the Estlander flap, this flap may reduce the aperture of the mouth. It also disrupts and displaces the modiolus. Finally, distortion of the lip and lack of neural supply can lead to severe aesthetic deformities and oral incompetence.

Karapandzic flap: Neurovascular rotational flap provides reconstruction with a competent oral sphincter. Similar to the Gillies and Estlander flaps, distortion and displacement of the modiolus occurs.

○ **What are the potential complications of lip reconstruction?**

The main complication post lip reconstruction is microstomia. Other complications, such as philtral or commissural obliteration, nerve injury and oral incompetence can also occur.

References

Burget GC and Menick FJ. Aesthetic restoration of one-half of the upper lip. Plast. Reconstr. Surg. 1986; 78(5): 586-593.

De Visscher JGAM, van der Waal I. Etiology of cancer of the lip. A review. Int. J. Oral Maxillofac. Surg. 1998; 27: 199-203.

De Visscher JGAM , Gooris PJJ, Vermey A, Roodenberg JLN. Surgical margins for resection of squamous cell carcinoma. Int. J. Oral Maxillofac. Surg. 2002; 31: 154-157.

Campbell JP. Surgical management of lip carcinoma. J. Oral Maxillofac. Surg. 1998; 56: 955-961.

Zide BM. Deformities of the lips and cheeks. In McCarthy JG (ed.).: Plastic Surgery. Philadelphia W.B. Saunders, 1990. pp. 2009-2037.

Schulte DL, Sherris DA, Kasperbauer JL. The anatomical basis of the Abbe flap. The Laryngoscope 2001; 111: 382-386.

McGregor IA. Reconstruction of the lower lip. Brit. J. Plast. Surg. 1983; 36: 40-47.

Tobin GR, O'Daniel TG. Lip reconstruction with motor and sensory innervated composite flaps. Clin. Plast. Surg. 1990; 17(4): 623-631.

Wei FC, Tan K, Chen IH, Hau SP, Liau CT. Mimicking lip features in free-flap reconstruction of lip defects. Br. J. Plast. Surg. 2001; 54: 8-11.

Godek CP. Weinzweig J. Bartlett SP. Lip reconstruction following Mohs' surgery: the role for composite resection and primary closure. Plast. Reconstr. Surg.. 2000;106(4):798-804.

TONGUE RECONSTRUCTION

Christiaan Schrag, BSc, MD, FRCS (C), and Fu-Chan Wei, MD, FACS

○ **Which portion of the tongue is described as the "oral tongue"?**

The anterior two thirds.

○ **What are other terms for the posterior third of the tongue?**

The pharyngeal tongue or tongue base.

○ **What separates the oral and pharyngeal portions of the tongue?**

The V-shaped sulcus terminalis.

○ **Where on the tongue is the foramen cecum?**

The center of the sulcus terminalis.

○ **During embryological development which structure migrates through the foramen cecum of the tongue?**

The thyroid.

○ **Which embryological structures fuse to form the tongue?**

The median tongue bud (tuberculum impar) and 2 distal tongue buds form the oral tongue. The hypobranchial eminence becomes the pharyngeal tongue.

○ **Describe the surface anatomy of the tongue.**

The oral tongue has an apex, which touches the incisors, a dorsum and a smooth ventral surface, which is contiguous with the oral floor and gums. The tongue base is more vertical in orientation and contiguous with the glossoepiglottic folds.

○ **What nerves provide general sensation to the tongue?**

Oral: lingual nerve (from V3). Pharyngeal: glossopharyngeal nerve.

○ **Which cranial nerves transmit taste sensation?**

Cranial nerves VII, IX and X all contain special sensory taste afferent fibers.

○ **What is the course of the chorda tympani nerve?**

The chorda tympani carries taste sensory fibers from the anterior 2/3rds of the tongue to the intratemporal facial nerve. With the lingual nerve the chorda tympani travels from the ventral surface of the tongue to the lingual sulcus, where it is caudal to the submandibular duct; Then superiorly, to the lingual border of the mandible near the third molar. The chorda tympani leaves the lingual nerve at the medial border of the lateral pterygoid and traverses the middle ear, joining CN VII in the facial canal.

○ **Where are taste buds located?**

Tongue, soft palate, palatoglossal arches, posterior surface of the epiglottis (CN X) and posterior oropharynx.

○ **How many taste buds are there on each papilla?**

Approximately three, 250 and 1200 taste buds are found on the fungiform, vallate and foliate papillae, respectively. Filiform papillae have no taste buds.

○ **What are the four types of taste?**

Salty, sweet, sour and bitter.

○ **Where on the tongue is salty taste sensed?**

The entire tongue surface can sense salty taste. There is a strong misconception that there is a "taste map". In fact every taste can be sensed in all regions of the tongue.

○ **What other sensation is important in recognizing flavors?**

Olfaction. Patients who cannot smell may complain of lack of taste sensation.

○ **Describe the musculature of the tongue.**

Four pairs of extrinsic muscles (excluding the palatoglossus) connect the tongue to the hyoid, mandible, and styloid process. These muscles position the tongue within the mouth. Four pairs of intrinsic muscles control the shape of the tongue.

○ **What are the most important functions of the tongue?**

Airway protection, swallowing (deglutition), tasting and speech. Chewing per se is not a tongue function, but adequate breakdown of food requires that it be presented over and over to the teeth by the tongue.

○ **Describe the phases of swallowing?**

Initially, in the voluntary (oral) phase of swallowing, the apex of the tongue is pressed against the palate. The intrinsic muscles move food posteriorly into the oropharynx by elevating sequential portions of the tongue to the palate. The tongue base is positioned superiorly and posteriorly, forming a food platform in readiness for the involuntary phase. Concurrently the hyoid bone is moved superiorly.

During the involuntary (pharyngeal) phase the palatopharyngeal sphincter seals the nasopharynx while the larynx and pharynx are elevated. The tongue base and pharyngeal constrictors force the food bolus inferiorly over the posteriorly arched epiglottis and closed laryngeal inlet.

○ **How are lingual cancers staged?**

The American Joint Committee on Cancer (AJCC) method for planning treatment, estimating prognosis and comparing research of oral and oropharyngeal cancers involves categorizing tumors according to the tumor size (Tis, T1, T2, T3, or T4), nodal metastases (N0, N1, N2, N3) and presence of distant metastases (M0, M1). Once the three tumor characteristics (TNM) are known the tumor can be given a stage I to IV. Oral tongue cancer staging differs from pharyngeal tongue only with respect to the T4 definitions, because the adjacent structures that might be invaded vary.

T1 = tumor ≤ 2 cm
T2 = 2 cm < tumor ≤ 4 cm
T3 = tumor > 4 cm
T4 = invades adjacent structures

○ **What are the priorities in lingual reconstruction?**

Immediate wound closure, prevention of orocervical fistula, obliteration of dead space lingual to the mandible, maintenance/restoration of tongue function and coverage of major vessels.

○ **What are secondary goals in tongue reconstruction?**

Aesthetic contouring of the neck following modified or radical neck dissection and reconstruction of any contiguous defects. The results should be stable over time, require minimal anesthesia time and have little donor site morbidity.

○ **How is residual tongue function maintained with reconstruction?**

The most important factor in preserving function is maintaining residual tongue mobility. Reconstruction methods that may lead to tethering of the residual tongue include primary closure, skin grafting or poorly designed regional or distant flaps. Correctly planned reconstructions provide sufficient flap size for coverage of the defect with the tongue in all ranges of movement.   In addition, the flap should cover adjacent floor of mouth, pharyngeal or palate defects as required.

○ **Why is the volume of a free flap important in reconstructing subtotal or total tongue defects?**

The presence of bulk in a flap supports the ventral tongue, preventing prolapse or contralateral shifting of the residual tongue. Bulk allows the tongue to contact the palate, which is important for speech and swallowing.

○ **What are the options for reconstructing lingual defects?**

Primary closure, skin grafts, and local, regional or distant flaps. Common free flaps for tongue reconstruction include radial/ulna forearm, lateral arm, TRAM, and anterolateral thigh.

○ **Which free flaps can be used to provide general sensation to the reconstructed tongue?**

Radial forearm, anterolateral thigh and lateral arm are three commonly used flaps for tongue reconstruction, which may be innervated to provide sensation.

○ **Do non-innervated flaps used for tongue reconstruction regain sensation?**

Yes. Ninety percent of non-innervated fasciocutaneous free flaps placed on an unscarred bed in the oral cavity regained at least some sensory modalities, likely the result of axonal sprouting into the flap. Sensory upgrading of the flap may occur secondary to the large cortical representation of the tongue in the sensory homonculus.

○ **Do innervated free flaps for tongue reconstruction regain normal sensation?**

No. Flaps are unable to taste because they lack taste buds. However, patients rarely complain about loss of taste (likely because taste buds are almost ubiquitous within the buccal cavity). General sensory function of an innervated free flap approaches that of the normal tongue and is superior to the donor site sensation.

○ **Do innervated flaps function better than non-innervated flaps?**

No studies to date have compared tongue function in innervated versus non-innervated flaps. Innervated flaps gain general sensation sooner post-operatively than non-innervated flaps. However, sensation may not be important for tongue function.

○ **What factors affect sensory recovery in flaps used for tongue reconstruction?**

Post-operative radiation and the use of a recipient nerve other than the lingual or inferior alveolar nerve negatively impact the sensory recovery of innervated free flaps for tongue reconstruction. Age, smoking and the size of the defect do not influence the return of sensation.

❍ **What is the effect of a palatal build-down prosthesis on tongue function?**

A prosthesis placed over the palate in an attempt to achieve tongue-palate contact has a negative impact on function because the patient will lose important sensory feedback from the palate. (Palatal sensation might explain how noninnervated flaps are able to function similarly to reinnervated flaps.)

❍ **What are the important determinates of functional outcome following tongue reconstruction?**

The primary predictor of post-operative function is defect size, with larger defects associated with poorer outcomes. Post-operative radiotherapy and midline defects correlate with worse functional results. Reconstructions that maintain tongue mobility and bulk give patients better speech and swallowing.

❍ **What are the advantages of the radial forearm free flap for tongue reconstruction?**

Large surface area available; thin, pliable tissue; long pedicle if required; technically easy to harvest; several useful variants: neurofasciocutaneous, osseofasciocutaneous, tendofasciocutaneous.

❍ **What are the disadvantages of the radial forearm free flap?**

Lack of bulk for large tongue defects and the donor site morbidity, which includes sensory changes and poor cosmesis.

❍ **What are the advantages of the suprafascial dissection for a radial forearm free flap?**

Fewer donor site complications: decreased rate of skin graft loss; less delayed healing; decreased incidence of tendon exposure.

❍ **What options exist for reconstructing total or subtotal tongue defects?**

Primarily free flaps: ALT, iliac crest/groin, TRAM, jejunum.

❍ **For total tongue defects can the tongue muscles be reconstructed?**

No. Currently, the tongue muscles are too complex to reconstruct. Functioning gracilis may be transferred in either a longitudinal or transverse orientation, with the goal of providing only elevation of the neotongue when required. Too few studies exist to comment on the utility of functioning muscle transfers in tongue reconstruction.

❍ **Are there problems associated with using muscle flaps for tongue reconstruction?**

Non-innervated muscle flaps undergo atrophy and over time may not provide enough bulk in reconstruction of large defects. The reinnervation of musculocutaneous flaps is worse than non-innervated fasciocutaneous flaps.

References

Avery CME, Pereira J, Brown AE. Suprafascial dissection of the radial forearm flap and donor site morbidity. Int J Oral Maxillofac Surg 2001; 30: 37-41.

Bannister LH. Alimentary system. In Williams PL , ed. Gray's Anatomy. 38th Edition. Toronto: Churchill-Livingstone, 1999, pp 1683-1733.

Bastian RW, Riggs LC. Role of sensation in swallowing function. Laryngoscope 1999; 109: 1974-1977.

Berry M, Bannister LH, Standring SM. Nervous system. In Williams PL, ed. Gray's Anatomy. 38th Edition. Toronto: Churchill-Livingstone, 1999, pp 901-1397.

Boyd B, Mulholland S, Gullane P, Irish J, Kelly L, Rotstein, Brown D. Reinnervated lateral antebrachial cutaneous neurosome flaps in oral reconstruction: are we making sense? Plast Reconstr Surg 1994; 93: 1350-1359.

Chang SCN, Miller G, Halbert CF, Yang KH, Chao WC, Wei FC. Limiting donor site morbidity by suprafascial dissection of the radial forearm flap. Microsurgery 1996; 17: 136-140.

Collins P. Embryology and Development. In Williams PL , ed. Gray's Anatomy. 38th Edition. Toronto: Churchill-Livingstone, 1999, pp 91-341.

de Bree R, Hartley C, Smeele LE, et al. Evaluation of donor site function and morbidity of the fasciocutaneous radial forearm flap. Laryngoscope 2004; 114(11):1973-6.

Evans GRD, Kroll SS. Intraoral soft tissue reconstruction. In Schusterman MA, ed. Microsurgical reconstruction of the cancer patient. Philadelphia: Lippincott-Raven Publishers, 1997:13-29.

Greene FL, Balch CM, Page DL et al AJCC Cancer Staging Handbook , 6th ed. New York: Springer-Verlag, 2002.

Haughey BH. Tongue reconstruction: concepts and practice. Laryngoscope 1993; 103: 1132-1141.

Huang CH, Chen HC, Huang YL, et al. Comparison of the radial forearm flap and the thinned anterolateral thigh cutaneous flap for reconstruction of tongue defects: an evaluation of donor-site morbidity. Plastic and Reconstructive Surgery 2004; 114(7):1704-10.

Imanishi Y, Isobe K, Nameki H, et al. Extended sigmoid-shaped free jejunal patch for reconstruction of the oral base and pharynx after total glossectomy with laryngectomy. British Journal of Plastic Surgery 2004; 57:195-202.

Kimata Y, Sakuraba M, Hishinuma S, Ebihara S, Hayashi R, Asakage T, Nakatsuka T, Harii K. Analysis of the relations between the shape of the reconstructed tongue and the postoperative functions after subtotal or total glossectomy. Laryngoscope 2003; 113: 905-909.

Kuriakose MA, Loree TR, Spies AS, Meyers S, Hicks WL. Sensate radial forearm free flaps in tongue reconstruction. Arch Otolaryngol Head Neck Surg 2001; 127: 1463-1466.

Kveton JF, Bartoshuk LM. Taste. In Bailey BJ, Calhoun KH eds. Head and Neck Surgery-Otolaryngology. Second edition. Philadelphia: Lippincott-Raven Publishers, 1998: 609-626.

McConnell FM. Analysis of pressure generation and bolus transit during pharyngeal swallowing. Laryngoscope 1988; 98: 718-724.

Murakami R, Tanaka K, Kobayashi K, Fujii T, Sakito T, Furukawa M, Kobayashi T, Shigeno K. Free groin flap for reconstruction of the tongue and oral floor. Journal of Reconstructive Microsurgery 1998; 14: 49-55.

Nakatsuka T, Harii K. Analysis of the relations between the shape of the reconstructed tongue and postoperative functions after subtotal or total glossectomy. Laryngoscope 2003; 113: 905-909.

Nicoletti G, Soutar DS, Jackson MS, Wrench AA, Robertson G. Chewing and swallowing after surgical treatment for oral cancer: functional evaluation in 196 selected cases. Plast Reconstr Surg 2004; 114: 329-338.

Nicoletti G, Soutar DS, Jackson MS, Wrench AA, Robertson G, Robertson C. Objective assessment of speech after surgical treatment for oral cancer: experience from 196 cases. Plast Reconstr Surg 2004; 113: 114-127.

Salibian AH, Allison GR, Armstrong WB, Krugman ME, Strelzow VV, Kelly T, Brugman JJ, Hoerauf P, McMicken BL. Functional hemitongue reconstruction with microvascular ulnar forearm flap. Plast Reconstr Surg 1999; 104: 654-660.

Salibian A, Allison GR, Rappaport I, et al. Total and subtotal glossectomy: function after microvascular reconstruction. Plast Reconstr Surg 1990; 85(4):513-524.

Santamaria E, Wei, FC, Chen IH, Chuang DCC. Sensation recovery on innervated radial forearm flap for hemiglossectomy reconstruction by using different recipient nerves. Plast Reconstr Surg 1999; 103: 450-457.

Soutar DS, McGregor IA. The radial forearm flap in intraoral reconstruction: the experience of 60 consecutive cases. Plast Reconstr Surg 1986; 78: 1-8.

Swartz, Banis. Intraoral reconstruction. In Swartz, Banis, Eds. Head and Neck Microsurgery. 1992

Urken ML, Moscoso JF, Lawson W, Biller HF. A systematic approach to functional reconstruction of the oral cavity following partial and total glossectomy. Arch Otolaryngol Head Neck Surg 1994; 120: 589-601.

Vriens JPM, Acosta R, Soutar DS, Webster MHC. Recovery of sensation in the radial forearm free flap in oral reconstruction. Plast Reconstr Surg 1996; 98: 649-656.

Yoleri L, Mavioglu H. Total tongue reconstruction with free functional gracilis muscle transplantation: a technical note and review of the literature. Annals of Plastic Surgery 2000; 45:181-186.

Yousif NJ, Dzwierzynski WW, Sanger JR, et al. The innervated gracilis musculocutaneous flap for total tongue reconstruction. Plast Reconstr Surg 1999; 104(4):916-921.

CHEST AND ABDOMINAL WALL RECONSTRUCTION

Alex Senchenkov, MD, and Craig H. Johnson, MD

Thoracic Reconstruction

○ **What are the common clinical problems that require intervention by a plastic surgeon?**

Chest wall defects related to tumor ablation, infection, radiation therapy, trauma, and congenital anomalies as well as bronchopleural fistula, chronic empyema, exposed grafts, implants, and hardware.

○ **What are the important principles in thoracic reconstruction?**

1) Complete extirpation of tumors and radiated ulcers or debridement of infection
2) Obliteration of intrathoracic dead space
3) Skeletal stabilization if >4 rib segments or >5 cm of the chest wall removed
4) Adequate soft tissue coverage with well-vascularized tissue
5) Creation of air-tight thoracic cavity

Medical and nutritional optimization and appropriate antibiotic coverage guided by tissue biopsies are important as well

○ **What is the most common reason for failed reconstruction?**

Inadequate debridement

○ **List the types of thoracotomies that are used.**

Sternotomy (most common approach in cardiac surgery) and anterolateral, posterolateral, axillary, muscle-sparing posterolateral, clam shell, open book type thoracotomies

○ **What reconstructive implications does sternotomy have?**

If performed for CABG, records need to be reviewed with regard to internal mammary artery use.

○ **What reconstructive implications does an anterolateral thoracotomy have?**

Anterolateral thoracotomy allows rapid exploration of pleural cavities, frequent indication is resuscitative or ER thoracotomy. LIMA is very frequently divided.

○ **What reconstructive implications does a posterolateral thoracotomy have?**

Posterolateral thoracotomy is most commonly performed approach to lungs, esophagus, posterior mediastinal structures, and thoracic spine. Latissimus dorsi muscle is divided as a part of exposure and cannot be used as a flap.

○ **What reconstructive implications does an axillary thoracotomy have?**

Axillary thoracotomy provides exposure for extended pulmonary resections including procedures involving chest wall resection. Pectoralis and latissimus muscles are left intact and the serratus anterior is divided in direction of its fibers. Serratus anterior vessels are divided and serratus anterior flap cannot be used.

❍ **What reconstructive implications does a muscle-sparing posterolateral thoracotomy have?**

This approach preserves the latissimus dorsi and serratus anterior muscles with only slight limitation of the intrathoracic exposure. The latissimus dorsi and serratus anterior can be used for reconstruction.

❍ **What reconstructive implications does a clam-shell thoracotomy have?**

This approach is a bilateral anterolateral thoracotomy with transverse division of sternum and both internal mammary arteries.

❍ **What reconstructive implications does an open-book thoracotomy have?**

This consists of a left anterolateral thoracotomy that is extended into sternotomy and continued superior to the clavicle. Usually performed on the left for emergent access to the left subclavian artery. Clavicle is sometimes removed for exposure. Left IMA is always divided and left thoracoacromial trunk may be transected.

❍ **What are the best choices for flap selection in chest wall reconstruction?**

- **First choice regional flaps:** pectoralis major, latissimus dorsi, serratus anterior, and rectus abdominis muscle flap
- **Second choice regional flap:** omental flap
- **Microvascular flaps:** contralateral latissimus dorsi, tensor fascia lata, free TRAM, free rectus abdominis

❍ **What is blood supply of the latissimus dorsi muscle flap?**

Subscapular vessels that give rise to thoracodorsal and circumflex scapular vessels; alternatively, a reverse flap can be based on 4 to 6 medial and 4 to 6 lateral perforating vessels from lumbar and posterior intercostal vessels, respectively (Type V).

❍ **Can this flap be utilized in the patients with prior ligation of thoracodorsal vessels?**

Yes. This flap can survive based on the retrograde flow from the serratus anterior artery and the vena comitantes

❍ **What are the options for skeletal stabilization of the chest wall?**

Autologous tissues: muscle and fascial flaps, rib and fascial grafts

Prosthetic materials: mesh (marlex, teflon, prolene, Gore-Tex) or composite mesh-methyl methacrylate sandwich.

❍ **What are advantages and disadvantages of autologous and prosthetic skeletal stabilization?**

Split rib grafts are technically difficult, frequently fail due to difficulty in stabilization, and involve donor site morbidity

Fascial grafts are not difficult, but do not provide rigidity and have donor site morbidity.

Mesh is without donor site morbidity and is easy to use, but is semirigid, and carries risk of mesh infection

Composite mesh-methyl methacrylate sandwich straightforward and rigid, but carries risk of mesh infection. For the clean chest wall defect, prosthetic reconstruction has largely supplanted the use of rib grafts

❍ **What is important when prosthetic materials are used for the chest wall reconstruction?**

Well-vascularized tissue coverage of the prosthetic materials is critical for successful reconstruction.

❍ **What is the main concern in prosthetic skeletal stabilization of the chest wall?**

Infection of the mesh (5% for Marlex mesh)

○ **What is the main reason for mesh infection?**

Ischemic failure of the overlying flap

○ **How do you approach infected chest wall mesh?**

Infected mesh generally needs to be removed; however, if the Marlex or composite mesh-methyl methacrylate sandwich is allowed to remain in place for 6 – 8 weeks, fibrous capsule that forms around the mesh will be rigid enough to prevent flailing of the reconstructed segment of the chest after the removal of the infested mesh.

○ **What is different in irradiated chest wall reconstruction?**

Radiation stiffens the chest wall that decreases the need in skeletal stabilization.

○ **What is oncologic implication of well-vascularized chest wall coverage?**

It allows postoperative radiation therapy.

○ **What is the main blood supply to the sternum?**

Perforators of IMA

○ **How do patients present with sternal wound infections?**

Early with sternal instability and wound drainage, late with draining fistula

○ **What is the etiology of sternal wound infection?**

It is both mechanical and infectious. Common risk factors are:
- Use of unilateral or bilateral internal mammary artery during CABG leads to sternal infection 0.03% and 2.4%, respectively; 0% when IMA spared
- Diabetes mellitus 5.7% vs 0.3% without DM
- Age 0.2% in <60, 1.6% in 60-70, and 3.1% in >60
- COPD
- Multiple re-operations

Risk is from 0.4 to 5.0% of cardiac operations

○ **What are the types of clinical presentation in sternal wound infection?**

Type I: Sternotomy wound dehiscence occurs within first three postoperative days without signs of active infection and with negative wound cultures.

Type II: It usually occurs 2-3 weeks postop and presents with purulent mediastinitis, osteomyelitis, and costochondritis.

Type III: Wound presents months to years after the operation with sinus tracts due to osteomyelitis and costochondritis.

○ **How are Type I sternal wound infections handled?**

Sternum is rewired after minimal debridement.

○ **When is the plastic surgeon involved in sternal wound infections?**

Plastic surgeons are usually involved with type II and III.

O   **How do you treat sternotomy infections?**

Meticulous and frequent debridement of all infected tissues and often cartilage down to the costochondral junctions. These procedures should be done in conjunction with a cardiac surgeon. Wet-to-wet dressings or VAC are commonly utilized. Only clean granulating wounds are amenable to flap reconstruction.

O   **Has one stage thorough debridement with immediate coverage with muscle flaps also been reported**?

Yes.

O   **Name the most common reasons for recurrence of post-reconstruction sternal infections.**

In the order of frequency, retained infected cartilage (most common), bone, and foreign body

O   **What is the flap of choice for sternal reconstruction?**

Pectoralis major muscle flap. Dual blood supply from thoracoacromial vessels and internal mammary vessels (Type V), which allow use as either advancement (based on thoracoacromial) or turnover (based on mammary system) flap. One or both muscles can be used.

O   **What are additional or alternative flaps that can be used for sternal reconstruction?**

Superiorly based **rectus abdominis** muscular or musculocutaneous flap is either alternative or adjunct to pectoralis major flap when additional bulk is required.

Omentum flap is a secondary option because it requires laparotomy. Omentum is used when other flaps are not available.

O   **What is blood supply of the rectus abdominis flap?**

It has dual blood supply from superior and inferior epigastric arteries each of which can sustain the flap (Type III). Superior epigastric artery originates from IMA.

O   **Can a superiorly based rectus abdominis flap be utilized after ipsilateral use of IMA for CABG?**

The superior part of the rectus abdominis can be raised on the eighth intercostal artery, but blood supply to the inferior third of the muscle is less reliable. IMA utilization for CABG does not usually interrupt IMA communication with eighth intercostal vessels and allows utilization of the ipsilateral rectus flap.

O   **Can a superiorly based rectus abdominis flap be used if the patient has a subcostal or chevron incision?**

Subcostal or chevron incisions interrupt the origin of the superior epigastric artery and preclude the use of a superiorly based rectus abdominis flap.

O   **Is radiation to the anterior chest wall and internal mammary lymph node basin a contraindication to the use of superiorly based rectus flap?**

No. The rectus abdominus flap is still useful in these patients

O   **When is there a concern about the patency of the IMA?**

Sternal resections, wide debridement of the infected tissues at the sternotomy site, sternal retention suture use, anterolateral thoracotomy, etc. If there is a question of the vascular integrity, **duplex** or **arteriography** should be performed.

○   **How do you manage sternal wound infections in children?**

Principles of treatment are the same. Debridement should be limited to only grossly infected or devitalized tissues.

○   **What are the indications for the use of muscle flaps in pleural diseases?**

Reinforcement of the bronchial closure of a bronchopleural fistula and obliteration of a persistent pleural space

○   **What is a bronchopleural fistula?**

Communication between a bronchus and the pleural cavity that is usually caused by necrotizing pneumonia, empyema, postoperative necrosis of the bronchial stump, or necrosis of bronchial wall secondary to radiation.

○   **How can postoperative bronchopleural fistula be prevented?**

- Avoid leaving a long bronchial stump during lobectomy or pneumonectomy because it collects secretions and leads to infection and dehiscence of the stump closure.
- Assure viability of the bronchial stump margins
- Cover the stump with well vascularized local tissues or muscle flap

○   **How do you treat bronchopleural fistulas?**

Re-exploration, debridement of the bronchial stump, and coverage with muscle flaps. Serratus anterior muscle is the most commonly used for this purpose, followed by latissimus dorsi, pectoralis major, and rectus abdominis muscles. Complete obliteration of the pleural space is not necessary.

○   **What is a thoracic empyema?**

A collection of frank pus within the pleural space.

○   **How do you treat empyema in various stages?**

Stage I: Exudative or simple parapneumonic effusion that usually resolves with antibiotics and thoracentesis or chest tube drainage

Stage II: Fibrinopurulent stage fluid is turbid. In late stage II, fibrin deposits lead to loculations making it a complex effusion treatment is surgical. VATS or open drainage are indicated to evacuate infectious material

Stage III: Organizing or chronic stage heralds with formation of an inelastic pleural peel, entrapping the lung. Presence of the peel or chronic organized hematoma are indications for decortication.

○   **What is the first stage of treating postpneumonectomy empyema?**

Frequently associated with bronchopleural fistula (BPF). Open pleural drainage, debridement, and closure of the BPF with muscle flap. In absence of BPF, flaps not used and the chest is packed open with antibacterial solutions. Packing changed every 6 hours. If flap is used to repair the BPF, dressing changes done in the OR every 2 days.

○   **What is the second stage of treating postpneumonectomy empyema?**

Obliteration of the pleural space and closure of the chest wall. After pleural space is clean and granulating, the cavity is filled with antibiotic solution and closed in layers in watertight manner.

○   **What is the treatment of late postpneumonectomy empyema?**

Obliteration with flaps since closure is unlikely to be successful.

❍   **How do you treat chronic empyema in a debilitated patient who cannot withstand a major reconstructive operation?**

An epithelialized tract in the form of an Eloesser skin flap of Clagett window can be constructed between the skin and pleural cavity for chronic drainage.

❍   **How do you obliterate the intrathoracic dead space?**

The ipsilateral latissimus dorsi, serratus anterior, pectoralis major muscle flaps and omentum flaps are used in this order of frequency. Several flaps may be required to fill the infected hemithorax.

❍   **How do you transpose the muscle flap into the chest?**

Through a double-rib-resection using a 4-5 cm incision. This window is created depending on the muscle flap design and its blood supply. Chest tubes are placed for drainage before closure of the chest.

❍   **How do you obliterate the postpneumonectomy empyema cavity in absence of available flaps?**

Thoracoplasty is staged removal of ribs to allow the hemithorax to collapse. This can be an alternative for obliteration of the hemithorax for post-pneumonectomy empyema as a last resort operation if flaps are not available or sufficient and infection is difficult to control.

❍   **What are the flaps that are useful in esophageal repairs?**

While elective esophageal operations usually do not require flap reconstruction, the repair of ruptured esophagus greatly benefit from flap utilization (used to reinforce the esophageal repair)
   • **Intercostal muscle flap** is raised and preserved in the beginning of the initial thoracotomy from the intercostal muscles (5th or 6th intercostal space)
   • **Thal flap** is a random diaphragmatic flap
   • **Pleural** and **pericardial flaps** are random flaps used to enforce esophageal closure in the presence of marked inflammation that causes hyperemia and vascular ingrowth

❍   **Describe flap selection in upper, middle and lower third back wound reconstruction.**

Trapezius muscle flap (upper), latissimus muscle flap (middle), gluteus muscle flap (lower)

❍   **What are the configurations of using the latissimus dorsi flap in back reconstruction?**

Standard unilateral latissimus dorsi flap, bilateral latissimus dorsi flap, "reverse" latissimus dorsi flap

❍   **What are pedicled perforator flaps used in back reconstruction?**

Large fasciocutaneous flaps raised based on the perforators and used for reconstruction of lumbosacral defects

❍   **What are examples of pedicled perforator flaps used in back reconstruction?**

Fourth lumbar perforator flap (skin territory from the posterior midline to the rectus muscle), superior or inferior gluteal artery flaps (preservation of the muscle on the involved side), intercostal artery flaps (9th and 10th intercostal perforators)

❍   **Describe the truncal features of Poland's syndrome.**

Absence of the sternal head of the pectoralis major muscle, aplasia or hypoplasia of the breast, nipple, subcutaneous fat, and axillary hair, ipsilateral muscular anomalies: absence of the entire pectoralis major, latissimus dorsi, serratus, pectoralis minor, supraspinatus, infraspinatus, and external oblique muscles

O **T/F: Poland's syndrome may involve lung herniation.**

True. Anomalies or absence of the anterior chest wall with lung herniation in extreme cases.

O **What are the upper extremity anomalies in Poland's syndrome?**

Anomalies of the ipsilateral arm: shortening, hypoplasia, brachysyndactyly, hypoplasia or complete absence of the middle phalanges

O **What is the most likely etiology of Poland's syndrome?**

Subclavian artery hypoplasia on the 6th week of gestation

O **How do you reconstruct the breast and chest wall deformity in Poland's syndrome?**

Latissimus dorsi flap with breast implant in a woman. Tissue expansion and contralateral mastopexy also an option. Skeletal stabilization of the chest wall in severe cases to avoid displacement of the breast prosthesis.

O **What is the indication for reconstruction in male patients?**

Aplasia or significant chest wall deformity

O **What is Mobius' syndrome?**

Bilateral facial dysplasia with associated cranial nerve palsies (CN III, IV, VI, IX, X, and XII) often combined with Poland's syndrome. Muscle and innervation of the lower lip is mysteriously preserved.

Reconstruction of the abdominal wall

O **What is the blood supply and innervation of the abdominal wall?**

The blood supply and innervation come from the 7th through 12th intercostal and 1st lumbar neurovascular bundles that run between the internal oblique and transverse abdominis muscles towards the rectus sheath.

O **What are the goals of abdominal wall reconstruction?**

Protect intra-abdominal organs, prevent hernia, and provide stable soft tissue coverage and an acceptable contour

O **How do you manage skin and partial-thickness soft tissue defects?**

Utilize the principle of "reconstructive ladder": primary closure, secondary closure, skin grafting, local and regional flaps, and free tissue transfer. Myofascial defects with intact skin are reconstructed with either tension free primary closure or prosthetic materials to restore fascial support of abdominal wall.

O **What is your approach to full-thickness abdominal wall defects?**

Tension free primary closure is the first choice, but rarely possible. Local tissue methods include components separation, fascial partition release, and tissue expansion. Reconstruction of complex full-thickness abdominal wounds can be staged with skin grafting over the abdominal viscera or omentum and thus converting it into elective secondary reconstruction

O **Describe "component separation" technique.**

The rectus muscle is separated from the posterior sheath. The external oblique aponeurosis is incised lateral to the rectus sheath and the external oblique muscle is elevated off internal oblique. This allows the composite flap consisting of the rectus muscle, the anterior rectus sheath, and the internal oblique and transverse abdominis muscles to advance towards the midline.

❍   What distances are gained with "components separation"?

On each side, an estimated length gain is 3-5 cm at the epigastrium, 7-10 cm at the umbilical region, and 1-3 cm at the suprapubic region.

❍   Describe "fascial partition release" technique.

There exists two sets of vertical relaxing incisions. The first incision is made through the transverse rectus abdominis muscle from the visceral side of the abdominal wall behind the rectus muscle, preserving the posterior leaflet of the aponeurosis of the internal oblique muscle. The second incision is made through the aponeurosis of the external oblique muscle lateral to the rectus sheath.

❍   What distances are gained with the "fascial partition" release?

These incisions permit advancement of the abdominal wall of 10 cm at the epigastrium, 20 cm at the umbilicus, and 6 cm at the suprapubic region.

❍   Where is a tissue expander placed in the abdominal wall?

The tissue expander is placed between the internal and transverse muscle to create an additional length of the innervated abdominal wall soft tissues.

❍   What are cons of abdominal wall tissue expansion?

Tissue expansion is not widely used. The disadvantages are prolonged expansion time, risk of infection and denervation of the abdominal muscles, and difficulty to expand the stiff fibrotic abdominal wall after multiple operations.

❍   What 7 muscle flaps can be used for abdominal wall reconstruction?

- The tensor fascia lata and rectus femoris (lateral femoral circumflex vessels) are used most frequently; good reach for supraumbilical defects.
- The gracilis and the vastus lateralis are second choice flaps.
- The extended rectus femoris muscle including posterolateral iliotibial tract fascia that reach the epigastrium has been described.
- The pedicled anterolateral thigh flap (based on descending brunch of lateral femoral circumflex vessels) extends from greater trochanter to just above patella and can reach 8 cm above the umbilicus
- The omentum is a very important coverage of the abdominal contents that is routinely utilized in abdominal reconstruction. Skin grafting over omentum provides durable coverage.

❍   Describe a staged approach to the open abdomen in a complex critically ill trauma patient.

Stage I is the placement of temporary mesh (Vicryl, Gor-Tex, or just a simple Bogotá bag from 3 L GU irrigation bag); minimizes loss of abdominal domain. As the edema of the viscera is decreasing the patient is taken back for irrigation of the abdomen and staged closure. **Stage II** is removal of temporary mesh 2-3 weeks later and often residual defect can be closed with skin flaps and converted into ventral hernia. **Stage III** is placement of the skin graft over granulating abdominal viscera. **Stage IV** is repair of the ventral hernia with either primary closure, prosthetic materials, components separation, or fascial partition release.

❍   How do you manage an enterocutaneous fistula in a major abdominal wall defect?

Provide meticulous care of an open abdomen to control infection and promote granulation followed by skin graft over bowel. Control fistula drainage with sump drain or Malecot catheter and with ostomy bag following skin graft.

In 6-12 months when skin graft separates from underlying bowel loops and adhesions, edema, and scarring have improved, operative closure of the fistula and abdominal wall reconstruction can be undertaken.

○ **Describe your reconstructive options for the ventral hernia on a contaminated case.**

Autologous tissue should be utilized because the use of prosthetic mesh is contraindicated. Fascia lata graft, regional flaps, components separation, fascial partition release can be considered.

○ **What is Alloderm?**

Acellular dermal matrix manufactured from human cadaveric dermis; new alternative to the fascial graft. Alloderm behaves as an autologous material and can incorporate into the tissues in a contaminated or dirty environment.

○ **What is the Stoppa repair?**

Repair of an incisional hernia with the mesh placed into a retroparietal, preperitoneal position. For the midline incisional hernia, placement of the mesh between the rectus abdominis muscle and its posterior sheath so that the mesh is held in place by intra-abdominal pressure; preoperative pneumoperitoneum to increase the abdominal domain.

○ **How is preoperative pneumoperitoneum performed for large hernias with loss of domain?**

Over 6 to 15 days preoperatively the patient is injected with air into the peritoneal cavity, starting with 500 cc and continuing to as much as 18,500 cc to achieve preoperative expansion of the abdominal cavity and to allow return of the abdominal contents into the abdomen without postoperative respiratory distress.

References

Maxwell GP, McGibbon BM, Hoopes JE. Vascular considerations in the use of a latissimus dorsi myocutaneous flap after a mastectomy with an axillary dissection. *Plast Reconstr Surg.* Dec 1979;64(6):771-780.

Arnold PG, Pairolero PC. Chest-wall reconstruction: an account of 500 consecutive patients. *Plast Reconstr Surg.* Oct 1996;98(5):804-810.

Kroll SS, Walsh G, Ryan B, King RC. Risks and benefits of using Marlex mesh in chest wall reconstruction. *Ann Plast Surg.* Oct 1993;31(4):303-306.

Cosgrove DM, Lytle BW, Loop FD, et al. Does bilateral internal mammary artery grafting increase surgical risk? *J Thorac Cardiovasc Surg.* May 1988;95(5):850-856.

Roth DA. Thoracic and abdominal wall reconstruction. In: Aston SJ, Beasley RW, Thorne CHM, eds. *Grabb and Smith's Plastic Surgery.* 5 ed. Philadelphia: Lippincott-Raven; 1997:1023-1029.

Pairolero PC, Arnold PG. Management of recalcitrant median sternotomy wounds. *J Thorac Cardiovasc Surg.* Sep 1984;88(3):357-364.

Pairolero PC, Arnold PG, Harris JB. Long-term results of pectoralis major muscle transposition for infected sternotomy wounds. *Ann Surg.* Jun 1991;213(6):583-589; discussion 589-590.

Stiegel RM, Beasley ME, Sink JD, et al. Management of postoperative mediastinitis in infants and children by muscle flap rotation. *Ann Thorac Surg.* Jul 1988;46(1):45-46.

Stahl RS, Kopf GS. Reconstruction of infant thoracic wounds. *Plast Reconstr Surg.* Dec 1988;82(6):1000-1011.

Arnold PG, Pairolero PC. Intrathoracic muscle flaps: a 10-year experience in the management of life-threatening infections. *Plast Reconstr Surg.* Jul 1989;84(1):92-98; discussion 99.

de Hoyos A, Sundaresan S. Thoracic empyema. *Surg Clin North Am.* Jun 2002;82(3):643-671, viii.

Miller JI, Mansour KA, Nahai F, Jurkiewicz MJ, Hatcher CR, Jr. Single-stage complete muscle flap closure of the postpneumonectomy empyema space: a new method and possible solution to a disturbing complication. *Ann Thorac Surg.* Sep 1984;38(3):227-231.

Conner CW. Trunk reconstruction. *Selected Readings in Plastic Surgery.* 2002;9(31):1-46.

Roche NA, Van Landuyt K, Blondeel PN, Matton G, Monstrey SJ. The use of pedicled perforator flaps for reconstruction of lumbosacral defects. *Ann Plast Surg.* Jul 2000;45(1):7-14.

Higgins JP, Orlando GS, Blondeel PN. Ischial pressure sore reconstruction using an inferior gluteal artery perforator (IGAP) flap. *Br J Plast Surg.* Jan 2002;55(1):83-85.

Rubin LR. Congenital facial paralysis, including Mobius' syndrome. In: Rubin LR, ed. *The Paralyzed Face.* St. Louis: Mosby - Year Book; 1991:80-86.

Ramirez OM, Ruas E, Dellon AL. "Components separation" method for closure of abdominal-wall defects: an anatomic and clinical study. *Plast Reconstr Surg.* Sep 1990;86(3):519-526.

Thomas WO, 3rd, Parry SW, Rodning CB. Ventral/incisional abdominal herniorrhaphy by fascial partition/release. *Plast Reconstr Surg.* May 1993;91(6):1080-1086.

Fabian TC, Croce MA, Pritchard FE, et al. Planned ventral hernia. Staged management for acute abdominal wall defects. *Ann Surg.* Jun 1994;219(6):643-650; discussion 651-643.

Silverman RP, Singh NK, Li EN, et al. Restoring abdominal wall integrity in contaminated tissue-deficient wounds using autologous fascia grafts. *Plast Reconstr Surg.* Feb 2004;113(2):673-675.

Hirsch EF. Repair of an abdominal wall defect after a salvage laparotomy for sepsis. *J Am Coll Surg.* Feb 2004;198(2):324-328.

Stoppa RE. The treatment of complicated groin and incisional hernias. *World J Surg.* Sep-Oct 1989;13(5):545-554.

Coelho JC, Brenner AS, Freitas AT, Campos AC, Wiederkehr JC. Progressive preoperative pneumoperitoneum in the repair of large abdominal hernias. *Eur J Surg.* Jun-Jul 1993;159(6-7):339-341.

Carlson GW, Bostwick Jr. Abdominal wall reconstruction. In: Auchauer BM, Eriksson E, Guyuron B, Coleman JJr, Russel RC, Vander Kolk CA, eds. *Plastic Surgery: Indications, Operations, and Outcomes.* Vol 1. St. Louis: Mosby; 2000:563-574.

STERNAL WOUND RECONSTRUCTION

Douglas M. Sammer, MD

○ **How frequently does dehiscence of median sternotomy wounds occur?**

1-5 percent of median sternotomy wounds will dehisce.

○ **What are the contributing causes of median sternotomy dehiscence?**

Infection, diabetes, use of the internal mammary artery for bypass grafting, multiple operations, and mechanical factors.

○ **What is the Pairolero classification of infected median sternotomies?**

A three group classification system for describing infected median sternotomies based upon duration and clinical findings.

○ **What is a Type I median sternotomy wound breakdown?**

Within 1-3 days after operation the wound develops breakdown, serosanguinous drainage, and instability. There is no soft tissue, cartilage, or bone infection. Debridement and rewiring of the sternum and reclosure of the wound is required.

○ **What is a Type II median sternotomy wound breakdown?**

Within 2-3 weeks after operation the wound develops cellulitis, osteomyelitis, and mediastinitis, often with purulent drainage. Treatment consists of aggressive debridement, IV antibiotics based on tissue cultures, and immediate or delayed wound closure, usually requiring a flap.

○ **What is a Type III median sternotomy wound breakdown?**

Many months or years after operation the patient develops instability of the sternal wound or a draining sinus tract secondary to osteomyelitis. There is usually not purulent mediastinitis and or cellulitis. Treatment consists of aggressive debridement, IV antibiotics based on tissue cultures, and wound closure, usually requiring a flap.

○ **What are the main goals of reconstruction of a sternal wound?**

Debridement and treatment of infection, obliteration of dead space, and soft tissue coverage. Skeletal stability is not required.

○ **What is the main cause of failure of reconstruction of a dehisced/infected median sternotomy wound?**

Insufficient debridement.

○ **Which is the first choice for flap coverage of sternal wounds?**

Pectoralis major muscle or myocutaneous flaps.

○ **What is the blood supply to the pectoralis major flap?**

It has a type V blood supply, with the primary pedicle being the pectoral branch of the thoracoacromial artery, and the segmental pedicle being the intercostal perforators.

○ **How is the pectoralis major flap used for sternal reconstruction?**

It is most often used as a muscle flap, based on the pectoral branch of the thoracoacromial artery. It is advanced unilaterally or bilaterally into the sternal wound. The insertion on the humerus can be freed, allowing greater advancement. It can also be used as bilateral myocutaneous flaps which are advanced medially to cover the wound.

○ **Can the pectoralis major be used based on its IMA perforators?**

Yes. The pectoralis major muscle can be based on perforators from the internal mammary artery. Its pectoral branch pedicle is divided. Its insertion on the humerus is freed and turned over into the sternal wound. This is contraindicated if the IMA has been used for bypass grafting.

○ **What is the second choice for flap coverage of sternal wounds?**

Rectus abdominis muscle flap.

○ **What is the blood supply to the rectus abdominis flap?**

It has a type III blood supply, with the superior deep and inferior deep epigastric arteries being the two main pedicles. These flaps are based superiorly, on the superior deep epigastric artery.

○ **What is the range of coverage of the rectus abdominis flap?**

It provides better coverage of the inferior aspect of a sternal wound than does the pectoralis major flap. It can reach the superior aspect of the sternal wound.

○ **What is a contraindication of use of a superiorly based rectus abdominis flap?**

A prior subcostal incision or a chevron incision. Any incision that divides the rectus abdominis muscle superiorly disrupts the superior deep epigastric artery, and the muscle cannot be used distal to that incision.

○ **Is the prior use or division of the IMA for bypass grafting a contraindication to using an ipsilateral rectus abdominis flap?**

No. The rectus abdominis has good collateral blood supply superiorly. Intercostal and subcostal arteries (T8 is the dominant one) supply the deep superior epigastric artery sufficiently if the IMA is divided.

○ **What is another good flap for sternal wounds?**

The omentum flap.

○ **What is the blood supply to the greater omentum?**

The left and right gastroepiploic arteries.

○ **When used as a pedicled flap to repair a sternal wound, what is the blood supply to the omentum?**

Often, the flap will reach to fill the defect if both the left and right gastroepiploic arteries are intact. However, it is sometimes necessary to divide the left gastroepiploic artery to gain more distance.

○ **When should a free flap be used for sternal reconstruction?**

Only when regional flaps are not possible or have already failed.

○   **What is the most common organism identified in sternal infections / mediastinitis?**

Staphylococcus species.

○   **Should debridement and flap coverage be performed in one stage, or should flap coverage be performed in a delayed fashion after debridement and dressing changes or closed drainage?**

Studies indicate that aggressive debridement and immediate flap coverage has a very high success rage (approximately 95%) and avoids the drawbacks of delayed closure, such as multiple operations and prolonged exposure of mediastinal contents.

○   **What are other advantages of flap closure of infected / dehisced sternal wounds?**

Decreased hospital stay and cost.

References

Cohen M. Reconstruction of the chest wall. In: Cohen M, ed. Mastery of Plastic and Reconstructive Surgery. Boston: Little, Brown and Company, 1994:1248-1267.

Rosenthal AH. Thoracic and abdominal reconstruction. In: Brown DL, Borschel GH, eds. Michigan Manual of Plastic Surgery. Philadelphia: Lippincott Williams&Wilkins, 2004:344-348.

Roth DA. Thoracic and abdominal wall reconstruction. In: Aston SJ, Beasley RW, Thorne CHM, eds. Grabb and Smith's Plastic Surgery. 5th ed. Philadelphia: Lippincott-Raven, 1997:1023-1029.

Seyfer AE. Chest wall reconstruction. In: Achauer BM, Eriksson E, eds. Plastic Surgery Indications, Operations, and Outcomes. St. Louis: Mosby, 2000:547-562.

LOWER EXTREMITY RECONSTRUCTION – SOFT TISSUE CONCEPTS

Robert E. H. Ferguson, Jr., MD and Lee Q. Pu, MD, Ph.D.

○ **What are the boundaries of the femoral triangle?**

- Proximally – inguinal ligament
- Laterally – sartorius
- Medially – adductor longus
- Floor – iliacus, psoas, pectineus, adductor longus

○ **What nerve innervates the anterior femoral (extensor group) muscles?**

Femoral nerve.

○ **The medial femoral (adductor group) muscles are primarily innervated by what nerve?**

Obturator nerve (the pectineus is innervated by the obturator nerve medially and the femoral nerve laterally; the adductor magnus is innervated by the obturator nerve and the tibial division of the sciatic nerve).

○ **What are the compartments of the lower extremity?**

- anterior
- lateral
- superficial posterior
- deep posterior

○ **Which muscles of the lower extremity are located in the superficial posterior compartment?**

- gastrocnemius (medial and lateral heads)
- plantaris
- soleus

○ **Deep posterior compartment?**

- flexor hallucis longus
- tibialis posterior
- flexor digitorum longus

○ **Lateral compartment?**

- peroneus brevis
- peroneus longus

○ **Anterior compartment?**

- tibialis anterior
- extensor digitorum longus
- extensor hallucis longus

○ **In which compartments do the trifurcated arteries travel in the lower extremity?**

Anterior tibial artery – anterior compartment.
Posterior tibial artery – deep posterior compartment
Peroneal artery – deep posterior compartment

○ **What nerve may accompany the lesser saphenous vein and what does it innervate?**

The **sural nerve** provides sensation to the skin over the posterolateral lower extremity, the lateral heel, and the lateral border of the foot.

○ **The plantar surface of the foot may be divided into four layers. Which muscles may be found in the most superficial layer?**

- flexor digitorum brevis
- abductor hallucis
- abductor digiti quinti

○ **What nerves provide sensation to the foot and what are their respective dermatomes?**

- Posterior tibial nerve – plantar midfoot and heel
- Sural nerve – lateral midfoot
- Saphenous nerve – medial ankle
- Superficial peroneal nerve – dorsal distal foot
- Deep peroneal nerve – first web space

○ **Which nerve of the lower extremity is the preferred donor nerve for grafting?**

Sural nerve.

○ **What findings are indicative of compartment syndrome?**

- paresthesia
- pain on passive extension
- pallor
- pulseless
- palpable tenseness
- compartmental pressures > 35 mmHg (or differential pressure < 30)

Keep in mind that absence of a pulse is a late finding as venous and lymphatic flow through the compartment will occlude prior to compression of arterial flow. A differential pressure is obtained by subtracting the compartmental pressure from the patient's diastolic pressure.

○ **How do you treat a compartment syndrome of the lower extremity?**

Fasciotomies. Medial and lateral longitudinal incisions should allow adequate exposure to incise intermuscular septae thereby releasing all four compartments. Remember that fasciotomies will also be appropriate for expected severe elevation in compartment pressures that are associated with crush injury, electrical burn, massive fluid resuscitation, and reperfusion injury.

○ **What is the procedure of choice for reconstruction of small to medium defects of the plantar surface of the foot?**

V-Y plantar advancement flap. The plantar skin and fascia should be incised congruently to maintain intact the vessels perforating the fascia from the medial and lateral plantar arteries.

○   **What would you do to reconstruct a more extensive defect of the plantar foot in an ambulatory patient?**

Provide soft tissue coverage that is durable and tolerant of shear forces experienced with ambulation. A muscle flap with a skin graft has been shown to perform well for such reconstructions.

○   **What additional measures should be considered when reconstructing the plantar surface of the foot?**

If the plantar surface is insensate, the patient should be educated on being vigilant and meticulous in caring for the foot. Custom orthotics with a metatarsal bar should decrease metatarsal head pressure and shearing and compression forces on the reconstructed foot.

○   **What is the Gustillo classification system for tibial injury?**

Gustillo Classification

I		Low energy, simple bone fracture, wound < 1 cm
II		Moderate comminution and contamination, wound > 1 cm, moderate soft tissue damage
III		High energy, comminution of the fracture, wound > 1 cm, extensive soft tissue damage
	A	Adequate soft tissue cover
	B	Inadequate soft tissue coverage, extensive periosteal stripping
	C	IIIB with associated arterial injury

○   **What is the Byrd classification system for tibial injury?**

Byrd Classification

I	Low-energy fracture, oblique or spiral fracture with clean-cut laceration < 1 cm
II	Medium-energy trauma, displaced or comminuted fracture with laceration > 2 cm, myocutaneous contusion
III	High-energy trauma, severely displaced or comminuted fracture, segmental fracture or bone defect, laceration > 2 cm, myocutaneous soft tissue loss
IV	High-energy bursting trauma, crushing or avulsion with arterial damage (that requires repair)

○   **What muscles can be used to reconstruct the soft tissue over the proximal 1/3 of the tibia?**

Medial gastrocnemius (medial sural artery and venae comitantes).
Lateral gastrocnemius (lateral sural artery and venae comitantes).

○   **What muscle can be used to reconstruct the soft tissue over the middle 1/3 of the tibia?**

Soleus (branches of the popliteal, posterior tibial, and peroneal arteries and their venae comitantes). Modifications of this muscle may be made, such as a hemisoleus for greater arc of rotation.

○   **What muscle can be used to reconstruct the soft tissue over the distal 1/3 of the tibia?**

Free muscle transfer. The choice of muscle will depend upon the extent of soft tissue injury, necessary pedicle length, and the surgeon's familiarity. While a free tissue transfer for a distal 1/3 open tibial fracture is the classic answer, there are possibilities of local flaps such as a distally-based hemisoleus flap.

○   **Within what timeframe should an osteocutaneous defect of the tibia receive definitive soft tissue reconstruction?**

Infection rates increase after 5 days and other major complications increase after 15 days. Given ideal circumstances, soft tissue reconstruction after adequate debridement should be within 5 days of the injury.

○   **A reverse-flow sural artery flap is used to reconstruct a calcaneous wound. To best preserve the vascularity of this flap, the distal dissection of the pedicle should terminate where?**

5 cm above the lateral malleolus

○   **When might amputation be recommended over lower extremity salvage?**

- insensate foot
- loss of plantar flexion
- ischemia time > 6 hours
- severe medical illness
- tibial loss > 8 cm (although some surgeons have reported successful reconstruction with free fibula transfer from the contralateral leg with defects larger than this).

References

Francel TJ, Vander Kolk CA, Hoopes JE, Manson PN, Yaremchuk MJ. Microvascular soft-tissue transplantation for reconstruction of acute open tibial fractures: timing of coverage and long-term functional results. Plast Reconstr Surg 1992: 89:478-87.

Gustilo RB, Mendoza RM, Williams DN. Problems in the management of type III (severe) open fractures: a new classification of type III open fractures. J Trauma 1987; 24:742-746.

Hasegawa M. The distally based superficial sural artery flap. Plast Reconstr Surg 1994; 93:1012-1014.

Kasabian AK, Karp NS. Lower extremity reconstruction. In: Aston SJ, Beasley RW, Thorne CH, eds. Grabb and Smith's Plastic Surgery. 5th ed. Philadelphia:Lippincott-Raven Publishers, 1997:1031-1048.

May Jr JW, Rohrich RJ. Foot reconstruction using free microvascular muscle flaps with skin grafts. Clin Plast Surg 1986; 13:681-689.

Thorne CH, Siebert JW, Grotting JC, et al. Reconstructive surgery of the lower extremity. In: McCarthy JG, ed. Plastic Surgery. Philadelphia: WB Saunders Co, 1990:4029-4092.

LOWER EXTREMITY RECONSTRUCTION – ORTHOPEDIC CONCEPTS

Gary Ross, MBChB, MRCS, MD

○ **What is the blood supply of the femur?**

a) Main supply is the trochanteric anastomsosis, (superior gluteal, inferior gluteal, medial circumflex and lateral circumflex)
b) also the nutrient artery passing along femoral neck beneath the capsule
c) connection between trochanteric anastomosis and cruciate anastomosis at level of lower trochanter.

○ **What is the blood supply of the tibia?**

Tibial endosteal artery enters from tibia posteriorly at the junction of the proximal and middle thirds and runs distally/obliquely for 5.5 cm then branches proximally and distally. Also metaphyseal artery and periosteal supply.

○ **What is the blood supply of the fibula?**

Nutrient pedicle from peroneal artery enters fibula posterior to the interosseous membrane 17cm below the styloid process in middle third of the fibula

○ **How many compartments exist in the thigh and leg. Which muscles, nerves and blood vessels lie in which compartments?**

Thigh

Compartment	Motor Nerve	Blood supply	Muscles
Anterior	Femoral (L2-4)	Femoral	Quadriceps Femoris, Sartorius Iliopsoas, Pectineus
Medial	Obturator (L2-4)	Profunda Femoris Obturator	Gracilis, Adductor Longus Adductor Brevis, Adductor Magnus, Obturator Externus
Posterior	Sciatic (L4-S3)	Profunda Femoris (branches)	Biceps Femoris, Semitendinosus Semimembranosus Adductor Magnus

Lower leg

Compartment	Motor Nerve	Blood Supply	Muscles
Anterior	Deep peroneal	Tibialis Anterior	Tibialis anterior Extensor digitorum longus Extensor hallucis longus Peroneus tertius
Lateral	Sup peroneal	Peroneal	Peroneus longus Peroneus brevis
Sup Posterior	Tibialis (branches)	Tibialis Posterior (branches)	Gastrocnemius Plantaris Soleus

Deep Posterior	Tibialis	Tibialis Posterior	Popliteus Flexor digitorum longus Flexor hallucis longus Tibialis posterior

❍   **Which nerves supply sensation to the foot?**

Dorsum:- superficial peroneal except the first web which is supplied by the deep peroneal
Sole:- medial and lateral plantar's from the posterior tibial

❍   **The classification using the mangled extremity severity score (MESS, Johansen 1990) classifies patients according to which 4 criteria?**

• shock
• ischemia
• age
• skeletal/soft tissue damage

❍   **For what MESS score is amputation recommended?**

7 or higher

❍   **What is Gustillo's classification of open tibial fractures as modified in 1998?**

I   "with cutaneous defect <1cm, clean, little soft tissue injury"
II   "laceration >1cm, no extensive soft-tissue injury, no flaps or avulsions"
           moderate crush injury & comminution of # & contamination
III   extensive soft tissue damage with muscle & sometimes n/vasc, high contamination "included are high
           energy, industrial, segmental & severe comminution"
IIIA   "extensive soft-tissue lacerations, high-energy injury but cover available"
IIIB   "soft-tissue loss & periosteal stripping, massive contamination, bone comminution or loss"
IIIC   any injury with arterial injury requiring repair regardless of soft tissue damage degree

❍   **What is the amputation rate for Gustillo grade IIIC tibial fracture?**

87%

❍   **What reconstructive options are available for coverage of knee defects/<u>upper third tibia</u> defects?**

• fasciocutaneous flaps
• muscle flaps
• free flaps
Medial head of gastrocnemius is the most popular.

❍   **What reconstructive options are available for <u>middle third tibial</u> defects?**

• fasciocutaneous
• soleus flap
• tibialis anterior flap
• free flap

❍   **What reconstructive options are available for <u>lower third tibial</u> defects?**

• distally based fasciocutaneous
• adipofascial turnover flap
• sural artery flap

- free flap

○ **What reconstructive options are available for ankle/heel defects?**

- distally based islanded fasciocutaneous
- sural artery flap
- free flap

Smaller defects can be covered by medial and lateral plantar flaps, dorsalis pedis.

○ **Which region of the lower limb are free flaps most commonly used for reconstruction?**

Ankle and lower third tibia

○ **According to Godina pts requiring free flap reconstruction for tibial coverage are classified as reconstructed <u>early</u> (<72hrs), <u>delayed</u> (>72hrs and <3 months) or <u>late</u> (>3 months).**
a) Microvascular failure and infection was commonest in which group?

Delayed group

a) Microvascular success and absence of infection was commonest in which group?

Early group

○ **For Gustillo 111b fractures what is the recommended form of fixation?**

Unreamed intramedullary nailing. External fixation may be required if nailing is not possible.

○ **Can a microvascular anastomosis be performed within the zone of injury?**

Although the anastomosis is preferred to be outside the zone of trauma, Kolker has shown the possibility of anastomosis within the zone of injury.

○ **What is the approach of splitting the gastrocnemius to posterior tibial artery called?**

Godina's posterior approach.

○ **A bone gap of over 10 cm exists in the tibia.**
a) What are the reconstructive options?

Acute shortening and subsequent lengthening using an Ilizarov frame or free vascularized bone.

b) Which vascularized bone would you use?

Free fibula flap from the contralateral leg.

○ **Ilizarov distraction osteogenesis distracts approximately at what rate?**

0.25mm distraction x4/day

○ **After the desired length of bone is achieved how long is the Ilizarov frame left on?**

For the same length of time as the distraction to allow <u>consolidation</u>.

○ **What is the ideal length of stump that should be preserved for a below knee amputation?**

10 – 15cm although modern prosthesis can be fitted with even shorter stumps

○ **What is a Lisfranc amputation?**

Amputation through the level of the transmetatarsal joints

○ **What is a Symes amputation?**

Amputation just above the ankle joint.

○ **What are the first signs in compartment syndrome?**

General pain and tingling in the limb out of proportion with the injury with **<u>pain on passive extension</u>** of the involved muscle groups.

○ **What is the normal tissue pressure?**

2-7mmHg

○ **At what tissue pressure is one concerned of compartment syndrome?**

>30mmHg

○ **What incisions would you use to perform fasciotomies to the lower leg?**

Two vertical incisions 2cm to either side of the subcutaneous border of the tibia.

○ **Through which of the above incisions would you decompress the posterior compartments?**

Usually the medial one

○ **Which compartments are released via the lateral incision?**

Anterior and lateral compartments

○ **What is the commonest organism associated with acute osteomyelitis?**

Staphylococcus aureus.

○ **In children which organism is commonly associated with acute osteomyelitis other than *Staphylococcus aureus*?**

Haemophilus influenzae.

○ **For free flap reconstruction of the lower limb what are the advantages of fasciocutaneous flaps over muscle flaps?**

They are thinner, may be sensate and revisional surgery is easier.

○ **For free flap reconstruction of the lower limb what are the advantages of muscle flaps over fasciocutaneous flaps?**

Fill cavities more effectively, and thought to be better at reducing infection.

○ **What are the common presenting complaints of a patient with chronic osteomyelitis?**

- pain
- pyrexia

- redness
- tenderness
- discharging sinus

○ **What are the typical X-ray appearances of a patient with chronic osteomyelitis?**

Bone rarefaction surrounded by sclerosis and sometimes sequestra.

PRESSURE SORE TREATMENT

Clark F. Schierle, MD, PhD

○ **What is the etiology of pressure sores?**

Tissue ischemia and hypoxia from prolonged pressure above the 32mm Hg of the capillary bed

○ **Where are the most common sites of pressure sores?**

The ischial tuberosity, the trochanter, and the sacrum.

○ **How are pressure sores graded?**

On a four stage scale

○ **What are the characteristics of a stage I pressure sore?**

Intact skin with non-blanching erythema

○ **What are the characteristics of a stage II pressure sore?**

Partial thickness skin loss.

○ **What are the characteristics of a stage III pressure sore?**

Full thickness skin loss with involvement of subcutaneous tissues extending down to but not including deep fascia

○ **What are the characteristics of a stage IV pressure sore?**

Involvement of deep structures including muscle, bone, joint capsules, etc…

○ **Why is the term decubitus ulcer to be avoided?**

Prolonged pressure irrespective of the patient's position (supine, lateral decubitus, sitting) leads to the development of sores through tissue ischemia and necrosis, not erosion as implied by the term ulcer.

○ **What are some basic principles guiding pressure sore treatment and reconstruction?**

Pressure relief: the etiology of the pressure sore must be identified and eliminated with more frequent turnings, elimination of pressure points, special mattresses. Nutrition: patients must achieve an anabolic state for optimum wound healing, supplementation with high protein shakes, vitamins or other supplements may be necessary. Debridement of nonvital tissue: thorough debridement of any nonvital or infected tissue is at least as critical as choice of flap for reconstruction.

○ **What is the gold standard test for osteomyelitis in association with pressure sores?**

Bone biopsy

○ **What other tests can assist in the diagnosis?**

Lytic bone changes on plain film or CT, or inflammation on MRI, as an elevated white count, erythrocyte sedimentation rate and C-reactive protein are all suggestive of osteomyelitis.

○ **What is appropriate treatment for osteomyelitis?**

Six to eight weeks of intravenous antibiotic therapy.

○ **What is the etiology of spasticity in paraplegics?**

Elimination of higher CNS suppression of spinal reflex arcs leading to hypertonia and hyperreflexia

○ **What is the significance of spasticity in pressure sore management?**

It can exacerbate pressure points, place tension on wound edges, and contribute to joint or muscle contracture.

○ **What are some treatments for spasticity?**

Systemic diazepam or baclofen, intrathecal baclofen, phenol or alcohol, neurosurgical treatment with cordotomy or rhizotomy.

○ **What are some reconstructive options for sacral and ischial pressure sores?**

Gluteus maximus musculocutaneous flap, superior gluteal artery perforator (SGAP) fasciocutaneous flap, lumbosacral perforator fasciocutaneous flap, gracilis musculocutaneous flap or muscle flap with skin graft, rectus femoris mycocutaneous flap. These are typically used as rotation or V-Y advancement flaps.

○ **What is the definitive treatment for trochanteric pressure sores with involvement of the hip joint?**

Girdlestone arthroplasty with vastus lateralis muscle flap ablation of the dead space.

○ **What is the blood supply to the gluteus maximus?**

It is a Mathes & Nahai type III muscle with dominant pedicles comprised of the superior and inferior gluteal arteries. The piriformis muscle serves as the anatomic landmark separating the two pedicles.

○ **What is the blood supply to the gracilis?**

It is a Mathes & Nahai type II muscle with its dominant pedicle supplied by the medial circumflex femoral artery which arises from the profunda femoris.

○ **What is the blood supply to the vastus lateralis?**

It is a Mathes & Nahai type II muscle with its dominant pedicle supplied by the descending branch of the lateral circumflex femoral artery which arises from the profunda femoris.

○ **What is the blood supply to the rectus femoris?**

It is a Mathes & Nahai type II muscle with its dominant pedicle supplied by the lateral circumflex femoral artery which arises from the profunda femoris.

References

Braden BJ, Bergstrom N. Clinical utility of the Braden scale for Predicting Pressure Sore Risk. Decubitus 1989;2(3):44-6, 50-1.

Evans GR, Lewis VL, Jr., Manson PN, Loomis M, Vander Kolk CA. Hip joint communication with pressure sore: the refractory wound and the role of girdlestone arthroplasty. Plast Reconstr Surg 1993;91(2):288-94.

Lewis VL, Jr., Bailey MH, Pulawski G, Kind G, Bashioum RW, Hendrix RW. The diagnosis of osteomyelitis in patients with pressure sores. Plast Reconstr Surg 1988;81(2):229-32.

Mathes SJ, Nahai F. Clinical atlas of muscle and musculocutaneous flaps. St. Louis: Mosby; 1979.

Mathes SJ, Nahai F. Clinical applications for muscle and musculocutaneous flaps. St. Louis: Mosby; 1982.

Mathes SJ, Nahai F. Reconstructive surgery : principles, anatomy & technique. New York St. Louis: Churchill Livingstone; Quality Medical Pub. 1997.

Norton D. Calculating the risk: reflections on the Norton Scale. 1989. Adv Wound Care 1996;9(6):38-43.

HIGH-YIELD
QUESTIONS/ANSWERS

Samuel J. Lin, MD

AESTHETIC AND BREAST SURGERY

○ **What is the Antia-Buch flap used for?**

Lesions located on the lateral rim; tissue used from postauricular skin to reconstruct the helical margin.

○ **Where on the avulsed pinna is anastomosis of the arteries most appropriate?**

The posterior surface; larger arteries enter the pinna on the posterior surface.

○ **What type of basal cell carcinoma requires additional excision by Moh's technique?**

Morpheaform; also known as sclerosing basal cell carcinoma.

○ **Compared to traditional transaxillary submuscular breast augmentation, endoscopic techniques are associated with a decreased rate of what?**

Malpositioning of the implant.

○ **Where does the common canaliculus enters the lacrimal sac posterior to?**

The medial canthal tendon.

○ **Breast ptosis results from elongation and laxity of what structure?**

Cooper's ligaments.

○ **With tumescence during suction lipectomy, what percentage total blood loss is to be expected of the total aspirate?**

1%.

○ **The wet technique?**

This technique utilizes 300 ml of fluid per region – 25 % blood in the aspirate.

○ **What branch of the facial nerve is injured most frequently during face lift?**

Buccal.

○ **What are the three zones of injury occurring in a nasal fracture?**

Upper vault (nasal bones, ethmoid, vomer, cephalic septal border); middle vault (upper lateral cartilages, septum, maxilla); lower vault (alar cartilages, inferior septum).

○ **What muscle is most commonly injured in blepharoplasty?**

Superior oblique; clinically may see tilting of head, and depression of chin.

○ **What effect do corticosteroids have on edema and ecchymosis following rhytidectomy?**

No change in both instance.

○ **What is the procedure required for a patient who exhibits a Jones I test without dye and a Jones II test with dye in the tear sac?**

Dacryocystorhinostomy.

○ **How is a Jones I test performed?**

Instill 2% fluoroscein dye into the conjunctival fornices; recovery of dye indicates a normal lacrimal system (or positive result); a negative result necessitates a Jones II test.

○ **How is a Jones II test performed?**

Dilation of the punta is performed first; fluid passing into the nose indicates that obstruction of the nasolacrimal duct is cleared.

○ **Complications from smoking arise in what percentage of patients undergoing abdominoplasty?**

50%.

○ **What period of time should be told to the smoking patient undergoing surgery?**

Discontinue smoking 4-8 weeks before surgery and 4 weeks after surgery.

○ **Mastectomy resulting in decreased bulk in the inferior and lateral portions of the right pectoral muscle is caused by denervation of what nerve?**

Medial pectoral; C8-T1 supplies lower and lateral sternal portion of pectoralis major and pectoralis minor muscle.

○ **What does the lateral pectoral nerve supply?**

Arises from C5-6, supplies the medial portion of the pectoralis muscle.

○ **How does one assess the status of the pectoralis muscle in post-mastectomy reconstruction?**

Have patient place hands on hips and contract chest muscles.

○ **What nerve supplies the sensation of the nipple-areola complex?**

The 4th intercostal nerve.

○ **What characterizes aponeurotic ptosis?**

Good levator function; elevation of eyelid crease, ability to visualize shadow of iris with eyelid closure (positive Nesi sign) or translucent upper eyelid.

○ **What are mechanisms of ptosis?**

Mechanical, myogenic, neurogenic.

○ **During breast augmentation, underfilling of the implants below the manufacturer's recommended minimum will most likely have what effect?**

Decreases longevity of the implant and leads to early rupture.

○ **What is the limit at which airway resistance increases in the internal nasal valve?**

Less than 10-12 degrees.

○ **What defines the internal nasal valve area?**

The caudal margin of the upper lateral cartilage, septum, nasal floor, and anterior edge of inferior turbinate.

○ **Treatment of an auricular hematoma by needle aspiration is likely to result in what?**

Seroma.

○ **In addition to contour irregularities, UAL is likely to cause what complication more frequently than SAL?**

Thermal injury.

○ **What adverse effect is lessened by endoscopic browlifting as opposed to conventional coronal browlifting?**

Scalp sensibility changes.

○ **What advantage does an extended latissimus dorsi flap have over a standard latissimus dorsi flap in the setting of breast reconstruction?**

A decreased need for adjuvant breast implantation.

○ **Secondary healing of what part of the nose is least likely to provide an acceptable cosmetic result?**

The nasal tip.

○ **What mammographic finding is seen 6 to 18 months following an inferior pedicle reduction mammoplasty?**

Parenchymal redistribution, nipple elevation, calcifications, oil cysts from localized fat necrosis.

○ **Breast reduction by liposuction is most useful in breasts with what percentage of fat?**

50%.

○ **What procedure will address lower eyelid skin laxity with 2mm of scleral show bilaterally?**

Lower lid blepharoplasty with lateral canthopexy.

○ **In a young patient undergoing MRM with postop radiation, what procedure will provide the best aesthetic reconstruction?**

Delayed reconstruction with autologous tissue.

○ **In a study comparing early and late complications in patients who underwent TRAM reconstruction followed by radiation vs. radiation treatment followed by TRAM reconstruction, what were the differences?**

The early complications did not differ, but the late complications were more frequent in the group undergoing immediate reconstruction.

O   **Following lower lid blepharoplasty, a woman exhibiting scleral show, round, sad looking eyes, photophobia, epiphora, what has anatomically occurred?**

Scarring between the orbital septum and the capsulopalpebral fascia, resulting in lower lid retraction (without lid eversion); other causes include lateral canthal tendon laxity, midface descent.

O   **A six year old boy with an obtuse concha-mastoid angle with a normal antihelical fold is best treated by what technique?**

Setback of the concha using concha-mastoid sutures.

O   **What are common causes of prominent ears?**

Enlarged conchal bowl, obtuse concha-mastoid angle, loss of the anti-helical fold.

O   **How is ear prominence corrected from loss of the antihelical fold?**

Abrading or scoring the antihelix and placing Mustarde sutures between the conchal and scaphoid eminence.

O   **A woman who has the BRCA-2 mutation has a lifetime incidence of what percentage of developing breast cancer?**

60%.

O   **Compared with primary rhytidectomy, distortion of the hairline is more or less frequent in secondary rhytidectomy?**

More likely to occur; if the same incisions are used, recession of the temporal hairline, obliteration of sideburn hair, and alopecia may occur.

O   **Are the risks of hematoma, hypertrophic scarring, and skin slough higher in the setting of secondary rhytidectomy?**

Typically not.

O   **What is the eyelid function in patients with Bell's palsy?**

Ectropion from dysfunction of the orbicularis muscle; inability to close the eye.

O   **Sharp dissection lateral to the lateral edge of the pectoralis muscle during augmentation mammaplasty may result in what complication?**

Numbness of the nipple-areola complex; the fourth and fifth anterolateral intercostal nerves provide sensation to the nipple-areola complex.

O   **In a patient with microgenia who has both bony deficiencies in the anteroposterior and vertical dimensions, what is the most appropriate treatment?**

Osseous genioplasty.

O   **How well does chin implantation correct vertical deficiency of the chin?**

It only corrects anteroposterior dimension.

❍ **What is consistently the best marking for the new nipple position during reduction mammaplasty?**

The inframammary fold.

❍ **What techniques have important roles in providing tip projection in addition to tip grafting?**

Suturing of the medial crura, placing a strut graft between the medial crura.

❍ **What effect occurs with resection of the lateral and medial crura and the nasal spine?**

Decrease of tip projection.

❍ **What effect does a complete transfixion incision have?**

Decreases projection secondary to weakening of nasal support.

❍ **Sensation to the nipple-areolar complex is derived from what?**

Anterolateral branches of the 3rd through 5th intercostal nerves (primarily the 4th nerve).

❍ **True or false: Suction lipectomy may be an effective procedure for management of axillary hyperhidrosis, HIV-associated lipodystrophy, lymphedema, and Madelung's disease.**

True.

❍ **What is Madelung's disease?**

Benign symmetric lipomatosis; diffuse growth of nonencapsulated lipomas, in neck, shoulders, posterior trunk.

❍ **T/F: The evaluation of the nasal airway should include the nasal dorsum.**

False.

❍ **T/F: Microtia and inner ear abnormalities may be closely related.**

False.

❍ **What is orbital auricular vertebral syndrome otherwise known as?**

Goldenhar syndrome (associated with microtia, cervical spine abnormalities, mandibular hypoplasia, preauricular pits/sinuses, hemifacial microsomia).

❍ **What nerve is typically involved in Frey's syndrome?**

Auriculotemporal nerve, a branch of V.

❍ **What is the nerve of Jacobson?**

The tympanic branch of IX, which provides sensation to the tympanic cavity.

❍ **In a patient with a negative Cottle maneuver, what procedure is likely to improve the nasal airway?**

Lateral strut graft of the crus.

❍ **What comprises the external nasal valve?**

Columella, ala, nasal sill.

○   **What comprises the internal nasal valve?**

Area of the angle between the upper lateral cartilage and septum.

○   **An 1:1 infiltrate to aspirate ratio during liposuction indicates which technique?**

Superwet.

○   **What defines tumescent technique during liposuction?**

2-3 cc wetting solution/1 cc of aspirate.

○   **What is the wet technique?**

Injecting 100-300 cc of wetting solution per area regardless of amount of aspirate removed.

○   **Transverse rhytids along the root of the nose are from which muscle group?**

Procerus (originates from upper lateral cartilage inserting into skin/glabella.

○   **What is the origin/insertion of the corrugator?**

Originate along periosteum/medial orbital rim inserting into dermis of upper eyelid.

○   **What develops from the first three hillocks of the ear during development?**

1st three hillocks are from the 1st arch; tragus, helical root, superior helix.

○   **What develops from the second three hillocks of the ear?**

Antitragus, antihelix, inferior helix and lobule; from the 2nd branchial arch.

○   **Define pseudoptosis of the breast.**

The nipple remains above the IMF, but the breast mass descends below the NAC.

○   **What is second degree ptosis?**

The nipple is located beneath the IMF, but is not the lowest point of the breast.

○   **What is first degree?**

The NAC descends to the level of the IMF.

○   **Following a face lift, an inability to raise the upper lip on one side is due to what complication?**

Injury to the buccal branch of the facial nerve (innervates levator labii oris).

○   **What does injury to the cervical branch of the facial nerve manifest as?**

Platysma weakening, or an asymmetric smile.

○   **What must be evaluated first during a consult for chin implantation?**

The patient's occlusion.

○ **Fullness of the lateral orbit noted during browlift may be due to what structure?**

A ptotic lacrimal gland.

○ **What is the treatment of a ptotic lacrimal gland?**

Suspension of the gland, not resection.

○ **What is the mechanism of greater dermal injury with the CO2 laser as compared with the Er:YAG laser?**

The Er:YAG laser has an affinity for water that is 10x greater; also the pulse rate is shorter than that of the CO2 laser.

○ **What may be done to improve excess scleral show and slowed retraction of a "snap-back" test following blepharoplasty?**

Lateral canthopexy.

○ **A painful vesicular rash in the days following CO2 laser treatment of facial rhytids is best treated by what method?**

Acyclovir (prophylactic treatment is important).

○ **Is isotretinoin used for premedicating laser patients?**

No; Accutane is contraindicated.

○ **How is vestibular stenosis treated?**

An alar base flap.

○ **In polymastia, where are accessory mammary structure most commonly found?**

The axilla.

○ **What is the treatment principle of cryptotia?**

Detaching the superior auricle from the temporal area and placing a skin graft in the retroauricular area.

○ **How is Stahl's ear treated?**

Advancing the 3rd crus of the antihelix.

○ **Placing sutures from the concha to the mastoid bowl and rasping the anterior surface of the antihelix has been described for what condition?**

Correction of prominent ears.

○ **How is the constricted ear treated?**

Partially detaching the helix from the scapha and suturing the helix.

○ **Reanimation of the lower face 3 years following Bell's palsy with resultant good eye coverage is best treated in what manner?**

Neurotized free muscle transfer using cross-facial grafts; facial muscle atrophy occurs after 18 months of absent innervation.

❍ **How is a "hanging" columella treated?**

Trimming of the caudal margin of the septum and medial crura of the lower lateral cartilage.

❍ **What is the most common complication following 30% TCA peeling?**

Hyperpigmentation.

❍ **What complication is associated with phenol peeling?**

Cardiac arrhythmias.

❍ **With laser treatments?**

HSV reactivation.

❍ **What approach is used for browlift in a 60 year old woman with a high hairline with brow descent under the level of the supraorbital rim?**

Open browlift through a hairline incision.

❍ **What may cause resorption of the malar fat pad following rhytidectomy?**

Disruption of the branches of the angular artery; significant in malar fat pad advancement greater than 2 cm.

❍ **What is the most common cause of asymmetric enlargement of a breast over a year with a palpable mass in a teenage girl?**

Fibroadenoma; treat with excision.

❍ **What is the treatment for an auricular implant (porous polyethylene) covered with a temporoparietal fascial flap with subsequent exposure of the implant?**

Dressing changes and secondary wound healing for at least six months.

❍ **What supplies sensation to the NAC?**

The LATERAL cutaneous branch from T4.

❍ **What supplies sensation to the upper breast?**

Cervical branches from the 3rd and 4th .

❍ **The medial and inferior breast?**

Branches from the anterior cutaneous branches.

❍ **How is a patient treated with 3.5 mm of ptosis and 10 mm levator function?**

Re-suturing of the levator aponeurosis.

❍ **What are the classifications of ptosis?**

Neurogenic, myogenic, mechanical, aponeurotic.

○ **When is eyebrow suspension used for ptosis treatment?**

Poor levator function (less than 4 mm) and greater than 3 mm of ptosis.

○ **When is the Fasanella-Servat procedure used?**

Good levator function and minimal ptosis (less than 2 mm).

○ **What procedure is used for levator function between 4 and 10 mm and 3mm ptosis?**

Levator resection.

○ **What agent is typically used in rejuvenating fine facial rhytids?**

TCA (15% to 35%).

○ **What is a critical factor in deciding breast contouring following implant removal?**

Preoperative ptosis (remains unchanged following removal).

○ **What best determines performing contouring and implant removal in the same setting?**

Thickness of residual breast (minimum thickness of 4 cm required).

○ **What is the treatment for bone resorption following chin implantation with chin asymmetry?**

Implant removal, bone graft, and sliding genioplasty.

○ **Numbness of the anterolateral thigh after abdominoplasty is due to what complication?**

Injury to the lateral femoral cutaneous nerve (becomes superficial 10 cm below the anterior superior iliac spine).

○ **What is the course of the lateral femoral cutaneous nerve?**

Arises from L2-3, passes 1 cm medial to the ASIS, superficial to the sartorius, and branches anteriorly and posteriorly.

○ **What does the genitofemoral nerve innervate?**

Sensation to skin of scrotum, mons pubis, labia and over the superior portion of the femoral triangle.

○ **What does the iliohypogastric supply?**

Sensation to the skin of the lateral buttocks and abdomen above the pubis.

○ **What does the ilioinguinal nerve supply?**

Sensation to the superomedial thigh and scrotum or mons pubis.

○ **The obturator nerve?**

Skin of the medial and lower thigh.

○ **What is the first treatment for nipple cyanosis following breast reduction?**

Releasing the sutures surrounding the NAC and return to the OR.

❍   **What are criterion for free nipple grafting?**

Reduction amount greater than 1500 grams, nipple transposition length greater than 25 cm, and a smoking or history of diabetes.

❍   **What is the treatment of 4 mm ptosis and 2 mm levator function in a 5 year old?**

Frontalis suspension.

❍   **What is associated with inadvertent blepharoptosis – Botox injection of the corrugator or lateral orbicularis?**

The corrugator.

❍   **What is the treatment of an obtuse cervicomental angle, marked fat pads in anterior neck, subcutaneous banding, and loose redundant skin in the neck?**

Removal of cervical fat and platysmaplasty.

❍   **Transcutaneous lower lid blepharoplasty is associated with what undesired finding most commonly?**

Malpositioned lower eyelids.

❍   **What may be done for asymmetrical lower eyelids following blepharoplasty?**

Conservative (taping, Frost stitches) treatment first; surgery for failed conservative treatment (tarsal strip, wedge tarsectomy).

❍   **What factors lead to a saddle nose deformity?**

Excessive dorsal or septal resection, nasal bone comminution during infracture, or a fracture of the perpendicular ethmoid plate.

❍   **What is the next step in a resection specimen following reduction mammaplasty containing invasive ductal carcinoma?**

Determine tumor margins; decide on completion mastectomy.

❍   **What findings are seen in Poland's syndrome?**

Pectoralis muscle sternal head hypoplasia, hypoplasia/aplasia of the breast, ipsilateral hand anomalies; males and females equally affected; chest wall anomalies.

❍   **What percentage of patients undergoing orbital floor fracture repair through a preseptal transconjunctival approach develop ectropion?**

Close to 0%.

❍   **What principle guides the Mustarde otoplasty approach?**

Using mattress sutures to bend the antihelix.

❍   **What is the Stenstrom technique?**

Using an otoabrader to bend the anterior antihelical surface.

○ **What is the Graham and Gault otoplasty technique?**

Endoscopic scoring and suture of the cartilage posteriorly.

○ **What is the Luckett procedure?**

Excision of a cresent shaped piece of skin/cartilage.

○ **What is the Furnas technique?**

Sutures spanning the concha to the mastoid.

○ **What is the relation of the temporal branch of the facial nerve to the superficial temporal fascia above the zygomatic arch?**

Deep to the superficial temporal fascia.

○ **What patients should Botox not be injected into?**

Egg/albumin sensitivity.

○ **What affects the quality of mammography with breast implants?**

Implant position, capsular contracture, native breast volume.

○ **What common medications may cause gynecomastia?**

Tagamet, Digoxin, Minocycline, spironolactone.

○ **What agents are administered before dermabrasion to prevent hyperpigmentation?**

Hydroquinones.

○ **Is tretinoin or isotretinoin used for skin preparation before dermabrasion?**

Tretinoin; Isotretinoin (Accutane) is contraindicated for 1 year before laser or dermabrasion due to risk of scarring and delayed healing.

○ **What specific technique has been shown to decrease the recurrence rate in thigh lifts?**

Superficial fascial system suspension; anchoring skin flap to Colles' fascia.

○ **What clinical findings are seen in levator aponeurosis dehiscence?**

Ptosis, elevated supratarsal crease, thinning of upper eyelid skin.

○ **What is typically done for levator aponeurosis dehiscence?**

Levator advancement.

○ **What is the most frequent rhytidectomy complication?**

Hematoma (0.3% to 8.1%).

❍   **What are risk factors for hematoma following rhytidectomy?**

Male patients and hypertension.

❍   **What vascular supply are the temporal scalp flap and Washio flap based upon?**

Posterior temporal branch of the superficial temporal artery.

❍   **What does the deep branch of the supraorbital nerve innervate?**

Central frontoparietal scalp.

❍   **What does the superficial branch of the supraorbital nerve innervate?**

Central forehead and hairline.

❍   **What supplies sensation to the nasal radix?**

The supratrochlear and infratrochlear nerves.

❍   **What supplies sensation to the temporal forehead?**

V2 and V3.

❍   **What supplies sensation to the temporal scalp?**

The occipital nerve.

❍   **What are key elements of the Lejour reduction mammaplasty?**

Central vertical gland excision and excision of skin in one direction; upper pedicle; more difficult to determine resection endpoint.

❍   **What supplies sensation to the nasal tip?**

External nasal branch of the anterior ethmoidal nerve; emerges from nasal bone and lateral nasal cartilage.

❍   **What part of the nose is innervated by the infraorbital nerve?**

Lower lateral half and skin of the columella.

❍   **What is supplied by the infratrochlear nerve?**

Superior portion of the nasal side wall and skin over the radix.

❍   **What is a likely cause of chronic lower lid deformity following ORIF of the orbital floor?**

Posterior lamella shortening; posterior lamella (capsulopalpebral fascia) comprised of tarsus, lower lid retractors, conjunctiva.

❍   **What is the most worrisome component of a secondary rhytidectomy regarding postoperative complications?**

Hairline distortion.

❍   **How does the vascular supply of the skin flap compare in a secondary rhytidectomy?**

Usually good or better due to the delay factor following the primary procedure; skin slough is less frequent.

○ **Where is a 1 cm defect on the nose most amenable to healing by secondary intention?**

Area of the medial canthus, glabella, nasolabial fold, and philtrum.

○ **What is considered the best reconstructive option for the breast in as a secondary procedure following mastectomy and irradiation?**

TRAM reconstruction; implant reconstruction associated with increased capsular contraction rate with prior irradiation.

○ **What is the next appropriate step for a woman preceding breast augmentation with milky discharge and regular menstrual cycles?**

Obtaining a serum prolactin level to rule out a pituitary lesion; thyroid function studies, medication history (eg. tricyclic antidepressants).

○ **What are the common descriptive findings in the prominent ear?**

Conchal valgus, cranioauricular angle greater than 40 degrees, antihelical underfolding; widened conchoscaphal angle (greater than 90 degrees).

○ **What are general options for correcting the prominent ear?**

Concha to scapha sutures, concha to mastoid sutures, scoring the cartilage anteriorly, conchal resection, postauricular skin resection.

○ **What is the most frequent complication following periareolar mastopexy?**

Areolar widening.

○ **What is the mechanism of outward pseudohernation of the buccal fat pad?**

Buccopharyngeal membrane attenutation.

○ **What is the most likely cause of death following liposuction?**

Thromboembolism; followed by abdominal wall perforation, anesthetic complication, infection.

○ **What is done for nasolacrimal duct obstruction?**

Dacryocystorhinostomy.

○ **What predisposing factors cause patients to have dry eye syndrome after blepharoplasty?**

Exophthalmos, scleral show, lower lid hypotonia, maxillary hypoplasia.

○ **What is the mechanism of Botox?**

Prevents acetylcholine uptake.

○ **What is the latency period and duration of effect of Botox?**

Onset beginning 3-7 days and lasting for 4-6 months.

❍   **What is the most frequent chronic complication following brachioplasty?**

Scar widening.

❍   **What is blepharochalasis?**

Recurrent episodes of painless edema of the eyelids; unclear etiology; caused by elastic tissue deficiency; leading to "baggy" appearance of lids.

❍   **What is dermatochalasis?**

Excess eyelid skin.

❍   **What is pachydermoperiostosis?**

Genetic syndrome resulting in enlarged hands, feet, eyelids, and toes.

❍   **What is the pattern of hair growth following hair transplant?**

One month of hair growth, loss of hair, and normal growth following three months; six months required for permanent hair growth into area.

❍   **What is the optimal timing for microtia surgery in a child?**

At 6-7 years of age; the ear is practically fully developed by age 7.

❍   **What is the ear canal typically created in microtia with respect to auricular reconstruction?**

Typically following the creation of the auricle.

❍   **What defines a tuberous breast?**

Constricted appearance of breast; unilateral narrowing of the breast; narrow breast diameter, superior displacement of the IMF; areola enlarged; breast hypoplasia.

❍   **How is a tuberous breast treated?**

Augmentation mammaplasty with IMF adjustment, radial scoring of the breast glandular tissue, areola reduction.

❍   **What is the mechanism of retinoids in regards to the skin?**

Decreased activity of metalloproteases from AP1 transcription inhibition.

❍   **What is the mechanism of tretinoin?**

Thinning the stratum corneum, epidermal thickening, atypia reversal, increased collagen synthesis.

❍   **What is the mechanism of topical vitamin C?**

Decreases free radical effects of UVB and increased collagen production.

❍   **What is the mechanism of alpha hydoxy acids?**

Increased desquamation from decreased corneocyte adhesion.

❍   **What is the mechanism of hydroquinones?**

Block conversion of dopamine to melanin; blocking tyrosinase.

❍ **What is the rate of additional procedures following breast implant augmentation?**

25% of patients requiring additional procedure within 13 years.

❍ **What is the rate of deflation after implant augmentation?**

1% annually.

❍ **What is the approximate rate of capsular contraction?**

20-25%.

❍ **What portion of breast parenchyma is affected after implant augmentation?**

Estimated 5% not entirely seen on mammography.

❍ **What is the initial management of the neonate with prominent ears?**

Molding with tape and splinting.

❍ **How long do maternal estrogens remain in the neonate?**

6 months, which allows for shaping of auricular cartilage.

❍ **What is the natural progression of Bell's palsy?**

85% have recovery spontaneously within 3 weeks.

❍ **What is the Stahl's ear deformity?**

A 3rd crus, antihelical flattening, scaphoid fossa deformity.

❍ **What is the constricted ear?**

Helical and scaphal hooding.

❍ **What is seen in cryptotia?**

Upper pole of the ear is buried beneath skin; absence of superior auriculocephalic sulcus missing.

❍ **What is the blepharophimosis syndrome?**

Genetic condition; telecanthus, ptosis, upper eyelid phimosis.

❍ **What is the most common form of acquired ptosis?**

Involutional; results from thinning of the levator aponeurosis; good levator function, elevated eyelid creases.

❍ **What level of dermis is dermabrasion performed at?**

Down to the upper third of the dermis.

❍ **What treatment is recommended for ice pick acne scars?**

Excision.

❍ **What nerve supplies the nipple-areola complex?**

The lateral branch of the fourth intercostals.

❍ **What factors are increased in smokers who undergo free TRAM breast reconstruction?**

Necrosis of the mastectomy skin, abdominal skin, and hernia rates.

❍ **What factors are not increased with smokers undergoing free TRAM breast reconstruction?**

Vessel thrombosis, fat necrosis, flap loss, or wound infection.

❍ **What surrounding nerves are at risk during abdominoplasty?**

Ilioinguinal, iliohypogastric and intercostals.

❍ **What are the grades of gynecomastia?**

I: mild enlargement without redundant skin
IIA: moderate enlargement without redundant skin
IIB: moderate enlargement with skin redundancy
III: marked enlargement with significant redundant skin

❍ **What are methods of treating gynecomastia?**

Suction lipectomy, excising a concentric circle of skin, amputation with free nipple grafting, glandular resection with liposuction.

❍ **What procedure is appropriate for a 33 year old patient who has lost 140 lbs. after a gastric bypass?**

Lower body lift.

❍ **What procedure is appropriate for a 40 year old patient with good skin tone and muscle tone with a localized area of excess fat?**

Suction lipectomy.

❍ **Is the umbilicus altered in mini-abdominoplasty?**

No.

❍ **What skin layer are hair follicles found at?**

The subcutaneous level.

❍ **What area of the incision is most at risk for necrosis after abdominoplasty?**

Area of the suprapubic region; lower midline flap is most at risk for ischemia.

❍ **A negative Jones I and positive Jones II test indicates what?**

Blockage of the nasolacrimal duct system.

❍ **What is the description of the mandible in Pierre-Robin sequence?**

Retrognathia; normal mandibular dimensions.

○ **What defines microgenia?**

Maldevelopment of the mental symphysis.

○ **What is the most appropriate next step for a smoker having undergone implant explantation with marked ptosis and less than 4 cm of breast thickness?**

Delayed mastopexy for 3 months at minimum.

○ **What are general indications for delayed mastopexy following implant explantation?**

Marked ptosis requiring nipple elevation of greater than 4 cm, breast mound less than 4 cm, smoking history.

○ **What is the procedure that should be done for grade II breast ptosis?**

For repositioning of the nipple-areola complex of 2-4 cm, a Wise pattern mastopexy may be performed.

○ **What procedure is recommended for pseudoptosis?**

Wedge excision from the inframammary fold.

○ **What treatment relieves burning and itching associated with keloids?**

Intralesional injection of steroid.

○ **What characterizes blepharophimosis syndrome?**

Type I: large epicanthal folds, epicanthus inversus, horizontal shortening of the eyelids, marked ptosis.
Type II: telecanthus, epicanthal fold absence, bilateral ptosis, no levator function, shortened eyelids.
Type III: missing epicanthal folds, telecanthus, antimongoloid slant; telecanthus.

○ **What treatment is done for blepharophimosis?**

Epicanthal fold repair, levator resection, medial canthoplasty, eyelid suspension.

○ **Skin laxity of the arms following massive weight loss is due to laxity of what structure?**

The clavipectoral fascia.

○ **What lasers are used for blue-green tattoos?**

Q-switched Nd:YAG and alexandrite lasers.

○ **What colors is the Nd:YAG laser used for?**

Red, brown, and orange.

○ **What is the Q-switched ruby laser used for?**

Tattoos with purple and violet pigments.

○ **What is the blood supply to the nasal tip during an open rhinoplasty?**

Lateral nasal artery which arises from the angular artery.

○ **What artery is divided during open rhinoplasty?**

The columellar branch of the superior labial artery.

○ **What vessels from the internal carotid artery supply the nasal skin?**

Dorsal nasal artery, external branch of the ethmoidal artery.

○ **What nerve supplies sensation to the superior cranial surface of the ear?**

Lesser occipital nerve.

○ **What nerve supplies sensation to the skin of the anterosuperior EAC?**

Lesser occipital nerve.

○ **What areas are supplied by the great auricular nerve?**

Inferior half of the lateral ear and inferior portion of the cranial surface of the ear.

○ **What area is supplied by the auriculotemporal nerve?**

Sensation to the anterosuperior surface of the external ear.

○ **What does Arnold's nerve supply?**

Sensation to the concha and posterior EAC.

○ **What defect is a dorsal nasal flap typically used for?**

A defect of the nasal tip up to 2 cm.

○ **What defines normal levator function?**

Greater than 10 mm of excursion.

○ **What degree of ptosis is the Fasanella-Servat procedure performed for?**

Mild ptosis.

○ **What is the polybeak deformity following rhinoplasty due to?**

Excessive reduction of the tip particularly in the setting of poor nasal tip projection.

○ **What is the treatment for alar collapse with inspiration and a pinched nasal tip?**

Grafting of the nasal tip with cartilage.

○ **What is the likely cause of increased show of the lower incisors following genioplasty?**

Inadequate repair of the mentalis muscle upon closure; lower lip drifts downward with healing.

○ **What muscle supplies blood to the anterior bony segment following a horizontal genioplasty?**

The anterior digastric.

○   **What is the most frequent complication of abdominoplasty combined with liposuction?**

Seroma formation.

○   **What is given for ptosis seen in Horner's syndrome?**

Phenylephrine eyedrops.

○   **At what trimester does maldevelopment occur and microtia result?**

First trimester between 4.5 weeks and 10 weeks.

○   **What is the most appropriate procedure for a patient with Hamilton class VI alopecia?**

Scalp reduction; followed by recreating the anterior hairline.

○   **What are features of Gorlin syndrome?**

Nevoid basal cell carcinoma syndrome; AD; multiple basal cell carcinomas; mandibular cysts; intracranial calcifications.

○   **What is the treatment for a complete upper auricular defect from a burn several years ago?**

Rib cartilage framework for the upper ear with temporoparietal fascia flap and skin graft.

○   **After bilateral TRAM elevation, what supplies the umbilicus primarily?**

Ligamentum teres.

○   **What normally supplies the umbilical skin?**

Vessels from the deep inferior epigastric arteries, ligamentum teres, and the medial umbilical ligament.

○   **What are the zones of the malar region?**

Zone I: 1st third of the zygomatic arch and malar bone.
Zone II: Middle third of the zygomatic arch.
Zone III: Paranasal.
Zone IV: Posterior third of the zygomatic arch.
Zone V: Submalar region.

○   **What is the largest zone?**

Zone I.

○   **Which malar zones are rarely augmented in aesthetic surgery?**

Zone III and Zone IV.

○   **What is the appearance with Zone V malar augmentation?**

Midface fullness, rounded appearance of the cheeks.

○   **Regarding hair growth phases, what characterizes male pattern alopecia?**

Lengthened telogen phase; shortened anagen phase.

❍   **What is the genetic transmission of male pattern alopecia?**

X-linked autosomal inheritance.

❍   **What is the result of increased 5-alpha reductase activity?**

Alopecia.

❍   **The stratification of Fitzpatrick skin types is important for what?**

Risk of pigmentary changes following chemical peeling.

❍   **What Fitzpatrick skin types are at risk for pigmentary changes after chemical peel?**

4, 5, 6.

❍   **What physiologic changes with collagen are seen with application of tretinoin for periorbital rhytids?**

Increased type III collagen over 6 to 12 months; up to 80% increase in collagen.

❍   **What changes are seen in the skin with tretinoin therapy?**

Thickened dermis; skin elasticity improves.

❍   **What is the treatment of choice 14 days after blepharoplasty in a patient with lagophthalmos?**

Corneal lubrication.

❍   **What growth phase of hair is active growth in?**

The anagen phase; lasts 3 years.

❍   **What is the likely cause of recurrent prominence of ears following otoplasty at 7 months?**

Suture failure at the antihelical fold.

❍   **What structure are the upper eyelid fat pads immediately posterior to?**

The orbital septum; the fat pads sit just anterior to the levator aponeurosis.

❍   **In the lower lids the fat pads are located just anterior to what structure?**

The inferior retractors.

❍   **What separates the medial and middle fat pads in the lower lid?**

The inferior oblique.

❍   **What is the management of an anterior platysmal band?**

Plication in the midline.

❍   **What is the greatest source of dissatisfaction following breast reduction?**

Noticeable scarring.

○ **What is the most important factor in facial reanimation following trauma?**

Length of time between injury and reconstruction; facial muscles are viable for 2 years following paralysis; after 2 years, free muscle transfer required.

○ **What is the likely cause of a supraumbilical bulge after abdominoplasty?**

Not placating the rectus muscle.

○ **Following reduction mammaplasty, what is the percentage of being able to breast feed?**

30%.

○ **What is the best treatment for multiple actinic keratoses of the face?**

Topical 5-FU treatment.

○ **What type of genioplasty should be performed in a patient with sagittal deficiency and vertical excess with class I occlusion?**

Jumping genioplasty.

○ **Where should the brow peak in a female patient undergoing browlifting?**

At the lateral limbus to lateral canthal area.

○ **What is the best flap to use for a defect of the lateral nasal ala?**

Nasolabial flap, superiorly based.

○ **What is the best flap to use for a nasal tip defect?**

Banner flap.

○ **What should be used for a defect of the lateral nasal wall above the ala?**

Cheek advancement flap.

○ **A defect of the caudal third of the nose centrally?**

Fronto-nasal flap.

○ **What skin characteristics negatively affect results after rhinoplasty?**

Thick skin with large sebaceous glands; skin envelope does not conform easily.

○ **Is smoking thought to have an effect on rhinoplasty?**

No; not a mild to moderate smoking history.

○ **What is the treatment for chronic ectropion and excessive scleral show after a chemical burn?**

Full thickness skin grafting.

○ **What is the mechanism of involutional ectropion?**

Laxity of the lower lid from the lower lid retractors becoming disinserted from the tarsal plate.

○   **What is the treatment for involutional ectropion?**

Lateral canthoplasty, lateral wedge excision, or excising of a full thickness wedge from the lateral canthal region.

CRANIOMAXILLOFACIAL SURGERY

○   **What findings are consistent with vertical maxillary excess (long face syndrome)?**

Gummy smile, long obtuse nasolabial angle, Class II Angle classification, obtuse nasolabial angle, lip incompetence, show of upper incisors with lips in repose; mentalis muscle strain.

○   **What is appearance of the chin in vertical excess syndrome?**

Chin is retruded; mandible appears retrognathic.

○   **What defines a "gummy" smile?**

Greater than 4 mm of incisor show at rest and greater than 2 mm with active movement.

○   **What is the lip-tooth relationship in long face syndrome?**

Lip-to-tooth relationship greater than 3 mm.

○   **What differentiates mandibular deficiency from vertical maxillary excess?**

SNB angle decreased with mandibular deficiency.

○   **What are characteristics of mandibular excess?**

Wide lower third of face, prominent lower lip, anterior crossbite, Class III angle classification, increased SNB angle.

○   **What are characteristics of vertical maxillary deficiency (short face syndrome)?**

Decreased facial height, absence of maxillary show with edentulous look, protruding chin, wide alar bases, class III Angle, normal or greater SNB.

○   **In patients younger than 2 years, when should mandibular distraction osteogenesis by performed?**

When there is tongue-based airway compromise secondary to mandibular hypoplasia which pulls the mandible forward relieving airway obstruction.

○   **Why should children younger than 2 with only selected congenital hypoplasia or aplasia of only selected portions of the mandible not undergo distraction osteogenesis?**

Risk for permanent dental injury in patients who do not have airway compromise.

○   **How reliably does distraction osteogenesis improve patients with laryngomalacia or tracheomalacia?**

It will not reliably improve airway obstruction.

○   **At what time is distraction osteogenesis initiated in patients with hemifacial microsomia?**

Older than 1 year.

○ **What is the treatment of patients with an acute open lock deformity of the mandible?**

Attempted closed reduction under sedation in the ED.

○ **What is the deformity in open lock deformity?**

Condyle slips into position anterior to the articular eminence.

○ **What is the treatment of a teenage girl with RA and mandibular retrusion and anterior open bite?**

Maxillary impaction (to close the open bite deformity), advancement genioplasty.

○ **35 year old man sustains nasal trauma resulting in a localized purplish mass on the left side of the septum – what is the next step in management?**

Immediate incision and drainage of the septal mass.

○ **What is a long term sequelae of septal hematoma?**

Septal perforation leading to saddle nose deformity.

○ **Application of an arch bar to the maxillary alveolus requires anesthesia of which nerves?**

Nasopalatine and anterior superior alveolar.

○ **What nerve trunk does the nasopalatine nerve originate from?**

V2.

○ **Which nerve provides sensation to the posterior palate?**

Greater palatine nerve.

○ **Following resection of a pleomorphic adenoma, a recurrent multinodular tumor requires what type of therapy next?**

XRT.

○ **In patients sustaining bilateral parasymphyseal fractures, which muscle exerts a distractive force on the anterior fracture segment?**

The geniohyoid.

○ **What is the function of the geniohyoid muscle?**

To depress and retract the mandible.

○ **What is the function of the posterior belly of the digastric muscle?**

Elevates the hyoid, has only a secondary effect on the anterior mandible.

○ **Which Tessier cleft has displacement of the medial canthus of the eyelid?**

No. 3 cleft is characteristic of having a medially displaced medial canthus; also referred to as a naso-ocular cleft (inferomedial wall is absent); nose is shortened, colobomas, NLD obstruction.

❍   **What are characteristics of a No. 1 cleft?**

Just lateral to midline, begins at cupid's bow and passes through dome of nostril; notching of alar dome; nasal bone may be absent; septum unaffected; hypertelorism and encephalocele may be associated.

❍   **A No. 4 cleft?**

Passes between the piriform aperture and infraorbital foramen; begins lateral to cupid's bow and philtrum; passes lateral to the nasal ala onto cheek; terminates in lower eyelid; medial canthal tendon unaffected.

❍   **A No. 5 cleft?**

Begins behind canine and extends through maxillary sinus to orbital floor; colobomas of lateral lower lids and clefting of upper lip medial to oral commissure associated.

❍   **Which cleft is the incomplete form of Treacher Collins syndrome?**

No. 6; passes inferior and lateral to the oral commissure, toward angle of mandible; colobomas of lateral lower eyelids; downward slant of palpebral fissures.

❍   **Which is the most common atypical cleft?**

No. 7; 1/3000 births; absent zygomatic arch.

❍   **Where does a no. 8 cleft extend?**

From lateral commissure of palpebral fissure to temporal region; colobomas also seen of lower eyelids.

❍   **Which cleft is the supraorbital extension of the no. 5 cleft?**

No. 9.

❍   **A patient sustaining a frontal sinus fracture in a MVA with CSF rhinorrhea and displacement of anterior/posterior sinus walls and injured nasofrontal ducts requires what operation?**

Cranialization of the frontal sinus in conjunction with neurosurgery.

❍   **What are the steps in cranialization?**

Bifrontal craniotomy to repair dura, removal of posterior wall of frontal sinus and associated mucosa; occlusion of nasofrontal duct with a pericranial flap or fat; burring down sharp edges; allowing the brain to expand into this new potential space.

❍   **Frontal sinus exenteration involves what?**

Removal of the anterior table of the frontal sinus only.

❍   **What is involved in frontal sinus obliteration?**

Removing all the mucosa within the frontal sinus; allowing the nasofrontal duct to occlude.

❍   **Which muscles produce side-to side grinding motions of the mandible?**

Medial and lateral pterygoid; rotation occurs around the vertical axis of the contralateral condyle.

❍   **What is the origin/insertion of the medial pterygoid? How does it function?**

Originates from the medial surface of the lateral pterygoid plate and tuberosity of maxilla and inserts into the medial surface of the mandibular angle/ramus; elevates and pulls mandible medially.

○ **What is the origin/insertion of the lateral pterygoid? Its function?**

Originates from the lateral surface of the lateral pterygoid plate (inferior head) and infratemporal surface of the greater wing of the sphenoid (superior head) and inserts into the mandibular condylar neck (inferior head) and articular disk of TMJ (superior head); protrudes the mandible forward and opens mouth.

○ **Simultaneous action of all four pterygoid muscles results in what motion of the mandible?**

Protrusion of the mandible.

○ **Where does the masseter originate/insert?**

Originates from zygomatic arch; inserts onto ramus.

○ **Where does the temporalis muscle insert?**

Originates from the temporal fossa and attaches to the coronoid process of the mandible; primarily elevates mandible, but also can retract mandible.

○ **Following a bilateral cleft lip repair, tightness of the upper lip with a wide hypoplastic philtrum with absence of muscle competence and redundant lower lip may be treated with what kind of flap?**

Abbe flap (to create a functional philtrum in patients with tightness of the upper lip following cleft lip repair.

○ **What are the dimensions of a reconstructed philtrum in the adult?**

No wider than 10 mm and no longer than 15 mm.

○ **What is the incidence of concomitant cervical spine injury with a mandibular fracture?**

10%.

○ **In a patient with VPI with central velopharyngeal closure and poor lateral wall motion, what procedure is indicated?**

Sphincter pharyngoplasty.

○ **What muscle is transposed in sphincter pharyngoplasty?**

Palatopharyngeus (incorporated into the posterior pharyngeal wall to create a sphincter).

○ **When is a pharyngeal flap indicated?**

Correction of deficits of the central palate with good lateral wall motion; the levator veli palatini is used as well in the palate for attachment of the posterior wall flap.

○ **Where is the tensor veli palatini muscle located relative to the levator veli palatini?**

The TVP is anterior to the LVP.

○ **Where are the palatoglossus muscles located – in the anterior or posterior tonsillar pillar?**

Anterior.

O   **A neonate with a 1.5 cm reddish mass adjacent to the nasal root with overlying telangiectasias that is firm, not compressible and nonpulsatile is most likely what type of mass?**

Glioma (rarely with bony defects, intracranial connections).

O   **What embryonic tissue derives nasal dermoids?**

Mesoderm and ectoderm (hair follicles, sebaceous glands, smooth muscle).

O   **What external nasal lesions transilluminate and are compressible?**

Encephaloceles (external, or sincipital) are soft, bluish, compressible, and pulsatile that transilluminate; Furstenberg's sign.

O   **What nerve innervates the oral commissures bilaterally?**

Buccal nerve, a branch of V3.

O   **What causes a 10 month old boy to tilt his head to the right who also has an uncorrected left coronal synostosis?**

Paresis of the ipsilateral superior oblique muscle (foreshortening of the orbital roof on the affected side; relative paresis of superior oblique occurs).

O   **In surgically correcting the patient with NOE fracture, what is the most appropriate management of the lacrimal system?**

Observation; generally low incidence of duct injury in patients undergoing ORIF without overlying lacerations.

O   **How does one evaluate persistent epiphora following surgery for a NOE fracture?**

Dacryocystography; followed by a DCR if required for treatment.

O   **What muscle courses around the pterygoid hamulus?**

The tensor veli palatini.

O   **Where does the levator veli palatini run relative to the hamulus?**

It passes posterior to the hamulus creating a muscular sling.

O   **A complete unilateral cleft lip is associated with what type of movement of the ala?**

Lateral, inferior, and posterior (the piriform rim is also deficient, which also supports the ala.

O   **Treacher Collins syndrome involves which Tessier cleft(s)?**

No. 6, 7, and 8 clefts.

O   **What is the class occlusion seen in Treacher Collins?**

Class II.

O   **What are the characteristics of the maxilla, palate, and mandible in Treacher Collins?**

Maxilla protrudes, palatal plane is moved upwards and posteriorly; micrognathia, decreased length of the ramus and body; hypoplastic or absent condyle; cleft in the inferolateral orbital floor also occurs; hypoplastic zygoma, maxilla, and mandible.

❍   **What type of synostosis is seen in Crouzon's?**

Bilateral coronal synostosis (acrocephalosyndactyly) forehead and superior orbital rim retrusion, proptosis, midface hypoplasia.

❍   **What type of occlusion is seen in Crouzon's?**

Angle's type III.

❍   **What abnormalities are seen in Goldenhar's?**

Oculoauriculovertebral dysplasia; subset of hemifacial microsomia, epibulbar dermoids and scapula/spine anomalies seen; may be bilateral; resemble a No. 7 cleft; mandibular hypoplasia.

❍   **What is Romberg's syndrome?**

Progressive hemifacial atrophy, appears initially as cutaneous pigmentation and progresses to destruction of facial soft tissues and skeleton.

❍   **What are the zones of distraction osteogenesis?**

Fibrous zone (central region of the distraction gap); transitional zone (adjacent to the fibrous zone, contains fibrous tissue undergoing ossification); zone of remodeling bone (surrounded by zone of mature bone).

❍   **What nerve supplies sensation to the buccal mucosa?**

The trigeminal nerve (V).

❍   **What are the clinical findings of a unilateral condylar fracture?**

Upward cant of mandible to the fractured side, early contact of molars on ipsilateral side; contralateral lateral open bite.

❍   **What are the clinical findings of a bilateral condylar fracture?**

Anterior open bite secondary to loss of posterior vertical height.

❍   **What is the malocclusion seen in a 6 year old who has undergone a unilateral cleft lip/palate previously with an unrepaired alveolar cleft?**

Posterior crossbite (an unrepaired alveolar cleft causes maxillary arch collapse, the arch will be deficient in the A-P, transverse, and vertical directions.

❍   **What is the clinical appearance of a posterior crossbite?**

Lower dentition is labial to the upper dentition.

❍   **What is the definition of Angle's class I?**

The mesiobuccal cusp of the 1st maxillary molar sits in the buccal groove of the 1st mandibular molar.

❍   **Define overbite and overjet.**

Overbite describes the distance between the mandibular and maxillary incisors in the vertical plane; overjet describes the distance between the incisors in the horizontal plane.

O   **What direction does the central mandibular segment move in a pt. sustaining bilateral vertically and horizontally unfavorable fractures adjacent to the canine roots?**

Downward and posterior (actions of the digastric and geniohyoid/genioglossus.

O   **What points of fixation are required in patients with zygomaticomaxillary complex fractures?**

Z-F suture, inferior orbital rim, and zygomaticomaxillary buttress.

O   **What is the most common type of nonsyndromic single-suture craniosynostosis?**

Sagittal (50% of patients with single suture fusions); elongated skull with frontal/occipital bossing.

O   **What is turribrachycephaly?**

Shortened, wide skull with increased vertical height at top of skull; from bilateral coronal synostosis.

O   **How common is lambdoid suture fusion?**

Extremely rare, in 1-2 % in pts. with craniosynostosis.

O   **What is trigonocephaly?**

Metopic suture fusion; leaves a prominent midline ridge in forehead; occurs in 10% of all single-suture fusions; triangularly shaped forehead.

O   **How often does single-suture squamosal synostosis occur?**

Isolated fusion does not occur.

O   **What areas are affected in auriculotemporal nerve paresis during superficial parotidectomy?**

Numbness of tragus, EAC, tympanum, and temporal skin; fibers also go to the parotid gland as secretomotor fibers and articular fibers to the TMJ.

O   **What branch is the auriculotemporal nerve from?**

V3, mandibular division of V.

O   **What nerve innervates the concha? The antihelix?**

Auricular branch of X.

O   **What areas are supplied by the great auricular nerve? The lesser occipital nerve?**

Both these nerves are derived from C2-3; the areas supplied are the helix and lobule.

O   **What procedure is most appropriate for a 15 year old with Apert's in need of 25 mm of midface advancement?**

Le Fort III with distraction osteogenesis for advancement; distraction osteogenesis preferred over bone grafting for greater than 10 mm.

❍ **In an infant with hemifacial microsomia, should macrostomia or deficiencies of the mandibular ramus/body be corrected first?**

Macrostomia; hemifacial microsomia associated with 1st and 2nd branchial arch anomalies and Tessier No. 7 cleft.

❍ **What nerve passes through foramen ovale?**

V3.

❍ **Where does V1 pass through?**

The superior orbital fissure.

❍ **What nerve passes through the foramen rotundum?**

V2.

❍ **What is the most likely diagnosis of a pt with a painless mass at the angle of the mandible for the past 10 years with a biopsy showing luminal ductal cells mixed with sheets of myoepithelial cells?**

A pleomorphic adenoma; most common benign tumor of the parotid; contains TWO populations of cells (epithelial and mesenchymal cells).

❍ **How does a myoepithelioma of the parotid differ from a pleomorphic adenoma?**

More rare, affects parotid or palate, histologically similar but also shows spindle cells.

❍ **What parotid tumor has a characteristic of being bilateral?**

Warthin's (papillary cystadenoma lymphomatosum); male smokers; 10% multicentric, 10% bilateral.

❍ **What structures arise from the lateral nasal processes?**

The nasal ala.

❍ **What structures arise from the medial nasal processes?**

The columella, nasal tip, philtrum, and premaxilla; this occurs during the sixth week of gestation.

❍ **What structures arise from the frontonasal processes?**

The bridge and root of the nose.

❍ **Which muscle of mastication pulls the mandible upward, medially, and forward?**

The medial pterygoid.

❍ **What is the origin/insertion of the anterior digastric muscle? The posterior digastric?**

Originates from the inside lower border of the symphysis and attaches to the lateral corner of the hyoid bone. Posterior belly extends between the hyoid and mastoid.

❍ **How does the digastric function in distracting the mandible in the setting of a fracture?**

The digastric pulls the anterior mandibular fragments postero-inferiorly.

❍   **What is the function of the mylohyoid?**

Elevates the tongue.

❍   **Abnormalities of the corpus callosum is most frequently associated with premature fusion of which cranial suture?**

The metopic suture (trigonocephaly); also associated with higher incidence of developmental delay.

❍   **What is the most appropriate initial step in evaluating an infant in respiratory distress with retrogenia and glossoptosis?**

Prone positioning; Pierre-Robin sequence occurs with a 50% incidence of high-arched clefts of the soft palate; hard palate clefting also occurs in some patients.

❍   **What are alternative treatments if prone positioning does not help the neonate with Pierre-Robin sequence?**

Lip-tongue adhesion, tracheostomy, mandibular distraction osteogenesis.

❍   **What cranial suture has the greatest incidence of synostosis associated with mutations in the loci for FGF receptors?**

Coronal; in both unilateral and bilateral.

❍   **What bony segments are moved together in a Le Fort I osteotomy?**

The entire alveolar process of the maxilla, vault of the palate, pterygoid processes.

❍   **What bony segments are included in a Le Fort II?**

A central maxillary segment is undisturbed; also included are portions of the medial orbital walls, orbital floor, and nasofrontal junction.

❍   **The external auditory canal develops from which embryologic structure?**

1st branchial groove.

❍   **Which hillocks does the first branchial arch give rise to?**

The first three hillocks.

❍   **What cranial nerve innervates the temporalis muscle?**

V3.

❍   **An anterior chamber hemorrhage of the eye is known as what?**

A hyphema.

❍   **What defines subconjunctival hemorrhage?**

Bleeding occurring in the bulbar or palpebral conjunctiva; from extravasation of conjunctival capillaries.

❍   **What is the most common complication of a sagittal split osteotomy?**

Loss of lower lip sensibility.

○ **Craniofacial microsomia is the most common major craniofacial anomaly – how is it transmitted?**

It does not demonstrate genetic transmission – likely an intrauterine event; eg. Hematoma.

○ **How are Apert's and Crouzon's differentiated clinically?**

Apert's patients have severe syndactyly of the middle three digits of the hands and feet; Crouzon's patients have normal extremities; both have craniosynostosis, exorbitism, and midface retrusion.

○ **How is Treacher-Collins transmitted?**

Autosomal Dominant.

○ **What are clinical characteristics of Treacher-Collins?**

Facial clefting, antimongoloid slant, colobomas, absence of eyelashes on medial portion of the lower eyelid, preauricular displacement of hair, micrognathia, malar/mandibular defects.

○ **What is the maximum bony defect (in mm) that will not require bone grafting?**

5 mm.

○ **What structures pass through the superior orbital fissure?**

III, IV, V_1, VI, sympathetic nerve fibers.

○ **What is the superior orbital fissure syndrome?**

Fractures that extend to the superior orbital fissure and orbital roof; vision is not affected.

○ **What is orbital apex syndrome?**

Injury to the optic nerve from extension of the fracture into the optic canal; loss of vision.

○ **Prominence of the ear is caused by effacement of what part of the ear?**

Superior crus of the antihelix; conchoscaphal angle is greater than 90 degrees; helix is greater than 12-15mm from the temporal skin.

○ **Prominence of the middle portion of the ear is caused by hypertrophy of what structure?**

Concha cavum; here the concha cavum has a depth of more than 1.5 cm.

○ **What soft tissue change is most likely seen following LeFort I advancement?**

Increased nasolabial angle, widened alar base; shortened upper lip, increased incisor show.

○ **How is upper lip shortening prevented during LeFort I advancement?**

V-Y advancement during closure.

○ **Regarding the chin, lower facial height, labiomental fold, and sagittal deficiency, alloplastic chin augmentation is best recommended in what setting?**

Symmetric chin, normal lower facial height, shallow labiomental fold, minimal sagittal deficiency.

❍ **How is velocardiofacial syndrome diagnosed?**

FISH analysis; for deletion of 22q11.2.

❍ **What are the components of velocardiofacial syndrome?**

AD; VPI, developmental delay, upward slanting of palpebral fissures, prominent nose with broad nasal root, aberrant carotid arteries; submucous cleft .

❍ **Define Angle class I.**

The mesiobuccal cusp of the 1st maxillary molar fits into the buccal groove of the 1st mandibular molar.

❍ **Define Angle class II, division 1.**

The mesiobuccal cusp of the 1st maxillary molar is anterior to the buccal groove of the 1st mandibular molar; division 1: lateral incisors angled labially.

❍ **Define Angle class II, division 2.**

Same previous Angle class II but the lateral incisors are angled lingually; retrognathic on appearance.

❍ **What are operative indications for TMJ pathology?**

Internal derangement associated with neoplasia, trauma.

❍ **What are surgical options for internal derangement?**

Intracapsular repositioning of the disk, excision of the disk, temporalis fascia flap placement.

❍ **A decreased SNA and normal SNB indicates what process of the maxilla?**

Maxillary retrusion.

❍ **What are normal values of SNA and SNB?**

SNA 82 degrees; SNB 80 degrees.

❍ **Normally how much incisor show appears at rest?**

2-3 mm.

❍ **What muscle causes the medial displacement of the condyle following a fracture?**

Lateral pterygoid.

❍ **What is the sequence of repair in a patient with midface fractures and bilateral condylar neck fractures?**

ORIF of condylar neck fractures followed by midface fractures.

❍ **What is the most common cause of an open bite deformity following LeFort I and bilateral sagittal split osteotomy in a patient?**

Centric relation not equaling centric occlusion, or having the condyles not seat properly in each respective glenoid fossa.

○ **What population of patients does progressive condyle resorption occur in?**

Young women; a late cause of open bite deformity causing shortening of the condyle and clockwise rotation of the mandible.

○ **What defines vertical maxillary deficiency?**

Decrease in vertical height, absence of maxillary incisor show, short/flat upper lip, protrusive chin, acute mandibular plane.

○ **During pediatric distraction osteogenesis, what techniques optimize bone formation?**

Lower energy corticotomy (minimizing central medullary bone trauma); less than 5mm of intraoperative immediate distraction; stable fixator placement.

○ **What passes through the stylomastoid foramen?**

The facial nerve and stylomastoid artery.

○ **What passes through the jugular foramen?**

IX, X, XI, and the internal jugular vein.

○ **What passes through foramen ovale?**

V3 and accessory meningeal artery.

○ **How is scaphocephaly treated?**

Cranial vault remodeling with barrel staving.

○ **What is scaphocephaly?**

Premature closure of the sagittal suture; skull is long, narrow and characteristically keel shaped.

○ **What procedures are done for unicoronal and bicoronal synostosis?**

Bilateral frontal craniotomy and bilateral fronto-orbital advancement.

○ **The buccal nerve is a branch of which nerve?**

V3; arises from surface of the buccinator. Supplies sensation to medial cheek.

○ **What is the dorsal nasal nerve a branch of?**

Nasociliary nerve, V1.

○ **What is the sensory territory of the infratrochlear nerve?**

The nasal root and medial eyelid.

○ **What is the zygomaticofacial nerve a branch of?**

V2; supplies zygomatic skin and upper portion of central cheek.

○   **What symptoms define Pierre-Robin sequence?**

Micrognathia, glossoptosis, respiratory distress, cleft palate.

○   **What is the initial management of a neonate with Pierre-Robin?**

Prone positioning; evaluation of the lower airway for synchronous anomalies; later, other interventions include distraction osteogenesis, tongue-lip adhesion, tracheotomy.

○   **What are symptoms of Binder syndrome?**

Nasomaxillary hypoplasia, low/flat nasal tip, absent nasal spine; Angle Class III malocclusion.

○   **What is Klippel-Feil syndrome?**

Shortened neck, low posterior hairline, hearing loss, cleft palate, facial abnormalities; fusion of cervical spine.

○   **What is Shprintzen's syndrome?**

Otherwise known as velocardiofacial syndrome; most common syndrome seen in cleft lip/palate; thymus/parathyroid glands absent; cardiac anomalies, velopharyngeal dysfunction.

○   **What is van der Woude's syndrome?**

Cleft lip/palate, LOWER lip pits (from accessory saliva glands); extremity anomalies.

○   **Does the medial or lateral pterygoid elevate the mandible?**

The medial.

○   **What action does the digastric muscle have on the mandible following a fracture?**

Pulls anterior mandibular segment posteriorly and inferiorly.

○   **What is the action of the lateral pterygoid in unilateral subcondylar fractures?**

The ipsilateral condylar head is pulled in anteriorly and medially; the contralateral lateral pterygoid continues to protrude the mandible, thus deviating the jaw to the fracture side.

○   **Embyrologically, what arises from the frontonasal process?**

The nasal bridge and root.

○   **What arises from the medial nasal processes?**

Columella, tip, philtrum, premaxilla.

○   **What arises from the lateral nasal processes?**

The alae.

○   **Which branchial arch gives rise to the stylopharyngeus muscle?**

The 3rd.

❍   **What muscles are derived from the 1ˢᵗ branchial arch?**

Muscles of chewing, anterior digastric, myelohyoid, tensor tympani.

❍   **What is the most appropriate next step for treatment of a naso-orbital-ethmoid fracture?**

ORIF and bone grafting.

❍   **What muscle travels around the hamulus in the mouth?**

The tensor veli palatini.

❍   **What bone does the hamulus arise from?**

The medial pterygoid plate.

❍   **A 5 month old with anterior displacement of the right ear and zygoma and right side of the forehead with flattening of the right side of the occiput has what process?**

Right sided posterior deformational plagiocephaly.

❍   **What are the most common causes of synostotic plagiocephaly?**

Unilateral coronal and lambdoidal craniosynostosis.

❍   **How frequent is deformational plagiocephaly?**

1/70 infants.

❍   **What findings are seen in posterior deformational plagiocephaly?**

Unilateral; parallelogram shaped head; ipsilateral flattening of the occiput with anterior displacement of ipsilateral ear.

❍   **What findings are seen in bilateral deformational plagiocephaly?**

Flattening of the occipital area, mastoid bulging bilaterally, biparietal eminence bossing.

❍   **What is seen in lambdoidal craniosynostosis?**

Ipsilateral occipital flattening with lambdoid suture ridging (from fusion of the suture); INFERIOR displacement of the ear.

❍   **What shape is the skull in lambdoidal craniosynostosis?**

Trapezoid-like.

❍   **Based on radiographic CT findings, what are operative indications for an orbital blowout fracture?**

Orbital floor defect greater than 2cm, low vertical height of the globe, co-existing other facial fractures.

❍   **What are clinical indications for operative intervention in orbital blowout fractures?**

Symptomatic diplopia, positive forced duction testing, failed resolution of extraocular muscle entrapment after 1 week.

❍   **Does the supraorbital artery derive its blood supply from the internal or external system? The supratrochlear artery?**

Both are branches of the ophthalmic artery, which branches from the internal carotid artery.

❍   **What is an important consideration when deciding whether to use an external or internal distraction device following a LeFort III?**

Using an external device allows for in-office removal, saving an operative procedure for the patient.

❍   **Nerve injury during osseous genioplasty most likely results in what symptom?**

Numbness of the lower lip (mental nerve).

❍   **In a teenage boy with Angle Class III, 12 mm of negative overjet, and normal SNB angle, what procedure is most appropriate for maxillary advancement?**

Distraction osteogenesis of the maxilla; LeFort I single stage advancement of more than 10 mm is considered unpredictable.

❍   **What is the procedure of choice in a patient to advance the maxilla who has had cleft lip/palate repair and pharyngeal flap with a 14 mm negative overjet?**

Maxillary distraction osteogenesis.

❍   **What environmental exposure has been linked to squamous cell carcinoma of the maxillary sinus?**

Nickel.

❍   **What is the most useful component to anatomically reduce in a ZMC fracture?**

The lateral orbital wall, alternatively, the sphenoid wing can be also used.

❍   **Where does the levator palpebrae superioris originate from?**

The lesser wing of the sphenoid.

❍   **Where do the superior oblique and rectus muscles originate from?**

The annulus tendineus communis.

❍   **What structure does the inferior oblique arise from?**

The maxilla.

❍   **Gustatory sweating following parotid surgery is due to malfunction of what nerve?**

Auriculotemporal.

❍   **What is the mechanism of Frey's syndrome?**

Aberrant connections between postganglionic parasympathetic fibers from the otic ganglion and postganglionic sympathetic fibers to sweat glands.

❍   **What effect does Botox have on Frey's syndrome?**

Intracutaneous administration blocks acetylcholine transmission and may improve symptoms for up to a year.

○ **What structure does the stapes derive from?**

The second branchial arch.

○ **A melanoma with a Clark level of IV and Breslow thickness of 2.8 mm with an in-transit metastasis has what stage?**

Stage III (T4, N0).

○ **How is vertical maxillary excess and a retruded chin treated?**

Typically by LeFort I with maxillary impaction and genioplasty.

○ **What is the appearance of the nose in vertical maxillary excess typically?**

Alar base constriction and an obtuse nasolabial angle.

○ **What are other signs of vertical maxillary excess?**

Lip incompetence, incisor show, mentalis strain

○ **Where does the nasolacrimal duct drain into the nasal cavity?**

Inferior meatus.

○ **What structures drain into the middle meatus?**

The frontal, anterior ethmoid, and maxillary sinuses.

○ **What areas of the mandible are fractured most commonly?**

The angle and body.

○ **What is most appropriate initial therapy for a child with a enlarging hemangioma of the eyelid?**

Oral steroids 2-3 mg/kg/day (low dose); surgical management if steroids are unsuccessful.

○ **What structure is incised during a preseptal transconjunctival approach to the orbital floor?**

The capsulopalpebral fascia.

○ **What nerve supplies the superior helix of the auricle?**

The auriculotemporal nerve (CN V).

○ **What nerves provide sensation to the ear?**

Auriculotemporal branch(V), VII, Jacobsen's nerve (IX), Arnold's nerve (X), lesser occipital nerve (C2), great auricular nerve (C2,3).

○ **What system controls pupillary constriction?**

Parasympathetics of the eye; travel with CN III and the inferior oblique.

❍   **What clinical finding is seen in direct trauma to the optic nerve?**

Afferent pupillary defect (Marcus-Gunn pupil).

❍   **What muscle of the tongue is supplied by CN X?**

The palatoglossus.

❍   **What is the appearance of the palpebral fissure following zygomatic fractures?**

Downward cant due to pulling of Whitnall's ligament inferiorly.

❍   **What finding during facial fracture causes rounding of the palpebral fissure?**

Lateral canthal ligament detachment or comminuted frontal process of the zygoma.

❍   **What structures travel through the superior orbital fissure?**

V1, III, IV, and VI.

❍   **What branches off CN V1?**

The frontal, nasociliary, and lacrimal nerves.

❍   **What syndrome has brachycephaly, hypertelorism, bregmatic prominence, maxillary hypoplasia, and bony syndactyly of toes and hands?**

Apert's.

❍   **Members of a family with frontal recession, maxillary retrusion, proptosis and exorbitism without extremity anomalies have what syndrome?**

Crouzon's.

❍   **What findings are seen in Carpenter's syndrome?**

Brachydactyly, syndactyly, polydactyly, cardiac disease, obesity, GU anomalies; AR.

❍   **What is seen in Nager syndrome?**

Acrofacial dysostosis; AR; cleft palate, orbital, zygomatic, maxillo-mandibular hypoplasia, pre-axial hypoplasia or agenesis; auricular defects, mental retardation; syndactyly of the second web space.

❍   **What is seen in Pfeiffer syndrome?**

Synostosis, acrocephalosyndactyly, broad thumbs, midface hypoplasia.

❍   **What procedure is done for horizontal deficiency and vertical excess of the chin?**

Jumping genioplasty.

❍   **What embryologic anomaly is responsible for primary cleft palate?**

Failed lateral and median palatine process fusion.

❍   **What causes secondary cleft palate?**

Failed lateral palatine process fusion to each other and the nasal septum.

O   **What causes cleft lip?**

Fusion of the medial nasal prominence and maxillary prominence.

O   **What causes macrostomia?**

Failed fusion of the maxillary and mandibular prominences.

O   **In a maxillary advancement for 1 cm of negative overjet, what primary factor is the most significant risk for VPI?**

Midface hypoplasia due to cleft palate repair (higher risk than other craniofacial syndromes such as microsomia or Crouzon's).

O   **What is the most common Tessier facial cleft?**

No. 7 (macrostomia, zygomatic arch absence).

O   **Which Tessier cleft includes the same position as a unilateral cleft lip?**

No. 3; also extends to affect nasal ala and medial canthus.

O   **What is the appropriate management of Romberg's hemifacial atrophy?**

Parascapular flap; deepithelialized and placed under skin flap.

O   **What is the most common cause of late enophthalmos following ORIF of an orbital floor and zygomatic arch fracture?**

Inadequate reduction.

O   **Where does a frontonasal encephalocele communicate intracranially?**

Foramen cecum.

O   **What is the metachronous incidence of squamous cell carcinoma in a pt. who continues to smoke?**

40%; those who stop tobacco have an incidence of 6%.

O   **What is the normal latency period in mandibular distraction in a 6 year old?**

1 week.

O   **What are symptoms of TMJ internal derangement?**

Anterior excursion of the meniscus with posterior and superior positioning of the condyle; jaw clicking; preauricular pain.

O   **What is the relationship of the condyle during an acute TMJ dislocation?**

Anterior excursion of the condyle past the eminence.

O   **What is the safest landmark for identifying the facial nerve during parotid surgery?**

Using the tympanomastoid suture line.

○   **Following a LeFort I, what provides vascularity to the maxillary segment?**

The ascending pharyngeal artery and ascending palatine artery (of the facial artery).

○   **What does the greater palatine artery supply?**

Palate and roof of mouth.

○   **What does the lesser palatine artery supply?**

Soft palate and palatine tonsils.

○   **What is cryptotia?**

Absence of the superior auriculocephalic sulcus; upper pole is buried beneath the scalp.

○   **What normally supplies blood to the maxilla?**

Internal maxillary artery by descending palatine, posterior superior alveolar, and infraorbital arteries.

○   **What is cup ear?**

Hooding of the scapha and helix and antihelical flattening.

○   **What is lop ear?**

Auricular protrusion and superior helical folding.

○   **What are characteristics of mandibular prognathism?**

Angle Class III, lower facial third prominence.

○   **What are characteristics of mandibular retrognathism?**

Anterior teeth protrusion, lip incompetence, deep labiomental crease.

○   **What treatment should be undertaken for an anterior frontal sinus fracture with a nondisplaced posterior wall fracture and patency of the nasofrontal duct?**

Repair of the anterior wall alone.

○   **What approach is undertaken if the nasofrontal duct is obstructed?**

Obliteration of the frontal sinus.

○   **What situation necessitates cranialization?**

Comminution of the posterior wall; concomitant CSF leak.

○   **What clinical symptoms define superior orbital fissure syndrome?**

Fracture affecting III, IV, V_1, and VI; extraocular muscle paralysis, levator palpebrae weakness, numbness of the forehead, eyebrow, upper eyelid.

○ **What is orbital apex syndrome?**

Superior orbital fissure syndrome with blindness (from optic nerve involvement).

○ **When do the permanent canine teeth erupt?**

Between 10 and 11 years of age.

○ **When do the permanent 1st molars erupt?**

6 -7 years of age.

○ **What nerve is the cause of Frey's syndrome?**

Aberrant regeneration of the auriculotemporal nerve.

○ **What is the mechanism of Frey's syndrome?**

Aberrant regeneration of the auriculotemporal nerve to sweat glands; test with Minor's starch-iodine test.

○ **What is the treatment of Frey's syndrome?**

Tympanic neurectomy, topical glycopyrrolate, and/or Prantal (diphemanil methyl sulfate) to control gustatory sweating.

○ **Where does the great auricular nerve travel within the neck?**

Exists on top of the SCM 9 cm from the caudal EAC and 6.5 cm inferior to the tragus.

○ **What type of mandible fracture is seen in a patient with chin deviation to the left, upward mandibular cant to the left, and right sided open bite deformity?**

Left condylar fracture; also with loss of posterior ramus height on left, chin deviated to left due to right lateral pterygoid.

○ **What growth factor has been associated with craniosynostosis in the animal model?**

TGF-beta in the posterior frontal suture line.

○ **When does the anterior fontanelle close?**

24 months.

○ **When does the posterior fontanelle close?**

2 months.

○ **What is the treatment for bilateral subcondylar fractures?**

ORIF through preauricular incisions.

○ **What is the most common craniofacial anomaly?**

Hemifacial microsomia.

○ **Fractures of what part of the mandible is most significant for growth in the child?**

Fractures of the condyle.

○   **What are late complications of frontal sinus fractures?**

Orbital abscess, mucocele, osteomyelitis.

○   **What are complications of frontal sinus fractures occurring within the first few weeks?**

Meningitis, mucocele, frontal sinusitis.

○   **What does the first branchial groove develop into?**

The EAC.

○   **What is the most common site of squamous cell carcinoma of the paranasal sinuses?**

The maxillary sinus (chronic exposure to nickel and wood working materials).

○   **What is most common cause of TMJ ankylosis?**

Trauma.

○   **What permanent tooth erupts first?**

The first molar (6 to 7 years of age).

○   **What are the commonly used cranial base planes?**

Frankfort horizontal, basion-nasion, sella-nasion.

○   **What are common maxillary planes used?**

Axis of the maxillary incisor, nasion to A point, occlusal, and palatal.

○   **What bones form the lateral orbital wall?**

Zygoma, greater wing of the sphenoid.

○   **What bones form the orbit?**

Greater wing of sphenoid, lacrimal, palatine, maxilla, ethmoid, frontal, lesser wing of the sphenoid.

○   **What structures drain into the middle meatus?**

The anterior ethmoid, maxillary, and frontal sinuses.

○   **What drains into the inferior meatus?**

The nasolacrimal duct.

○   **What is the primary action of the superior oblique?**

Depression; also abduction and intorsion; innervated by the trochlear nerve.

○   **What is the percentage of coexisting spine injuries with panfacial MVC trauma?**

10%.

○ **What muscle is used in sphincter pharyngoplasty for reconstruction?**

Palatopharyngeus.

○ **What is the blood supply to the sternocleidomastoid muscle?**

Occipital, superior thyroid, and thyrocervical trunk.

○ **What metal on CT scan exhibits the greatest amount of scatter?**

Stainless steel; titanium and vitallium have the least scatter.

○ **What suture line is broken in Lefort III but not monobloc advancement?**

Frontozygomatic suture and nasofrontal junction.

○ **What muscles are important for closure of the velum?**

Levator veli palatini, uvulus, palatopharyngeus, and superior pharyngeal constrictors; (NOT the tensor veli palatini).

○ **What is the mechanism of velopharyngeal insufficiency with the levator veli palatini in cleft palate?**

The levator inserts on the posterior hard palate; repair reproduces the sling required for closure.

○ **What is the role of the tensor veli palatini?**

Tenses the soft palate; important for Eustachian tube function.

○ **What attaches to Whitnall's tubercle?**

Lateral rectus fascial extension, lateral check ligament, lateral levator aponeurosis horn, and lateral palpebral ligaments.

○ **What is the suspensor ligament of Lockwood composed of?**

Fascia from the inferior rectus and inferior oblique.

○ **What is the most frequent site of mandible fractures?**

Angle (35%), parasymphyseal region (24%), body (18%).

○ **What premature fusion causes brachycephaly?**

Bilateral coronal synostosis; cranial vault is shortening in A-P dimension; frontal skull is flat and wide.

○ **What is lambdoid synostosis known as?**

Occipital or posterior plagiocephaly; oblique and posterior flattening.

○ **What is the condition present with a normal SNA and decreased SNB?**

Mandibular retrusion.

○ **What is the Landes angle?**

Frankfort horizontal and N-A plane; normal value 88 degrees.

○   **What is the likely cause of a gradual bony enlargement of the left fronto-orbital region in a 9 year old?**

Fibrous dysplasia.

○   **What is McCune Albright's syndrome?**

Polyostotic fibrous dysplasia, hyperthyroidism, abnormal pigmentation, sexual precocity.

○   **In a patient with mandibular prognathism and maxillary hypoplasia, what is the required treatment?**

LeFort I with sagittal split osteotomy.

○   **What is the likely cause of enophthalmos after trauma?**

Bony orbital volume increase.

○   **What is the next course of treatment following a LeFort I with a unilateral posterior open bite deformity?**

Removal of hardware and disimpaction of the maxillary fracture.

○   **What is Binder's syndrome?**

Midface hypoplasia, flat nasal dorsum, retracted columella, anterior nasal spine absence; Angle class III occlusion.

○   **What do the first 3 hillocks give rise to?**

The tragus, root of the helix, and superior helix.

○   **What do the second 3 hillocks give rise to?**

The antihelix, antitragus, and lobule.

○   **What does Meckel's cartilage form?**

Malleus, incus, mandible, sphenomandibular ligament.

○   **What does Reichert's cartilage form?**

Stapes, styloid process, stylohyoid ligament, lesser cornu of the hyoid, part of the hyoid body.

○   **What is the first structure to be released during treatment of a retrobulbar hematoma?**

The lateral canthal tendon.

○   **Where is Tenon's capsule located?**

It covers the globe and extraocular muscles; lower portion constitutes Lockwood's ligament.

○   **What is the study of choice in patients with painless jaw clicking after trauma?**

MRI to rule out internal derangement.

○   **What Tessier cleft is associated with macrostomia?**

No. 7.

○ **Which cleft is associated with absence of the zygomatic arch?**

Also No. 7.

○ **What is the likelihood of malignant transformation in acinic cell carcinoma of the parotid?**

Infrequent; bilateral or multicentric lesion.

○ **What is the most common malignant tumor of the parotid?**

Mucoepidermoid carcinoma.

○ **What is the layer underneath which is used for the Gillies approach to a zygomatic arch fracture?**

Deep layer of the deep temporal fascia.

○ **What is the mechanism of action of the TMJ during the last portion of jaw opening?**

Upper joint space translation.

○ **What is the sequence of events in TMJ opening?**

Rotation (condyle in lower joint space), rotation/translation, translation within the joint (condyle in upper joint space).

○ **What innervates the tensor veli palatini?**

Cranial nerve V.

○ **What innervates the levator veli palatini?**

The superior laryngeal branch of CN X.

○ **What innervates the stylopharyngeus?**

CN IX.

○ **What innervates the palatopharyngeus?**

CN X.

○ **What supplies vascularity to the trapezius flap?**

The transverse cervical artery; secondary source occipital artery; type II muscle flap.

○ **What supplies sensation to the lobule and posterior 2/3 of the ear?**

The great auricular nerve.

○ **What supplies sensation to the posterior ear and EAC?**

Arnold's nerve (branch of X).

○ **What supplies sensation to the anterior superior helix and tragus?**

Auriculotemporal nerve (branch of V).

○   **What supplies sensation to the posterior auricle and concha?**

Posterior auricular nerve, lesser occipital nerve.

○   **What is the rate of distraction osteogenesis in the pediatric mandible?**

1 mm/day.

○   **What process causes the changing of recipient mesenchymal cells into osteoprogenitor cells from BMP stimulation?**

Osteoinduction.

○   **What is osteoconduction?**

Bone ingrowth into grafted material.

○   **What structures should be inspected following nasal trauma regarding septal deviation?**

Septal cartilage, perpendicular plate of the ethmoid, vomer.

○   **What is the first line treatment for nasopharyngeal carcinoma?**

Radiation therapy.

○   **What is the likely response to a 2 cm squamous cell carcinoma of the lower lip to radiotherapy?**

90% complete response.

○   **What permanent teeth have the longest roots?**

The cuspids (canines); 27 mm height.

○   **What bone mainly comprises the medial orbital wall?**

Ethmoid bone.

○   **The lingual nerve is a branch of what nerve?**

The mandibular branch of CN V.

○   **What are main branches of the mandibular division of CN V?**

Lingual nerve, inferior alveolar nerve, long buccal branch, mental nerve, auriculotemporal branch.

○   **What does the auriculotemporal nerve innervate?**

Sensation to the anterior auricle, temporal region, and portion of EAC and TMJ.

○   **What are the main branches of the maxillary division of CN V?**

Infraorbital nerve, nasopalatine nerve, posterosuperior alveolar nerve, posterosuperior nasal nerve.

○   **What structure is the likely cause of ectropion following an orbital floor fracture reduction through a subciliary incision?**

Scarring of the orbital septum.

○   **What structure is avoided when making an incision into the first lower eyelid crease during an orbital floor fracture case?**

This incision preserves the innervation of the pretarsal portion of the orbicularis oculi; normal lid tone is preserved.

○   **The mental nerve located in relation to what tooth of the mandible?**

The second bicuspid.

○   **Where is Stensen's duct located relative the maxillary teeth?**

Opposite the second molar..

○   **What muscle contributes to medial displacement of the condyle following a fracture?**

Lateral pterygoid.

○   **The Frankfort horizontal passes through which points?**

The porion and orbitale.

○   **What is the treatment for a unilateral nondisplaced coronoid fracture?**

Short term mandibulomaxillary fixation.

○   **What is the treatment for a mandibular osteogenic sarcoma?**

Wide excision, followed by radiation/chemotherapy.

○   **Where do the most minor salivary gland tumors arise in the mouth?**

The palate.

○   **What is the histological subtype of most minor salivary gland tumors?**

Adenoid cystic carcinoma.

○   **In an edentulous patient, what can be used for maxillomandibular fixation?**

Intraoral splints that are custom made; fixed to the maxilla or mandible using wires/screws.

○   **What is advocated for first-line treatment for a chylous fistula in the neck?**

Medium chain triglyceride diet with closed drainage on suction.

○   **Which side is a chylous fistula usually associated on?**

Injury to the thoracic duct on the left.

○   **What are the physical findings associated with a unilateral cleft lip?**

Rotation of the premaxilla and outward projection; collapsed lateral maxillary segment; shortened columella, attenuation of the lower lateral cartilage; alar base rotated outward; shortened philtrum.

○   **What direction are the septum and cartilage deviated towards in a unilateral cleft lip?**

Towards the non-cleft side.

HAND and EXTREMITIES

○   **What tendon transfer is most appropriate in a child with spastic cerebral palsy with mental retardation and a clenched fist with ulnar palmar maceration?**

FDS to FDP; this will lengthen and weaken the finger flexors; may also arthrodese wrist rather than transferring to wrist extensors.

○   **When is texture discrimination appropriate for children with CP?**

Age 2-3 years.

○   **Trauma to the dorsalis pedis artery in the lower leg is most likely associated with what neuropraxia?**

Decreased deep peroneal nerve function; first web space decreased sensation.

○   **What innervates the dorsal aspect of the foot?**

Superficial peroneal nerve.

○   **What innervates the lateral foot?**

Sural nerve.

○   **Medial?**

Saphenous nerve.

○   **Which of these nerves travels with an artery?**

Deep peroneal nerve.

○   **What innervates the plantar surface?**

Tibial nerve; travels with PT.

○   **What is the immediate treatment for Hydrofluoric acid burns?**

Calcium gluconate gel application (prevention of hypocalcemia, hypomagnesemia, hyperkalemia).

○   **What is given for phenol burns?**

Mineral oil.

○   **What is given for creosol burns?**

Polyethylene glycol.

○ **What is the most common primary benign tumor of the hand?**

Enchondroma (benign cartilaginous tumor).

○ **What signifies pain in the absence of fracture with enchondroma?**

Malignant degeneration.

○ **What is the radiographic finding in enchondroma?**

Scalloped, lytic lesion within the medullary canal.

○ **What is Ollier disease?**

Multiple enchondromatosis.

○ **What is Maffucci syndrome?**

Multiple enchondromas with subcutaneous hemangiomas.

○ **How often do chondromyxoid fibromas occur in the upper extremity?**

Rarely .

○ **How often do giant cell tumors occur in the distal upper extremity?**

Only 2-5% in hand; radius is third most commonly affected site.

○ **How often do osteoid osteomas cause pain?**

Frequently, at night, give NSAIDS.

○ **What defines the midpalmar space?**

Flexor tendons, metacarpal bone and interosseous fascia, septum from third metacarpal to FDP, superficial aponeurosis (deep to the flexor tendon to fascia over $2^{nd}/3^{rd}$ volar interossei and $3^{rd}/4^{th}$ metacarpals).

○ **What is the thenar space?**

Radial to vertical septum between third MC and FDP of long finger; extends to radial edge of abductor pollicis brevis.

○ **What tendons are ruptured most commonly in RA?**

EPL (treat with ECRL transfer) and EDQ.

○ **How do extensor tendon ruptures progress in the RA patient?**

Ulnar to radial progression (Vaughn-Jackson progression); EDQ then EDC to small, ring, then long fingers.

○ **What is a Mannerfeldt lesion?**

Rupture of FPL over a scaphoid spur (flexor ruptures far less frequently, usually affecting radial digits)

○ **What prevents closed reduction of the little finger in a volar dislocation of the PIP joint?**

Extensor tendon; when condyle has pushed through the extensor tendon and acts as sling.

○   **What is more common – volar or dorsal dislocations of the PIP?**

Dorsal.

○   **What may prevent dorsal dislocations of the PIP from adequate closed reduction?**

Volar plate and flexor tendons, though rarely.

○   **What is the most common primary blood supply to the great toe in toe to thumb transfer?**

1st dorsal metatarsal artery from DP; may travel dorsal or plantar to interosseous muscle.

○   **What hand tumor has an affinity for immunosuppressed patients?**

Keratoacanthoma (thought to be a variant of SCCa); appears as red papule, expands rapidly over several weeks.

○   **What is the likelihood for future siblings to be affected with constriction band syndrome?**

No genetic transmission; 4th most common congenital hand anomaly.

○   **What are the three most common congenital hand anomalies?**

Polydactyly, syndactyly, and trigger thumb.

○   **What other anomalies are seen with amniotic band syndrome?**

Club foot, cleft lip/palate, craniofacial defects, hemangioma, meningocele.

○   **What is the most appropriate treatment for radial nerve palsy after a humeral ORIF 6 months later?**

Tendon transfers.

○   **What transfers are performed for radial nerve palsy?**

Pronator teres to ECRB for wrist extension.

○   **What transfers are performed for finger extension?**

FCR, FCU, FDS(3,4) to EDC.

○   **What transfers are performed for thumb extension?**

PL or FCR to EPL.

○   **What is the best option for reconstruction of volar skin of the index when dorsal skin of the long finger is not available?**

Thenar flap (for tips of index/long fingers); these fingers flex easily into the thenar crease.

○   **What option is there for ring and small finger volar skin defects?**

Hypothenar flaps.

○   **What procedure may be used for volar pad defects of the thumb?**

Moberg flap; volar advancement flap; composed completely of palmar thumb skin.

○ **With a SLAC wrist what procedure is most appropriate in a dock worker?**

SLAC wrist, with DISI and radioscaphoid arthrosis is best treated with scaphoid excision and 4 corner arthrodesis (lunate, capitate, hamate, triquetrum) in a dock worker.

○ **How is SLAC wrist classified?**

Stage I: radioscaphoid
Stage II: radial midcarpal
Stage III: ulnar midcarpal
Stage IV: pancarpal

○ **What structure defines the growth and differentiation of the new limb during embryologic development?**

Apical ectodermal ridge (which arises from the Wolffian ridge, protruding from the main trunk).

○ **What structure defines anterior-posterior morphology of the limb?**

Zone of polarizing activity.

○ **When do the upper extremities begin to develop?**

At 4 weeks; by the 5th week, the hand is recognizable; the apical ectodermal ridge becomes flattened; hand appears initially as paddle.

○ **When are the fingernails identifiable?**

At the 17th week of gestation.

○ **What is the first step in a patient with a 2cm gap in the ulnar nerve following trauma?**

Ulnar nerve transposition (provides up to 4 cm of length; 2 cm of length at distal forearm and wrist).

○ **PIP contractures in fifth finger Dupuytren's is most likely caused by what structures?**

Central, lateral, and spiral cords.

○ **What other fascial structures may contribute to flexion contractures?**

Grayson's, Cleland's, lateral digital sheath, natatory ligament, pretendinous and spiral bands, superficial transverse ligament.

○ **What does the central cord arise from?**

The pretendinous band.

○ **What is the lateral cord from?**

Central digital sheath.

○ **What is the spiral cord composed of?**

Pretendinous and spiral bands, lateral digital sheath, and Grayson's ligament.

❍   **Contraction of the spiral cord has what effect on the neurovascular bundle?**

Medial and superficial displacement of the bundle.

❍   **What causes contracture of the MP joint?**

Action from the pretendinous cord (which does not contribute to PIP contracture).

❍   **What does the natatory cord cause?**

Adduction contractures of the digits (passes transversely across palm at level of web spaces).

❍   **What is the most common organism causing septic arthritis of the hand/wrist?**

Staph. aureus. Streptococcus is next.

❍   **What organism will likely be cultured from a human bite wound?**

Eikenella corrodens.

❍   **What is the best option for a distal third defect following trauma with exposed bone?**

Fasciocutaneous flap.

❍   **What defects will a gastrocnemius flap cover in the leg?**

Upper, some middle third of the leg defects.

❍   **How is onychomycosis treated?**

6 weeks of terbinafine or itraconazole .

❍   **Is terbinafine associated with any side effects?**

Stevens-Johnson, neutropenia, hepatic failure.

❍   **What is lumbrical plus deformity?**

Extension of the PIP on attempting to make a fist (occurs following repair; secondary to release of FDP of index).

❍   **How is lumbrical plus treated?**

Division of the lumbrical (with attempted flexion lumbrical exerts tension through lateral band).

❍   **When is transfer of the interosseous muscle performed?**

Correction of rheumatoid ulnar drift.

❍   **What is the acceptable limit of before surgical correction is necessary in a pediatric patient with camptodactyly?**

30 degrees of extension of the PIP.

❍   **How are minimal extension deficits corrected in camptodactyly?**

Transfer lumbrical tendon into central slip.

❍ **How are extension deficits greater than 30 degrees treated?**

Release of abnormal lumbrical and superficialis tendons; release of accessory collateral ligaments to volar plate; FTSG.

❍ **What is the Zancolli-lasso procedure?**

Portions of FDS brought through A2 pulley; for correction of ulnar palsy digital clawing.

❍ **What are Kanavel's signs?**

Fusiform swelling, partial flexed posturing of finger, tenderness over flexor tendon sheath, pain with passive extension; open and irrigate flexor sheath.

❍ **Where are incisions made for flexor tenosynovitis?**

Palm incision to inspect proximal A1 pulley and distal incision to visualize A4, A5 at minimum.

❍ **What is the best postoperative dressing for an infant following simple complete syndactyly release of the 3rd web space?**

Long arm cast.

❍ **What zone of flexor tendon repair is associated with the best prognosis?**

Zone 5.

❍ **Which finger has the most lacerations of the nail bed?**

The long finger.

❍ **How are nail bed lacerations classified?**

Simple, stellate, crush, amputated, avulsion.

❍ **Following a ring avulsion replantation failure, what is the next step in management?**

Ray amputation with most or all of the metacarpal.

❍ **What is the Littler flap?**

A neurovascular island flap based on the digital nerve/vascular bundle of long or ring.

❍ **What is the Shaw flap?**

SIEA flap; can be used for coverage of hand/forearm.

❍ **Where are the landmarks of the superficial inferior epigastric artery?**

Intersection of inguinal ligament and femoral artery; travels superiorly and laterally towards anterior axilla.

❍ **What is the arterial supply of the groin flap?**

SCIA.

❍ **What are landmarks for the SCIA?**

Originates from femoral artery, travels parallel to inguinal ligament, 1cm deep to the ligament.

○ **What is the best treatment of trapeziometacarpal DJD in factory worker?**

Arthrodesis.

○ **When is reconstruction of the palmar (oblique) ligament performed?**

Situations of prearthritic instability with pain of CMC joint.

○ **How are lunate dislocations classified?**

Midcarpal lunocapitate, complete lunate, and perilunate .

○ **How is a complete lunate injury differentiated from a perilunate injury?**

Presence of radiolunate joint dislocation concurrently.

○ **What other bony structures are involved in greater arc injury?**

High energy trauma; radial styloid, scaphoid, capitate, hamate, triquetrum, ulnar styloid fractures.

○ **What structures are involved in lesser arc injury?**

SL, LT, lunocapitate intervals.

○ **What is a collar button abscess?**

Pus communicating from volar web space to dorsal hand by palmar fascia or lumbrical canal.

○ **What is a characteristic finding of a collar button abscess?**

Finger abduction.

○ **Where is Parona's space?**

Between pronator quadratus and FDP tendons; communicates with radial and ulnar palmar bursa and midpalmar space.

○ **What area of swelling is associated with Parona's space infection?**

Volar wrist proximal to distal flexion crease.

○ **How is the scaphoid vascularized?**

Perforators enter distally and supply most proximal part last; high risk of avascular necrosis of proximal pole fractures.

○ **What nerve is typically decompressed during Volkman's contracture reconstruction with a muscle free flap?**

Median nerve at all points of compression.

○ **What forearm muscles are affected most often in compartment syndrome?**

FPL, FDP; in severe cases, FDS, FCU, FCR.

○ **What areas of compression are important in decompressing the median nerve?**

Lacertus fibrosus, two heads of pronator teres, proximal arch of FDS, carpal canal; ligament of Struthers (band between supracondylar humeral process and medial epicondyle).

○ **Does Volkman's ischemic contracture involve the anterior interosseous nerve?**

No.

○ **What is ectrodactyly?**

Partial or total absence of fingers suggesting central hand deficiency.

○ **What is typical central hand deficiency?**

Absence of third ray; usu. bilateral, cleft lip/palate, congenital heart disease, syndactyly and foot involvement common.

○ **What is atypical central deficiency?**

Usu. with several deficient rays unilaterally; known as symbrachydactyly; sporadic inheritance; syndactyly/foot involvement not common.

○ **What is camptodactyly?**

Nontraumatic flexion deformity of PIP; usually bilateral; involves small finger.

○ **What is hypothenar hammer syndrome?**

Ulnar artery thrombosis; symptoms include pain, paresthesia, temperature decrease, numbness of ulnar digits.

○ **What is the treatment of a neuroma in continuity in the extremity?**

Neuroma excision and nerve grafting (e.g. with sural nerve).

○ **What influences the success of a replanted digit?**

Most importantly mechanism of injury (crush, avulsion lower success rates) ; cooling of amputated part improves success.

○ **What differentiates complex and simple syndactyly?**

Complex: skin and bones are fused.

○ **When do infants with syndactyly undergo release?**

Typically by 18 months.

○ **What is the best diagnostic study for a high flow vascular malformation in the extremity?**

MRA.

○ **What symptoms accompany ulnar nerve compression at Guyon's canal?**

Weakness of grip, limited abduction/adduction of fingers, difficulty crossing fingers, decreased sensation over ulnar sided digits.

❍ **What is the significance of dorsoulnar sensation of the hand?**

Sensation to this area is supplied by ulnar nerve fibers arising 6 cm PROXIMAL to Guyon's canal.

❍ **What are the most common sites of compression of the ulnar nerve?**

Band of Osborne (cubital tunnel), Guyon's canal, arcade of Struther's (thin aponeurotic band from medial triceps head to medial intermuscular septum), origin of the FCU.

❍ **What describes the arcade of Struther's?**

fascial bands extending from the medial intermuscular septum that can compress the ulnar nerve.

❍ **What is another name for the deep branch of the radial nerve?**

Posterior interosseous nerve.

❍ **What are compression sites of the radial nerve?**

Arcade of Froshe (band over supinator), vascular leash of Henry (radial recurrent vessels that cross the nerve), ECRB, proximal supinator, distal supinator.

❍ **What is the most appropriate treatment for split nail deformity?**

Full thickness nail grafting from the toe; injured nail bed does not carry growth of new nail plate.

❍ **What are the likely anatomic causes of failed closed reduction of a dorsal dislocation of the MP joint of the index finger?**

Lumbrical muscle, volar plate, FDP.

❍ **What is the mechanism of failed closed reduction in this case?**

MC head protrudes volar between lumbrical and flexor tendons; volar plate is folded within the joint.

❍ **What are symptoms of complex regional pain syndrome I?**

Otherwise known as RSD; pain, stiffness, vasomotor instability; hyperhidrosis, osteoporosis may occur.

❍ **How is RSD diagnosed?**

Stellate ganglion blocks; thermography has also been used.

❍ **What is causalgia?**

Otherwise known as complex regional pain syndrome II; persistent pain following trauma with a known nerve injury.

❍ **What is most appropriate treatment following transverse nonhealing fractures of the 4th and 5th metacarpal shafts?**

Open reduction, miniplate fixation.

❍ **What is the most common mode of inheritance in typical cleft hand?**

Autosomal dominant.

○ **What are characteristics of typical cleft hand?**

V shaped cleft, absence of central digit, syndactyly of ulnar sided digits; associated with syndromes (EEC: ectrodactyly, ectodermal dysplasia, cleft lip/palate); cleft foot.

○ **What are characteristics of atypical cleft hand?**

U shaped hand that is broad; sometimes termed symbrachydactyly.

○ **What is the common cause of swan neck deformities in rheumatoid arthritis?**

Intrinsic tendon tightness.

○ **What procedures are recommended for swan neck deformities?**

MP arthroplasty, intrinsic releases, centralizing extrinsic extensor tendons; Zancolli-FDS reconstruction.

○ **What muscle harvested with a distally based posterior interosseous flap will maintain blood supply of the ulna?**

Muscle to the EPL.

○ **What fascial structures normally surround the neurovascular bundle in the finger?**

Cleland's, Grayson's ligaments, lateral digital sheet, retrovascular band.

○ **Where do EDC ruptures occur in RA?**

At level of distal ulna; must differentiate from extensor subluxation.

○ **Can FDS ruptures cause swan neck deformities in RA?**

Yes, less commonly.

○ **What is Cleland's ligament?**

Fascial structure lying deep and dorsal to neurovascular bundle; originates from side of phalanges and travels obliquely to skin.

○ **What is Grayson's ligament?**

Superficial to neurovascular bundle; arises from tendon sheath and goes to the skin; travel volar to the neurovascular bundle; thought to be involved in Dupuytren's.

○ **What is the lateral digital sheath?**

Composed of superficial fascia on both sides of the phalanges; fibers from the natatory ligament and spiral band contribute as well.

○ **What is the most appropriate time for correction of syndactyly?**

12-18 months for 3rd web space; earlier for 1st or 4th web space syndactyly.

○ **What defines complete syndactyly?**

Inclusion of the entire web space.

○   **What supplies the sartorius muscle flap?**

The superficial circumflex iliac and superficial femoral arteries.

○   **What potential flaps are supplied by the lateral circumflex femoral artery?**

Rectus femoris, TFL, vastus lateralis.

○   **What is a pincer nail deformity?**

Otherwise known as trumpet nail deformity; excess transverse nail curvature; pinching of the soft tissue of the fingertip.

○   **How is trumpet nail deformity treated?**

Lateral nail matrix elevation and dermal grafting.

○   **In neonatal brachial plexus palsy, complete recovery is likely if activity is seen in the deltoid and biceps by what week?**

Week 8.

○   **What is Dupuytren's diathesis?**

An early, aggressive form of Dupuytren's involving knuckles, plantar fascia, and Peyronie's disease.

○   **What digits are involved in Dupuytren's disease? In Dupuytren's diathesis?**

In Dupuytren's the ulnar digits; in diathesis the radial digits.

○   **What distinguishes the location of Heberden's and Bouchard nodes?**

Both seen in OA; Heberden's affects the DIP; Bouchard affects the PIP.

○   **What response is sometimes seen following surgery for Dupuytren's disease?**

A flare response (type of localized RSD).

○   **What is hypothenar hammer syndrome?**

Trauma to hand causing crushing of the ulnar artery at Guyon's canal resulting in a true aneurysm sending emboli to the digits.

○   **What upper extremity findings are seen in thoracic outlet syndrome?**

Sensorimotor findings in C8-T1; numbness in fingers (particularly small finger); test with Roos, Adson's tests.

○   **What patient population is Buerger's disease seen in?**

Middle aged smokers.

○   **What incision is used for compartment syndrome of the hand in releasing the adductor pollicis and interossei?**

Dorsal incision over the second metacarpal.

○ **What compartments are released in a hand compartment syndrome?**

4 dorsal, 3 volar interossei, adductor pollicis, and thenar/hypothenar eminences.

○ **What incisions are made for releasing all of the hand compartments?**

All dorsal incisions over the 2nd and 4th metacarpals; ulnar 5th metacarpal, radial 1st metacarpal.

○ **What is the best means of reducing a dorsal dislocation of the MP joint of the index?**

Wrist flexion with placing pressure distally and volarly; traction places the volar plate more dorsally preventing the MP joint from being reducible and tightens lumbricals and flexor tendons.

○ **What is the likely cause of point tenderness of the base of the nail that is sensitive to cold and painful on palpation?**

Glomus tumor; bright lesion on T2 MRI.

○ **What are the 2 most common tumors of the hand?**

Ganglions, followed by giant cell tumors

○ **Where are giant cell tumors usually found?**

Palmar surfaces of the wrist and hand.

○ **What is Vaughn-Jackson progression?**

Extensor tendon rupture from ulnar to radial sided digits.

○ **What is caput ulna?**

Prominence and dorsal subluxation of the ulna causing tendon ruptures.

○ **What is done for extensor tendon ruptures in RA?**

Transfer to radial extensors; centralized over MP joints.

○ **What comprises tendon transfers for radial nerve palsy?**

Pronator teres to ECRB, FCU to EDC, palmaris longus to EPL.

○ **What is done in the Boyes sublimis transfer?**

FDS(3) transferred to the EDC(3,4,5); FDS(4) to EIP and EPL; and FCR to adductor longus and EPB.

○ **What is seen on radiographs of the hand in scleroderma?**

Calcium deposits in the soft tissue; treat with calcium channel antagonists, NSAIDS, penicillamine.

○ **What is clinically seen in the hands in hypoparathyroidism?**

Carotenemia on the palms and soles.

○ **What is pronator syndrome?**

Compression proximally of the median nerve; sensory symptoms in the median nerve distribution; decreased palm sensation.

O   **What maneuvers reproduce pronator syndrome?**

Elbow flexion with elbow in pronation, resisted elbow flexion, resisted pronation with wrist flexion.

O   **What are compression points of the median nerve?**

The supracondylar process and ligament of Struthers (from supracondylar humeral process and medial epicondyle, lacertus fibrosis (fascia of aponeurosis from biceps tendon to flexor mass), pronator teres, FDS arch.

O   **What is anterior interosseous syndrome?**

Pain in proximal forearm; weakness/paralysis of FDP of index and long, FPL, and pronator quadratus.

O   **Where is the anterior interosseous nerve compressed potentially?**

Deep head of the pronator teres, FDS(4) tendinous origin, origin of FCU, accessory FPL, palmaris profundus.

O   **What is cubital tunnel syndrome?**

Compression of the ulnar nerve at the elbow; pain over proximal forearm; weakness of FDP of ring and small and 1st dorsal interosseous and abductor digiti minimi; numbness/tingling of ring/small fingers; sensory deficit of ring/small.

O   **What is posterior interosseous syndrome?**

Motor deficits without sensory deficits; weakness of wrist/thumb/thumb abduction/digit extensors; radial deviation of the wrist (ECRL innervated proximally); initially weakness and pain in forearm.

O   **What likely is the site of compression of the posterior interosseous nerve?**

Arcade of Frohse.

O   **Where do most patients have compression with radial tunnel syndrome?**

At the arcade of Frohse (band over deep radial nerve entering supinator); also vascular leash, ECRB tendon.

O   **What is the primary symptom seen in radial tunnel?**

Pain rather than numbness or weakness over the mobile wad with extension, resisted supination, or passive flexion/pronation of the wrist.

O   **What motor or sensory loss is seen with radial tunnel syndrome?**

None.

O   **What is the most appropriate step for avascular necrosis of the proximal pole of the scaphoid following ORIF?**

Bone pedicle flap; based on perforators from neighboring extensor compartments.

O   **What percentage of nondisplaced scaphoid fractures heal by casting alone?**

90%.

○ **What is the incidence of complete healing in scaphoid fractures displaced by more than 1 mm?**

55% have nonunion; 50% have eventual avascular necrosis.

○ **What is Kienbock's disease?**

Avascular necrosis of the lunate.

○ **What most likely prevents closed reduction in PIP dislocations?**

FDP tendon (flexion causes entrapment of the proximal phalangeal condyles); volar plate also is a potential cause of failed reduction.

○ **What is the treatment for extrinsic tendon tightness of the PIP following a old burn injury?**

Central slip release.

○ **What is treatment for intrinsic tendon tightness?**

Release of the lateral bands.

○ **What is the sequence of replantation for a five finger amputation?**

Thumb, followed by long or ring, with index least in order of importance.

○ **What is the sequence of reconstructing the structures of an amputated digit?**

First bone/tendon, then vein/artery, then nerves last.

○ **What position on the metacarpal is most appropriate for a index to long finger transposition?**

At the level of the metacarpal base.

○ **What is the likely effect on power grip and key pinch following a ray resection of the index finger?**

20% decrease; loss of supination strength.

○ **What is the treatment for an acute scapholunate tear?**

Open repair through a dorsal incision; Blatt capsulodesis further secures the repair.

○ **What are Mayfield's classification of perilunate instability patterns?**

I: SL instability or tearing of SL and volar radioscaphoid ligaments
II: dislocation of the capitate
III: LT separation
IV: lunate dislocation

○ **What encompasses greater arc injuries in the setting of perilunate dislocations?**

Fractures of the radial styloid, capitate, triquetrum, ulnar styloid.

○ **When is scaphoidectomy recommended?**

In scaphoid nonunion advanced collapse; progressive chronic arthritis in conjunction with a proximal row carpectomy or four corner arthrodesis.

❍   **What artery courses through the triangular space?**

The circumflex scapular.

❍   **What are the boundaries of the triangular space?**

The long head of the triceps, teres major and teres minor.

❍   **Where is the quadrangular space in relation to the triangular space?**

Immediately lateral.

❍   **What comprises the quadrangular space?**

Surgical humeral neck, lateral head of the triceps, teres major, teres minor.

❍   **What passes through the quandrangular space?**

The axillary nerve and posterior humeral circumflex artery.

❍   **What is the period of immobilization for a nondisplaced scaphoid waist fracture?**

10 to 14 weeks in a thumb spica cast.

❍   **What is the lumbrical plus deformity?**

Occurs following transection of the FDP tendon; in flexion, the lumbrical through the radial lateral band causes paradoxical PIP extension.

❍   **What is the treatment of lumbrical plus deformity?**

Division of the lumbrical tendon or releasing the radial lateral band.

❍   **What flexor tendon ruptures are seen most frequently in RA?**

FPL and FDP of the index due to bony spurs over the distal scaphoid.

❍   **What is intersection syndrome?**

Second dorsal compartment tenosynovitis; near intersection of 1st and 2nd extensor compartments; pain and swelling 4 cm proximal to wrist; proximal to Lister's tubercle.

❍   **What is Wartenberg syndrome?**

Compression of the dorsal sensory branch of the radial nerve between the brachioradialis and ECRL tendons; pain, numbness of dorsoradial wrist following wearing a bracelet.

❍   **What length of bone is provided by the fibula free flap?**

More than 20 cm.

❍   **What procedure may be done for a 1.5 cm diameter defect of the volar distal thumb?**

Moberg flap (palmar advancement flap).

❍   **What is the most appropriate treatment for a full thickness burn of the forearm?**

Early tangential excision to punctate bleeding and coverage with split thickness skin grafts.

❍ **What joints are affected in osteoarthritis of the thumb?**

CMC, STT, radiocarpal joints; initially, there is volar beak ligament failure.

❍ **What are felons?**

Infections of the pulp space usually caused by Staph A.

❍ **What is the mechanism in congenital clasp thumb?**

Absence of the EPB and/or EPL; MP flexion and thumb adduction.

❍ **Where does the first dorsal metacarpal artery travel in relation to the 1ˢᵗ dorsal interosseous muscle?**

Within the fascia of the muscle; communicates with perforators from the superficial arch near the MP joint.

❍ **What is a Stener lesion?**

Palpable mass on the ulnar metacarpal head; comprised of adductor pollicis fascia interposed between torn ulnar collateral ligament and MP joint of thumb.

❍ **What muscle may cause carpal tunnel syndrome in a heavy laborer?**

Lumbrical. The lumbrical inserts into radial sagittal band and aids in extension of the interphalangeal joints as well as flexion of MP joints.

❍ **What is the appropriate treatment of a chronic paronychia of the finger?**

Usually due to *Candida*; if topical/oral antifungals are not successful, eponychial marsupialization.

❍ **What are associated syndromes of radial club hand?**

VATER, Holt-Oram, Fanconi anemia, TAR syndrome (thrombocytopenia-absent radius syndrome).

❍ **What test is performed to detect Fanconi anemia?**

Mitomycin testing to prevent pancytopenia complications.

❍ **What structures are involved in Dupuytren's contractures of the PIP joint?**

Central, lateral, retrovascular, and spiral cord (pretendinous band, vertical band, spiral band, Grayson's ligaments, lateral digital sheath contribute to the spiral cord).

❍ **What are the subtypes of the thumb-in-palm deformity in cerebral palsy?**

Type I: simple adduction contracture.
Type II: type I with MP flexion deformity.
Type III: adduction with hyperextension deformity and/or MP instability.
Type IV: type I with FPL spasticity.

❍ **What level of amputation should be done for a subungual melanoma?**

At the DIP joint.

❍ **What manipulations of the upper extremity will increase median and ulnar nerve length during repair?**

Shoulder abduction and elbow flexion.

❍ **What is the best treatment for a 30 year old steelworker with CMC arthritis?**

Trapeziometacarpal arthrodesis.

❍ **What are characteristics of juvenile RA?**

Exhibit wrist flexion with loss of wrist extension; carpal bone and metacarpals are deviated ulnarly, loss of IP flexion, loss of MP flexion and radial deviation of MP joints.

❍ **How common are tendon ruptures seen in juvenile RA?**

Rare.

❍ **In adult RA, what direction does the carpus tend towards?**

Radial deviation and supination.

❍ **What is the guiding principle in zone II flexor tendon repairs to ensure greatest motion?**

Immediate early active flexion.

❍ **What spatial relation does the ulnar motor group have with respect with the sensory group in the wrist?**

Ulnar and dorsal to the sensory group; at Guyon's the motor fascicles become dorsal and radial.

❍ **What is the treatment for a type IV mallet injury?**

Closed reduction and pin fixation; 30% of the articular surface of the phalanx has been avulsed.

❍ **What is the treatment for a type I mallet injury?**

Stack splinting; immobilizes DIP joint in extension.

❍ **What is the quadriga effect?**

Excessive distal pull by one FDP tendon; leaves other digits with decreased flexion.

❍ **What is the treatment for a CMC dislocation of the thumb?**

Closed reduction by axial traction and pronation with application of pressure to the metacarpal base and pinning.

❍ **What is normal total active motion for an index finger?**

90 (MP) +110 (PIP) +70 (DIP) = 270 degrees.

❍ **What is the appropriate treatment for the 3ʳᵈ MP joint of a piano player with severe OA?**

Silicone implant arthroplasty.

❍ **What is the best way to correct a supination defect in a quadriplegic?**

Redirection of the biceps tendon through the interosseous membrane.

○ **What is a Moberg flap used for?**

Volar defects of the thumb; 2 arteries and 2 nerves are included; may be advanced 1-1.5 cm.

○ **What are common causes of the lumbrical plus deformity?**

Distal amputations, lengthy FDP interposition grafts; excessive profundus lengthening procedures.

○ **What is the local muscle flap used for antecubital fossa wounds?**

Brachioradialis flap; based on the radial recurrent artery.

○ **What is the lateral arm flap based on?**

Perforating branches of the profunda brachii artery.

○ **What nerve palsy is occasionally seen in tourniquet usage during hand surgery?**

Radial nerve palsy.

○ **What is arthrogryposis?**

Multiple joint contractures seen at birth.

○ **What is Madelung's deformity?**

Radial shortening, palmar subluxation of the carpus, ulnar head prominence; slowed growth of the ulnar distal radius.

○ **What is the treatment of most Salter fractures?**

Closed reduction with pin fixation.

○ **What is the first step in managing an above elbow amputation five hours later?**

Arterial shunting.

○ **What is a longitudinally bracketed epiphysis?**

Causes angular deformity of the finger; longitudinal growth is delayed on one side while the other side of the phalanx grows normally; associated with delta phalanx.

○ **What is Secretan's disorder?**

Peritendinous fibrosis following minor work related trauma; may be associated with lymphedema.

○ **Where do the perforators arise to supply the osteocutaneous radial forearm flap?**

Between the brachioradialis and flexor carpi radialis.

○ **What is the appearance of an enchondroma on plain films?**

Radiolucent neoplasm; thinning and expansion of the bony cortex.

○ **What is the risk of multiple enchondromas?**

Degeneration to chondrosarcomas.

○   **Following a Gustillo IIIB injury, what pulse lavage agent is likely to preserve cellular function while cleaning the wound?**

1% surgical soap.

○   **What is the earliest clinical sign of upper extremity compartment syndrome?**

Worsening pain with passive muscle stretching.

○   **What organism is associated with medicinal leech therapy during antibiotic prophylaxis?**

Aeromonas hydrophila.

○   **What sensation is detected by Pacinian corpuscles?**

Vibration.

○   **What skin component detects burning pain?**

Free endings of C fibers

○   **What detects moving 2 point discrimination?**

Meissner's corpuscles.

○   **What detects static 2 point discrimination?**

Merkel cells.

○   **What web space is most frequently affected in syndactyly?**

The 3rd web space

○   **What is the inheritance of syndactyly?**

Sporadic.

○   **What is Carpenter's syndrome?**

Simple syndactyly, brachydactyly, broad thumbs, craniosynostosis.

○   **What is Pfeiffer's syndrome?**

Partial syndactyly, broad thumbs, midface hypoplasia.

○   **What is a traumatic boutonniere deformity?**

Central slip disruption at the PIP joint with volar migration of the lateral bands; PIP flexion causes DIP extension.

○   **What causes PIP contractures in Dupuytren's?**

Central cord most likely cause; lateral and spiral cords can also cause contractures.

○   **What is the clinical finding of a natatory cord?**

Loss of finger abduction.

○ **What cord causes contractures of the DIP joint?**

The retrovascular cord; dorsal to the neurovascular bundle and palmar to Cleland's ligament.

○ **What contractures do pretendinous cords cause?**

MP contractures.

○ **What can be used for coverage for a dorsal exposed IP joint of the thumb?**

Kite flap.

○ **What is the kite flap based upon?**

1st or 2nd dorsal metacarpal artery; dorsal skin of the respective proximal phalanx is taken with the flap; superficial radial sensory nerve branch may be used for sensation.

○ **Where is the origin of the 1st dorsal metacarpal artery located?**

Just proximal to the bifurcation of the dorsal radial artery into the princeps pollicis and deep palmar arch.

○ **What congenital deformity is seen with a delta phalanx?**

Clinodactyly.

○ **What causes camptodactyly?**

Skin deficit, volar plate shortening, central slip deficiency, shortening of the sublimis tendon.

○ **What is the most frequent finding in late Volkmann's contractures?**

Flexor muscle fibrosis.

○ **In what population of patients do Volkmann's contractures occur?**

Children who have supracondylar fractures (brachial artery compromise).

○ **What nerve is most commonly involved in Volkmann's?**

Median nerve neuropathy most common.

○ **What is the typical clinical appearance of the hand in Volkmann's contracture?**

Wrist flexion, flexion/adduction of the thumb, MP extension, PIP/DIP flexion.

○ **What characterizes intrinsic plus deformities?**

Intrinsic muscle contracture; MP flexion, PIP extension.

○ **What is a Stener lesion?**

The ulnar collateral ligament of the thumb MP joint tears and retracts proximally; the adductor aponeurosis intercedes the space and prevents healing.

❍   **What treatment is done for a Stener lesion?**

Open reduction, internal fixation.

❍   **What is the treatment principle behind patients with RA regarding order of progression?**

Proximal to distal sequence (i.e. elbow arthroplasty before wrist arthrodesis before MP joint arthroplasties).

❍   **What diagnosis should be considered with rapid onset of psoriatic arthritis or Reiter's syndrome (arthritis, conjunctivitis, uveitis)?**

HIV infection.

❍   **What forearm muscles lie the deepest when considering sequelae of compartment syndrome?**

The FDP and FPL.

❍   **What are known as the superficial flexors of the forearm?**

FDS, FCR, FCU, pronator teres.

❍   **What are the deep extensors?**

EPL, EPB, APL, EIP.

❍   **What are the superficial extensors?**

Brachioradialis, ECRL, ECRB, EDC, ECU.

❍   **What are the more aggressive subtypes of basal cell carcinoma?**

Infiltrative, ulcerative, sclerosing, morpheaform.

❍   **For a subungual melanoma of the thumb, what is the most appropriate level of amputation?**

The diaphysis of the proximal phalanx.

❍   **What prevents a Clark level from being assigned in subungual melanomas?**

Absence of subcutaneous tissue in the nailbed.

❍   **What maneuvers are done to preserve web space and function following a proximal phalanx amputation of the thumb?**

Z-plasty, 1st dorsal interosseous tendon detachment, more proximally reattaching the adductor pollicis.

❍   **What structures may be released to improve PIP motion following a severe pilon fracture?**

Collateral ligaments, volar plate, capsule, check rein ligaments; capsulectomy to improve finger motion.

❍   **What borders the lunula of the nailbed?**

Sterile matrix distally and germinal matrix proximally.

❍   **What percentage of people do not have a plantaris muscle on one side?**

15%.

O   **What clinical finding may be seen with a glomus tumor of the nailbed?**

Blue discoloration of the nailbed and distal phalanx erosion.

O   **Where are giant cell tumors of the hand found?**

Palmar wrists, hands, fingers.

O   **Where are mucous cysts typically located in the hand?**

They are ganglions of the DIP joint; Heberden's nodes associated.

O   **What study is typically done for evaluating osteomyelitis of the calcaneus?**

MRI.

O   **What procedure may be done for osteomyelitis of the proximal phalanx of the thumb following EPL repair?**

Decortication and removal of all affected bone; IV antibiotics.

O   **What is next appropriate step for a 2 year old child with a functional thumb but adactyly of the other digits at the level of the MP joint?**

Second toe to hand transfer.

O   **What is Kienbock's disease?**

Avascular necrosis of the lunate.

O   **What is the end stage result of scapholunate dissociation?**

SLAC wrist.

O   **What does the lunate appear like with perilunate dislocation?**

Triangular shaped on A-P.

O   **What are characteristics of scleroderma of the hand?**

Joint stiffness, "shiny" edema of the hands; also may be associated with dysphagia.

O   **What components form CREST syndrome?**

Calcinosis, Raynaud's, esophageal dysfunction, sclerodactyly, telangiectasias.

O   **A laceration over the MP joint of the thumb is likely in what extensor zone?**

V; EPL likely injured.

O   **What is the role of the intrinsics in thumb extension?**

Able to extend thumb IP joint to a neutral position.

О   **What is the treatment for a volar dislocation of the PIP joint with middle phalanx volarly subluxed?**

Lateral band and central slip repair; classically described as irreducible by closed means.

О   **What structures are injured in a volar dislocation of the PIP joint?**

Volar plate, collateral ligament, accessory collateral ligament; may attempt reduction by flexing the MP and PIP joints.

О   **What is the treatment for unstable dorsal dislocations of the PIP joint?**

Volar plate arthroplasty.

О   **What are the borders of the anatomic snuffbox?**

Volar (APL and EPB) and dorsal border (EPL).

О   **How does C7 nerve compression present?**

Weakness in the muscles supplied by the radial nerve (including triceps) and muscles in median nerve distribution (pronator teres, FCR, FDS, FPL).

О   **What is the next step in treating gangrene of the distal tip in a patient with severe peripheral vasculitis?**

Venous bypass; amputation only as a last resort.

О   **What tendon transfer may be done for severe carpal tunnel syndrome with difficulty opposing the thumb in all positions?**

Palmaris longus (Camitz) to aid the abductor pollicis longus; this is an abductorplasty.

О   **What is done for a pit viper bite to the hand?**

Fasciotomy, IV antibiotics, antivenin.

О   **What does the Bunnell opponensplasty involve?**

Transfer of the ring FDS.

О   **What does a Huber opponensplasty involve?**

Abductor digiti minimi.

О   **A Phalen-Miller?**

Transfer of the ECU tendon.

О   **A Burkhalter opponensplasty?**

Transfer of the EIP tendon.

О   **What is the treatment principle of the ulna in radial club hand surgery?**

Centralization of the ulna.

О   **What is the status of the thumb in type IV radial club hand?**

Absence of the thumb with absence of the radius; scaphoid and trapezium usually absent; index pollicization may be performed.

○ **What other common syndromes are associated with radial club hand?**

VATER, Holt-Oram, TAR.

○ **What is a flag flap used for?**

Defects of the proximal or MP joints of the digits; not used for the thumb.

○ **Following a distal radius fracture ORIF, thumb pain and numbness may be due to what?**

Acute carpal tunnel syndrome; release the carpal tunnel.

○ **What procedure may be done for severe ischemic peripheral vascular disease before amputation?**

Distal venous arterialization bypass.

○ **What is the mechanism of a boutonniere deformity of the PIP joint?**

Extensor mechanism (central slip, transverse and oblique retinacular ligaments, lateral bands) becomes imbalanced; central slip injured.

○ **What is the management for a stage I boutonniere deformity?**

Splinting the PIP joint at 0 degrees.

○ **What is the likely cause of recurrent paronychia?**

Candida albicans.

○ **What do radiographs show in giant cell tumors of the hand?**

Radiolucent expansile lesions of the epiphysis; multifocal tumor.

○ **What nerve graft may be used for a 2.7 cm defect of a digital nerve?**

Terminal branch of the posterior interosseous nerve.

○ **Where is the posterior interosseous nerve located?**

Deep to the extensors at the wrist; lies in the floor of the 4th compartment radially; ulnar and deep to the EPL.

○ **What findings on radiographs are seen in pantrapezial arthritis?**

CMC and STT joint narrowing and arthritic changes .

○ **What is the length of advancement that is able to be accomplished using a Moberg flap?**

1.5 cm.

○ **What prevents being able to use a Moberg-type advancement flap in the digits?**

The digits do not have a dual arterial supply like the thumb.

❍ **What are the earliest carpal bones visible on radiographs?**

The capitate and hamate; appositional growth occurs in the carpal bones.

❍ **What is the last carpal bone to be seen on xray?**

The pisiform, at 6.5 years.

❍ **What nonoperative management exists for Dupuytren's?**

Collagenase, cortisone, skeletal traction, extension splinting.

❍ **What is a thenar flap used for?**

Coverage of defects of the index and middle finger tips.

INTEGUMENT

❍ **What is the recurrence rate of keloids following simple excision?**

At least 55% and reported even higher.

❍ **What is the most likely result of axillary silicone granulomas following breast augmentation?**

They are a known tissue response to the presence of foreign material and should be resected when present.

❍ **What is the optimal treatment for carbonaceous material imbedded in the face?**

ND:YAG laser treatment (also used for road asphalt, amateur tattoo ink).

❍ **What artery does the saphenous artery arise from?**

Descending genicular artery.

❍ **What does the superficial femoral art become at the knee?**

Popliteal artery.

❍ **What does the lateral circumflex femoral artery arise from?**

The profunda femoris artery.

❍ **What medication is most appropriate to treat heterotopic ossification?**

Etidronate.

❍ **How often may heterotopic ossification occur in spinal cord injury patients?**

40 %.

❍ **What agent most readily decreases the depth of a phenol peel?**

Using liquid soap.

❍ **What effects do antibiotic ointment and taping have on phenol peel?**

Increasing the depth.

❍ **What is the most appropriate treatment for a patient exhibiting a dark bluish discoloration of a TRAM flap following free TRAM reconstruction with signs of venous congestion?**

Operative intervention.

❍ **What clinical appearance characterizes the endpoint of dermabrasion at the level of the superficial reticular dermis?**

Confluent bleeding with a coarse tissue background.

❍ **When does re-epithelialization begin following dermabrasion?**

Seven to 10 days.

❍ **What clinical appearance occurs with dermabrasion to the superficial papillary dermis?**

Sparse punctate bleeding.

❍ **What theoretical gain in length is achieved with a z-plasty angle of 60 degrees?**

75 %.

Z-plasty	Length gain (%)
30	25
45	50
60	75
75	100

❍ **What is the mechanism of Botox?**

Inhibition of acetylcholine release at the neuromuscular junction.

❍ **What age group characterizes keratoacanthomas?**

Men older than 50 years.

❍ **What clinical appearance describes keratoacanthomas?**

Umbilicated center with a keratin plug.

❍ **Where do cylindromas form?**

They are found firm, fleshy tumors of the scalp, rarely solitary.

❍ **What cutaneous lesion is characteristically found on the lower extremities of young adults?**

Dermatofibroma (fibrous popular lesion).

❍ **Where do syringomas form?**

In females during adolescence occurring only on the lower eyelids.

❍ **For treatment of a sacral pressure sore, what is the highest level at which bony debridement may be done without entering the dural space?**

S2-3.

○   **At what level does the conus medullaris lie?**

L2.

○   **What organisms are typically isolated in patients with hidradenitis?**

Staph. aureus and *Streptococcus viridans*.

○   **Which sweat glands are affected in hidradenitis?**

The apocrine sweat glands.

○   **Lesions around the nostrils that are culture negative but demonstrate noncaseating granulomas are indicative of what likely process?**

Sarcoidosis.

○   **What systemic process is lupus pernio associated with?**

Sarcoidosis.

○   **What is appropriate treatment of sarcoidosis?**

Intralesional steroids, oral hydroxychloroquine or methotrexate.

○   **What is rhinosporidiosis?**

A chronic fungal condition of the nose caused by Rhinosporidium seeberi bacteria; cultures may be negative.

○   **What is Apligraf composed of?**

Bilayer of neonatal epidermal keratinocytes and dermal fibroblasts within a matrix of bovine collagen.

○   **What is Alloderm composed of?**

Lyophilized cellular cadaveric dermis.

○   **What is Biobrane composed of?**

Nylon and silicone fabric coated with porcine collagen.

○   **Integra?**

Dermal matrix of bovine collagen and shark derived chondroitin sulfate covered by bilayer of silastic epidermis; silicone layer is removed and skin graft placed on underlying dermal matrix.

○   **Transcyte?**

Neonatal dermal fibroblasts cultured onto a thin membrane of silicone bonded to nylon mesh and bovine collagen.

○   **What are common characteristics of von Hippel-Lindau disease?**

Hemangiomas affecting the retina and hemangioblastomas of the cerebellum/visceral organs; seizures/mental retardation.

❍ **What are common characteristics of Klippel-Trenaunay syndrome?**

Port wine stain (usually over one extremity) and overlying venous/lymphatic malformations; limb hemihypertrophy (usually the leg).

❍ **What is Parkes-Weber syndrome?**

Similar to Klippel-Trenaunay syndrome but distinguished by presence of A-V fistulas; also hypertrophy of upper extremity.

❍ **What is Osler-Weber-Rendu syndrome?**

Hereditary hemorrhagic telangiectasia; AD; multiple ecstatic vessels; epistaxis, hematuria, hematemesis.

❍ **What is Sturge-Weber syndrome?**

Port wine stain in distribution of V1 & V2; may be associated with seizures, intracranial calcifications, hemiparesis, glaucoma; leptomeningeal venous malformations.

❍ **What blood level is increased in calciphylaxis?**

Parathyroid hormone; protein C is decreased.

❍ **What surgical interventions may be beneficial in patients with calciphylaxis?**

Debridement, skin grafting, subtotal thyroidectomy.

❍ **What finding is more likely to occur in patients undergoing with the Erbium:YAG laser than with the CO_2 laser?**

Transudative wound.

❍ **What laser currently is felt to be the treatment of choice for ablative resurfacing of the skin?**

Er:YAG laser (absorbs water within the epidermis a minimum of 10 times more efficiently than the CO2 laser); photomechanical rather than photothermal process.

❍ **How frequent is permanent hypopigmentation with Er:YAG vs. CO_2?**

Less than 5% with Er:YAG and as great as 40% in CO_2.

❍ **What physiologic changes occur in acute burn injury?**

Decreased cardiac output, decreased plasma volume, increased systemic vascular resistance , decreased capillary pressure.

❍ **What characterizes the anagen and telogen phases in male pattern alopecia?**

Decreased anagen (active phase of hair follicle), increased telogen phase(resting phase).

❍ **Follicles changing from terminal to villous fibers are seen in what process?**

Male pattern alopecia.

❍ **How is the Parkland formula administered?**

Lactated Ringer's solution (4 ml/kg/% TBSA [second and third degree only]) administered during the first 24 hours. Half administered during the first eight hours and the second half administered during the remaining 16 hours.

O **What distinguishes the long duration of bupivacaine compared to lidocaine?**

Protein binding.

O **What factor determines the potency of a local anesthetic?**

Lipid solubility – higher solubility leads to higher potency.

O **Local anesthetics with a higher pKa have what characteristic onset of action?**

Slower onset of action.

O **What pigmented nevus is classified as a hamartoma?**

Becker nevus (has epidermal and dermal elements); males more frequently involved; brown patches on upper trunk; hypertrichosis ; underlying smooth muscle hamartoma present.

O **Where are acral nevi typically located?**

Palmar or plantar surfaces (typically junctional or compound).

O **What terms also describe a dysplastic nevus?**

Clark's nevus, atypical nevus, or atypical mole (precursor to malignant melanoma).

O **What is a Sutton's nevus?**

Otherwise known as a halo nevus; central melanocytic nevus surrounded by halo of hypopigmented skin.

O **What patients do Spitz nevi form in?**

In children; benign proliferation of melanocytes on face, trunk, or extremities; characterized by irregular growth phase; difficult to distinguish from malignant melanoma.

O **What is the most likely adverse effect from topical silver sulfadiazine?**

Neutropenia.

O **What adverse effect occurs with silver nitrate?**

Hyponatremia; penetrates tissue poorly.

O **Sulfamylon (mafenide acetate)?**

Metabolic acidosis and pain; excellent penetration of burn eschar.

O **What type of vascular malformation changes in size with body position?**

Venous malformation, due to its compressibility and propensity to fill with blood.

O **What characterizes the bone adjacent to lymphatic malformations?**

Bony overgrowth.

○   **How often will squamous cell carcinoma develop in actinic keratoses?**

20 %.

○   **What is Bowen's disease?**

Intraepithelial squamous cell carcinoma; solitary lesions with red discoloration; potentially caused by UV, arsenic, viral infections, chronic trauma.

○   **Why do keratoacanthomas require excision?**

Keratoacanthomas grow rapidly over weeks and regress spontaneously; in rare instances progress to carcinoma; initially firm, flesh-colored then progress to dome-shaped nodules with umbilicated center with keratin plug.

○   **Where do keratoacanthomas typically occur?**

Face, neck and dorsal aspect of arms.

○   **What defines a T3 melanoma?**

Tumor with a Breslow thickness of 1.5 to 4 mm.

○   **What laser wavelength has the greatest affinity for water?**

2940 nm.

○   **Which laser is used for cutaneous vascular lesions?**

585 nm pulsed dye laser.

○   **What is the double Q-switched Nd:YAG laser used for?**

Has a 1064 nm wavelength; used for hair removal or tattoos.

○   **What is the millisecond pulsed Nd:YAG laser used for?**

Treatment of vascular lesions.

○   **What is the wavelength of the CO_2 laser?**

10,600 nm; mechanism of photothermal injury.

○   **Which cell type is predominantly involved in wound contracture?**

Fibroblast; TGF-beta may also contribute to wound contracture.

○   **What is the time frame for wound contracture?**

Begins 4-5 days after initial injury and continues until at least 21 days after injury.

○   **Which vascular lesion is characterized by an arteriole central vessel?**

Spider angioma (arteriolar malformation).

○   **Where do spider angiomas occur?**

On face in both children and adults. Treat with laser or electrocautery.

○   **Where are macular stains seen?**

On skin of neonates, not true vascular nevi.

○   **Are pyogenic granulomas true vascular malformations?**

No. they receive their blood from capillaries.

○   **What type of vascular malformation is a strawberry hemangioma?**

Venous malformation; do not grow commensurately with the child.

○   **Where is the most appropriate donor site for hair from the scalp?**

The occipital region. (donor dominance greatest in the occipital region)

○   **How long must a person's hands be splinted following toxic epidermal necrolysis syndrome?**

These patients have skin sloughing at the dermal epidermal junction; injury only to level of superficial dermis; skin will heal without contracture.

○   **What are long term complications of toxic epidermal necrolysis syndrome in the integument?**

Changes in skin pigmentation, complications involving eyes and fingernails.

○   **What is the mechanism of action of silicone sheeting in scar maturation?**

Increasing the static electronegative field inducing favorable wound effects.

○   **Has silicone sheeting been shown to decrease wound tension, affect contact inhibition, or regulate intracellular integrins?**

No.

○   **How is a 8 mm by 8 mm traumatic defect of the alar margin treated most commonly?**

Composite graft from the ear.

○   **What is the effect of skin treatment with topical tretinoin (retinoic acid)?**

Thinning of the stratum corneum; thickening of epidermis; inhibits binding of AP1 transcription factor to DNA by 70% (decreases collagenase).

○   **What is the recurrence rate of an ischial pressure sore after undergoing debridement/coverage?**

80% within 9 -18 months.

○   **What is the advantage of using Integra for coverage of full-thickness burns?**

Allowing for use of thinner autografts; Integra revascularized in 2-3 weeks.

○   **What is Integra?**

Synthetic bilaminar membrane with dermal matrix of bovine collagen cross linked with chondroitin sulfate covered by temporary silastic epidermis.

❍ **What requirement is needed before injection of bovine collagen (Zyderm)?**

Test dose 4 weeks prior to injection (3%) allergic reaction.

❍ **What supplies the secondary pedicle of the gracilis muscle flap?**

Superficial femoral artery/vein.

❍ **What type of flap is the gracilis?**

Type II muscle flap (one dominant and one secondary pedicle); dominant pedicle is ascending branch of the medial femoral circumflex artery.

❍ **What pedicle supplies the rectus femoris flap?**

Lateral femoral circumflex.

❍ **What supplies the vastus lateralis?**

The lateral femoral circumflex.

❍ **What is the recurrence rate of a BCC less than 2 cm following initial treatment?**

10%.

❍ **Where is recurrence of BCC highest?**

In periorbital, periauricular, perinasal regions.

❍ **What particular BCC is prone to recurrence?**

Morpheaform BCC.

❍ **Which benign lesion has been shown to result from sun exposure?**

Lentigines (benign pigmented macules); do not fade in absence of sun exposure.

❍ **What are ephelides?**

Common pigmented freckles not related to sun exposure.

❍ **What is xanthelasma?**

Multiple soft yellow orange plaques occurring around eyes as a result of deposition of lipid laden macrophages.

❍ **Name two type III muscle flaps.**

Gluteus maximus and rectus abdominis (dual dominant pedicles).

❍ **What are type I muscle flaps?**

One dominant pedicle (gastrocnemius, TFL, vastus lateralis).

○ **What are type II muscle flaps?**

One dominant pedicle and secondary pedicle (gracilis, trapezius).

○ **What is a type IV muscle flap?**

Segmental blood supply (external oblique, sartorius).

○ **Type V?**

dominant pedicle and multiple secondary segmental pedicles (latissimus, pectoralis major).

○ **What is an absolute contraindication for VAC therapy?**

Presence of exposed blood vessels.

○ **What auricular lesion is painful and is associated with the side down when the patient sleeps?**

Chondrodermatitis nodularis helices; painful erythematous nodule on helix or antihelix; treatment is excision.

○ **What are acrochordons?**

Skin tags.

○ **What is the most appropriate treatment following blepharoptosis after Botox?**

Use of alpha adrenergic agonist eyedrops; ocular decongestion (naphazoline); contract Mueller's.

○ **What are known complications of Botox?**

Diplopia, retrobulbar hemorrhage, globe perforation, lagophthalmos, photophobia, epiphora, ectropion, exposure keratitis.

○ **What are the immune responses in a 60% TBSA burn in a young healthy adult?**

Impairment of cell-mediated immunity; impairment of T lymphocyte function; suppression of circulating T cells; activation of T helper lymphocytes; decrease in Ig; marked decrease in IgG; increased IL-7.

○ **What is contained in Jessner's solution?**

Resorcinol, salicylic acid, lactic acid, ethanol.

○ **What is Jessner's solution often used for?**

Hyperpigmentation.

○ **What is the histopathologic exam of a proliferating hemangioma going to show?**

Increased collagenase, increased mast cells, multilaminate BM, plump endothelial cells, increased levels of circulating 17 beta estradiol.

○ **What do the mast cells in hemangiomas produce?**

Heparin, stimulating capillary endothelial cell migration.

○ **What properties do vascular malformations exhibit in the endothelium and basement membrane?**

Flattening of endothelium, thinning of BM, normal quantity of mast cells.

❍ **Following a partial thickness burn, what antimicrobial dressing is applied to the wound without having to consider patient allergy?**

Acticoat

❍ **Do Biobrane and Transcyte have antimicrobial activity?**

No.

❍ **What is the procedure of choice in an ambulatory patient with a grade IV sacral pressure sore?**

Superior gluteal artery perforator flap (unilateral).

❍ **What is the mechanism of finasteride?**

Inhibition of 5-alpha reductase (which converts testosterone into dihydroxytestosterone).

❍ **What is the most frequently seen problem with fat grafting?**

Undercorrection.

❍ **Where is the greatest amount of "take" for a fat graft in the face?**

Along the nasolabial folds.

❍ **Thromboxane B2 and prostaglandin F2a are thought to have what effect on tissues?**

Induction of microvascular thrombosis.

❍ **What effects do prostaglandin I2 and E2 have?**

Antiplatelet activity, causing vasodilation.

❍ **What is the ratio of type I collagen to type III in hypertrophic scars?**

2:1, normally 4:1.

❍ **Where is type I collagen found?**

In 90% of the tissues (bone, tendon, skin).

❍ **Where is type II found?**

Hyaline cartilage and eye tissue.

❍ **Where is type III found?**

Skin, arteries, uterus, intestinal wall, fetal wound collagen; hypertrophic and immature scar can contain up to 30% type III.

❍ **Where is type IV found?**

Basement membranes.

❍   **What is the effect of deep mechanical massage on the skin?**

Collagen band accumulation in the middle and deep subcutaneous regions.

❍   **What is Fitzpatrick type II skin characterized by?**

Usually burns, rarely tans.

Skin type	Skin Color	Characteristics
I	White	Always burns, never tans
II	White	Usu. burns, rarely tans
III	White	Sometimes burns, tans average
IV	White	Rarely burns, tans more than average
V	Brown	Rarely burns, tans profusely
VI	Black	Never burns, deep pigmentation

❍   **What is the main concern for using autologous cartilage grafting?**

Risk of warping.

❍   **During burn physiology, monoclonal antibodies limit the depth of injury in which zone?**

The zone of stasis.

❍   **Going from superficial to deep, what are the zones of burn injury?**

Zone of coagulation, zone of stasis (microthrombi, neutrophil adherence, vasoconstriction), zone of hyperemia (vasodilation and vasoactive mediator release).

❍   **What humoral factor has been shown to stimulate collagen producing fibroblasts?**

TGF-beta.

❍   **What factor increases the ability of cartilage to survive as a graft prior to placement?**

Proteoglycan matrix (composed of type II collagen).

❍   **What is the required concentration of factor VIII before major surgery is undertaken?**

Hemophilia A requires 80% of normal factor VIII levels.

❍   **What is the most likely finding following flap coverage of one ischial pressure sore?**

Development of a pressure sore on the opposite side from transfer of weight to contralateral side.

❍   **What is a Marjolin's ulcer?**

Malignant degeneration of a chronic wound edge to carcinoma.

❍   **What are clinical findings of systemic inflammatory response syndrome?**

Body temp lower than 96.8 or greater than 101.5, pulse greater than 90, RR greater than 20, leukocyte count less than 4000 or greater than 12000.

❍   **Wound sepsis occurs in what concentration of organisms per gram of tissue?**

10^5 per gram of tissue.

○ **Rhinophyma in an older male patient is best treated by what means?**

Tangential excision with healing by secondary intention.

○ **What mechanism occurs during tissue expansion of random skin flaps?**

Increased survival; secondary to delay-type phenomenon.

○ **What is seen histologically with the dermis and epidermis during tissue expansion?**

Total collagen content increased; thinning of the dermis, thickening of the stratum spinosum (epidermis).

○ **Following a burn injury, what is the time limit after which secondary healing will lead to hypertrophic scarring?**

After 3 weeks, open wounds have a higher chance of hypertrophic scarring.

○ **How is embolization used in AVM treatment?**

Used to target the center of the AVM.

○ **What is the distal limit of the reversed sural artery flap when raising the pedicle?**

Pivot the pedicle at least 5 cm above the lateral malleolus (to decrease risk of disruption of the peroneal perforators).

○ **Where is the sural nerve located with respect to the short saphenous vein?**

The nerve is lateral to both the superficial sural artery and short saphenous vein.

○ **What have studies indicated regarding pain control in DIEP vs. free TRAM breast reconstruction?**

Less use of analgesia postoperatively in DIEP flaps.

○ **What flap has greater abdominal wall morbidity?**

Free TRAM.

○ **What flap has greater fat necrosis?**

DIEP.

○ **What is likely to occur with trunk flexion following a DIEP harvest?**

Decrease in flexion strength.

○ **Which laser is used most frequently for treating lymphatic malformations?**

Erbium (2910 nm).

○ **What are the alexandrite (755 nm) and diode (810 nm) lasers used for?**

Removing hair, blue/green pigments.

○ **What are the Nd:YAG (532 nm) and pulsed dye (585 nm) lasers used for?**

Small vascular lesions.

○   **What is the Nd:YAG (1064 nm) used for?**

Tattoo pigments (blue, black); 2-6 mm skin penetration.

○   **What is the most appropriate treatment for a burn to the dorsum of the hand?**

Early excision and split thickness grafting.

○   **What occurs to the bone surrounding cervical lymphatic malformations?**

Hypertrophy of the bone (typically the maxilla and mandible, causing open bite deformity, prognathism, and malocclusion).

○   **What premalignant skin condition is associated with melanoma?**

Xeroderma pigmentosum (AR).

○   **What is the likelihood of malignancy with actinic keratoses?**

They harbor a 10% chance of developing into squamous cell carcinoma; treat actinic keratoses with 5-FU or excision.

○   **What is Bazex's syndrome?**

X linked; hypotrichosis, hypohidrosis, multiple basal cell carcinomas.

○   **What is the Erythroplasia of Queyrat?**

Otherwise known as Bowen's disease/ squamous cell in situ affecting the penis.

○   **Where does the nevus sebaceous of Jadassohn occur?**

Head and neck; 10% may develop basal cell carcinoma.

○   **Of the more frequently known genetic collagen disorders (eg. Ehlers-Danlos), which is a candidate for rhytidectomy?**

Cutis laxa (nonfunctioning elastase inhibitor); aneurysms and hernias prone to develop.

○   **What is the mechanism behind Ehlers-Danlos syndrome?**

Lysyl oxidase deficiency; joint hypermobility, thin skin.

○   **What is progeria?**

Hutchinson-Gilford syndrome; AR; growth retardation, cardiac disease, skin laxity, premature aging.

○   **What are characteristics of Werner's syndrome?**

Premature facial aging, short stature, alopecia, arteriosclerosis; cataracts; AR.

○   **What is Restylane composed of?**

Hyaluronic acid.

❍ **What is Isolagen composed of?**

Autologous agent from human skin cells with an extracellular matrix.

❍ **What does the deep inferior epigastric artery arise from?**

The external iliac.

❍ **What are calcium alginate dressings most useful for during pressure sore treatment?**

Absorbing exudate; also may trap debris and microorganisms, but no inherent antimicrobial activity.

❍ **What is most important for growth of a reconstructed ear in microtia repair?**

Perichondrium.

❍ **What are copper vapor lasers used for?**

Absorbed by red and brown pigment.

❍ **The lateral thigh flap is supplied by what arterial supply?**

The 3rd branch of the profunda femoris artery.

❍ **Name the deep adductor muscles from superior to inferior.**

The pectineus, adductor brevis, adductor longus, adductor magnus.

❍ **What supplies the gracilis?**

The medial circumflex artery.

❍ **Name common examples of a type I flap.**

TFL, gastrocnemius, vastus lateralis.

❍ **Name examples of a type II flap.**

Gracilis, abd digiti minimi, soleus.

❍ **Name examples of a type III flap.**

Rectus abdominis, gluteus maximus serratus.

❍ **Name examples of a type IV flap.**

Sartorius, extensor hallucis longus, tibialis anterior.

❍ **Name examples of a type V flap.**

Latissimus dorsi, pectoralis major.

❍ **What defines a giant congenital nevus?**

Larger than 20 cm in diameter, twice the size of the patient's palm.

○   **What is a range of melanoma risk in giant congenital nevi?**

4-8% (though controversial).

○   **What is the laser most appropriate for large capillary vascular malformations of the eyelid?**

The flashlamp pumped pulsed dye laser (585 nm).

○   **What vitamin has been shown to reverse the negative effects of steroid use?**

Vitamin A counteracts the negative effect on wound healing by restoring monocytic activity.

○   **What are the effects of smoking on free TRAM breast reconstruction regarding fat necrosis and vessel thrombosis?**

Generally not believed to increase the rate of fat necrosis or vessel necrosis; however, hernia, mastectomy skin flap and abdominal skin flap necrosis may occur at increased rates.

○   **Preoperative delay of smoking for what period of time is recommended before surgery?**

Four weeks.

○   **What factors are associated with nonmelanocytic skin malignancy?**

Frequency of lifetime sunburns, sun exposure during adolescence/childhood, exposure at irregular intervals.

○   **What is the relationship of depth of sunburn and development of skin malignancy?**

No association.

○   **What is the type of UV radiation emitted by tanning beds?**

UVA.

○   **What are proposed mechanisms of dextran?**

Decreased factor VIII and von Willebrand factor, increased electronegativity, modification of fibrin, volume expansion, inhibits alpha-2 antiplasmin.

○   **What are general characteristics of vascular malformations?**

Present at birth, do not regress, grow with child.

○   **What are general characteristics of hemangiomas?**

True neoplasms; develop by 1 year then may regress spontaneously.

○   **What findings are seen with Klippel Feil syndrome?**

Short neck, lower posterior hairline, cervical vertebral fusion.

○   **What is seen with Maffucci syndrome?**

Multiple enchondromas (mostly in hand) and venous malformations; deformities of fingers and toes; chondrosarcoma risk.

❍   **What are common characteristics of venous malformations?**

Dark lesions that become enlarged with dependency and change with position.

❍   **What treatments are advocated for venous malformation?**

Laser treatment and wedge resection if small enough, sclerotherapy and excision for larger lesions.

❍   **What protein has been implicated in breast capsule formation?**

Fibrinogen.

❍   **What is cutis aplasia?**

Absence of the skin and scalp at birth; also may include the bone.

❍   **What is the treatment for cutis aplasia?**

Maintaining a clean, moist wound environment; silver sulfadiazine dressing changes.

❍   **What muscle is the gracilis immediately posterior to during harvest?**

Adductor longus.

❍   **What muscle is posterior to the gracilis?**

Adductor magnus.

❍   **What relative levels of ATP are typically found in keloid and hypertrophic scars?**

Increased.

❍   **What is the general rule in using a groin flap regarding the vascularity of the superficial circumflex iliac artery?**

The superficial circumflex iliac (SCIA) and superficial inferior epigastric arteries have separate origins in 40% of the time; the SCIA is from the common femoral artery and travels parallel to the inguinal ligament 2-3 cm inferior to the ligament.

❍   **What is the Parkland formula?**

4 ml/kg/%TBSA burned given within the first 24 hours; half is given within the first 8 hours and the remainder given over 16 hours.

❍   **What margins are required for treatment of Merkel cell carcinoma in the head and neck?**

Wide 3 cm margins with primary neck dissection.

❍   **When should a delay procedure be performed for a pedicled TRAM?**

In patients with risk factors for flap loss: obesity, smokers, prior radiation, or large breast volume needed.

❍   **What is the treatment of a hydrofluoric acid burn?**

Administration of 10% calcium gluconate gel and local injection.

O **What is used for phosphorus burns?**

Copper sulfate irrigation.

O **What is used for phenol burns?**

Polyethylene glycol or vegetable oil.

O **What is the most common adverse effect with Alloderm lip augmentation?**

Resorption of the graft.

O **Why should halo nevi be excised?**

Melanoma similarity; melanomas can develop in an incomplete halo; the pigmentary change or "halo" surrounding the nevus (leukoderma) not painful usually.

O **What is the likely process seen with brown recluse spider bite treatment (dapsone)?**

Hemolysis; there is no antivenin.

O **What is the most effective means of detecting silicone implant rupture?**

MRI; one report stated 13.4 years as the mean age; one report stated half of patients with implants 7-10 years with rupture or hemorrhage on MRI.

O **What is Muir-Torre syndrome?**

AD; multiple cutaneous malignancies (BCC, SCCa, keratoacanthomas) as well as malignancies of colon, bladder, ovary, and kidneys.

O **What is Proteus syndrome?**

Partial gigantism of the extremities; hemifacial hemihypertrophy, macrocephaly; subcutaneous lipomas; vascular anomalies (capillary, lymphatic, venous malformations).

O **What forms of basal cell carcinoma are prone to recurrence?**

Sclerosing and morpheaform types.

O **What area of the face is at increased risk for fat embolism and blindness during fat injection?**

The glabellar region; ophthalmic artery communicates with this region.

O **What is the likely physiologic change seen in vitamin C deficiency?**

Decreased hydroxylation of lysine and proline; decreased collagen cross-linking.

O **What are physiologic effects seen with vitamin A deficiency?**

Decreased fibronectin production and monocyte activation.

O **What are the physiologic changes seen with a large second/third degree burn?**

Decreased leukocyte function, T helper lymphocyte production and immunoglobulins decreased, complement activation and T suppressor lymphocytes are increased; circulating complement decreased; decreased B lymphocyte activity.

○ **How resistant are cultured epithelial autografts to infection?**

Low resistance; 100 to 1000 colonies/cm^3 are required for infection.

○ **How resistant are STSGs to infection?**

10^4 to 10^5 colonies/cm^3 for infection.

○ **What fraction of hemangiomas are noted in the first month?**

4/5.

○ **How frequent are cutaneous horns associated with malignancy?**

May contain malignant cells; 20% seen with premalignant conditions.

○ **What is the best placement of Alloderm for lip augmentation?**

Submucosally along the dry/wet vermilion border.

○ **Where are Spitz nevi located in children?**

The head and neck region; in adults, these are found on the extremities.

○ **What is a Hutchinson's freckle?**

Otherwise known as lentigo maligna melanoma; only located within epidermal layers; invasive melanoma occurring 5-30%.

○ **What substance has been shown to reverse premalignant skin conditions?**

Retinoids (topical application).

○ **What arteries supply the gastrocnemius muscle flap?**

Medial and lateral sural arteries.

○ **What is the treatment of scorpion stings?**

Observation and cold compresses in adults usually; in children hospitalization with monitoring for arrhythmias, muscle spasms, airway control.

○ **What is the mechanism of cellular growth in hemangiomas?**

Hyperplasia.

○ **What characterizes amateur tattoos?**

Irregular placement of dye in the superficial dermis; small pigment particles (professional tattoos are of larger pigment sizes).

○ **What is the most frequent cause of infectious secondary lymphedema?**

Wuchereria bancrofti.

❍ **What is Kasabach-Merritt syndrome?**

Marked thrombocytopenia with single or multiple hemangiomas; treat with embolization, compression, interferon, steroids, or radiation.

❍ **What distinguishes ester and amide local anesthetics?**

Amides have an "I" in the prefix before the "caine" (eg. bupivacaine, lidocaine, mepivacaine); amides are more stable and cause fewer allergic reactions.

❍ **What are the phases of wound healing and the predominant cells in each phase?**

Inflammation (PMNs, macrophages; 1st week); proliferative (fibroblasts; 1 week to 5 weeks); maturation (cross linking of collagen; 5 weeks to 2 years).

❍ **In a 3 year old with an oral commissure electrical burn, what is the length of time required for splinting?**

6 months to prevent microstomia.

❍ **What free flap provides bone as well as a sensate skin paddle for the floor of the mouth?**

Lateral arm; radial collateral artery and posterior brachial cutaneous nerve (C5-6).

❍ **What topographic portion of the humerus is used in the lateral arm flap?**

The postero-lateral portion.

❍ **What is the blood supply of the parascapular flap?**

The circumflex scapular artery.

❍ **What characterizes the toxin of the black widow spider?**

Neurotoxin; treat with IV calcium gluconate and diazepam.

❍ **What characterizes the toxin of the brown recluse spider?**

Dermonecrotic.

❍ **What is Wolff's law of bone grafting?**

Stress is important for survival of grafted bone.

❍ **Do membranous or endochondral bone grafts last longer?**

Membranous bone grafts.

❍ **What type of skin grafts grow commensurately with a child?**

Full thickness grafts.

❍ **What is the main drawback with unilaminar skin substitutes?**

Poor mechanical protection.

❍ **What are advantages with unilaminar skin substitutes?**

Helpful in wound debridement, fluid absorption, decreasing bacterial count, and stimulating granulation.

○ **Bovine collagen is best injected into what skin layer?**

The dermis.

○ **What characterizes the bone formation with hydroxyapatite cement?**

Osteoconduction; peripheral ingrowth of new bone.

○ **What is the mechanism of silicone sheeting in improving scars?**

Static electronegative field increase.

○ **What is the venous drainage for the reversed radial forearm flap?**

Radial venae comitantes.

○ **What flap may be used for a ischial pressure sore and prior ligation of the profunda femoris artery on the same side?**

Gluteal thigh flap; based on the inferior gluteal artery.

○ **What is the blood supply for the rectus femoris?**

Descending branch of the lateral circumflex.

○ **What is the blood supply of the gracilis muscle?**

Ascending branch of the medial circumflex.

○ **What is the supply of the TFL?**

Ascending branch of the lateral circumflex.

○ **What is Milroy's disease?**

X linked dominant; primary lymphedema; unilateral pitting edema; normal bone growth, no hemihypertrophy.

○ **What best describes the status of the shell of a subglandular breast implant placed a decade ago?**

Loss of shell strength as compared to preimplantation.

○ **What skin lesion is found in the distribution of CN V?**

Nevus of Ota (V_1 and V_2); 80% in females.

○ **What is an epelis?**

Pigmented freckle with normal number of melanocytes and high concentration of melanin.

○ **What areas are the nevus of Ito seen?**

In the areas of the lateral brachiocutaneous and supraclavicular nerves.

○ **Where is the nevus of Jadassohn seen?**

On the scalp and face.

○ **What is the malignant potential of the nevus of Jadassohn?**

15% develop into BCC.

○ **What is the treatment of a hemangioma of the upper lid that is obstructing the visual axis?**

Excision; ambylopia may develop in as short as 1 week.

○ **What is the percentage of hair growth if 2/3 of the hair shaft is transplanted?**

Growth in 30% of the time; hair bulb is not required for growth.

○ **What head and neck free flap allows the greatest movement of skin in relation to the bone?**

The scapular free flap.

○ **What supplies vascularity to the inferior pole of the scapula?**

Angular branch of the thoracodorsal artery.

○ **Skin grafts of what type are used for dorsal burn contractures of the hand?**

Full thickness.

○ **What population of people have Merkel cell carcinoma?**

Most frequently seen in the head and neck region of elderly women.

○ **What area of the body is most frequently affected by sebaceous carcinoma?**

Eyelid; meibomian gland.

○ **For what defects of the scalp is tissue expansion most appropriate?**

Greater than 15%.

○ **Can rhytidectomy be performed in a patient with pseudoxanthoma elasticum?**

Disorder of premature skin laxity, calcium deposition within the elastic fibers; yes, rhytidectomy may be performed.

○ **What bony landmarks are used for locating the superior gluteal artery?**

A third of the way down starting from the PSIS along a line drawn from the PSIS to the trochanter.

○ **What is the most common cause of death in paraplegics with pressure sores?**

Renal failure due to amyloid disease.

○ **What effect on epithelialization does isotretinoin have?**

Decreases epithelialization; otherwise known as Accutane); thinning of the stratum corneum.

○ **What retinoid is often used as a pretreatment for chemical peeling and laser?**

Tretinoin.

○ **What supplies motor innervation to the gracilis?**

Anterior branch of the obturator nerve; travels between the adductor longus and adductor brevis.

○ **What nerve supplies the rectus femoris?**

Femoral nerve.

○ **What supplies motor innervation to the TFL?**

Inferior branch of the superior gluteal nerve.

○ **The erythroplasia of Queyrat has squamous cell carcinoma affecting what site?**

The penis; part of Bowen's disease; 15% of Bowen's disease becomes invasive SCCa.

○ **Where are keloids likely to form?**

Face, cheek, ear, shoulder, upper arm, anterior chest.

○ **What is the best treatment for a 1 cm skin defect of the upper eyelid in a 75 year old woman?**

Skin graft from the contralateral side.

○ **What skin cream provides protection against UVA(long and short wave) and UVB?**

Zinc oxide.

○ **SPF rating is limited by what fact?**

It only rates UVB protection, not UVA.

○ **What microbe is associated with leech therapy?**

Aeromonas hydrophila; treat with bactrim or fluoroquinolones.

○ **What happens to glucose concentration after a burn injury?**

Increases; glucose should not be added to the resuscitation fluids.

○ **What happens to cardiac output after a burn injury?**

Decreases; decreased plasma volume, increased SVR.

○ **A purple "cobblestone" lesion in an adult is likely what type of vascular malformation?**

A capillary malformation; usually in distribution of the VI and VII nerves.

○ **What is the Branham sign?**

Decreased heart rate after compression of an AVM (causing a baroreceptor response).

○ **What histologic change is seen with tretinoin use?**

Compact stratum corneum which causes smoothing of the skin; increase in hyaluronic acid, increase in epidermal thickness, increase in dermal mucin, decreased melanin production.

○ **What adverse effects are seen with tretinoin use?**

Retin-A has been associated with erythema, crusting, and sun-sensitivity.

○ **What type of antibodies are formed in a reaction to bovine collagen?**

IgG antibodies; 3% of all patients may have a reaction.

○ **What is the collagen makeup of Zyderm?**

95% type I and 5% type II.

○ **What characteristic of full thickness skin grafts has the most effect on inhibiting wound contraction?**

The fraction of grafted dermis.

○ **What dressings are typically used for burns of the ear?**

Mafenide acetate dressing changes; in preventing suppurative chondritis.

○ **During wound healing, collagen synthesis and breakdown reach a steady state at what time?**

21 days.

○ **What is an appropriate method of reconstructing the scalp following a 35% burn wound?**

Tissue expansion.

○ **What has a higher rate of infection when applied to the donor site of a skin graft – Duoderm or Biobrane?**

Biobrane.

○ **What is the best choice of flap for a 1.7 cm defect of the columella?**

Nasolabial flap.

References

Ablove RH, et al. The physiology and technique of skin grafting. *Hand Clin*. 1997;13:163-173.

Abrahams JJ, et al. Diagnostic radiology of the cranial base. *Clin Plast Surg*. 1995;22:373-405.

Achauer BM, et al. Burn reconstruction. In: Achauer BM, Eriksson E, Guyuron B, et al, eds. *Plastic Surgery: Indications, Operations, and Outcomes*. Saint Louis, Mo: Mosby - Year Book, Inc; 2000;1:431-432.

Achauer BM, et al. Electrical burn injury of the upper extremity. *Br J Plast Surg*. 1994;47:331-340.

Achauer BM, et al. Vascular lesions. *Clin Plast Surg*. 1982;69:412-420.

Achauer BM. Reconstructing the burned face. *Clin Plast Surg*. 1992;19:623-636.

Achauer BM. Scalp. In: *Burn Reconstruction*. New York, NY: Thieme Medical Publishers, Inc; 1991:13-22.

Achauer BM. The burned hand. In: Green DP, Hotchkiss RN, Pederson WC, eds. *Operative Hand Surgery*. 4th ed. New York, NY: Churchill Livingstone, Inc; 1999;2:2045-2060.

Acland RD. The free iliac flap: a lateral modification of the free groin flap. *Plast Reconstr Surg*. 1979;64:30.

Adams WP Jr, et al. Lipid infiltration as a possible biologic cause of silicone gel breast implant aging. *Plast Reconstr Surg*. 1998;101:64.

Adams WP Jr. Discussion - the role of plastic surgery in congenital cutis laxa: a 10-year follow-up. *Plast Reconstr Surg*. 1999;104:1179.

Adamson GJ, et al. Amputations. In: Achauer BM, Eriksson E, Guyuron B, et al, eds. *Plastic Surgery: Indications, Operations, and Outcomes*. Saint Louis, Mo: Mosby - Year Book, Inc; 2000;4:1831-1843.

Adamson JE, et al. The growth pattern of the external ear. *Plast Reconstr Surg*. 1965;36:466-470.

Adani R, et al. The "kite flap" for dorsal thumb reconstruction. *Acta Chir Plast*. 1995;37:63-66.

Adcock D, et al. Analysis of cutaneous and systemic effects of Endermologie in the porcine model. *Aesthetic Surg J*. 1998;18:414.

Adcock D, et al. Analysis of the effect of deep massage in the porcine model. *Plast Reconstr Surg*. 2001;108:233.

Agur AM, et al. The neck. In: Gardner JN, ed. *Grant's Atlas of Anatomy*. 9th ed. Baltimore, Md: Williams & Wilkins; 1995;7:556-557.

Akin S, et al. Osteocutaneous posterior interosseous flap for reconstruction of the metacarpal bone and soft-tissue defects in the hand. *Plast Reconstr Surg*. 2002;109:982.

Aldrete JA, et al. Evaluation of intracutaneous testing for investigation of allergy to local anesthetic agents. *Anesth Analg*. 1970;49:173.

Alexander CS. Craniofacial anomalies and principles of their correction. In: Georgiade GS, Riefkohl R, Levin LS, eds. *Textbook of Maxillofacial and Reconstructive Surgery*. 3rd ed. Baltimore, Md: Williams & Wilkins; 1997:273-296.

Allcroft RA, et al. Cartilage grafts for head and neck augmentation and reconstruction. *Otolaryngol Clin North Am*. 1994;27:69.

Allen RJ, et al. Deep inferior epigastric perforator flap for breast reconstruction. *Ann Plast Surg*. 1994;32:32-38.

Allison GR, et al. Prevention of Frey's syndrome with superficial musculoaponeurotic system interpretation. *Am J Surg*. 1993;166:407.

Allison GR. Anatomy of the auricle. *Clin Plast Surg*. 1990;17:209-212.

Almeida MF, et al. Reverse-flow island sural flap. *Plast Reconstr Surg*. 2002;109:583.

Alster TS, ed. *Manual of Cutaneous Laser Techniques*. Philadelphia, Pa: Lippincott Williams & Wilkins; 2000:33-51, 119-134.

Alster TS, et al. An overview of cutaneous laser resurfacing. *Clin Plast Surg*. 2001;28:37-52.

Alster TS, et al. Erbium:YAG cutaneous laser resurfacing. *Dermatol Clin*. 2001;19:453.

Alster TS, et al. Treatment of scars: a review. *Ann Plast Surg*. 1997;39:418-432.

Alster TS. Cutaneous resurfacing with CO2 and erbium:YAG lasers: preoperative, intraoperative, and postoperative complications. *Plast Reconstr Surg*. 1999;103:619-634.

Alster TS. Q-switched alexandrite laser treatment (755nm) of professional and amateur tattoos. *J Am Acad Dermatol*. 1995;33:69-73.

Alter BP. Arm anomalies and bone marrow failure may go hand in hand. *J Hand Surg.* 1992;17A:566-571.

Alvi A, et al. Malignant tumors of the salivary glands. In: Myers EN, Suen JY, eds. *Cancer of the Head and Neck.* Philadelphia, Pa: WB Saunders Co; 1996:525-527.

Amadio PC, et al. Fractures of the carpal bones. In: Green DP, Hotchkiss RN, Pederson WC, eds. *Operative Hand Surgery.* 4th ed. New York, NY: Churchill Livingstone, Inc; 1999;1:809-864.

Amadio PC, et al. Reflex sympathetic dystrophy syndrome: consensus report of an ad hoc committee of the American Association of Hand Surgery on the definition of reflex sympathetic dystrophy syndrome. *Plast Reconstr Surg.* 1991;87:371.

American Joint Committee on Cancer: Manual for Staging of Cancer. 4th ed. Philadelphia, Pa: JB Lippincott Co; 1992.

Aminoff M. Nervous system. In: Tierney LM Jr, McPhee SJ, Papadakis MA, eds. *Medical Diagnosis and Treatment.* 38th ed. Stamford, Conn: Appleton & Lange; 1999:932.

Anderson JE, ed. *Grant's Atlas of Anatomy.* 8th ed. Baltimore, MD: Williams & Wilkins; 1983.

Anderson RL, et al. Aponeurotic ptosis surgery. *Arch Ophthalmol.* 1979;97:1123-1128.

Andreason TJ, et al. Massive infectious soft tissue injury: diagnosis and management of necrotizing fasciitis and purpura fulminans. *Plast Reconstr Surg.* 2001;107:1025-1034.

Angel MF. Beneficial effects of staphage lysate in treatment of chronic recurrent hidradenitis suppurativa. *Surg Forum.* 1987;38:111.

Angelides AC. Ganglions of the hand and wrist. In: Green DP, Hotchkiss RN, Pederson WC, eds. *Operative Hand Surgery.* 4th ed. New York, NY: Churchill Livingstone, Inc; 1999;2:2171-2183.

Angrigiani C, et al. Posterior interosseous reverse forearm flap: experience with 80 consecutive cases. *Plast Reconstr Surg.* 1993;92:285.

Anthony JP, et al. The muscle flap in the treatment of chronic lower extremity osteomyelitis: results in patients over 5 years after treatment. *Plast Reconstr Surg.* 1991;88:311-324.

Anthony JP, et al. Update on chronic osteomyelitis. *Clin Plast Surg.* 1991;18:515-523.

Antia NH, et al. Chondrocutaneous advancement flap for the marginal defect of the ear. *Plast Reconstr Surg.* 1967;39:472.

Antonyshyn O. Principles in management of facial injuries. In: Georgiade GS, Riefkohl R, Levin LS, eds. *Textbook of Maxillofacial and Reconstructive Surgery.* 3rd ed. Baltimore, Md: Williams & Wilkins; 1997:339-350.

Apesos J, et al. Autologen. *Clin Plast Surg.* 2000;27:507-513.

Apfelberg DB, et al. Decorative and traumatic tattoo biophysics and removal.

Arca E, et al. An open, randomized, comparitive study of oral fluconazole, itraconazole and terbinafine therapy in onychomycosis. *J Dermatol Treatment.* 2002;13:3-9.

Arey LB, ed. *Developmental Anatomy.* 26th ed. Philadelphia, Pa: WB Saunders Co; 1970.

Argenta LC, et al. Advances in tissue expansion. *Clin Plast Surg.* 1985;12:159.

Argenta LC, et al. Refinements in reconstruction of congenital breast deformities. *Plast Reconstr Surg.* 1985;76:73-82.

Argenta LC, et al. Vacuum-assisted closure: a new method for wound control and treatment: clinical experience. *Ann Plast Surg.* 1997;38:563-577.

Ariyan S, et al. Radiation effects: biologic and surgical considerations. In: McCarthy JG, ed. *Plastic Surgery.* Philadelphia, Pa: WB Saunders Co; 1990;1:831.

Ariyan S. Sternocleidomastoid muscle and musculocutaneous flap. In: Strauch B, Vasconez LO, Hall-Findlay EJ, eds. *Grabb's Encyclopedia of Flaps*. Boston, Mass: Little, Brown & Co; 1990;1:485-491.

Armstrong MB, et al. Free-tissue transfer for lower-extremity reconstruction in the immunosuppressed diabetic transplant recipient. *J Reconstr Microsurg*. 1997;13:1-5.

Arnaud E, et al. Postoperatice mental and morphological outcome for nonsyndromic brachycephaly. *Plast Reconstr Surg*. 2002;110:6-12.

Arnold J. Pursuing the perfect strip: harvesting donor strips with minimal hair transection. *Internat J Aesthet Restorative Surg*. 1995;3:148-153.

Aronson J, et al. Experimental healing of distraction osteogenesis comparing metaphyseal with diaphyseal sites. *Clin Orthop*. 1994;301:25-30.

Aronson J. Experimental and clinical experience with distraction osteogenesis. *Cleft Palate Craniofac J*. 1994;3:473-482.

Aronson J. Mechanical induction of osteogenesis: the importance of pin rigidity. *J Ped Orthop*. 1988;8:396-401.

Aronson J. Principles of distraction osteogenesis: the orthopedic experience. In: McCarthy JG, ed. *Distraction of the Craniofacial Skeleton*. New York, NY: Springer-Verlag; 1999:55-56.

Arturson MG. The pathophysiology of severe thermal injury. *J Burn Care Rehabil*. 1985;6:129-146.

Ash MM, et al. Clinical occlusion. In: Ash MM, Ramfjord S, eds. *Occlusion*. 4th ed. Philadelphia, Pa: WB Saunders Co; 1995:50-62.

Aspestos J, et al. Autologen. *Clin Plast Surg*. 2000;27:507-513.

Athanasian EA, et al. Giant cell tumors of the bones of the hand. *J Hand Surg*. 1997;22A:91-98.

Athanasian EA. Bone and soft tissue tumors. In: Green DP, Hotchkiss RN, Pederson WC, eds. Operative Hand Surgery. 4th ed. New York, NY: Churchill Livingstone, Inc; 1999;3:2223-2253.

Atiyeh BS, et al. Perinipple round-block technique for correction of tuberous/tubular breast deformities. *Aesthetic Plast Surg*. 1998;22:284-288.

Attinger C, et al. Soft tissue reconstruction for calceneal fractures or osteomyelitis. *Ortho Clin North Am*. 2001;32:135-170.

Ausprunk DH, et al. Migration and proliferation of endothelial cells in preformed and newly formed blood vessels during tumor angiogenesis. *Microvasc Res*. 1977;14:53.

Austad ED. Breast implant-related silicone granulomas: the literature and litigation. *Plast Reconstr Surg*. 2002;109:1724.

Availability of new rabies vaccine for human use. *MMWR Morb Mortal Wkly Rep*. 1998;47:12, 19.

Ayliffe P, et al. Nasoethmoid fractures. In: Booth PW, Schendel SA, Hausamen JE, eds. *Maxillofacial Surgery*. London, England: Churchill Livingstone, Inc; 1999;1:141-159.

Back SM. Two new cutaneous flaps: the medial and lateral thigh flaps. *Plast Reconstr Surg*. 1983;71:354.

Bafaqeeh SA, et al. Simultaneous open rhinoplasty and alar base excision: is there a problem with the blood supply of the nasal tip and columellar skin? *Plast Reconst Surg*. 2000;105:344.

Bahr W, et al. Comparison of transcutaneous incisions used for exposure of the infraorbital rim and orbital floor: a retrospective study. *Plast Reconstr Surg*. 1992;90:585-591.

Bailey AJ, et al. Characteristics of the collagen of human hypertrophic and normal scars. *Biochem Biophys Acta*. 1975;405:412.

Baird WL, et al. Maxillofacial trauma. In: Jurkiewicz JM, Krizek TJ, Mathes SJ, et al, eds. *Plastic Surgery: Principles and Practice*. Philadelphia, Pa: Mosby - Year Book, Inc; 1990;1:231-270.

Baker DC, et al. Avoiding facial nerve injuries in rhytidectomy. *Plast Reconstr Surg*. 1979;64:781-795.

Baker DC, et al. The physiologic treatment of nasal obstruction. *Clin Plast Surg*. 1977;4:121.

Baker DC. Complications of cervicofacial rhytidectomy. *Clin Plast Surg*. 1983;10:543-562.

Baker DC. Facial paralysis. In: McCarthy JG, ed. *Plastic Surgery*. Philadelphia, Pa: WB Saunders Co; 1990;3:2237-2319.

Baker JL. A practical guide to ultrasound-assisted lipoplasty. *Clin Plast Surg*. 1999;26:363-368.

Baker TJ, et al. Chemical peeling and dermabrasion: injectable collagen. In: McCarthy JG, ed. *Plastic Surgery*. Philadelphia, Pa: WB Saunders Co; 1990;1:781-784.

Baker TJ, Stuzin JM, Baker TM, eds. *Facial Skin Resurfacing*. Saint Louis, Mo: Quality Medical Publishing, Inc; 1998.

Baker TM. Dermabrasion: as a complement to aesthetic surgery. *Clin Plast Surg*. 1998;25:81.

Balakrishnan A, et al. Lymphangioma of the tongue: a review of pathogenesis, treatment, and the use of surface laser photocoagulation. *J Otolaryngol Otol*. 1991;105:924.

Bang H, et al. Palmar advancement flap with the V-Y closure for thumb tip injuries. *J Hand Surg*. 1992;17A:933-941.

Bannister LH. Alimentary system. In: Bannister LH, et al, eds. *Gray's Anatomy*. New York, NY: Churchill Livingstone, Inc; 1995:1683-1812.

Baran NK, et al. Growth of skin grafts, flaps, and scars in young minipigs. *Plast Reconstr Surg*. 1972;50:487-496.

Barber HD, et al. Mandibular fractures. In: Fonseca RJ, Walker RV, eds. *Oral and Maxillofacial Trauma*. 2nd ed. Philadeplhia, Pa: WB Saunders Co; 1997;1:473-489.

Barfred T. The hypogastric (Shaw) skin flap. In: Strauch B, Vasconex LO, eds. *Grabb's Encyclopedia of Flaps*. Boston, Mass: Little, Brown & Co; 1990;2:1101-1104.

Barker JR, et al. Magnetic resonance imaging of severe frostbite injuries. *Ann Plast Surg*. 1997;38:275-279.

Barnett MP. Labial incompetence: a marker for progressive bone resorption in Silastic chin augmentation. *Plast Reconstr Surg*. 1997;100:553-554.

Barnhill RL. Malignant melanoma, dysplastic nevi, and Spitz tumoprs: histologic classification and characteristics. *Clin Plast Surg*. 2000;27:331-360.

Barnum M, et al. Radial tunnel syndrome. *Hand Clin*. 1996;12:679-689.

Barrera A. Micrograft and minigraft megasession hair transplantation results after a single session. *Plast Reconstr Surg*. 1997;100:1524-1530.

Barrera A. The use of micrografts and minigrafts for the treatment of burn alopecia. *Plast Reconstr Surg*. 1999;103:581-584.

Barrie KA, et al. The role of multiple strands and locking sutures on gap formation of flexor tendon repairs during cylindrical loading. *J Hand Surg*. 2000;25A:714-720.

Bartlett SP, et al. Craniosynostosis syndromes. In: Aston SJ, Beasley RW, Thorne CH, eds. Grabb & Smith's Plastic Surgery. 5th ed. Philadelphia, Pa: Lippincott-Raven; 1997:295-304, 325-326.

Bartlett SP, et al. Mandibulofacial dysostosis. In: Lin KY, Ogle RC, Jane JA, eds. *Craniofacial Surgery: Science and Surgical Technique*. Philadeplhia, Pa: WB Saunders Co; 2002:288.

Bartlett SP, et al. The surgical management of orbitofacial dermoids in the pediatric patient. *Plast Reconstr Surg*. 1993;91:1208-1215.

Barton FE Jr, et al. Acquired deformities of the nose. In: McCarthy JG, ed. *Plastic Surgery*. Philadelphia, Pa: 1990;3:1924-2008.

Barton FE Jr. Aesthetic aspects of nasal reconstruction. *Clin Plast Surg.* 1988;15:155-166.

Barton FE, et al. Direct fixation of the malar pad. In: Menick FJ, ed. *Facial Aesthetic Surgery.* Philadelphia, Pa: WB Saunders Co; 1997:329-355.

Barton FE. Rhytidectomy and the nasolabial fold. *Plast Reconstr Surg.* 1992;90:601.

Bass LS. Understanding laser-tissue interactions helps predict clinical effects (letter). *Plast Reconstr Surg.* 1995;95:607.

Basset CL, et al. Clinical implications of cell function in bone grafting. *Clin Orthop.* 1972;87:49.

Bauer BS, et al. Congenital deformities of the ear. In Bentz, ed. *Pediatric Plastic Surgery.* Stamford, Conn: Appleton & Lange; 1998:359.

Baum Ra, et al. Multicenter trial to evaluate vascular magnetic resonance angiography of the lower extremity. *JAMA.* 1995;274:875.

Baumann A, et al. Use of preseptal transconjunctival approach in orbit reconstruction surgery. *J Oral Maxillofac Surg.* 2001;59:287-291.

Baylis HI, et al. Complications of lower blepharoplasty. In: Putterman AM, ed. *Cosmetic Oculoplastic Surgery.* 2nd ed. Philadelphia, Pa: WB Saunders Co; 1993:356-363.

Bays RA. Surgery for internal derangement. In: Bays RA, Quinn PD, eds. *Oral and Maxillofacial Surgery.* Philadelphia, Pa: WB Saunders Co; 2000:275-300.

Beahrs OH, et al. *Manual for Staging of Cancer - American Joint Committee on Cancer.* 3rd ed. Philadelphia, Pa: JB Lippincott; 1988:27-32.

Becker GD, et al. Nonsurgical repair of perinasal skin defects. *Plast Reconstr Surg.* 1991;88:764.

Bednar MS, et al. Osteoid osteoma of the upper extremity. *Hand Clin.* 1995;11:211-221.

Beekman WH, et al. Imaging signs and radiologists' jargon of ruptured breast implants. *Plast Reconstr Surg.* 1998;102:1281-1289.

Beekman WH, et al. Life span of silicone gel-filled mammary prostheses. *Plast Reconstr Surg.* 1997;100:1723-1726.

Beer GM, et al. A new technique for the treatment of lacrimal gland prolapse in blepharoplasty. *Aesthet Plast Surg.* 1994;18:65-69.

Beimer E, et al. Total thumb reconstruction: a one-stage reconstruction using an osteocutaneous forearm flap. *Br J Plast Surg.* 1983;36:52.

Bell ML. Scalp reduction. *Clin Plast Surg.* 1982;9:269-278.

Berde CB, et al. Local anesthetics. In: *Anesthesia.* 5th ed. New York, NY: Churchill Livingstone, Inc; 2000;516.

Berdoll MS, et al. *Toxic Shock Syndrome.* Boston, Mass: CRC Press; 1991;33-45.

Berger RA, et al. Arthroplasty in the hand and wrist. In: Green DP, Hotchkiss RN, Pederson WC, eds. *Operative Hand Surgery.* 4th ed. New York, NY: Churchill Livingstone, Inc; 1999;1:147-191.

Bergman RA, et al. *Compendium of Human Anatomic Variation.* 1998:12-27.

Berman B, et al. The treatment of hypertrophic scars and keloids. *Eur J Dermatol.* 1998;8:591-595.

Bernard SL. Reconstruction of the burned nose and ear. *Clin Plast Surg.* 2000;27:97-112.

Bessette RW, et al. Temporomandibular joint dysfunction. In: Aston SJ, Beasley RW, Thorne CH, eds. *Grabbe & Smith's Plastic Surgery.* 5th ed. Philadephia, PA: Lippincott-Raven; 1997:345.

Betts NJ, et al. Soft tissue changes associated with orthognathic surgery. In: *Modern Practice in Orthognathic and Reconstructive Surgery*. Philadelphia, Pa: WB Saunders Co; 1992;2170-2209.

Bhandari M, et al. The efficacy of low-pressure lavage with different irrigating solutions to remove adherent bacteria from bone. *J Bone Joint Surg*. 2001;83:412-419.

Bhandari PS. Total ear reconstruction in post burn deformity. *Burns*. 1998;24:661-670.

Bhawan J, et al. Histological evaluation of the long term effects of tretinoin on photodamaged skin. *J Dermatol Sci*. 1996;11:177.

Binder WJ. Submalar augmentation, an alternative to face lift surgery. *Arch Otolaryngol Head Neck Surg*. 1981;115:797-802.

Bishop AT, et al. Flexor mechanism reconstruction and rehabilitation. In: Peimer CA, ed. *Sirgery of the Hand and Upper Extremity*. 1996;2:1139.

Bite U, et al. Orbital volume measurements in enophthalmos using 3-D CT imaging. *Plast Reconstr Surg*. 1985;75:502.

Blackburn WD Jr, et al. Lack of evidence of systemic inflammatory rheumatic disorders in symptomatic women with breast implants. *Plast Reconstr Surg*. 1997;99:1054-1060.

Blackman JR. Spider bites. *J Am Board Fam Pract*. 1995;8:288-294.

Blaisdell FW, et al. Revascularization of severely ischemic extremities with an arteriovvenous fistula. *Am J Surg*. 1966;112:166.

Blatt G, et al. Scapholunate injuries. In: Lichtman DM, Alexander AH, eds. *The Wrist and Its Disorders*. Philadelphia PA: WB Saunders Co; 1997:268-306.

Blondeel PN. Refinements in free flap breast reconstruction: the free bilateral deep inferior epigastric perforator flap anastamosed to the internal mammary artery. *Br J Plast Surg*. 1997;50:322.

Blondeel PN. The sensate free superior gluteal artery perforator (S-GAP) flap: a valuable alternative in autologous breast reconstruction. *Br J Plast Surg*. 1999;52:185.

Boles DS, et al. Pyogenic flexor tenosynovitis. *Hand Clin*. 1998;14:567-576.

Boon LM, et al. Complications of systemic corticosteroid therapy for problematic hemangioma. *Plast Reconstr Surg*. 1999;104:1616-1623.

Bosker FS, et al. Postoperative mydriasis after repair of orbital floor fracture. *Am J Ophthalmology*. 1993;115:372-375.

Bostwick J III, ed. *Plastic and Reconstructive Breast Surgery*. Saint Louis, Mo: Quality Medical Publishing; 1990.

Botte MJ, et al. Compartment syndrome and Volkmann's contracture. In: Peimer CA, ed. *Surgery of the Hand and Upper Extremity*. New York, NY: McGraw-Hill, Inc; 1996;2:1539-1558.

Botte MJ, et al. Volkmann's ischemic contracture of the upper extremity. *Hand Clin*. 1998;14:483-497.

Boussen H, et al. Chemotherapy of metastatic and/or recurrent undifferentiated nasopharyngeal carcinoma with cisplatin, bleomycin, and fluorouracil. *J Clin Oncol*. 1991;9:1675-1681.

Boutin RD, et al. Update on imaging of orthopedic infections. *Orthop Clin North Am*. 1998;29:41-66.

Bove A, et al. Facial nerve palsy: which flap? Microsurgical, anatomical, and functional considerations. *Microsurg*. 1998;18:286-289.

Bovet JL, et al. The vastus lateralis musculocutaneous flap in the repair of trochanteric pressure sores: technique and indications. *Plast Reconstr Surg*. 1982;69:830.

Bowers WH, et al. Treatment of chronic disorders of the distal radioulnar joint. In: Lichtman DM, ed. *The Wrist and Its Disorders*. 2nd ed. Philadelphia, Pa: WB Saunders Co; 1997:438.

Bowers WH. The distal radioulnar joint. In: Green DP, Hotchkiss RN, Pederson WC, eds. *Operative Hand Surgery*. 4th ed. New York, NY: Churchill Livingstone, Inc; 1999;1:1019-1021.

Boyd J, et al. Lip cancer. In: Medina JE, et al. *Clinical Practice Guidelines for the Diagnosis and Management of Cancer of the Head and Neck*. AmericanSociety for Head and Neck Surgeons; 1996:17-25.

Boyd JB, et al. Skeletal changes associated with vascular malformations. *Plast Reconstr Surg*. 1984;74:789-797.

Boyer MI, et al. Complications of the operative treatment of Dupuytren's disease. *Hand Clin*. 1999;15:161-166.

Boyer MI, et al. Microvascular surgery in the reconstruction of congenital hand anomalies. *Hand Clin*. 1998;14:135-142.

Boyes JH, ed. *Bunnell's Surgery of the Hand*. 5th ed. Philadelphia, Pa: JB Lippincott Co; 1970:653.

Bradley PJ. Tumors of the salivary gland. In: Jones AS, Phillips DE, Hilgers FJ, eds. *Diseases of the Head and Neck, Nose and Throat*. London: Arnold; 1998:329-346.

Brashear A, et al. Intramuscular injection of botulinum toxin for treatment of wrist and finger spasticity after a stroke. *N Engl J Med*. 2002;347:395-400.

Braunstein GD, et al. Gynecomastia. *Curr Ther Endocrinol Metab*. 1997;6:401-404.

Braunwald E, et al. *Harrison's Principles of Internal Medicine*. 15th ed. New York, NY: McGraw-Hill, Inc; 2001;2:2036-2037.

Brcic A. Primary tangential excision for hand burns. *Hand Clin*. 1990;6:211-219.

Brent B. Reconstruction of the auricle. In: McCarthy JG, ed. *Plastic Surgery*. Philadelphia, Pa: WB Saunders Co; 1990;3:2094-2152.

Brent B. Repair and grafting of cartilage in perichondrium. In: McCarthy JG, ed. *Plastic Surgery*. Philadelphia, Pa: WB Saunders Co; 1990;1:559-582.

Brent B. Technical advances in ear reconstruction with autogenous rib cartilage grafts: personal experience with 1200 cases. *Plast Reconstr Surg*. 1999;104:319-334.

Brink RR. Management of true ptosis of the breast. *Plast Reconstr Surg*. 1993;91:657-662.

Britton EN, et al. Acute flexor tendon injury: repair and rehabilitation. In: Peimer CA, ed. *Surgery of the Hand and Upper Extremity*. New York, NY: McGraw-Hill, Inc; 1996;1:1113-1132.

Brody GA, et al. Digital replantation applying the leech Hirudo medicinalis. *Clin Orthop*. 1989;245:133-137.

Brody GS. On the safety of breast implants. *Plast Reconstr Surg*. 1997;100:1309-1313.

Brody GS. Silicone technology for the plastic surgeon. *Clin Plast Surg*. 1988;15:517-520.

Brody HJ. Complications of chemical resurfacing. *Dermatol Clin*. 2001;19:427-438.

Brody HJ. Update on chemical peels. *Adv Dermatol*. 1992;7:275.

Brown EZ. Skin grafts. In: Green DP, ed. *Operative Hand Surgery*. 3rd ed. Ndew York, NY: Churchill Livingstone, Inc; 1993;2:1711-1740.

Brown EZ. Skin grafts. In: Green DP, Hotchkiss RN, Pederson WC, eds. *Operative Hand Surgery*. 4th ed. New York, NY: Churchill Livingstone, Inc; 1999;2:1759-1782.

Brown MD, et al. A cohort study of breast cancer risk in breast reduction patients. *Plast Reconstr Surg*. 1999;103:1674.

Brushart TM. Nerve repair and grafting. In: Green DP, Hotchkiss RN, Pederson WC, eds. *Operative Hand Surgery*. 4th ed. New York, NY: Churchill Livingstone, Inc; 1999;2:1381-1403.

Brushart TM. Peripheral nerve biology. In: *Hand Surgery Update*. Englewood, Co: American Society for Surgery of the Hand; 1994;1:20-21.

Brzozowski D, et al. Breast-feeding after inferior pedicle reduction mammaplasty. *Plast Reconstr Surg*. 2000;105:530-534.

Bucky LP, et al. Reduction of burn injury by inhibiting CD18-mediated leukocyte adherence in rabbits. *Plast Reconstr Surg*. 1994;93:1473-1480.

Budny PJ, et al. Salvage of prosthetic grafts and joints in the lower extremity. *Clin Plast Surg*. 1991;18:583-591.

Bujia J, et al. Class II antigenicity of human cartilage: relevance to the use of homologous cartilage grafts for reconstructive surgery. *Ann Plast Surg*. 1991;26:541.

Burch JM, et al. Trauma. In: Schwartz SI, ed. *Principles of Surgery*. New York, NY: McGraw-Hill, Inc; 1999:212-213.

Burge P. Closed cast treatment of scaphoid fractures. *Hand Clin*. 2001;17:541-551.

Burget GC, et al. Nasal reconstruction: seeking a fourth dimension. *Plast Reconstr Surg*. 1986;77:824.

Burget GC. *Aesthetic Reconstruction of the Nose*. Saint Louis, Mo: CV Mosby Co; 1992.

Burget GC. Aesthetic reconstruction of the tip of the nose. *Dermatol Surg*. 1995;21:419.

Burget GC. Aesthetic restoration of the nose. *Clin Plast Surg*. 1985;12:463.

Burggasser G, et al. The temporalis: blood supply and innervation. *Plast Reconstr Surg*. 2002;109:1862-1869.

Burkhart CG, et al. Calciphylaxis: a case report and review of the literature. *Wounds*. 1999;11:58-61.

Burns AJ, et al. Cutaneous vascular anomalies, hemangiomas, and malformations. In: Georgiade GS, Riefkohl R, Levin LS, eds. *Textbook of Plastic, Maxillofacial and Reconstructive Surgery*. 3rd ed. Baltimore, Md: Williams & Wilkins; 1997:178-197.

Burstein FD, et al. The use of hydroxyapatite cement in secondary craniofacial reconstruction. *Plast Reconstr Surg*. 1999;104:1270-1275.

Burt JD, et al. Cleft lip: unilateral primary deformities. *Plast Reconstr Surg*. 2000;105:1043.

Burton RI, et al. Extensor tendons - late reconstruc tion. In: Green DP, Hotchkiss RN, Pederson WC, eds. *Operative Hand Surgery*. 4th ed. New York, NY: Churchill Livingstone, Inc; 1999;2:1988-2021.

Burwell RG. Osteogenesis in cancellous bone grafts: considered in terms of its cellular changes, basic mechanisms, and the perspective of growth control and its possible aberrations. *Clin Orthop*. 1965;40:35-47.

Byrd HS, et al. The deep temporal lift: a multiplanar, lateral brow, temporal, and upper face lift. *Plast Reconstr Surg*. 1996;97:928-937.

Caballero E, et al. Diabetic foot infections. *J Foot Ankle Surg*. 1998;37:248-251.

Calkins ER. Nosocomial infections in hand surgery. *Hand Clin*. 1998;14:531-545.

Callan JP, et al. Actinic keratoses. *J Am Acad Dermatol*. 1997;36:650.

Calloway DM, et al. Changing concepts and controversies in the management of mandibular fractures. *Clin Plast Surg*. 1992;19:59-69.

Campion D. Electrodiagnostic testing in hand surgery. *J Hand Surg*. 1996;21A:947-956.

Canady KW. Evaluation of nasal obstruction in rhinoplasty. *Plast Reconstr Surg*. 1994;94:555.

Caouette-Laberge L, et al. Otoplasty: anterior scoring technique and results in 500 cases. *Plast Reconstr Surg*. 2000;105:504-515.

Cardenas-Camarena L, et al. Laboratory and histopathologic comparative study of internal ultrasound-assisted lipoplasty and tumescent lipoplasty. *Plast Reconstr Surg*. 2002;110:1158-1164.

Cardenas-Camarena L, et al. Large-volume liposuction and extensive abdominoplasty: a fewasible alternative for improving body shape. *Plast Reconstr Surg*. 1998;102:1698.

Carels RA, et al. Acute management of patients bitten by poisonous snakes. *Ned Tijdschr Geneeskd*. 1998;142:2773-2777.

Carlotti AE, et al. Facial changes associated with surgical advancement of the lip and maxilla. *J Oral Maxillofac Surg*. 1986;44:593-596.

Carlson GW. Oncologic and reconstructive principles. In: Achauer BM, Eriksson E, Guyuron B, et al, eds. *Plastic Surgery: Indications, Operations, and Outcomes*. Saint Louis, Mo: Mosby - Year Book, Inc; 2000;3:1067-1092.

Carlton JM, et al. Skin grafts and pedicle flaps. In: Peimer CA, ed. *Surgery of the Hand and Upper Extremity*. New York, NY: McGraw-Hill, Inc; 1996;2:1819-1844.

Carraway JH, et al. Reoperative blepharoplasty. In: Grotting JC, ed. *Reoperative Aesthetic & Reconstructive Surgery*. Saint Louis, Mo: Quality Medical Publishing, Inc; 1995:205-244.

Carraway JH, et al. The prevention and treatment of lower lid ectropium following blepharoplasty. *Plast Reconstr Surg*. 1990;85:971-981.

Carraway JH. Reconstruction of the eyelids and correction of ptosis of the eyelid. In: Aston SJ, Beasley RW, Thorne CH, eds. *Grabb & Smith's Plastic Surgery*. 5th ed. Philadelphia, Pa: Lippincott-Raven; 1997:529-544.

Carroll RE. Squamous cell carcinoma of the nail bed. *J Hand Surg*. 1976;1A:92-97.

Cassidy C, et al. Tendon dysfunction in systemic arthritis. In: Peimer CA, ed. *Surgery of the Hand and Upper Extremity*. New York, NY: McGraw-Hill, Inc; 1996;2:1645-1676.

Cassileth LB, et al. Clinical characteristics of patients with unicoronal synostosis and mutations of fibroblast growth factor receptor 3: a preliminary report. *Plast Reconstr Surg*. 2001;108:1849-1854.

Casson P, et al. Dysplastic and congenital nevi. *Clin Plast Surg*. 1993;20:105-113.

Casson PR, et al. Tumors of the maxilla. In: McCarthy JG, ed. *Plastic Surgery*. Philadelphia, Pa: WB Saunders Co; 1990;5:33317-3335.

Chan SW, et al. Rehabilitation of hand injuries. In: Cohen M, ed. *Mastery of Plastic and Reconstructive Surgery*. Boston, Mass: Little, Brown & Co; 1994;3:1745-1763.

Chang C, et al. Q-switched ruby laser treatment of oculodermal melanosis (nevus of ota). *Plast Reconstr Surg*. 1996;98:784.

Chang D, et al. Autologous breast reconstruction with the extended latissimus dorsi flap. *Plast Reconstr Surg*. 2002;110:751-761.

Chang DW, et al. Effect of smoking on complications in patients undergoing free TRAM flap breast reconstruction. *Plast Reconstr Surg*. 1996;12:467.

Chao KS, Perez CA, Brady LW, eds. *Radiation Oncology: Management Decisions*. Philadelphia, Pa: Lippincott-Raven; 1999:221-234.

Chaplin D, et al. Wrist and finger deformities in juvenile rheumatoid arthritis. *Acta Rheumatoid Scand*. 1969;15:206-223.

Chen CT, et al. The blood supply of the reverse temporalis muscle flap: anatomic study and clinical applications. *Plast Reconstr Surg*. 1999;103:1181-1188.

Chen YR, et al. Treatment of craniomaxillofacial fibrous dysplasia: how early and how extensive? *Plast Reconstr Surg*. 1990;86:835-842.

Cheng JT, et al. Collagen and injectable fillers. *Otolaryngol Clin North Am*. 2002;35:73-85.

Chidyllo SA, et al. The application of dental splints in regard to the modern techniques of rigid fixation. *J Craniofac Surg.* 1994;5:136-141.

Childers BJ, et al. Long-term results of irradiation for basal cell carcinoma of the skin of the nose. *Plast Reconstr Surg.* 1994;93:1169-1173.

Chin M, et al. Distraction of the midface. In: McCarthy JG, ed. *Distraction of the Craniofacial Skeleton.* New York, NY: Springer-Verlag; 1999:349-377.

Chin M, et al. Le Fort III advancement with gradual distraction using internal devices. *Plast Reconstr Surg.* 1997;100:819-832.

Chiu DT, et al. Repair and grafting of dermis, fat, and fascia. In: McCarthy, ed. *Plastic Surgery.* Philadelphia, Pa: WB Saunders Co; 1990;1:519-520.

Choe Ks, et al. Chin augmentation. *Facial Plast Surg.* 2000;16:45-54.

Choi M, et al. Preventing the infiltration of leukocytes by monoclonal antibodies blocks the development of progressive ischemia in rat burns. *Plast Reconstr Surg.* 1995;96:1177-1185.

Choi PD, et al. Iatrogenic injury to the ilioinguinal and iliohypogastric nerves in the groin: a case report, diagnosis, and management. *Ann Plast Surg.* 1996;37:60-65.

Chuinard RS, et al. Tendon transfers for radial nerve palsy: use of superficialis tendons for digital extension. *J Hand Surg.* 1978;3A:560.

Chung KC, et al. Decision-analysis methodology in the work-up of women with suspected silicone breast implant rupture. *Plast Reconstr Surg.* 1998;102:689-695.

Cioffi WG, et al. Leukocyte responses to injury. *Arch Surg.* 1993;128:1260-1267.

Cioffi WG. What's new in surgery: burns and metabolism. *J Am Coll Surg.* 2001;192:241-254.

Clark CP III. New directions in skin care. *Clin Plast Surg.* 2001;28:745-750.

Clark CP III. Office-based skin care and superficial peels: the scientific rationale. *Plast Reconstr Surg.* 1999;104:854.

Clark HM, et al. An approach to obstetrical brachial plexus injuries. *Hand Clin.* 1995;11:563-581.

Clayman MA, et al. Use of AlloDerm as a barrier to treat chronic Frey's syndrome. *Otolaryngol Head Neck Surg.* 2001;124:687.

Clemente CD, ed. *Gray's Anatomy of the Human Body.* 30th ed. Philadelphia, Pa: Lea & Febiger; 1985.

Clemente CD. *Anatomy: A Regional Atlas of the Human Body.* 2nd ed. Baltimore, Md: Urban & Schwartzenberg; 1981.

Clemente CD. *Anatomy: A Regional Atlas of the Human Body.* 4th ed. Baltimore, Md: Williams & Wilkins; 1997:435-576, 730, 735-736, 739, 748-750, 782, 845, 859, 866, 872, 888, 895, 896.

Cody DT, et al. Neoplasms of the nasal cavity. In: Cummings CW, Frederickson JM, Harker LA, et al, eds. *Otolaryngology Head and Neck Surgery.* 3rd ed. Saint Louis Mo: Mosby - Year Book, Inc; 1998;2:883-901.

Cohen M, ed. *Mastery of Plastic and Reconstructive Surgery.* Boston, Mass: Little, Brown & Co; 1994;3:1997.

Cohen SR, et al. Internal craniofacial distraction with biodegradable devices: early stabilization and protected bone regeneration. *J Craniofac Surg.* 2000;11:354-366.

Cohen SR, et al. Midface distraction. In: Samchukov ML, Cope JB, Cherkashin AM, eds. *Craniofacial Distraction Osteogenesis.* Saint Louis, Mo: Mosby - Year Book, Inc; 2001:520-530.

Cohen SR. Genioplasty. In: Achauer BM, Eriksson E, Guyuron B, et al, eds. *Plastic Surgery: Indications, Operations, and Outcomes.* Saint Louis, Mo; Mosby - Year Book, Inc; 2000:2563-2582, 2683-2703.

Cohen SR. Midface distraction. *Sem Orthodont.* 1999;5:52-58.

Cole JK, et al. Early excision and grafting of face and neck burns in patients over 20 years. *Plast Reconstr Surg*. 2002;109:1266.

Coleman JJ III. The bipedicled osteocutaneous scapula flap: a new subscapular system free flap. *Plast Reconstr Surg*. 1991;87:682-692.

Coleman JJ III. The pharynx. In: Achauer BM, Eriksson E, Guyuron B, et al, eds. *Plastic Surgery: Indications, Operations, and Outcomes*. Saint Louis, Mo: Mosby Year - Book, Inc. 2000;3:1289-1310.

Coleman SR. Facial recontouring with lipostructure. *Clin Plast Surg*. 1997;24:347-367.

Coleman SR. Long-term survival of fat transplants: controlled demonstrations. *Aesthetic Plastic Surg*. 1995;19:421.

Colen SR. Pressure sores. In: McCarthy JG, ed. *Plastic Surgery*. Philadelphia, Pa: WB Saunders Co; 1990;6:3797.

Commons GW, et al. Large-volume liposuction: a review of 631 consecutive cases over 12 years. *Plast Reconstr Surg*. 2001;108:1753-1763.

Concannon MJ, Hurov J, eds. *Hand Pearls*. Philadelphia, Pa: Hanley & Belfus, Inc; 2002;104, 141-145, 146-149.

Concannon MJ. Common hand problems. In: *Common Hand Problems in Primary Care*. Philadelphia, Pa: Hanley & Belfus, Inc; 1999;8:161.

Concannon MJ. Infections of the hand. In: *Common Hand Problems in Primary Care*. Philadelphia, Pa: Hanley & Belfus, Inc; 1999;7:127-132.

Connell BF, et al. Skin and SMAS flaps for facial rejuvination. In: Achauer BM, Eriksson E, Guyuron B, et al, eds. *Plastic Surgery: Indications, Operations, and Outcomes*. Saint Louis, Mo: Mosby - Year Book, Inc; 2000:2583-2607.

Conrad MH, et al. Pharmacologic optimization of microsurgery in the new millennium. *Plast Reconstr Surg*. 2001;108:2088.

Constantian M. Primary rhinoplasty: basic techniques. In: Cohen M, ed. *Mastery of Plastic and Reconstructive Surgery*. Boston, Mass: Little, Brown & Co; 1994;2:1999-2020.

Constantian MB. The incompetent external nasal valve: pathophysiology and treatment in primary and secondary thinoplasty. *Plast Reconstr Surg*. 1994;93:919.

Constantino PD, et al. Synthetic bone graft substitutes. *Otolaryngol Clin North Am*. 1994;27:1037-1074.

Cook TF, et al. Unusual cutaneous malignancies. *Semin Cutan Med Surg*. 1998;17:114-132.

Coons MS, et al. Boutonniere deformity. *Hand Clin*. 1995;11:387-402.

Cooper JS, et al. Recursive partitioning analysis of 2105 patients treated in Radiation Therapy Oncolgy Group studies of head and neck cancer. *Cancer*. 1996;77:1905-1911.

Cordeiro PG, et al. Reconstruction of the mandible with osseous free flaps: a 10-year experience with 150 consecutive patients. *Plast Reconstr Surg*. 1999;104:1314.

Coscarella E, et al. Subfascial and submuscular methods of temporal muscle dissection and their relationship to the frontal branch of the facial nerve: technical note. *J Neurosurg*. 2000;92:877-880.

Courtiss EH, et al. The fate of breast implants with infections around them. *Plast Reconstr Surg*. 1979;63:812.

Cowin DJ, et al. Long-term complications of snake bites to the upper extremity. *J South Orthop Assoc*. 1998;7:205-211.

Cram AE. Split thickness skin grafts. In: Blair WF, ed. *Techniques in Hand Surgery*. Baltimore, Md: Williams & Wilkins; 1996:8-12.

Cramer SF. The melanocyte differentiation pathway in spitz nevi. *Am J Dermatopath*. 1998;20:555-570.

Crawford F, et al. Oral treatments for toenail onychomycosis: a systematic review. *Arch Dermatol*. 2002;138:811-816.

Crawley WA, et al. Fractures of the mandible. In: Ferraro JW, ed. *Fundamentals in Maxillofacial Surgery*. New York, NY: Springer-Verlag; 1997:192-202.

Crawley WA, et al. Midface, upper face, and panfacial fractures. In: Ferraro JW, ed. *Fundamentals in Maxillofacial Surgery*. New York, NY: Springer-Verlag; 1997:203-214.

Cricker A, et al. Does intermittent sun exposure cause basal cell carcinoma. Case control study in Western Australia. *Int J Cancer*. 1995;60:489.

Cricker A, et al. Pigmentary and cutaneous risk factors for nonmelanocytic skin cancer: a case control study. *Int J Cancer*. 1991;48:650.

Cronin TD, et al. Deformities of the cervial region. In: McCarthy JG, ed. *Plastic Surgery*. Philadelphia, Pa: WB Saunders Co; 1990;3:2057-2077.

Cruz MJ et al. Pierre Robin sequence: secondary respiratory difficulties and intrinsic feeding abnormalities. *Laryngoscope*. 1999;109:1632-1636.

Cruz-Korchin N, et al. Macromastia: how much of it is fat? *Plast Reconstr Surg*. 2002;109:64-68.

Cunningham BL, et al. Saline-filled breast implant safety and efficacy: a multicenter retrospective review. *Plast Reconstr Surg*. 2000;105:2143-2149.

Cutting CB, et al. Repair and grafting of bone. In: McCarthy JG, ed. *Plastic Surgery*. Philadelphia, Pa: WB Saunders Co; 1990;1:583-629.

Czitrom AA, et al. The viability of articular cartilage in fresh osteochondral allografts after clinical transplantation. *J Bone Joint Surg*. 1990;72A:574.

Dagley S, et al. Inhibition and growth of bactaerogenes: the mode of action of phenols, alcohol, and ethyl acetate. *J Bacteriol*. 1950;60:369.

Daluiski A, et al. The molecular control of upper extremity development: implications for congenital hand anomalies. *J Hand Surg*. 2001;26A:8-22.

Daniel RK, ed. *Aesthetic Plastic Surgery: Rhinoplasty*. Boston, Mass: Little, Brown & Co; 1993:3-39, 99, 298.

Danikas D, et al. Mammographic findings following reduction mammoplasty. *Aesthetic Plast Surg*. 2001;25:283-285.

Dantzer E, et al. Reconstructive surgery using an artificial dermis (Integra): results with 39 grafts. *Br J Plast Surg*. 2001;54:659-664.

Dardour JC. Treatment of male pattern baldness and postoperative temporal baldness in men. *Clin Plast Surg*. 1991;775-790.

Davis GM, et al. Reduction mammaplasty: long-term efficacy, morbidity, and patient satisfaction. *Plast Reconstr Surg*. 1995;96:1106-1110.

Dawson D, Hallett M, Millender L, eds. *Entrapment Neuropathies*. Boston, Mass: Little, Brown & Co; 1990:97-100, 136-144, 201-208.

Dayan SH, et al. The forehead lift: endoscopic versus coronal approaches. *Aesthetic Plast Surg*. 2001;25:35-39.

De Cordier BC, et al. Endoscopic forehead lift: review of technique, cases, and complications. *Plast Reconstr Surg*. 2002;110:1558-1568.

Deitch EA, et al. Hypertrophic burn scars: analysis of variables. *J Trauma*. 1983;23:895.

Deitch MA, et al. Dorsal fracture dislocations of the proximal interphalangeal joint: surgical complications and long-term results. *J Hand Surg*. 1999;24A:914-923.

Delay E, et al. Autologous latissimus breast reconstruction: a 3-year clinical experience with 100 patients. *Plast Reconstr Surg*. 1998;102:1461.

Delgado R, et al. Osteosarcome of the jaw. *Head Neck*. 1994;16:246-252.

Della Rocca RC, et al. Nasolacrimal disorders and their treatment. *Clin Plast Surg*. 1988;15:195-207.

Dellon AL. Peripheral nerve injuries. In: Georgiade GS, Riefkohl R, Levin LS, eds. *Textbook of Plastic, Maxillofacial and Reconstructive Surgery*. Baltimore, Md: Williams & Wilkins; 1997:1011-1013.

DeLustro F, et al. Reaction to injectable collagen: results in animal models and clinical use. *Plast Reconstr Surg*. 1987;79:581-594.

Demling RH. Burns: fluid and electrolyte management. *Crit Care Clin*. 1985;1:27-45.

Demling RH. Fluid resuscitation. In: Bostwick JA, ed. *The Art and Science of Burn Care*. Rockville, Md: Aspen Publishers; 1987.

Denny AD, et al. Mandibular distraction osteogenesis in very young patients to correct airway obstruction. *Plast Reconstr Surg*. 2001;108:302-311.

deShazo RD, et al. An approach to the patient with a history of local anesthetic hypersensitivity: experience with 90 patients. *J Allergy Clin Immunol*. 1979;63:387.

Dhar SC, et al. The delay phenomenon: the story unfolds. *Plast Reconstr Surg*. 1999;104:2079-2091.

Diao E, et al. Total collateral ligament excision for contractures of the proximal interphalangeal joint. *J Hand Surg*. 1993;18A:395.

Dillerud E. Suction lipoplasty: a report on complications, undesired results, and patient satisfaction based on 3511 procedures. *Palst Reconstr Surg*. 1991;88:239-246.

Dinehart SM, et al. Cancer of the skin. In: Myers EN, Suen JY, eds. *Cancer of the Head and Neck*. Philadelphia, Pa: WB Saunders Co; 1996:143-159.

Dingman RO, et al. Surgical anatomy of the mandibular ramus of the facial nerve based on the dissection of 100 facial halves. *Plast Reconstr Surg*. 1962;29:266-272.

Dingman RO, et al. The clinical management of facial injuries and fractures of the facial bones. In: Converse JM, ed. *Reconstructive Plastic Surgery*. Philadelphia, Pa: WB Saunders Co; 1977.

Dingman RO, Natvig P. S*urgery of Facial Fractures*. Philadelphia, Pa: WB Saunders Co; 1964.

Dinner MI, et al. The tubular/tuberous breast syndrome. *Ann Plast Surg*. 1987;19:414-419.

Disa J, et al. Evaluation of combined sodium alginate and bio-occlusive membrane dressing in the management of split thickness donor sites. *Ann Plast Surg*. 2001;46:405-408.

Disa JJ, et al. Efficacy of magnetic resonance angiography in the evaluation of vascular malformations of the hand. *Plast Reconstr Surg*. 1997;99:136.

Disa JJ, et al. Efficacy of operative cure in pressure sore patients. *Plast Reconstr Surg*. 1992;89:272-278.

Disa JJ, et al. Mandible reconstruction with microvascular injury. *Semin Surg Oncol*. 2000;19:226.

Dobyns JH, et al. Congenital hand deformities. In: Green DP, ed. *Operative Hand Surgery*. New York, NY: Churchill Livingstone, Inc; 1993;1:251-548.

Doi K, et al. Free vascularized bone graft for nonunion of the scaphoid. *J Hand Surg*. 2000;25A:507-519.

Dolezal J. Jessner's solution. In: Rubin MG, ed. *Manual of Chemical Peels, Superficial and Medium Depth*. Philadelphia, Pa: JB Lippincott Co; 1992.

Dolezal RF. Fractures of the nose. In: Cohen M, ed. *Mastery of Plastic and Reconstructive Surgery*. Boston, Mass: Little, Brown & Co; 1994;2:1126-1135.

Dolynchuk K, et al. Orbital volumetric analysis: clinical application in orbitozygomatic complex injuries. *J Craniofac Trauma.* 1996;2:56-63.

Donald PJ, et al. Facial fractures. In: Snow JB Jr, Ballenger JJ, eds. *Ballenger's Otorhinolaryngology Head and Neck Surgery.* 16th ed. Hamilton, Ontario: BC Decker; 2003:900-950.

Donelan MB. Reconstruction of the burned hand and upper extremity. In: McCarthy JG, ed. *Plastic Surgery.* Philadelphia, Pa: WB Saunders Co; 1990;8:5473-5476.

Dowden RV, et al. Breast implant overfill, optimal fill, and the standard of care. *Plast Reconstr Surg.* 1999;104:1185.

Dowden RV, et al. The vastus lateralis muscle flap: technique and applications. *Ann Plast Surg.* 1980;4:396.

Dowden RV. Saline breast implant fill issues. *Clin Plast Surg.* 2002;28:445-450.

Doyle JR. Constriction ring reconstruction. In: Blair WF, ed. *Techniques in Hand Surgery.* Baltimore, Md: Williams & Wilkins; 1996:1106-1111.

Doyle JR. Extensor tendons - acute injuries. In: Green DP, Hotchkiss RN, Pederson WC, eds. *Operative Hand Surgery.* 4th ed. New York, NY: Churchill Livingstone, Inc; 1999;2:1851-1897.

Doyle JR. Sliding bone graft technique for arthrodesis of the trapeziometacarpal joint of the thumb. *J Hand Surg.* 1991;16A:363.

Dray GJ, et al. Dislocations and ligament injuries in the digits. In: Green DP, ed. *Operative Hand Surgery.* 3rd ed. New York, NY: Churchill Livingstone, Inc; 1982:773-774.

Drug Facts and Comparisons 2000. Saint Louis, Mo: Facts & Comparisons, Inc; 1999:1621.

Ducic I, et al. Outcome of patients with toxic epidermal necrolysis syndrome revisited. *Plast Reconstr Surg.* 2002;110:768-773.

Duffy M, et al. The superficial plane rhytidectomy revisited. *Plast Reconstr Surg.* 1994;93:1392.

Dufresne CR, et al. Pediatric facial trauma. In: McCarthy JG, ed. *Plastic Surgery.* Philadelphia, Pa: WB Saunders, Co; 1990;2:1142-1187.

Duguid IM. Ophthalmic injuris. In: Williams JL, ed. *Rowe and Williams' Maxillofacial Injuries.* 2nd ed. Edinburgh, Scotland: Churchill Livingstone, Inc; 1994;2:827-843.

Durham JW. Thumb metacarpophalangeal ulnar collateral ligament repair with local tissues. In: Blair WF, ed. *Techniques in Hand Surgery.* Baltimore, Md: Williams & Wilkins; 1996:533-537.

Dziewulski P. Burn wound healing. *Burns.* 1992;18:466-478.

Earley MJ. The arterial supply of the thumb first web space and index finger in its surgical application. *J Hand Surg.* 1986;11B:163-170.

Eaton CJ, et al. Treatment of skin and soft-tissue loss of the thumb. *Hand Clin.* 1992;8:71.

Echavez MI, et al. Effects of steroids on mood, edema, and ecchymosis in facial plastic surgery. *Arch Otolaryngol Head Neck Surg.* 1994;120:1137-1141.

Edgerton BW, et al. Dorsal cross-finger flaps. In: Strauch B, Vasconez LO, Hall-Findlay EJ, eds. *Grabb's Encyclopedia of Flaps.* 2nd ed. Philadelphia, Pa: Lippincott-Raven; 1998.

Eklund GW, et al. Improved imaging of the augmented breast. *Am J Radiol.* 1988;151:469-473.

El Deeb M, et al. Complications of orthognathic surgery. *Clin Plast Surg.* 1989;16:825.

Eliezri YD, et al. Lymphangioma circumscriptum: review and evaluation of carbon dioxide laser vaporization. *J Dermatol Surg Oncol.* 1988;14:357.

Elliot LF, et al. Scalp and calvarium. In: Jurkiewicz MJ, Mathes SJ, Krizek TJ, et al, eds. *Plastic Surgery: Principles and Practice*. Saint Louis, Mo: CV Mosby Co; 1990:419-440.

Elsahy NI. Acquired ear defects. *Clin Plast Surg*. 2002;29:175-186.

Elsahy NI. Reconstruction of the ear after skin and cartilage loss. *Clin Plast Surg*. 2002;29:201-212Elster AD. Quadriplegia after minor trauma in the Klippel-Feil syndrome. *J Bone Joint Surg*. 1984;66A:1473.

Enjolras O, et al. Facial port-wine stains and Sturge-Weber syndrome. *Pediatrics*. 1985;76:48.

Enjolras O, et al. Management of alarming hemangiomas in infancy: a review of 25 cases. *Pediatrics*. 1990;85:491-498.

Erickson SJ, et al. MR imaging of the ankle and foot. *Radiol Clin North Am*. 1997;35:163-192.

Erlich P, et al. The effects of vitamin A and glucocorticoids upon repair and collagen synthesis. *Ann Surg*. 1973;177:22.

Evans GR, ed. *Operative Plastic Surgery*. New York, NY: McGraw-Hill, Inc; 2000;166.

Evans GR, et al. Reconstruction of the irradiated breast: is there a role for implants? *Plast Reconstr Surg*. 1995;96:1111.

Evans GR, et al. Surgical correction of pressure ulcers in an urban center: is it efficacious? *Adv Wound Care*. 1994;7:40-46.

Eversmann WW Jr. Entrapment and compression neuropathies. In: Green DP, ed. *Operative Hand Surgery*. 3rd ed. New York, NY: Churchill Livingstone, Inc; 1982:1341-1385.

Ezaki M, et al. Congenital hand deformities. In: Green DP, Hotchkiss RN, Pederson WC, eds. *Operative Hand Surgery*. 4th ed. New York, NY: Churchill Livingstone, Inc; 1999;1:325-551.

Ezaki M. Amnion disruption sequence. In: Green DP, Hotchkiss RN, Pederson WC, eds. *Operative Hand Surgery*. 4th ed. New York, NY: Churchill Livingstone, Inc; 1999;1:429-431.

Ezaki M. Syndactyly. In: Green DP, Hotchkiss RN, Pederson WC, eds. *Operative Hand Surgery*. 4th ed. New York, NY: Churchill Livingstone, Inc; 1999;1:426.

Fagien S, et al. Primary and adjunctive use of botulinum toxin type A (Botox) in facial aesthetic surgery: beyond the glabella. *Clin Plast Surg*. 2001;28:127-148.

Fagien S. Botox for the treatment of dynamic and hyperkinetic facial lines and furrows: adjunctive use in facial aesthetic surgery. *Plast Reconstr Surg*. 1999;103:701-713.

Fagien S. Facial soft-tissue augmentation with injectable autologous and allogeneic human tissue collagen matrix (autologen and dermalogen). *Plast Reconstr Surg*. 2000;105:362-375.

Failla JM. Differential diagnosis of hand pain: tendonitis, ganglia, and other syndromes. In: Peimer CA, ed. *Surgery of the Hand and Upper Extremity*. New York, NY: McGraw-Hill, Inc; 1996;1:1223-1249.

Fara M. Anatomy and arteriography of cleft lips in stillborn children. *Plast Reconstr Surg*. 1968;42:29.

Fara M. The musculature of cleft lip and palate. In: McCarthy JG, ed. *Plastic Surgery*. Philadelphia, Pa: WB Saunders Co; 1990;4:2612.

Farhadieh RD, et al. Effect of distraction rate on biomechanical, mineralization, and histologic properties of an ovine mandible model. *Plast Reconstr Surg*. 2000;105:889.

Farmer KL, et al. Prevention of nonmelanoma skin cancer: standard and investigative approaches. *Clin Plast Surg*. 1997;24:663-671.

Feinberg S, et al. Reconstruction of the temporomandibular joint with pedicled temporalis muscle flaps. In: Bell WH, ed. *Modern Practice in Orthognathic and Reconstructive Surgery*. Philadelphia, Pa: WB Saunders Co; 1992:733.

Feinendegen DL, et al. Autologous fat injection for soft tissue auagmentation in the face: a safe procedure? *Aesthetic Plast Surg*. 1998;22:163-167.

Feinstein FR, et al. Fractures of the zygoma and zygomatic arch. In: *Surgery of Facial Bone Fractures*. New York, NY: Churchill Livingstone, Inc; 1987:136.

Feldman DL. Which dressing for split thickness skin graft donor sites? *Ann Plast Surg*. 1991;27:288-291.

Feldmann JJ. Corset platysmaplasty. *Clin Plast Surg*. 1992;19:369-382.

Feldon P, et al. Rheumatoid arthritis and other connective tissue diseases. In: Green DP, Hotchkiss RN, Pederson WC, eds. *Operative Hand Surgery*. 4th ed. New York, NY: Churchill Livingstone, Inc; 1999;2:1651-1739.

Ferlic DC. Rheumatoid flexor tenosynovitis and rupture. *Hand Clin*. 1996;12:561-572.

Fernandez DL, et al. Fractures of the distal radius. In: Green DP, Hotchkiss RN, Pederson WC, eds. *Operative Hand Surgery*. 4th ed. New York, NY: Churchill Livingstone, Inc; 1999;1:979.

Ferraro JW. Cephalometry and cephalometric analysis. In: Ferraro JW, ed. *Fundamentals in Maxillofacial Surgery*. New York, NY: Springer-Verlag; 1997:233-245.

Ferraro JW. Local anesthesia and infiltration techniques. In: Ferraro JW, ed. *Fundamentals in Maxillofacial Surgery*. New York, NY: Springer-Verlag; 1997:158-168.

Ferraro JW. Mandibular excess and deficiency. In: Ferraro JW, ed. *Fundamentals in Maxillofacial Surgery*. New York, NY: Springer-Verlag; 1997:270-283.

Ferraro JW. Oral anatomy. In: Ferraro JW, ed. *Fundamentals in Maxillofacial Surgery*. New York, NY: Springer-Verlag; 1997:127-157.

Fingeret M, et al. Jones Dye tests 1 and 2. In: *Atlas of Primary Eyecare Procedures*. Norwalk Ct: Appleton & Lange; 1990:120-121.

Fink JA, et al. Nonmelanotic malignant skin tumors of the hand. *Hand Clin*. 1995;11:255-264.

Fink MP. The role of cytokines as mediators of the inflammatory response. In: Townsend CM Jr, ed. *Sabiston's Textbook of Surgery*. 16th ed. Philadelphia, Pa: WB Saunders Co; 2001:41.

Fink SC, et al. Craniofacial syndromes. In: Bentz ML, ed. *Pediatric Plastic Surgery*. Stamford, Conn: Appleton & Lange; 1998;1:1-43.

Finley RK III, et al. Subungual melanoma: an eighteen-year review. *Surgery*. 1994;116:96-100.

Finn MC, et al. Congenital vascular lesions: clinical application of a new classification. *J Pediatr Surg*. 1983;18:894.

Fischer K, et al. Injuries associated with mandible fractures sustaines in motor vehicle collisions. *Plast Reconstr Surg*. 2001;108:328-331.

Fitzpatrick TB. The validity and practicality of sun reactive types I-IV. *Arch Dermatol*. 1988;124:869.

Fix RJ, et al. Fasciocutaneous flaps in reconstruction of the lower extremity. *Clin Plast Surg*. 1991;18:571-582.

Flatt AE. Digital artery sympathectomy. *J Hand Surg*. 1987;12A:391-400.

Flatt AE. *The Care of Congenital Hand Anomalies*. 2nd ed. Saint Louis, Mo: Quality Medical Publishing, Inc; 1994:292-316.

Flatt AE. *The Care of Congenital Hand Anomalies*. Saint Louis, Mo: CV Mosby Co; 1977.

Flatt AE. *The Care of the Arthritic Hand*. Saint Louis, Mo: Quality Medical Publishing, Inc; 1995.

Fleegler EJ, et al. Tumors of the perionychium. *Hand Clin*. 1990;6:113-135.

Fleegler EJ. Skin tumors. In: Green DP, Hotchkiss RN, Pederson WC, eds. *Operative Hand Surgery*. 4th ed. New York, NY: Churchill Livingstone, Inc; 1999;2:2184.

Fleming ID, et al. *AJCC Cancer Staging Manual*. 5th ed. Philadelphia, Pa: Lippincott-Raven;1997:163-170.

Floros C, et al. Complications and long-term results following abdominoplasty: a retrospective study. *Br J Plast Surg*. 1991;44:190-194.

Flowers R, et al. Blepharoplasty and periorbital aesthetic surgery. In: Aston SJ, Beasley RW, Thorne CH, eds. *Grabb & Smith's Plastic Surgery*. 5th ed. Philadelphia, Pa: Lippincott-Raven; 1997:617.

Flowers RS. Optimal procedure in secondary blepharoplasty. *Clin Plast Surg*. 1993;20:225-237.

Floyd WE III, et al. Benign cartilaginous lesions of the upper extremity. *Hand Clin*. 1995;11:119-132.

Floyd WE, et al. Acute and chronic sepsis. In: Peimer CA, ed. *Surgery of the Hand and Upper Extremity*. New York, NY: McGraw-Hill, Inc; 1996;2:1731-1762.

Fodor PB. Endermologie (LPG): does it work? *Aesthetic Plast Surg*. 1997;21:68.

Ford T, et al. Umbilical keloid: an early start. *Ann Plast Surg*. 1990;25:214-215.

Foucher G, et al. Digital reconstruction with island flaps. *Clin Plast Surg*. 1997;24:1-32.

Foucher G, et al. Island flaps based on the first and second dorsal metacarpal artery. In: Levin E, Germann G, eds. *Local Flaps about the Hand: Atlas of the Hand Clinics*. Philadelphia, Pa: WB Saunders Co; 1998.

Foucher G, et al. Neurovascular skin kite flap from the index finger. In: Strauch B, Vasconez LO, Hall-Findlay EJ, eds. *Grabb's Encyclopedia of Flaps*. 2nd ed. Philadelphia, Pa: Lippincott-Raven; 1998.

Fox SA. A modified Kuhnt-Szymanowski procedure for ectropion and lateral canthoplasty. *Am J Ophthalmol*. 1966;62:533.

Frank DH, et al. Human antibody response following multiple injections of bovine collagen. *Plast Reconstr Surg*. 1991;87:1080-1088.

Freeland AE. *Hand Fractures: Repair, Reconstruction, and Rehabilitation*. New York, NY: Churchill Livingstone, Inc; 2000:14-65.

Freidrich KL, et al. Changing trends with mandibular fractures: a review of 1,067 cases. *J Oral Maxillofac Surg*. 1992;50:586-589.

Freund RM, et al. Correlation between brow lift outcomes and aesthetic ideals for eyebrow height and shape in females. *Plast Reconstr Surg*. 1996;97:1343.

Friedlaender GE. Current concepts review: bone grafts. *J Bone Joint Surg. 1987;69A:786*.

Friedman HI, et al. Recurrent basal cell carcinoma in margin-positive tumors. *Ann Plast Surg*. 1997;38:232-235.

Friedman M, et al. Malignant tumors of the major salivary glands. *Otolaryngol Clin North Am*. 1986;19:625-636.

Friedman PM, et al. Comparative study of the efficacy of four topical anesthetics. *Dermatol Surg*. 1999;25:950-954.

Friedman S, et al. Breast secretions in normal women. *Am J Obstet Gynecol*. 1969;104:846.

Fuchs PC, et al. Synovial histology in carpal tunnel syndrome. *J Hand Surg*. 1991;16A:753-758.

Fuente del Campo A, et al. Treacher Collins syndrome (mandibulofacial dysostosis). *Clin Plast Surg*. 1994;21:613-623.

Fulton JE, et al. Fat grafting. *Dermatol Clin*. 2001;19:523.

Furnas D. The correction of prominent ears by concha-mastoid sutures. *Plast Reconstr Surg*. 1968;42:189.

Furnas DW. Complications of surgery of the external ear. *Clin Plast Surg*. 1990;17:305-318.

Furnas DW. External Ear. In: Jurkiwqicz MJ, Krizek TJ, Mathes SJ, et al, eds. *Plastic Surgery: Principles and Practice*. Saint Louis, Mo: CV Mosby Co; 1990:191-194.

Furnas DW. Otoplasty for prominent ears. *Clin Plast Surg*. 2002;29:273-288.

Furnas DW. Otoplasty for protruding ears, cryptotia, or Stahl's ear. In: Evans GR, ed. *Operative Plastic Surgery*. New York, NY: McGraw-Hill Inc; 2000:417.

Fusco FJ. The aging face and skin: common signs and treatment. *Clin Plast Surg*. 2001;28:1-12.

Gabel GT. Nerve entrapment. In: Herndon JH, ed. *Surgical Reconstruction of the Upper Extremity*. Stamford, Conn: Appleton & Lange; 1999:367-390.

Gagnon NB, et al. Facial reinnervation after facial paralysis: is it ever too late? *Arch Otorhinolaryngol*. 1989;246:303.

Garcia VF, et al. Reconstruction of congenital chest-wall deformities. *Surg Clin North Am*. 1989;69:1103-1118.

Garcia-Elias M. Carpal instabilities and dislocations. In: Green DP, Hotchkiss RN, Pederson WC, eds. *Operative Hand Surgery*. 4th ed. New York, NY: Churchill Livingstone, Inc; 1999;1:865-928.

Garfin SR, et al. Treatment of rattlesnake bites. *J Hand Surg*. 1980;5A:619-621.

Garza JR, et al. Secondary deformities of the cleft lip and nose. In: Bentz ML, ed. *Pediatric Plastic Surgery*. Stamford, Conn: Appleton & Lange; 1998:81.

Gasparro FP. P53 and dermatology. *Arch Dermatol*. 1998;134:1029-1032.

Gasser H. Delayed union and pseudoarthritis of the carpal navicular: treatment by compression screw osteosynthesis: a preliminary report on 20 fractures. *J Bone Joint Surg*. 1965;47A:249.

Gayle LB, et al. Treatment of chronic osteomyelitis of the lower extremities with debridement and microvascular muscle transfer. *Clin Plast Surg*. 1992;19:895-903.

Georgiade NG, et al. Esthetic breast surgery. In: McCarthy JG, ed. *Plastic Surgery*. Philadelphia, Pa: WB Saunders Co; 1990;6:3839-3896. Georgiade S. Hypermastia and ptosis. In: Georgiade GS, Riefkohl R, Levin LS, eds. *Plastic, Maxillofacial and Reconstructive Surgery*. Baltimore, Md: Williams & Wilkins; 1997:752.

Ger E, et al. The management of trigger thumb in children. *J Hand Surg*. 1991;16A:944-947.

Ger R, et al. Transmetatarsal amputation of the toe: an analytic study of ischemic complications. *Clin Anat*. 1999;12:407-411.

Gerber GS. Carcinoma in situ of the penis. *J Urol*. 1994;151:829-833.

Gersoff WK, et al. The effect of tourniquet pressure on muscle function. *Am J Sports Med*. 1989;17:123-127.

Gerwin M. Cerebral palsy. In: Green DP, Hotchkiss RN, Pederson WC, eds. *Operative Hand Surgery*. 4th ed. New York, NY: Churchill Livingstone, Inc; 1999;1:259-285.

Gherardini G, et al. Congenital syndromes associated with nonmelanoma skin cancer. *Clin Plast Surg*. 1997;24:649-661.

Gibson T, et al. The distortion of autologous grafts: its cause and prevention. *Br Plast Surg*. 1958;10:257.

Gilbert A. Long-term evaluation of brachial plexus surgery in obstetrical palsy. *Hand Clin*. 1995;11:583-595.

Gilbert DN, et al. *The Sandford Guide to Antimicrobial Therapy*. 29th ed. Antimicrobial Therapy, Inc; 1999.

Gillies H, et al. Operative correction by osteotomy of recessed malar maxillary compund in a case of oxycephaly. *Br J Plast Surg*. 1951;3:123.

Gilman S, Newman SW, eds. Ascending and descending pathways. In:*Manter and Gatz's Essentials of Clinical Neuroanatomy and Neurophysiology*. Philadelphia, Pa: FA Davis Co; 1996.

Gilula LA. *The Traumatized Hand and Wrist: Radiographic and Anatomic Correlation*. Philadelphia, Pa: WB Saunders Co; 1992.

Gingrass MK, et al. The treatment of nail deformities secondary to ganglions of the distal interphalangeal joint. *J Hand Surg*. 1995;20A:502-505.

Giovannitti JA, et al. Assessment of allergy to local anesthetics. *J Am Dent Assoc*. 1979;98:701.

Glat PM, et al. Distraction of the mandible: experimental studies. In: McCarthy JG, ed. *Distraction of the Craniofacial Skeleton*. New York, NY: Springer-Verlag; 1999:67-79.

Glat PM, et al. Management considerations for melanonychia striata and melanoma of the hand. *Hand Clin*. 1995;11:183-189.

Glat PM, et al. Wound Healing. In: Aston SJ, Beasley RW, Thorne CH, eds. *Grabb & Smith's Plastic Surgery*. 5th ed. Philadelphia, Pa: Lippincott-Raven; 1997:3-12.

Glickel SZ, et al. Dislocations and ligament injuries in the digits. In: Green DP, Hotchkiss RN, Pederson WC, eds. *Operative Hand Surgery*. 4th ed. New York, NY: Churchill Livingstone, Inc; 1999;1:772-808.

Glickel SZ. Metacarpophalangeal and interphalangeal joint injuries and instabilities. In: Peimer CA, ed. *Surgery of the Hand and Upper Extremity*. New York, NY: McGraw-Hill, Inc; 1996;1:1043-1067.

Goitz RJ, et al. Soft-tissue defects of the digits: coverage consideration. *Hand Clin*. 1997;13:189-205.

Goldberg DP. Assessment and surgical treatment of basal cell skin cancer. *Clin Plast Surg*. 1997;24:673-686.

Goldberg NS, et al. Periorbital hematomas. *Dermatol Clin*. 1992;10:653-661.

Goldner RD, et al. Replantation proximal to the wrist. *Hand Clin*. 1992;8:413-415.

Goldner RD, et al. Replantation. In: Green DP, Hotchkiss RN, Pederson WC, eds. *Operative Hand Surgery*. 4th ed. New York, NY: Churchill Livingstone, Inc; 1999;1:1139-1157.

Goldstein JA. Fixation principles. In: Achauer BM, Eriksson E, Guyuron B, et al, eds. *Plastic Surgery: Indications, Operations, and Outcomes*. Saint Louis, Mo: Mosby Year - Book, Inc. 2000;2:651-655.

Goodrich JJ, et al. *Craniofacial Anomalies: Growth and Development from a Surgical Perspective*. New York, NY: Thieme Medical Publishers, Inc; 1995.

Gordon L. Toe-to-thumb transplantation. In: Green DP, Hotchkiss RN, Pederson WC, eds. *Operative Hand Surgery*. 4th ed. New York, NY: Churchill Livingstone, Inc; 1999;2:1299-1326.

Gorlin RJ, et al. Multiple nevoid basal cell epithelioma, jaw cysts, and bifid ribs: a syndrome. *N Engl J Med*. 1960;262:908.

Gorlin RJ, et al. *Syndromes of the Head and Neck*. New York, NY: Oxford University Press; 1990:740-742.

Gorney M. Sucking fat: an 18-year statistical and personal retrospective. *Plast Reconstr Surg*. 2001;107:608-613.

Gosain AK, et al. A prospective study of the relationship between strabismus and head posture in patients with frontal plagiocephaly. *Plast Reconstr Surg*. 1996;97:881-891.

Gosain AK, et al. Biomechanical evaluation of titanium, biodegradable plate and screw, and cyanoacrylate glue fixation systems in craniofacial surgery. *Plast Reconstr Surg*. 1998;101:582-591.

Gosain AK, et al. Embryology of the head and neck. In: Aston SJ, Beasley RW, Thorne CH, eds. *Grabb & Smith's Plastic Surgery*. 5th ed. Philadelphia, Pa: Lippincott-Raven; 1997:223-236.

Gosain AK, et al. Giant congenital nevi: a 20-year experience and an algorithm for their management. *Plast Reconstr Surg*. 2001;108:622-631.

Gosain AK, et al. Midface distraction following Le Fort III and monobloc osteotomies: problems and solutions. *Plast Reconstr Surg*. 2002;109:1797-1808.

Gosain AK, et al. Use of tissue glue: current status. *Perspectives in Plastic Surgery*. 2001;15:129-145.

Gosain AK. Distraction osteogenesis of the craniofacial skeleton. *Plast Reconstr Surg*. 2001;107:278-280.

Gottlieb LJ, et al. Pediatric burn reconstruction. In: Bentz ML, ed. *Pediatric Plastic Surgery*. Stamford, Ct: Appleton & Lange; 1998;619-633.

Gould J. Arthroplasty of the metacarpophalangeal and interphalangeal joints of the digits and thumb. In: Peimer CA, ed. *Surgery of the Hand and Upper Extremity*. New York, NY: McGraw-Hill, Inc; 1996;2:1677-1689.

Graham GF. Cryosurgery. *Clin Plast Surg*. 1993;20:131-147.

Granick MS, et al. Salivary gland tumors. In: Aston SJ, Beasley RW, Thorne CH, eds. *Grabb & Smith's Plastic Surgery*. 5th ed. Philadelphia, Pa: Lippincott-Raven; 1997:453-457.

Gray H. *Gray's Anatomy*. 37th ed. Edinburgh, Scotland: Churchill Livingstone, Inc; 1989.

Gray H. The respiratory system. In: Goss CM, ed. *Anatomy of the Human Body*. Philadelphia, Pa: Lea & Febinger; 1973:1111-1140.

Grayson BH. Cephalometric analysis for the surgeon. *Clin Plast Surg*. 1989;16:633-644.

Grazer FM, et al. Fatal outcomes from liposuction: census survey of cosmetic surgeons. *Plast Reconstr Surg*. 2000;105:436.

Grazer FM, et al. Suction-assisted lipectomy. In: Achauer BM, Eriksson E, Guyuron B, et al, eds. *Plastic Surgery Indications, Operations, and Outcomes*. Saint Louis, Mo: Mosby - Year Book Inc; 2000:2859-2887.

Grazer FM. Abdominoplasty. In: McCarthy JG, ed. *Plastic Surgery*. Philadelphia, Pa: WB Saunders Co; 1990;6:3929-3963.

Grazer FM. Body contouring. In: McCarthy JG, ed. *Plastic Surgery*. Philadelphia, Pa: WB Saunders Co; 1990;6:3964.

Green DP. Radial nerve palsy. In: Green DP, Hotchkiss RN, Pederson WC, eds. *Operative Hand Surgery*. 4th ed. New York, NY: Churchill Livingstone, Inc; 1999;2:1481-1496.

Green H. Cultured cells for the treatment of disease. *Sci Am*. 265:96-102.

Green HA, et al. Aging, sun damage, and sunscreens. *Clin Plast Surg*. 1993;20:1-8.

Green RK, et al. A full nasal skin rotation flap for closure of soft-tissue defects in the lower one-third of the nose. *Plast Reconstr Surg*. 1996;98:163.

Greenbaum SS. Chemical peeling, injectable collagen implants and dermabrasion. In: Aston SJ, Beasley RW, Thorne CH, eds. *Grabb & Smith's Plastic Surgery*. 5th ed. Philadelphia, Pa: Lippincott-Raven; 1997:597-608.

Greenberg MF, et al. Ocular plagiocephaly: ocular torticollis with skull and facial asymmetry. *Ophtalmology*. 2000;107:173-178.

Greene RM, et al. Craniofacial embryology. In: Cohen M, ed. *Mastery of Plastic and Reconstructive Surgery*. Boston, Mass: Little, Brown & Co; 1994:459-470.

Greenwald D, et al. An algorithm for early aggressive treatment of frostbite with limb salvage directed by triple-phase scanning. *Plast Reconstr Surg*. 1998;102:10669-1074.

Greenwald DP, et al. Mechanical analysis of explanted silicone breast implants. *Plast Reconstr Surg*. 1996;98:269.

Gregory RO. Overview of lasers in plastic surgery. *Clin Plast Surg*. 2000;27:167.

Greider JL. Trigger thumb and finger release. In: Blair WF, ed. *Techniques in Hand Surgery*. Baltimore, Md: Williams & Wilkins; 1996;567-573.

Greinwald JH Jr, et al. An update on the treatment of hemangiomas in children with interferon alfa-2a. *Arch Otolaryngol Head Neck Surg*. 1999;125:21-27.

Greuse M, et al. Breast sensitivity after vertical mammaplasty. *Plast Reconstr Surg*. 2001;107:970-976.

Grodstein F, et al. A prospective study of incident squamous cell carcinoma of the skin in the nurses' health study. *J Natl Cancer Inst*. 1995;87:1061.

Grolleau JL, et al. Brest base anomalies: treatment strategy for tuberous breasts, minor deformities, and asymmetry. *Plast Reconstr Surg*. 1999;104:2040-2048.

Gross BG. Cardiac arrhythmias during phenol face peeling. *Plast Reconstr Surg*. 1984;73:590.

Gross MP, et al. The use of leeches for treatment of venous congestion of the nipple following breast surgery. *Aesthet Plast Surg*. 1992;16:343.

Grossman KI. Facial scars. *Clin Plast Surg*. 1000;27:627-642.

Grossman MC, et al. Cutaneous laser surgery. In: Aston SJ, Beasley RW, Thorne CH, eds. *Grabb & Smith's Plastic Surgery*. 5th ed. Philadelphia, Pa: Lippincott-Raven; 1997:205-219.

Grossman MD, et al. Ophthalmic aspects of orbital injury: a comprehensive diagnostic and management approach. *Clin Plast Surg*. 1992;19:71.

Gruss J, et al. Acute facial fractures and secondary facial deformity. In: Bell W, ed. *Modern Practice in Orthognathic and Reconstructive Surgery*. Philadelphia, Pa: WB Saunders Co; 1992:1012-1055.

Gruss JS, et al. The pattern and incidence of nasolacrimal injury in naso-orbital-ethmoid fractures: the role of delayed assessment and dacryocystorhinostomy. *Br J Plast Surg*. 1985;38:116-121.

Guerra JJ, et al. Equipment malfunction in common hand surgical procedures: complications associated with the pneumatic tourniquet and with the application of casts and splints. *Hand Clin*. 1994;10:45-52.

Guides to the Evaluation of Permanent Impairment. 4th ed. Chicago, Ill: American Medical Association; 1995:18-20.

Gundlach K. Fractures of the mandible. In: Cohen M, ed. *Mastery of Plastic and Reconstructive Surgery*. Boston, Mass: Little, Brown & Co; 1994;2:1165-1180.

Gunter JP, et al. Aesthetic analysis of the eyebrows. *Plast Reconstr Surg*. 1997;99:1808.

Gunter JP, et al. Correction of the pinched nasal tip with alar spreader grafts. *Plast Reconstr Surg*. 1992;90:821.

Gunter JP, et al. Lateral crural strut graft: technique and clinical applications in rhinoplasty. *Plast Reconstr Surg*. 1997;99:943-952.

Gunter JP, et al. Management of the deviated nose: the importance of septal reconstruction. *Clin Plast Surg*. 1988;15:43.

Gunter JP, et al. The classification and correction of alar-columellar discrepancies. *Plast Reconstr Surg*. 1996;97:643.

Guyuron B, et al. Ear projection and the posterior auricular muscle insertion. *Plast Reconstr Surg*. 1997;100:457-460.

Guyuron B, et al. Forehead rejuvenation. In: Achauer BM, Eriksson E, Guyuron B, et al, eds. *Plastic Surgery: Indications, Operations, and Outcomes*. Saint Louis, Mo: Mosby - Year Book, Inc; 2000:2563-2582.

Guyuron B, et al. Problems following genioplasty: diagnosis and treatment. *Clin Plast Surg*. 1997;24:507-514.

Guyuron B. Blepharoplasty and ancillary procedures. In: Achauer BM, Eriksson E, Guyuron B, et al, eds. *Plastic Surgery: Indications, Operations, and Outcomes*. Saint Louis, Mo: Mosby - Year Book, Inc; 2000:2539-2543.

Guyuron B. Combined maxillary and mandibular osteotomies. *Clin Plast Surg*. 1989;16:795-802.

Guyuron B. Genioplasty. In: Ferraro JW, ed. *Fundamentals of Maxillofacial Surgery*. New York, NY: Springer-Verlag; 1997:250-269.

Guyuron B. Nasal osteotomy and airway changes. *Plast Reconstr Surg*. 1998;102:856-863.

Guyuron B. Secondary rhytidectomy. *Plast Reconstr Surg.* 1997;100:1281-1284.

Haagensen CD. *Disease of the Breast.* Philadelphia, Pa: WB Saunders Co; 1971:1-28.

Habal M, et al. *Bone Grafts and Bone Substitutes.* Philadelphia, Pa: WB Saunders Co; 1992.

Hachulla E, et al. Digital arteritis, thrombosis and hypereosinophilic syndrome: an uncommon complication. *Rev Med Interne.* 1995;16:434-436.

Hackler RH, et al. Urethral complications following ischiectomy in spinal cord patients: a urethral pressure study. *J Urol.* 1987;137:253-255.

Hagan KF, et al. Trapezius muscle and musculocutaneous flaps. In: Strauch B, Vasconez LO, Hall-Findlay EJ, eds. *Grabb's Encyclopedia of Flaps.* 2nd ed. Philadelphia, Pa: Lippincott-Raven;1998:496-511.

Haimovici H, et al. Congenital microarteriovenous shunts: angiographic and Doppler ultrasonographic identification. *Arch Surg.* 1986;121:1065-1070.

Hall CD, et al. The initial management of patients with facial trauma. In: Cohen M, ed. *Mastery of Plastic and Reconstructive Surgery.* Boston, Mass: Little, Brown & co; 1994:1060-1068.

Hamdi M, et al. Breast sensation after superior pedicle versus inferior pedicle mammaplasty: anatomical and histological evaluation. *Br J Plast Surg.* 2001;54:43-46.

Hamilton JB. Male hormone stimulation is a prerequisite and an incitant in common baldness. *Am J Anat.* 1942;71:451.

Hamra ST. Correcting the unfavorable outcomes following face lift surgery. *Clin Plast Surg.* 2001;28:621-638.

Handel N, et al. Factors affecting mammographic visualization of the breast after augmentation mammaplasty. *JAMA.* 1993;269:987-988.

Hanke CW, et al. Risk assessment of polymyositis/dermatomyositis after treatment with injectable bovine collagen implants. *J Am Acad Dermatol.* 1996;34:450-454.

Hanke WC, et al. Merkel cell carcinoma. *Arch Dermatol.* 1989;125:1096-1100.

Hanna EY, et al. Neoplasms of the salivary glands. In: Cummings CW, Fredrickson JM, Harker LA, et al, eds. *Otolaryngology Head & Neck Surgery.* 3rd ed. Saint Louis, Mo: Mosby - Year Book, Inc; 1998;3:1255-1302.

Hansbrough JF, et al. Skin replacements. *Clin Plast Surg.* 1998;25:407-423.

Hardesty RA, et al. Craniofacial onlay bone grafting: a prospective evaluation of graft morphology, orientation, and embryonic origin. *Plast Reconstr Surg.* 1990;85:5.

Harmon CB. Dermabrasion. *Dermatol Clin.* 2001;19:439-442.

Harris AO, et al. Nonepidermal and appendageal skin tumors. *Clin Plast Surg.* 1993;20:115-130.

Harris L, et al. Is breast feeding possible after reduction mammaplasty? *Plast Reconstr Surg.* 1992;89:836-839.

Harrison BJ. Recurrence after surgical treatment of hidradenitis suppurativa. *Br Med J.* 1987;294:487.

Hasegawa M. The distally based superficial sural artery flap. *Plast Reconstr Surg.* 1994;93:1012-1014.

Haskell R. Applied Surgical Anatomy. In: Williams JL, ed. *Rowe and Williams' Maxillofacial Injuries.* 2nd ed. Edinburgh, Scotland: Churchill Livingstone, Inc; 1994;1:1-14.

Haug RH, et al. Management of maxillary fractures. In: Peterson LJ, ed. *Oral and Maxillofacial Surgery.* Philadelphia, Pa: JB Lippincott Co; 469-489.

Haugh M, et al. Terbinafine in fungal infections of the nails: a meta-analysis of randomized clinical trials. *Br J Dermatol.* 2002;147:118-121.

Haywood, et al. Treament of traumatic tattoos with the Nd:YAG laser: a series of nine cases. *Br J Plast Surg*. 199;52:97-98.

Heaton KM, et al. Surgical management and prognostic factors in patients with subungual melanoma. *Ann Surg*. 1994;219:197-204.

Hebert TJ. Open volar repair of acute scaphoid fractures. *Hand Clin*. 2001;17:589-599.

Heggers JP, et al. Cold induced injury: frostbite. In: Herndon DN, ed. *Total Burn Care*. Philadelphia, Pa: WB Saunders Co; 1996:408-414.

Heithoff SJ, et al. Median epicondylectomy for treatment of ulnar nerve compression in the elbow. *J Hand surg*. 1990;15A:22-29.

Helliwell TR, et al. Pathology of the head and neck. In: Jones AS, Phillips DE, Hilgers FJ, eds. *Diseases of the Head and Neck, Nose and Throat*. London: Arnold; 1998:24-42.

Helm KF, et al. Juvenile melanoma (Spitz nevus). *Cutis*. 1996;58:35-39.

Hensel JM, et al. An outcomes analysis and satisfaction survey of 199 consecutive abdominoplasties. *Ann Plast Surg*. 2001;46:357-363.

Hentz VR, et al. The nerve gap dilemma: a comparison of nerves repaired end to end under tension with nerve grafts in a primate model. *J Hand Surg*. 1993;18A:417-425.

Herford AS, et al. Reconstruction of superficial skin cancer defects of the nose. *J Oral Maxillofac Surg*. 2001;59:760-767.

Hester TR Jr, et al. Poland's syndrome: correction with latissimus muscle transposition. *Plast Reconstr Surg*. 1982;69:226-233.

Hewitt RG. Manifestations of human immunodeficiency virus infection in the upper extremity. In: Peimer CA, ed. *Surgery of the Hand and Upper Extremity*. New York, NY: McGraw-Hill, Inc; 1996;2:1787-1796.

Hidalgo DA, et al. Current trends in breast reduction. *Plast Reconstr Surg*. 1999;104:806.

Higgins JP, et al. Ischial pressure sore reconstruction using an inferior gluteal artery perforator (IGAP) flap. *Br J Plast Surg*. 2002;55:83.

Hilburn J. General principles and use of electrodiagnostic studies in carpal and cubital tunnel syndromes. *Hand Clin*. 1996;12:205-221.

Hinder F, et al. Pathophysiology of the systemic inflammatory response syndrome. In: Herndon DN, ed. *Total Burn Care*. Philadelphia, Pa: WB Saunders Co; 1996:207-216.

Hirshowitz B, et al. Static-electric field induction by a silicone cushion for the treatment of hypertrophic scars. *Plast Reconstr Surg*. 1998;101:1173-1183.

Hobar PC, et al. Cleft palate repair and velopharyngeal insufficiency. In: Aston SJ, Beasley RW, Thorne CH, eds. *Grabb & Smith's Plastic Surgery*. 5th ed. Philadelphia, Pa: Lippincott-Raven; 1997:263.

Hochman M. Reconstruction of midfacial and anterior skull base defects. *Otolaryngol Clin North Am*. 1955;28:1269-1277.

Hoffer MM. Cerebral palsy. In: Green DP, ed. *Operative Hand Surgery*. 3rd ed. New York, NY: Churchill Livingstone, Inc; 1982:215-223.

Hojer J, et al. Topical treatments for hydrofluoric acid burns: a blind controlled experimental study. *J Toxicol Clin Toxicol*. 2002;40:861-866.

Hold JE, et al. Reconstruction of the lacrimal drainage system. *Arch Otolaryngol*. 1984;110:211-220.

Holder LE, et al. Nuclear medicine, contrast angiography, and magnetic resonance imaging for evaluating vascular problems in the hand. *Hand Clin*. 1993;9:85-113.

Hollander JE, et al. Risk factors for infection in patients with traumatic lacerations. *Acad Emerg Med*. 2001;8:716-720.

Hollinshead WH, ed. *Anatomy for Surgeons*. Philadelphia, Pa: Harper & Row; 1982:93-155, 285, 307.

Hollinshead WH, et al. Head and neck anatomy. In: *Textbook of Anatomy*. 4th ed. Philadelphia, Pa: Harper & Row, Inc; 1985;895-899.

Holmes RE. Alloplastic implants. In: McCarthy JG, ed. *Plastic Surgery*. Philadelphia, Pa: WB Saunders Co; 1990;1:698-731.

Holmes RE. Alloplastic materials. In: McCarthy JG, ed. *Plastic Surgery*. Philadelphia, Pa: WB Saunders Co; 1990;1:698.

Honig SF. Incidence, trends, and the epidemiology of breast cancer. In: Spear SL, ed. *Surgery of the Breast: Principles and Art*. Philadelphia, Pa: Lippincott-Raven; 1998:3-21.

Hopkins R. Mandibular fractures: treatment by closed reduction and indirect skeletal fixation. In: Williams JL, ed. *Rowe and Williams' Maxillofacial Injuries*. 2nd ed. Edinburgh, Scotland: Churchill Livingstone, Inc; 1994;1:283-285.

Horn MA, et al. Modified autogenous latissimus breast reconstruction and the box top nipple. *Plast Reconstr Surg*. 2000;106:763.

Horton CE, et al. Treatment of a lacrimal bulge in blepharoplasty by repositioning the gland. *Plast Reconstr Surg*. 1978;61:701.

Hotchkiss RN. Elbow contracture. In: Green DP, et al, ed. *Operative Hand Surgery*. New York, NY: Churchill Livingstone, Inc; 1999;1:668-669, 679-681.

House F. Disorders of the thumb in cerebral palsy, stroke, and tetraplegia. In: Strickland JW, ed. *The Thumb*. New York, NY: Churchill Livingstone, Inc; 1994.

Howard BK, et al. The effects of ultrasonic energy on peripheral nerves: implications for ultrasound-assisted liposuction. *Plast Reconstr Surg*. 1999;103:984-989.

Howard BK, et al. Understanding the nasal airway: principles and practice. *Plast Reconstr Surg*. 2002;109:1128-1146.

Howard PS, et al. Endoscopic transaxillary submuscular augmentation mammaplasty with textured saline breast implants. *Ann Plast Surg*. 1996; 37:12-17.

Howard PS. The role of endoscopy and implant texture in transaxillary submuscular breast augmentation. *Ann Plast Surg*. 1999;42:245-248.

Hoyen HA, et al. Atypical hand infections. *Hand Clin*. 1998;14:613-634.

Huang AB, et al. Osteomyelitis of the pelvis/hips in paralyzed patients: accuracy and clinical utility of MRI. *J Comput Assist Tomog*. 1998;22:437.

Huang MH, et al. The differential diagnosis of posterior plagiocephaly: true lamboid synostosis versus potential molding. *Plast Reconstr Surg*. 1996;98:765.

Hudson DA. Some thoughts on choosing a Z-plasty: the Z made simple. *Plast Reconstr Surg*. 2000;106:665-671.

Huger WE Jr. The anatomic rationale for abdominal lipectomy. *Am Surgeon*. 1979;45:612-617.

Human rabies - Virginia, 1998. *MMWE Morb Mortal Wkly Rep*. 1999;48:95-97.

Hurst L, et al. Dupuytren's disease. In: Peimer CA, ed. *Surgery of the Hand and Upper Extremity*. New York, NY: McGraw-Hill, Inc; 1996;2:1601-1615.

Hurst LC, et al. Nonoperative treatment of Dupuytren's disease. *Hand Clin*. 1999;15:97-107.

Hurwitz S, ed. *Clinical Pediatric Dermatology: A Textbook of Skin Disorders of Childhood and Adolescence*. Philadelphia, Pa: WB Saunders Co; 1993:208-290.

Hyakusoku H, et al. Heel coverage with a T-shaped distally based sural island fasciocutaneous flap. *Plast Reconstr Surg*. 1994;93:872.

Hynes D, et al. Compression neuropathies: radial. In: Peimer CA, ed. *Surgery of the Hand and Upper Extremity.* New York, NY: McGraw-Hill, Inc; 1996;2:1291-1305.

Hynes DE. Neurovascular pedicle and advancement flaps for palmar thumb defects. *Hand Clin.* 1997;13:207-216.

Hynes W. Pharyngoplasty by muscle transplantation. *Br J Plast Surg.* 1950;3:128.

Idler RS, et al. Complications of replantation surgery. *Hand Clin.* 1992;8:427-451.

Ilizarov GA. The tension-stress effect on the genesis and growth of tissues: part I: the influence of stability of fixation and soft-tissue preservation. *Clin Orthop.* 1989;238:249-281.

Imbriglia JE, et al. Radial nerve reconstruction. In: Peimer CA, ed. *Surgery of the Hand and Upper Extremity.* New York, NY: McGraw-Hill, Inc; 1996;2:1361-1397.

Imbriglia JE. Four-corner arthrodesis. In: Blair WF, ed. *Techniques in Hand Surgery.* Baltimore, Md; Williams & Wilkins; 1996:865-871.

Incaudo G, et al. Administration of local anesthetics to patients with a history of prior adverse reaction. *J Allergy Clin Immunol.* 1978;61:339.

Inigo F, et al. Recovery of facial palsy after crossed facial nerve grafts. *Br J Plast Surg.* 1994;47:312.

Itoh Y, et al. The deep inferior epigastric artery free skin flap: anatomic study and clinical application. *Plast Reconstr Surg.* 1993;91:853-856.

Jackson DM. The diagnosis of the depth of burning. *Br J Surg.* 1953;40:588.

Jackson GL, et al. Role of parotidectomy for skin cancer of the head and neck. *Am J Surg.* 1981;142:464-469.

Jackson IT, et al. Hemangiomas, vascular malformations, and lymphovenous malformations: classification and methods of treatment. *Plast Reconstr Surg.* 1993;91:1216.

Jackson IT, et al. Orthognathic surgery. In: *Atlas of Craniomaxillofacial Surgery.* Saint Louis, Mo: CV Mosby Co; 1982:83.

Jackson IT, et al. Tumors of the craniofacial skeleton, including the jaws. In: McCarthy JG, ed. *Plastic Surgery.* Philadelphia, Pa: WB Saunders Co; 1990;5:3336-3411.

Jackson IT. Anatomy of the buccal fat pad and its clinical significance. *Plast Reconstr Surg.* 1999;103:2061.

Jackson IT. Intraoral tumors and cervical lymphadenectomy. In: Aston SJ, Beasley RW, Thorne CH, eds. *Grabbe & Smith's Plastic Surgery.* 5th ed. Philadephia, PA: Lippincott-Raven; 1997:439-452.

Jackson IT. Sphincter pharyngoplasty. *Clin Plast Surg.* 1985;12:711.

Jackson LE, et al. Controversies in the management of inferior turbinate hypertrophy: a comprehensive review. *Plast Reconstr Surg.* 1999;103:300-312.

Jackson T. Intraoral tumors and cervical lymphadenectomy. In: Aston SJ, Beasley RW, Thorne CH, eds. *Grabbe & Smith's Plastic Surgery.* 5th ed. Philadephia, PA: Lippincott-Raven; 1997:439-452.

Jacobovicz J, et al. Endoscopic repair of mandibular subcondylar fractures. *Plast Reconstr Surg.* 1998;101:437-441.

Jacobs JS, et al. The application of dental splints in regard to modern techiques of rigid fixation. In: Ferraro JW, ed. *Fundamentals of Maxillofacial Surgery.* New York, NY: Springer-Verlag; 1996:327-333.

Jacobs JS, et al. Traumatic deformities and reconstruction of the temporomandibular joint. In: Ferraro JW, ed. *Fundamentals of Maxillofacial Surgery.* New York, NY: Springer-Verlag; 1996:307-320.

Janfaza P, et al. Oral cavity. In: Janfaza P, Nadol JB, Galla RJ, et al, eds. Surgial Anatomy of the Head and Neck. Philadelphia, Pa: Lippincott Williams & Wilkins; 2001.

Janfaza P, et al. Scalp, cranium and brain. In: Janfaza P, Nadol JB, Galla RJ, et al, eds. *Surgical Anatomy of the Head and Neck*. Philadelphia, Pa: Lippincott Williams & Wilkins; 2001.

Jansen DA, et al. Breast cancer in reduction mammaplasty: case reports and a survey of plastic surgeons. *Plast Reconstr Surg*. 1998;101:361-364.

Jaques B, et al. Treatment of mandibular fractures with rigid osteosynthesis: using the AO system. *J Oral Maxillofac Surg*. 1997;55:1402-1406.

Jebson PJ, et al. Radial tunnel syndrome: long-term results of surgical decompression. *J Hand Surg*. 1997;22A:889-896.

Jebson PJ. Deep subfascial space infections. *Hand Clin*. 1998;14:557-566.

Jebson PJ. Infections of the fingertip. *Hand Clin*. 1998;14:547-555.

Jelks G, et al. Blepharoplasty. In Peck GC, ed. *Complications and Problems in Plastic Sugery*. New York, NY: Gower Medical Publishing; 1992:1-31.

Jelks GW, et al. Preoperative evaluation of the blepharoplasty patient: bypassing the pitfalls. *Clin Plast Surg*. 1993;20:213.

Jelks GW, et al. Reconstruction of the eyelids and associated structures. In: McCarthy JG, ed. *Plastic Surgery*. Philadelphia, Pa: WB Saunders Co; 1990;2:1671-1784.

Jelks GW, et al. The influence of orbital and eyelid anatomy on the palpebral aperture. *Clin Plast Surg*. 356-363.

Jobe R. Gold lid loads in Bell's palsy. *Plast Reconstr Surg*. 1974;53:29.

Johnson IT, et al. Management of complications of head and neck surgery. In: Myers EM, Suen JY, eds. *Cancer of the Head and Neck*. Philadelphia, Pa: WB Saunders Co; 1996;693-711.

Johnson MC, et al. Embryogenesis of cleft lip and palate. In: McCarthy JG, ed. *Plastic Surgery*. Philadelphia, Pa: WB Saunders Co; 1990;4:2525.

Johnson MC. Embryology of the head and neck. In: McCarthy JG, ed. *Plastic Surgery*. Philadelphia, Pa: WB Saunders Co; 1990;4:2451-2495.

Johnson TM, et al. Mohs' surgery for cutaneous basal cell and squamous cell carcinoma. In: Weber RS, Miller MJ, Goepfert H, eds. *Basal and Squamous Cell Cancers of the Head and Neck*. Baltimore, Md: Williams & Wilkins; 1996:147-155.

Johnston MC. Embryology of the head and neck. In: McCarthy JG, ed. *Plastic Surgery*. Philadelphia, Pa: WB Saunders Co; 1990;4:2491.

Jones I, et al. A buide to biological skin substitutes. *Br J Plast Surg*. 2002;55:185-193.

Jones KJ, et al. Thoracic outlet syndrome. In: Green DP, Hotchkiss RN, Pederson WC, eds. *Operative Hand Surgery*. 4th ed. New York, NY: Churchill Livingstone, Inc; 1999;2:1448-1465.

Jones NF, et al. Free skin and composite flaps. In: Green DP, Hotchkiss RN, Pederson WC, eds. *Operative Hand Surgery*. 4th ed. New York, NY: Churchill Livingstone, Inc; 1999;1:1159-1200.

Jones NF. Intraoperative and postoperative monitoring of microsurgical free tissue transfers. *Clin Plast Surg*. 1992;19:783-797.

Jones NF. Ischaemia of the hand. In: Peimer CA, ed. *Surgery of the Hand and Upper Extremity*. New York, NY: McGraw-Hill, Inc; 1996;2:1705.

Jones NF. Ischemia of the hand in systemic disease. *Clin Plast Surg*. 1989;16:547-556.

Jonsson CE, et al. Early excision and skin grafting of selected burns of the face and neck. *Plast Reconstr Surg*. 1991;88:88-92.

Jordan RB, et al. Splints and scar management for acute and reconstructive burn care. *Clin Plast Surg*. 2000;27:71-85.

Juliano PT, et al. Limited open sheath irrigation in the treatment of pyogenic flexor tenosynovitis. *Ortho Res*. 1991;20:1065-1069.

Kaban LB, Pogrel MA, Perrot DH, eds. *Complications in Oral and Maxillofacial Surgery*. Philadelphia, Pa: WB Saunders Col 1997:209.

Kahout MP, et al. Arteriovenous malformations of the head and neck: natural history and management. *Plast Reconstr Surg*. 1998;102:643-654.

Kane WJ, et al. The uremic gangrene syndrome: improved wound healing in spontaneously forming wounds following subtotal parathyroidectomy. *Plast Reconstr Surg*. 1996;98:671-678.

Kao CC, et al. Acute burns. *Plast Reconstr Surg*. 2000;105:2482-2492.

Karabulut AB, et al. Forehead lift: a combined approach using subperiosteal and subgaleal dissection planes. *Aesthetic Plast Surg*. 2001;25:378-381.

Karmo FR, et al. Blood loss in major liposuction procedures: a comparison study using suction-assisted versus ultrasonically assisted lipoplasty. *Plast Reconstr Surg*. 2001;108:241-247.

Karmo, et al. Blood loss in major liposuction procedures: a comparison study using suction-assisted versus ultrasonically assisted lipoplasty. *Plast Reconstr Surg*. 2001;108:241-247.

Karp NS, et al. Membranous bone lengthening: a serial histological study. *Ann Plast Surg*. 1992;29:2-7.

Kasabian AK, et al. Salvage of traumatic below-knee amputation stumps utilizing the filet of foot free flap: critical evaluation of six cases. *Plast Reconstr Surg*. 1995;96:1145-1153.

Kasabian AK, et al. Use of a multiplanar distracter for the correction of a proximal interphalangeal joint contracture. *Ann Plast Surg*. 1998;40:378-381.

Kasdan ML, et al. Outcomes of surgically treated mucous cysts of the hand. *J Hand Surg*. 1994;19A:504-507.

Kato T, et al. Epidemiology and prognosis of subungual melanoma in 34 Japanese patients. *Br J Dermatol*. 1996;134:383-387.

Katsaros J. Indications for free soft-tissue flap transfer to the upper limb and the role of alternative procedures. *Hand Clin*. 1992;8:479-507.

Kawamoto HK Jr, et al. Atypical facial clefts. In: Bentz ML, ed. *Pediatric Plastic Surgery*. Stamford, Conn: Appleton & Lange; 1998;175-225.

Kawamoto HK Jr. Craniofacial clefts. In: Aston SJ, Beasley RW, Thorne CH, eds. *Grabbe & Smith's Plastic Surgery*. 5th ed. Philadephia, PA: Lippincott-Raven; 1997:349-63.

Kawamoto HK Jr. Rare craniofacial clefts. In: McCarthy JG, ed. *Plastic Surgery*. Philadelphia, Pa: WB Saunders Co; 1990;4:2945-2951.

Kay SP, et al. Toe to hand transfers in children, part I: technical aspects. *J Hand Surg*. 1996;21B:723-734.

Kay SP, et al. Toe to hand transfers in children, part II: functional and psychological aspects. *J Hand Surg*. 1996;21B:735-745.

Kay SP. Cleft Hand. In: Green DP, Hotchkiss RN, Pederson WC, eds. *Operative Hand Surgery*. 4th ed. New York, NY: Churchill Livingstone, Inc; 1999;1:402-413.

Keeling CA. Range of motion measurement in the hand. In: Hunter JM, Mackin EJ, Callahan AD, eds. *Rehabilitation of the Hand: Surgery and Therapy*. Saint Louis, Mo: Mosby - Year Book, Inc; 1995;1:93-107.

Keleher AJ, et al. Breast cancer in reduction mammaplasty specimens: case reports and guidelines. *Breast J*. 2003;9:120-125.

Kelly KJ. Pediatric facial trauma. In: Vander Kolk CA, ed. *Plastic Surgery: Indications, Operations, and Outcomes*. Saint Louis, Mo: Mosby - Year Book, Inc; 2000;2:941-969.

Kemp ED. Bites and stings of the arthropod kind: treating reactions that can range from annoying to menacing. *Postgrad Med.* 1998;103:88-90.

Kenny P. The management of platysmal bands. *Plast Reconstr Surg.* 1996;98:99.

Kessler I. Centralization of the radial club hand by gradual distraction. *J Hand Surg.* 1989;14B:37-42.

Kiefhaber TR. Phalangeal dislocations/periarticular trauma. In: Peimer CA, ed. *Surgery of the Hand and Upper Extremity.* New York, NY: McGraw-Hill, Inc; 1996;1:939-972.

Kikkawa DO, et al. Orbital and eyelid anatomy. In: Dortzbach RK, ed. *Ophthalmic Plastic Surgery: Prevention and Management of Complications.* New York, NY: Raven Press; 1994:1-29.

Kilmer SL, et al. The Q-switched Nd:YAG laser effectively treats tattoos: a controlled, dose-response study. *Arch Dermatol.* 1993;129:971.A607Kim CK, et al. Regrowth of grafter human scalp hair after removal of the bulb. *Dermatol Surg.* 1995;21:312-313.

King GM. Microvascular ear transplantation. *Clin Plast Surg.* 2002;29:233-248.

Kitay GS, et al. Compression neuropathies. In: Peimer CA, ed. *Surgery of the Hand and Upper Extremity.* New York, NY: McGraw-Hill, Inc; 1996;2:1339-1362.

Klatsky SA. Blepharoplasty. In: Cohen M, ed. *Mastery of Plastic Surgery.* Boston, Mass: Little, Brown & Co; 1994;2:1920-1940.

Klein AW. Skin filling: collagen and other injectables of the skin. *Dermatol Clin.* 2001;19:491-508.

Klein JA. Tumescent technique for local anesthesia improves safely in large-volume liposuction. *Plast Reconstr Surg.* 1993;92:1085-1100.

Klein JA. Tumescent technique for regional anesthesia permits lidocaine doses of 35 mg/kg for liposuction. *J Dermatol Surg Oncol.* 1990;16:248-263.

Klein L, et al. H-collagen turnover in skin grafts. *Surg Gyn Obstet.* 1972;135:49-57.

Kleinman WB, et al. Thumb reconstruction. In: Green DP, Hotchkiss RN, Pederson WC, eds. *Operative Hand Surgery.* 4th ed. New York, NY: Churchill Livingstone, Inc; 1999;2:2068-2170.

Kligman AM, et al. Topical tretinoin for photoaged skin. *J Am Acad Dermatol.* 1986;15:836.

Klimo GF, et al. The treatment of trapeziometacarpal arthritis with arthrodesis. *Hand Clin.* 2001;17:261-270.

Kline DG, et al. *Atlas of Peripheral Nerve Surgery.* Philadelphia, Pa: WB Saunders Co; 2001:135-144, 145-150.

Kline DG. Timing for exploration of nerve lesions and evaluation of neuroma-in-continuity. *Clin Ortho.* 1982;163:42.

Klinert HE, et al. Etiology and treatment of the so-called mucous cyst of the finger. *J Bone Joint Surg.* 1992;54A:1955-1958.

Klinert HE, et al. Radial nerve entrapment. *Orthop Clin North Am.* 1996;27:305-315.

Klingman AM, et al. Topical tretinoin for photoaged skin. *J Am Acad Dermatol.* 1986;15:836.

Knize DM. A study of the supraorbital nerve. *Plast Reconstr Surg.* 1995;96:564-569.

Knize DM. An anatomically based study of eyebrow ptosis. *Plast Reconstr Surg.* 1996;97:1321.

Knize DM. Limited incisions of mental lipectomy and platysma plasty. *Plast Reconstr Surg.* 1998;101:473.

Knize DM. Limited-incision forehead lift for eyebrow elevation to enhance upper blepharoplasty. *Plast Reconstr Surg.* 1994;93:1392.

Knize DM. Reassessment of the coronal incision and subgaleal dissection for foreheadplasty. *Plast Reconstr Surg.* 1996;97:1334-1342.

Kobayashi S, et al. Correction of the hypoplastic nasal ala using an auricular composite graft. *Ann Plast Surg*. 1996;37:490-494.

Kobayashi S, et al. Recent advance in vasculitis syndrome. *Nippon Rinsho*. 1999;57:388-392.

Kobayashi, et al. Lymphedema. *Clin Plast Surg*. 1987;14:303-313.

Koh WL. When to worry about spider bites: inaccurate diagnosis can have serious, even fatal, consequences. *Postgrad Med*. 1998;102:235-236, 243-244, 249-250.

Kohout MP, et al. Arteriovenous malformations of the head and neck: natural history and management. *Plast Reconstr Surg*. 1998;102:643.

Koman LA, et al. Cerebral palsy: management of the upper extremity. *Clin Ortho*. 1990;253:62-74.

Koman LA, et al. RSD after wrist injury. In: Levin LS, ed. *Problems in Plastic and Reconstructive Surgery: the Wrist*. Philadelphia, Pa: JB Lippincott; 1992:300-321.

Koman LA, et al. Vascular disorders. In: Green DP, Hotchkiss RN, Pederson WC, eds. *Operative Hand Surgery*. 4th ed. New York, NY: Churchill Livingstone, Inc; 1999;2:2254-2302.

Koman LA, et al. Venous grafts for ulnar artery thrombosis. In: Blair WF, ed. *Techniques in Hand Surgery*. Baltimore, Md: Wiliams & Wilkins; 1996:1155-1163.

Koshima I, et al. The free or pedicled saphenous flap. *Ann Plast Surg*. 1988;21:369.

Kottke-Marchant K, et al. Effect of albumin coating on the in vitro blood compatibility of Dacron arterial prostheses. *Biomaterials*. 1989;10:147-155.

Koury ME, et al. The use of rigid internal fixation in mandibular gractures complicated by osteomyelitis. *J Oral Maxillofac Surg*. 1994;52:1114-1119.

Koury ME. Complications of mandibular fractures. In: Kaban LB, Pogrel MA, Perrott DH, eds. *Complications in Oral and Maxillofacial Surgery*. Philadelphia, Pa: WB Saunders Co; 1997:121-145.

Kramer GC, et al. Pathophysiology of burn shock and burn edema. In: Herndon DN, ed. *Total Burn Care*. 2nd ed. Philadelphia, Pa: WB Saunders Co; 2002:79-85.

Kroll SS, et al. Postoperative morphine requirements of free TRAM and DIEP flaps. *Plast Reconstr Surg*. 2001;107:338.

Krueger JK, et al. Clearing the smoke: the scientific rationale for tobacco abstention with plastic surgery. *Plast Reconstr Surg*. 2001;108:1063-1073.

Kulwin DR, et al. Blepharoplasty and brow elevation. In: Dortzbach RK, ed. *Ophthalmic Plastic Surgery: Prevention and Management of Complications*. New York, NY: Raven Press;1994:91-112.

Kumagai N, et al. Clinical application of autologous cultured epithelia for the treatment of burn wounds and burn scars. *Plast Reconstr Surg*. 1988;82:99-110.

Kumar S, et al. Cutis laxa. *J Dermatol*. 1996;23:721.

Kurihara K. Congenital deformities of the external ear. In: Cohen M, ed. *Mastery of Plastic and Reconstructive Surgery*. Boston, Mass: Little, Brown & Co; 1994;1:776-779.

Kurokawa M, et al. The use of microsurgical planing to treat traumatic tattoos. *Plast Reconstr Surg*. 1994;94:1069.

Laclerca C, et al. Hand and wrist injuries in young athletes. *Hand Clin*. 2000;16:525-527.

Ladin DA. Understanding dressings. *Clin Plast Surg*. 1998;25:433-441.

Lambert PR, et al. Anatomy and embryology of the auditory and vestibular systems. In: Canalis RF, Lambert PR, eds. *The Ear: Comprehensive Otology*. Philadelphia, Pa: Lipincott Williams & Wilkins; 2000:17-53.

Landau M, et al. Cutaneous manifestations of systemic diseases. In: Parish LC, Brenner S, Ramos-e-Silva M, eds. *Women's Dermatology- From Infancy to Maturity*. Pearl River, NY: The Parthenon Publishing Group; 2001:243-250.

Langstein HN, et al. Coverage of skull base defects. *Clin Plast Surg*. 2001;28:375.

Larsen DL. Management of the recurrent, benign tumor of the parotid gland. *Plast Reconstr Surg*. 2001;108:734.

Larson PE. Traumatic injuries of the condyle. In: Peterson LJ, ed. *Oral and Maxillofacial Surgery*. Philadelphia, Pa: JB Lippincott Co; 1992;1:435-469.

Laskawi R, et al. Frey's syndrome. Treatment with botulinum toxin. *Curr Probl Dermatol*. 2002;30:170-177.

Lassus C. A 30-year experience with vertical mammaplasty. *Plast Reconstr Surg*. 1996;97:373Lawrence WT. Physiology of the acute wound. *Clin Plast Surg*. 1998;25:321-340.

Lazova R, et al. Under the microscope: surgeons, pathologists, and melanocytic nevi. *Clin Plast Surg*. 2000;27:323-329.

Le TB, et al. Hand and wrist injuries in young athletes. *Hand Clin*. 2000;16:597-607.

Leana-Cox J, et al. Familial DiGeorge/velocardiofacial syndrome with deletions of chromosome 22q11.2: report of five families with review of the literature. *Am J Med Genet*. 1996;65:309-316.

Leber D. Ear reconstruction. In: Georgiade GS, Riefkohl R, Levin LS, eds. *Textbook of Plastic, Maxillofacial and Reconstructive Surgery*. Baltimore, Md: Williams & Wilkins; 1997:497.

Leclercq C, et al. Treatment of fingertip amputations. In: Peimer CA, ed. *Surgery of the Hand and Upper Extremity*. New York, NY: McGraw-Hill, Inc; 1996;1:1069-1100.

Lee C, et al. Endoscopic subcondylar fracture repair: functional, aesthetic, and rediographic outcomes. *Plast Reconstr Surg*. 1998;102:1434-1443.

Lee DH, et al. Sudden unilateral visual loss and brain infarction after autologous fat injection into nasolabial groove. *Br J Ophthalmol*. 1996;80:1026-1027.

Lee KJ. Thyroid and parathyroid glands. In: *Essential Otolaryngology Head & Neck Surgery*. 7th ed. Stamford, Conn: Appleton & Lange; 1995:574-575.

Lee WP, et al. Transplant biology and applications to plastic surgery. In: Aston SJ, Beasley RW, Thorne CH, eds. *Grabbe & Smith's Plastic Surgery*. 5th ed. Philadephia, PA: Lippincott-Raven; 1997:27-38.

LeFlore I, et al. Keloid formation on palmar surface of hand. *J Natl Med Assoc*. 1991;83:463-464.

Lejour M. Applied anatomy for vertical mammaplasty. In: *Vertical Mammaplasty and Liposuction*. Saint Louis, Mo: Quality Medical Publishing, Inc; 1994:53.

Lejour M. Evaluation of fat in breast tissue removed by vertical mammaplasty. *Plast Reconstr Surg*. 1997;99:386-393.

Lejour M. Vertical mammaplasty. *Plast Reconstr Surg*. 1993;92:985-986.

Le Roy JL Jr, et al. Infections requiring hospital readmission following face lift surgery: incidence, treatment, and sequelae. *Plast Reconstr Surg*. 1994;93:533.

Leslie BM. Rheumatoid extensor tendon ruptures. *Hand Clin*.1989;5:191.

Lettieri S, et al. Craniofacial syndromes. In: Weinzweig J, ed. *Plastic Surgery Secrets*. Philadelphia, Pa: Hanley & Belfus, Inc; 1999:96-99.

Lettieri S. Facial trauma. In: Achauer BM, Eriksson E, Guyuron B, et al, eds. *Plastic Surgery: Indications, Operations, and Outcomes*. Saint Louis, Mo: Mosby - Year Book, Inc; 2000;2:923-940.

Levine VJ, et al. Tattoo removal with the Q-switched Nd:YAG laser: a comparative study. *Cutis*. 1995;55:291.

Levy HJ. Ring finger ray amputation: a 25-year follow-up. *Am J Orthop*. 1999;28:359-360.

Lewis VL Jr. The diagnosis of osteomyelitis in patients with pressure sores. *Plast Reconstr Surg*. 1988;81:229.

Leyden JJ. Treatment of photodamaged skin with topical tretinoin: an update. *Plast Reconstr Surg*. 1998;102:1667-1671.

Lie JT. Histopathologic specificity of systemic vasculitis. *Rheum Dis Clin North Am*. 1995;21:883-909.

Light TR, et al. The longitudinal epiphyseal bracket: implications for surgical correction. *J Pediatr Orthop*. 1981;1:299-305.

Light TR. Congenital anomalies: syndactyly, polydactyly, and cleft hand. In: Peimer CA, ed. *Surgery of the Hand and Upper Extremity*. New York, NY: McGraw-Hill; 1996;2:2111-2144.

Lim B, et al. Digital replantations including fingertip and ring avulsions. *Hand Clin*. 2001;419-431.

Lin HW, et al. The health impact of solar radiation and prevention strategies: report of the Environment Council, American Academy of Dermatology. *J Am Acad Dermatol*. 1999;41:81-99.

Lin TM, et al. Continuous intra-arterial infusion therapy in hydrofluoric acid burns. *J Occup Environ Med*. 2000;42:892-897.

Linares M, et al. Subungual melanoma of the hand: unusual clinical presentation: case report. *Scand J Plast Reconstr Surg Hand Surg*. 1998;32:347-350.

Lineaweaver WC, et al. *Aeromonas hydrophilia* infections following use of medicinal leeches in replantation and flap surgery. *Ann Plast Surg*. 1992;29:238.

Linger TE, et al. Salivary tumors experience 30 years. *Clin Otolaryngol*. 1997;4:247.

Lisman RD, et al. Blepharoplasty: postoperative considerations and complications. In: Rees TD, LaTrenta GS, eds. *Aesthetic Plastic Surgery*. 2nd ed. Philadelphia, Pa: WB Saunders Co; 1994;2:597-599.

Lisman RD, et al. Complication of blepharoplasty. *Clin Plast Surg*. 1988;15:309.

Liss FE, et al. Capsular injuries of the proximal interphalangeal joint. *Hand Clin*. 1992;8:755-768.

Lister G, ed. *The Hand: Diagnosis and Indications*. 3rd ed. Edinburgh, Scotland: Churchill Livingstone, Inc; 1993;459-512.

Lister GD, et al. Skin flaps. In: Green DP, Hotchkiss RN, Pederson WC, eds. *Operative Hand Surgery*. 4th ed. New York, NY: Churchill Livingstone, Inc; 1999;2:1783-1850, 1973-1976.

Lister GD. Skin flaps. In: Green DP, ed. *Operative Hand Surgery*. 3rd ed. New York, NY: Churchill Livingstone, Inc; 1993;2:1741-1822.

Liszka TG, et al. Iliohypogastric nerve entrapment following abdominoplasty. *Plast Reconstr Surg*. 1994;93:181.

Lockwood T. Brachioplasty with superficial fascial skin suspension. *Plast Reconstr Surg*. 1995;96:912-920.

Lockwood T. Contouring of the arms, trunk, and thighs. In: Achauer BM, Eriksson E, Guyuron B, et al, eds. *Plastic Surgery: Indications, Operations, and Outcomes*. Saint Louis, Mo: Mosby - Year Book, Inc; 2000;5:2839-2857.

Lockwood T. Lower body lift with superficial fascial suspension. *Plast Reconstr Surg*. 1993;92:1112-1115.

Lockwood T. Reduction with superficial fascial skin suspension. *Plast Reconstr Surg*. 1999;103:1411-1419.

Lockwood T. Superficial fascial system (SFS) of the trunk and extremities: a new concept. *Plast Reconstr Surg*. 1991;87:1009-1018.

Lockwood T. The role of excisional lifting in body contour surgery. *Clin Plast Surg*. 1996;23:695-712.

Longaker MT, et al. Microvascular free-flap correction of severe hemifacial atrophy. *Plast Reconstr Surg*. 1995;96:800-809.

Lorenz HP, et al. Primary and secondary orbit surgery: the transconjunctival approach. *Plast Reconstr Surg*. 1999;103:1124-1128.

Losken HW, et al. Craniosynostosis. In: Bentz ML, ed. *Pediatric Plastic Surgery*. Stamford, Conn: Appleton & Lange; 1998:129-132.

Louis DS, et al. Amputations. In: Green DP, ed. *Operative Hand Surgery*. 3rd ed. New York, NY: Churchill Livingstone, Inc; 1982;62-72.

Louis DS, et al. Amputations. In: Green DP, Hotchkiss RN, Pederson WC, eds. *Operative Hand Surgery*. 4th ed. New York, NY: Churchill Livingstone, Inc; 1999;1:48-94.

Low DW. Modified chondrocutaneous advancement flap for ear reconstruction. *Plast Reconstr Surg*. 1998;102:174-177.

Lowen RM, et al. *Aeromonas hydrophilia* infection complicating digital replantation and revascularization. *J Hand Surg*. 1989;14A:714-718.

Lubahn JD. Dupuytren's fasciectomy: open palm technique. In: Blair WF, ed. *Techniques in Hand Surgery*. Baltimore, Md: Williams & Wilkins; 1996.

Luce EA. Frontal sinus fractures: guidelines to management. *Plast Reconstr Surg*. 1987;80:500-510.

Lupo G. The history of aesthetic rhinoplasty: special emphasis on the saddle nose. *Aesthetic Plast Surg*. 1997;21:309-327.

Lutz BS, et al. Microsurgical reconstruction of the buccal mucosa. *Clin Plast Surg*. 2001;28:339.

Mackinnon SE, Dellon AL, eds. *Surgery of the Peripheral Nerve*. New York, NY: Thieme Medical Publishers, Inc; 1988:171, 197-216, 226, 289-303.

MacKinnon SE, et al. A technique for the treatment of neuroma-in-continuity. *J Reconstr Microsurg*. 1992;8:379.

Mackinnon SE. Nerve injuries: primary repair and reconstruction. In: Cohen M, ed. *Mastery of Plastic and Reconstructive Surgery*. Boston, Mass: Little, Brown & Co; 1994;3:1598-1624.

MacLennan SE, et al. Free tissue transfer for limb salvage in purpura fulminans. *Plast Reconstr Surg*. 2001;107:1437-1442.

Maddi R, et al. Evaluation of a new cutaneous topical anesthesia preparation. *Reg Anesth*. 1996;15:109-112.

Magee KL, et al. Human papilloma virus associated with keratoacanthoma. *Arch Dermatol*. 1989;125:1587-1589.

Manassa EH, et al. Wound healing problems in smokers and nonsmokers after 132 abdominoplasties. *Plast Reconstr Surg*. 2003;111:2082-2087.

Mancoll JS, et al. Pressure sores. In: Aston SJ, Beasley RW, Thorne CH, eds. *Grabb & Smith's Plastic Surgery*. 5th ed. Philadelphia, Pa: Lippincott-Raven; 1997:1083.

Mannerfelt L, et al. Rupture of the extensor pollicis longus tendon after Colles' fracture and by rheumatoid arthritis. *J Hand Surg*. 1990;15B:49.

Mannick JA, et al. The immunologic response to injury. *J Am Coll Surg*. 2001;193:237-244.

Manson P. Management of midfacial fractures. In: Georgiade GS, Riefkohl R, Levin LS, eds. *Plastic, Maxillofacial and Reconstructive Surgery*. Baltimore, Md: Williams & Wilkins; 1997:351-376.

Manson PN, et al. Management of blow out fractures of the orbital floor. *Surg Ophthalmol*. 1991;35:280-292.

Manson PN, et al. Mechanisms of global support and posttraumatic enophthalmos I: the anatomy of the ligament sling and its relation to intramuscular cone orbital fat. *Plast Reconstr Surg*. 1986;77:193.

Manson PN, et al. Midface fractures: advantages of immediate extended open reduction and bone grafting. *Plast Reconstr Surg*. 1985;76:1.

Manson PN, et al. Studies on enophthalmos II: the measurement of orbital injuries and their treatment by quantitative computed tomography. *Plast Reconstr Surg*. 1986;77:203-214.

Manson PN. Facial fractures. In: Aston SJ, Beasley RW, Thorne CH, eds. *Grabbe & Smith's Plastic Surgery*. 5th ed. Philadephia, PA: Lippincott-Raven; 1997:383-412.

Manson PN. Facial injuries. In: McCarthy JG, ed. *Plastic Surgery*. Philadelphia, Pa: WB Saunders Co; 1990; 2:867-1141.

Manson PN. Reoperative facial fracture repair. In: Grotting JC, ed. *Reoperative Aesthetic and Reconstructive Plastic Surgery*. Saint Louis, Mo: Quality Medical Publishing, Inc; 1995;1:677-759.

Marchac D, et al. Craniosynostosis and craniofacial dysostosis. In: Cohen M, ed. *Mastery of Plastic and Reconstructive Surgery*. Boston, Mass: Little, Brown & Co; 1994;1:499-515.

Marchac D, et al. The axial frontonasal flap revisited. *Plast Reconstr Surg*. 1985;76:686.

Marieb EN, ed. Overview of the digestive system. In: *Human Anatomy and Physiology*. Redwood City, Ca: Benjamin/Cummings Publishing; 1995.

Mark R, et al. Osteosarcoma of the head and neck: the UCLA experience. *Arch Otolaryngol Head Neck Surg*. 1991;117:761-766.

Markiewitz AD, et al. Carpal fractures and dislocations. In: Lichtman DM, Alexander AH, eds. *The Wrist and Its Disorders*. Philadelphia, Pa: WB Saunders Co; 1997:206-211.

Markley JM Jr, et al. The composite neurovascular skin island graft in surgery of the hand. *Atlas Hand Clin*. 1998;59-76.

Marks R, et al. Malignant transformation of solar keratoses to squamous cell carcinoma. *Lancet*. 1998;1:795.

Marshall DR, et al. Breastfeeding after reduction mammaplasty. *Br J Plast Surg*. 1994;47:167-169.

Martin D, et al. Reconstruction of the hand with forearm island flaps. *Clin Plast Surg*. 1997;24:33-35.

Martin JJ Jr, et al. Acquired prosis: dehiscences and disinsertions - are they real or iatrogenic? *Ophthal Plast Reconstr Surg*. 1992;8:130-132.

Mason ME, et al. Revision orthognathic surgery. In: Booth PW, Schendel SA, Hausamen JE, eds. *Maxillofacial Surgery*. London, England: Churchill Livingstone, Inc; 1999;2:1321-1334.

Masquelet AC, et al. Skin island flaps supplied by the vascular axis of the sensitive superficial nerves: anatomic study and clinical experience in the leg. *Plast Reconstr Surg*. 1994;93:872.

Matarasso A, et al. Botulinum A exotoxin for the management of platysma bands. *Plast Reconstr Surg*. 1999;103:645-652.

Matarasso A. Abdominoplasty. In: Achauer BM, Eriksson E, Guyuron B, et al, eds. *Plastic Surgery: Indications, Operations, and Outcomes*. Saint Louis, Mo: Mosby - Year Book, Inc; 2000;5:2783-2821.

Matarasso A. Buccal fat pad excision: aesthetic improvement of the midface. *Ann Plast Surg*. 1991;26:413.

Matarasso A. Liposuction as an adjunct to a full abdominoplasty revisited. *Plast Reconstr Surg*. 2000;106:1197.

Matarasso A. Liposuction as an adjunct to a full abdominoplasty. *Plast Reconstr Surg*. 1995;5:829-836.

Matarasso A. Pseudoherniation of the buccal fat pad: a new clinical syndrome. *Plast Reconstr Surg*. 1997;100:723-730.

Matarasso SL. Complications of botulinum A exotoxin for hyperfunctional lines. *Dermatol Surg*. 1998;24:1249-1254.

Mathes SJ, et al. Classification of the vascular anatomy of muscles: experimental and clinical correlation. *Plast Reconstr Surg*. 1981;67:177.

Mathes SJ, et al. Superficial inferior epigastric artery (SIEA) flap. In: *Reconstructive Surgery*. New York, NY: Churchill Livingstone, Inc; 1997;2:1095-1103.

Mathes SJ, et al. The principles of muscle and musculocutaneous flaps. In: McCarthy JG, ed. *Plastic Surgery*. Philadelphia, Pa: WB Saunders Co; 1990;1:379-411.

Mathes SJ, Nahai F, eds. *Reconstructive Surgery: Principles, Anatomy and Technique*. Saint Louis, Mo: Quality Medical Publishing, Inc; 1997:29-31, 477-679, 617-642, 729-746, 965-984, 1005, 1043, 1161-1307, 1353-1370.

Mathes SJ. Muscle flaps and their blood supply. In: Aston SJ, Beasley RW, Thorne CH, eds. *Grabb & Smith's Plastic Surgery*. 5th ed. Philadelphia, Pa: Lippincott-Raven; 1997:61-72.

Matsuo K, et al. Nonsurgical correction of congenital auricular deformities. *Clin Plast Surg*. 1990;17:383-395.

Matteucci BM, et al. Systemic arthritic conditions of the upper extremities - inflammatory. In: Peimer CA, ed. *Surgery of the Hand and Upper Extremity*. New York, NY: McGraw-Hill, Inc; 1996;2:1617-1631.

Mattison C. *The Encyclopedia of Snakes*. United Kingdom: Blanford; 1995.

Maxwell GP, et al. Management of complications following augmentation mammoplasty. In: Georgiade GS, Riefkohl R, Levin LS, eds. *Textbook of Plastic, Maxillofacial and Reconstructive Surgery*. Baltimore, Md: Williams & Wilkins; 1997:736.

May JW, et al. Micro neurovascular free transfer of the big toe. In: Strauch B, Vasconez LO, Hall-Findlay EJ, eds. *Grabb's Encyclopedia of Flaps*. 2nd ed. Philadelphia, Pa: Lippincott-Raven;1998: 1013-1018.

Mayfield JK, et al. Carpal dislocations, pathomechanics and progressive perilunate instability. *J Hand Surg*. 1980;5A:226.

McCarroll HR. Congenital anomalies: a 25-year overview. *J Hand Surg*. 2000;25A:1007-1037.

McCarroll HR. Congenital anomalies: radial dysplasia. In: Peimer CA, ed. *Surgery of the Hand and Upper Extremity*. New York, NY: McGRaw-Hill, Inc; 1996;2:2075-2093.

McCarthy JG, et al. A surgical system for the correction of bony chin deformity. *Clin Plast Surg*. 1991;18:139-152.

McCarthy JG, et al. Craniofacial microsomia. In: McCarthy JG, ed. *Plastic Surgery*. Philadelphia, Pa: WB Saunders Co; 1990;4;2491,3106,3054-3055.

McCarthy JG, et al. Craniofacial syndromes. In: McCarthy JG, ed. *Plastic Surgery*. Philadelphia, Pa: WB Saunders Co; 1990;4:3101-3160.

McCarthy JG, et al. Craniosynostosis. In: McCarthy JG, ed. *Plastic Surgery*. Philadelphia, Pa: WB Saunders Co; 1990;3013-3055.

McCarthy JG, et al. Distraction osteogenesis of the craniofacial skeleton. *Plast Reconstr Surg*. 2001;107:1812-1827.

McCarthy JG, et al. Principles of craniofacial surgery. In: McCarthy JG, ed. Plastic Surgery. Philadelphia, Pa: WB Saunders Col 1990;5:2974-3012.

McCarthy JG, et al. Rhinoplasty. In: McCarthy JG, ed. *Plastic Surgery*. Philadelphia, Pa: WB Saunders Co; 1990;3:1804.

McCarthy JG, et al. Surgery of the jaws. In: McCarthy JG, ed. *Plastic Surgery*. Philadelphia, Pa: WB Saunders Col 1990;2:1187, 1188-1474.

McCarthy JG, et al. Velopharyngeal function following maxillary advancement. *Plast Reconstr Surg*. 1979;64:180-189.

McCarthy JG. Craniofacial microsomia. In: Aston SJ, Beasley RW, Thorne CH, eds. *Grabbe & Smith's Plastic Surgery*. 5th ed. Philadephia, PA: Lippincott-Raven; 1997:305-319.

McCarthy JG. Introduction to plastic surgery. In: McCarthy JG, ed. *Plastic Surgery*. Philadelphia, Pa: WB Saunders Co; 1990;1:28, 68.

McCauley RL. Correction of burn alopecia. In: Herndon DN, ed. *Total Burn Care*. Philadelphia, Pa: WB Saunders Co; 1996:499-502.

McClinton MA. Tumors and aneurysms of the upper extremity. *Hand Clin*. 1993;9:151-169.

McComb H. Primary correction of unilateral cleft lip nasal deformity: a 10-year review. *Plast Reconstr Surg.* 1985;75:791-799.

McCord CD. *Eyelid Surgery: Principles and Techniques.* Philadelphia, Pa: Lippincott-Raven; 1995.

McCord CD. The evaluation and management of the patient with ptosis. *Clin Plast Surg.* 1988;15:169-184.

McCraw JB, Arnold PG, eds. *McCraw and Arnold's Atlas of Muscle and Musculocutaneous Flaps.* Norfold, Va: Hampton Press Publishing Co; 1988;89-91.

McCraw JB, et al. The value of fluorescein in predicting the viability of arterialized flaps. *Plast Reconstr Surg.* 1977;60:710-719.

McDowell CL, et al. Tetraplegia. In: Green DP, Hotchkiss RN, Pederson WC, eds. *Operative Hand Surgery.* 4th ed. New York, NY: Churchill Livingstone, Inc; 1999;2:1594.

McFarlane R. Patterns of diseased fascia in the fingers of Dupuytren's contracture. *Plast Reconstr Surg.* 1974;54:31.

McFarlane RM, et al. The anatomy and treatment of camptodactyly of the small finger. *J Hand Surg.* 1992;17A:35-44.

McFarlane RM. Dupuytren's contracture. In: Green DP, ed. *Operative Hand Surgery.* 3rd ed. New York, NY: Churchill Livingstone, Inc; 1982:563-591.

McFarlane RM. Dupuytren's disease. In: McCarthy JG, ed. *Plastic Surgery.* Philadelphia, Pa: WB Saunders Co; 1990;8:5061.

McFarlane RM. The anatomy of Dupuytren's contracture. *Bulletin Hosp Jt Dis Orthop Inst.* 1984;44:318-337.

McGrath MH. Benign tumors of the teenage hand. *Plast Reconstr Surg.* 2000;105:218.

McGrath MH. Infections of the hand. In: McCarthy JG, ed. *Plastic Surgery.* Philadelphia, Pa: WB Saunders Co; 1990;8:5229-5556.

McGregor IA. Major salivary glands. In: McGregor IA, Howard DJ, eds. *Rob & Smith's Operative Surgery: Head and Neck.* 4th ed. Oxford, England: Butterworth-Heinmann Ltd; 1992:326-340.

McGrouther DA. Dupuytren's contracture. In: Green DP, Hotchkiss RN, Pederson WC, eds. *Operative Hand Surgery.* 4th ed. New York, NY: Churchill Livingstone, Inc; 1999;1:563-591.

McGuirt WF, et al. Mandubular fractures: their effect on growth and dentition. *Arch Otolaryngol Head Neck Surg.* 1987;113:257.

McKee NH. Amputation stump management and function preservation. In: McCarthy JG, ed. *Plastic Surgery.* Philadelphia, Pa: WB Saunders Co; 1990;7:4329-4339.

McKinney P, et al. Prevention of injury to the great auricular nerve during rhytidectomy. *Plast Reconstr Surg.* 1980;66:675-679.

McLeish WM, et al. Cosmetic eyelid surgery and the problem eye. *Plast Reconstr Surg.* 1992;19:357-368.

McMahon JD, et al. Lasting success in teenage reduction mammaplasty. *Ann Plast Surg.* 1995;35:227-231.

McNamara MG, et al. Ischaemia of the index finger and thumb secondary to thrombosis of the radial artery in the anatomical snuffbox. *J Hand Surg.* 1998;23B:28-32.

Meara JG, et al. Tuberous breast deformity: principles and practice. *Ann Plast Surg.* 2000;45:607-611.

Medina JE, et al. Malignant melanoma of the head and neck. In: Myers EN, Suen JY, eds. *Cancer of the Head and Neck.* 3rd ed. Philadelphia, Pa: WB Saunders Col 1996:160-183.

Mendes D, et al. Traumatic deformities and reconstruction of the temporomandibular joint. In: Cohen M, ed. *Mastery of Plastic Surgery.* Boston, Mass: Little, Brown & Co; 1994;2:1220-1229.

Menick FJ. Anatomic reconstruction of the nasal tip cartilages in secondary and reconstructive rhinoplasty. *Plast Reconstr Surg.* 1999;104:2187-2201.

Mercer D, et al. Merkel cell carcinoma: the clinical course. *Ann Plast Surg.* 1990;25:136-141.

Messina A, et al. The contiguous elongation treatment by the TEC device for Dupuytren's contracture of the fingers. *Plast Reconstr Surg.* 1993;92:84-90.

Meyer K, et al. Secondary rhinoplasty. In: Daniel RK, ed. *Aesthetic Plastic Surgery: Rhinoplasty.* Boston, Mass: Little, Brown & Co; 1993:819-820.

Meyerson MD, et al. Nager acrofacial dysostosis: early intervention and long-term planning. *Cleft Palate J.* 1977;14:35-40.

Michelow BJ, et al. The natural history of obstetrical brachial plexus palsy. *Plast Reconstr Surg.* 1994;93:675-681.

Michie DD, et al. Influence of occlusive and impregnated gauze dressings on incisional healing: a prospective, randomized, controlled study. *Ann Plast Surg.* 1994;32:57-64.

Millard DR Jr. Unilateral cleft lip deformities. In: McCarthy JG, ed. *Plastic Surgery.* Philadelphia, Pa: WB Saunders Co; 1990;4:2627.

Miller LM, et al. Vasospastic disorders: etiology, recognition and treatment. *Hand Clin.* 1993;9:171-187.

Minamikawa Y. Extensor repair and rehabilitation. In: Peimer CA, ed. *Surgery of the Hand and Upper Extremity.* New York, NY: McGraw-Hill, Inc; 1996;1:1163.

Mitchnick MA, et al. Microfine zinc oxide (Z-cote) as a photostable UVA/UVB sunblock agent. *J Am Acad Dermatol.* 1999;40:85-90.

Mladick RA. Body contouring of the abdomen, thighs, hips and buttocks. In: Georgiade GS, Riefkohl R, Levin LS, eds. *Textbook of Plastic, Maxillofacial and Reconstructive Surgery.* Baltimore, Md: Williams & Wilkins; 1997:674-684.

Moffat CJ, et al. Assessing a calcium alginate dressing in management of pressure sores. *J Wound Care.* 1992;1:22-44.

Molina F, et al. Maxillary distraction: aesthetic and functional benefits in cleft lip-palate and prognathic patients during mixed dentition. *Plast Reconstr Surg.* 1998;101:951.

Monaco JL, et al. Acute wound healing an overview. *Clin Plast Surg.* 2003;30:1.

Moore KE, et al. The contributing role of condylar resorption to skeletal relapse following mandibular advancement surgery: report of five cases. *J Oral Maxillofac Surg.* 1991;49:448-460

Moore KL, Dalley AF, eds. *Clinically Oriented Anatomy.* 4th ed. Philadelphia, Pa: Lippincott Williiams & Wilkins; 1999:574, 845, 899, 937-939, 1082-1086.

Moore KL, ed. *Clinically Oriented Anatomy.* 3rd ed. Baltimore, Md: Williams & Wilkins; 1992:862.

Moore KL, ed. *The Developing Human.* 4th ed. Philadelphia, Pa: WB Saunders Co; 1988:170-206.

Moore KL, ed. *The Developing Human.* 6th ed. Philadelphia, Pa: WB Saunders Co; 1998:170, 220.

Moore KL, et al. Summary of cranial nerves. In: Moore KL, Dalley II AF, eds. *Clinically Oriented Anatomy.* 4th ed. Philadelhia, Pa: Lippincott Williams & Wilkins; 1999:1082-1096.

Moran JF. Surgical treatment of pulmonary tuberculosis. In: Sabiston DC, ed. *Testbook of Surgery.* Philadelphia, Pa: EB Saunders Co; 1991:1729-1737.

Morganroth GS, et al. Nonexcisional treatment of benign and premalignant cutaneous lesions. *Clin Plast Surg.* 1993;20:91-104.

Morykwas MJ, et al. Vacuum-assisted closure: a new method for wound control and treatment: animal studies and basic foundation. *Ann Plast Surg.* 1997;38:553-562.

Moscona RR, et al. An unusual late reaction to Zyderm I injections: a challenge for treatment. *Plast Reconstr Surg.* 1993;92:331-334.

Motoki DS, et al. The healing of bone and cartilage. *Clin Plast Surg.* 1990;17:527.

Moy OJ, et al. Microsurgical methods and replantation. In: Peimer CA, ed. *Surgery of the Hand and Upper Extremity*. New York, NY: McGraw-Hill, Inc; 1996:1845-1874.

Mubarak SJ, et al. Acute compartment syndromes. *Surg Clin North Am*. 1983;63:539-565.

Mueller BU, et al. The infant with a vascular tumor. *Semin Perinatol*. 1999;23:332.

Muhling J. Surgical treatment og craniosynostosis. In: Booth PW, Schendel SA, Hausamen JE, eds. *Maxillofacial Surgery*. London, England: Churchill Livingstone, Inc; 1999;2:877-888.

Mullaney PB, et al. Corneal keloid from unusual penetrating trauma. *J Pediatr Ophthalmol Strabismus*. 1995;32:331-332.

Mulliken JB, et al. Analysis of posterior plagiocephaly. *Plast Reconstr Surg*. 1999;103:371.

Mulliken JB, et al. Hemangiomas and vascular malformations in infants and children: a classification based on endothelial characteristics. *Plast Reconstr Surg*. 1982;69:412-422.

Mulliken JB, et al. Induced osteogenesis: the biological principle and clinical applications. *J Surg Res*. 1984;37:487.

Mulliken JB, et al. The anatomy of cupid's bow in normal and cleft lip. *Plast Reconstr Surg*. 1993;92:395.

Mulliken JB, Young AE, eds. *Vascular Birthmarks: Hemangiomas and Malformations*. Philadelphia, Pa: WB Saunders Co; 1988.

Mulliken JB. Cutaneous vascular anomalies. In: McCarthy JG, ed. *Plastic Surgery*. Philadelphia, Pa: WB Saunders Co; 1990;5:3191-3274.

Mulliken JB. Cutaneous vascular lesions in children. In: Serafin D, Georgiade NG, eds. *Pediatric Plastic Surgery*. Saint Louis, Mo: CV Mosby Co; 1984:137-154.

Mullins JB, et al. Complications of the transconjunctival approach: a review of 400 cases. *Arch Otolaryngol Head Neck Surg*. 1997;123:385-388.

Munro IR, et al. Craniofacial syndromes. In: McCarthy JG, ed. *Plastic Surgery*. Philadelphia, Pa: WB Saunders Co; 1990;4:3101-3123.

Munro IR, et al. Maxillonasal dysplasia (Binder's syndrome). *Plast Reconstr Surg*. 1979;63:657.

Munser AM. Alteration of the immune system in burns and implications for therapy. *Eur J Pediatr Surg*. 1994;4:231-242.

Murray J. Cold, chemical and irradiation injuries. In: McCarthy, ed. *Plastic Surgery*. Philadelphia, Pa: WB Saunders Co; 1990;7:5431-5440.

Murray JF, et al. Transmetacarpal amputation of the index finger: a clinical assessment of hand strength and complications. *J Hand Surg*. 1977;2A:471-481.

Murray PM. Septic arthritis of the hand and wrist. *Hand Clin*. 1998;14:579-587.

Mustarde J. The correction of prominent ears using mattress sutures. *Br J Plast Surg*. 1963;16:170.

Mustarde JC. The treatment of prominent ears by buried mattress sutures: a ten year survey. *Plast Reconstr Surg*. 1967;39:382.

Mustoe T, et al. Carcinoma in chronic pressure sores: a fulminant disease process. *Plast Reconstr Surg*. 1986;77:116-121.

Nagata S. Microtia: auricular reconstruction. In: Achauer BM, Eriksson E, Guyuron B, et al, eds. *Plastic Surgery: Indications, Operations, and Outcomes*. Saint Louis, Mo: Mosby - Year Book, Inc; 1023-1056.

Nahas FX, et al. The role of plastic surgery in congenital cutis laxa: a 10-year follow-up. *Plast Reconstr Surg*. 1999;104:1174-1178.

Nakajima T, et al. One-stage repair of blepharophimosis. *Plast Reconstr Surg*. 1991;87:24.

Nath RK, et al. Antibody to transforming growth factor beta reduces collagen production in injured peripheral nerve. *Plast Reconstr Surg.* 1998;102:1100.

Natvig K, et al. Relationship of intraoperative rupture of pleomorphic adenomas to recurrence: an 11-25 year follow-up study. *Head Neck.* 1994;16:213-217.

Naumann M. Evidence-based medicine: botulinum toxin in focal hyperhidrosis. *J Neurol.* 2001;248:31-33.

Nelson BR, et al. Sebaceous carcinoma. *J Am Acad Dermatol.* 1995;33:1-15.

Nelson RD, et al. Mechanisms of loss of human neutrophil chemotaxis following thermal injury. *J Burn Care Rehabil.* 1987;8:496.

Nesi FA, et al. Correction of traumatic ptosis of the eyelid and reconstruction of the lacrimal system. In: Cohen M, ed. *Mastery of Plastic and Reconstructive Surgery.* Boston, Mass: Little, Brown & Co; 1994;2:1105-1108.

Nesi FA, et al. Instrumentation in ophthalmic plastic surgery. In: *Smith's Ophthalmic Plastic and Reconstructive Surgery.* 2nd ed. Saint Louis, Mo: Mosby - Year Book, Inc; 1998:117-118.

Nesi Fa. *Smith's Ophthalmic Plastic and Reconstructive Surgery.* Saint Louis, Mo: Mosby - Year Book, Inc; 1998:375, 511.

Netscher D, et al. Benign and premalignant skin conditions. In: Achauer BM, Eriksson E, Guyuron B, et al, eds. *Plastic Surgery: Indications, Operations, and Outcomes.* Saint Louis, Mo: Mosby - Year Book, Inc; 2000;1:293-324.

Netscher DT, et al. Premalignant skin tumors, basal cell carcinoma, and squamous cell carcinoma. In: Cohen M, ed. *Mastery of Plastic and Reconstructive Surgery.* Boston, Mass: Little, Brown & Co; 1994;1:309-332.

Netscher DT. Congenital hand problems. *Hand Clin.* 1998;25:544.

Netter FH, ed. *Atlas of Human Anatomy.* 2nd ed. East Hanover, NJ:Novart/Hoechstetter Printer Co, Inc; 1997:18-21, 47-49.

Netter FH, ed. *Atlas of Human Anatomy.* 3nd ed. New York, NY: Novartis Medical Education; 2003.

Netter FH, ed. *Atlas of Human Anatomy.* Summit, NJ: Ciba-Geigy Corporation; 1989:19, 34, 36-37, 113-115, A436122, 491, 506, 508, 510.

Neuman JF. Evaluation and treatment of gynecomastia. *Am Fam Physician.* 1997;55:1835-1844, 1849-1850.

Neumeister MW, et al. Calcinosis of the hand in scleroderma: a case report. *Can J Plast Surg.* 1999;7:241-244.

Neviaser RJ. Acute infections. In: Green DP, Hotchkiss RN, Pederson WC, eds. *Operative Hand Surgery.* 4th ed. New York, NY: Churchill Livingstone, Inc; 1999;2:1033-1047.

Nguyen PN, et al. Advances in the management of orbital fractures. *Clin Plast Surg.* 1992;19:87-98.

Niessen FB, et al. On the nature of hypertrophic scars and keloids: a review. *Plast Reconstr Surg.* 1999;104:1435-1458.

Norris RL Jr. Envenomations. In: *Intensive Medicine.* Boston, Mass: Little, Brown & Co; 1996;1585-1590.

O'Brien CJ, et al. Neck dissection and parotidectomy. In: Balch CM, Houghton AN, Sober AJ, et al, eds. *Cutaneous Melanoma.* 3rd ed. Saint Louis, Mo: Quality Medical Publishing, Inc; 1998:245-257.

O'Connor WJ, et al. Merkel cell carcinoma. *Dermatol Surg.* 1996;22:262-267.

Ogawa R, et al. Postoperative electrin-beam irradiation therapy for keloids and hypertrophic scars: retrospective study of 147 cases followed for more than 18 months. *Plast Reconstr Surg.* 2003;111:547-555.

Ogose A, et al. Malignant melanoma extending along ulnar, median, and musculocutaneous nerves: a case report. *J Hand Surg.* 1998;23A:875-878.

Ohlms LA, et al. Interferon alfa-2a therapy for airway hemangiomas. *Ann Otol Rhinol Laryngol.* 1994;103:1-8.

Ohmori K. Application of microvascular free flaps to burn deformities. *World J Surg*. 1978;2:193-202.

Ohtsuka H, et al. Clinical experience with nasolabial flaps. *Ann Plast Surg*. 1981;6:207.

Oikarinen KS. Clinical management of injuries of the maxilla, mandible, and alveolus. *Dent Clin N Am*. 1995;39:113-130.

Oishi SN, et al. The difficult scalp and skull wound. *Clin Plast Surg*. 1995;22:51-59.

Olbricht SM. Treatment of malignant cutaneous tumors. *Clin Plast Surg*. 1993;20:167-180.

Olehnik WK, et al. Median nerve compression in the proximal forearm. *J Hand Surg*. 1994;19A:121-126.

O'Neal D, et al. Transient compartment syndrome of the forearm resulting from venous congestion from a tourniquet. *J Hand Surg*. 1989;14A:894-896.

Opperman LA, et al. TGF-beta 1, TGF-beta 2, and TGF-beta 3 exhibit distinct patterns of expression during cranial suture formation and obliteration in vivo and in vitro. *J Bone Miner Res*. 1997;12:301.

Orentreich N, et al. Biology of scalp hair growth. *Clin Plast Surg*. 1982;9:197.

Orentreich N, et al. Dermabrasion: as a complement to dermatology. *Clin Plast Surg*. 1998;25:63-80.

Ortiz-Monasterio F, et al. Advancement of the orbits and the midface in one piece, combined with frontal repositioning, for the correction of Crouzon's deformities. *Plast Reconstr Surg*. 1978;61:507.

Osburn K, et al. Congenital pigmented and vascular lesions in newborn infants. *J Am Acad Dermatol*. 1987;16:788.

Osler T. Antiseptics in surgery. In: *Surgical Infections*. Boston, Mass: Little, Brown & Co; 1994:119.

Ostad A, et al. Tumescent anesthesia with a lidocaine dose of 35 mg/kg is safe. *Dermatol Surg*. 1996;22:921-927.

O'sullivan ST, et al. Immunosuppression following thermal injury: pathogenesis of immunodysfunction. *Br J Plast Surg*. 1997;50:615.

Owen C, et al. Keratoacanthoma. In: Lebwohol MG, ed. *Treatment of Skin Disease: Comprehensive Therapeutic Strategies*. Philadelphia, Pa: Mosby - Year Book, Inc; 2002:315.

Owsley JQ, et al. Does steroid medication reduce facial edema following face lift surgery? A prospective, randomized study of 30 consecutive patients. *Plast Reconstr Surg*. 1996;98:1-6.

Ozyazgan I, et al. Eicosanoids and the inflammatory cells in frostbitten tissue: prostacyclin, thromboxane, polymorphonuclear leukocytes, and mast cells. *Plast Reconstr Surg*. 1998;101;1881-1886.

Padwa BL, et al. Cervicofacial lymphatic malformation: clinical course, surgical intervention, and pathogenesis of skeletal pathology. *Plast Reconstr Surg*. 1995;951-960.

Pakiam AI. Reversed dermis flap. In: Strauch B, Vasconez LO, Hall-Findlay EJ, eds. *Grabb's Encyclopedia of Flaps*. 2nd ed. Philadelphia, Pa: Lippincott-Raven; 1998.

Park C, et al. An analysis of 123 temporoparietal fascial flaps: anatomic and clinical considerations in total auricular reconstruction. *Plast Reconstr Surg*. 1999;104:1295-1306.

Park C, et al. Arterial supply of the anterior ear. *Plast Reconstr Surg*. 1992;90:38-44.

Parkes A. The "lumbrical plus" finger. *Hand*. 1970;2:164-165.

Parsa FD. How to avoid eyelid ptosis when injecting botulinum toxin into the corrugators. *Plast Reconstr Surg*. 2000;105:1564-1565.

Pasyayan HM, et al. Clinical experience with the Robin sequence. *Cleft Palate J*. 1984;21:270-276.

Pasyk KA, et al. Elecrton microscopic evaluation of guinea pig skin and soft tissues "expanded" with a self-inflating silicone implant. *Plast Reconstr Surg*. 1982;70:37.

Patel MR. Chronic infections. In: Green DP, Hotchkiss RN, Pederson WC, eds. *Operative Hand Surgery*. 4th ed. New York, NY: Churchill Livingstone, Inc; 1999;2:1783-1850.

Patipa M. The evaluation and management of lower eyelid retraction following cosmetic surgery. *Plast Reconstr Surg*. 2000;106:438-453.

Patrice SJ, et al. Pyogenic granuloma (lobular capillary hemangioma): a clinicopathologic study of 178 cases. *Pediatr Dermatol*. 1991;8:267-276.

Peacock EE, Jr, et al. Wound healing. In: McCarthy JG, ed. *Plastic Surgery*. Philadelphia, Pa: WB Saunders Co; 1990;1:161-185.

Pearl RM. Treatment of enophthalmos. *Clin Plast Surg*. 1992;19:99.

Peck G. Nasal tip projection: goals and maintenance. In: Rees TD, ed. *Rhinoplasty: Problems and Controversies*. Saint Louis, Mo; CV Mosby Co; 1988:10.

Peck GC, et al. Unfavorable results in rhinoplasty. In: Goldwyn RM, ed. *The Unfavorable Results in Plastic Surgery*. Boston, Mass: Little, Brown & Co; 1984;2:539-561.

Peck GP, et al. Secondary rhinoplasty. In: Georgiade GS, Riefkohl R, Levin LS, eds. *Plastic, Maxillofacial and Reconstructive Surgery*. Baltimore, Md: Williams & Wilkins; 1997:646-656.

Pederson E, et al. Cancer of respiratory origins among workers at a nickel refinery in Norway. *Int J Cancer*. 1973;12:32.

Pederson WC. Lymphedema of the extremities. In: Aston SJ, Beasley RW, Thorne CH, eds. *Grabb & Smith's Plastic Surgery*. 5th ed. Philadelphia, Pa: Lippincott-Raven; 1997:1124-1130Peer LA. The fate of autogenous human bone grafts. *Br J Plast Surg*. 1950;3:233.

Pegington J. The side of the mouth and parapharynx. In: Pegington J, ed. *Clinical Anatomy In Action - The Head and Neck*. Edinburgh, Scotland: Churchill Livingstone, Inc; 1986;2:143-150.

Peimer CA, et al. Hand function following single ray amputation. *J Hand Surg*. 1999;24:1245-1248.

Peimer CA, et al. Tumors of bone and soft tissue. In: Green DP, ed. *Operative Hand Surgery*. 3rd ed. New York, NY: Churchill Livingstone, Inc; 1993;3:2225-2250.

Pelc NJ, et al. Pigmentary changes in the skin: an introduction for surgeons. *Clin Plast Surg*. 1993;20:53-65.

Pellegrini VD Jr. The basal articulations of the thumb: pain, instability and osteoarthritis. In: Peimer CA, ed. *Surgery of the Hand and Upper Extremity*. New York, NY: McGraw-Hill, Inc; 1996:1019-1042.

Peng YP, et al. Comparison of first carpometacarpal joint arthrodesis with contralateral excision arthroplasty in a patient with bilateral saddle arthritis: a case report. *Ann Acad Med Singapore*. 1999;28:451-454.

Pensler JM, et al. Craniofacial gliomas. *Plast Reconstr Surg*. 1996;98:27-30Perez CA, et al. Carcinoma of the nasopharynx: factors affecting prognosis. *Int J Radiat Oncol Biol Phys*. 1992;23:271-280.

Perrott DH, et al. Acute management of orbitozygomatic fractures. *Oral Maxillofac Surg Clin North Am*. 1993;5:475-493.

Peterson RA, et al. Facile identification of the facial nerve branches. *Clin Plast Surg*. 1987;14:785-788.

Petri WA. Antimicrobial agents. In: Hardman JG, Limbirg LE, Gilman AG, eds. *The Pharmacological Basis of Therapeutics*. New York, NY: McGraw-Hill, Inc; 2001:1171-1192.

Phillips JW, et al. Strength of silicone breast implants. *Plast Reconstr Surg*. 1996;97:1215.

Phillips LG, et al. Pressure ulcerations. In: Jurkiewicz MJ, Krizek TJ, Mathes SJ, et al, eds. *Plastic Surgery: Principles and Practice*. Saint Louis, Mo: CV Mosby Co; 2:1223-1251.

Physicians' Desk Reference. Montvale, NJ: Medical Economics Co; 2000:638.

Physicians' Desk Reference. Montvale, NJ: Medical Economics Co; 2003:2825.

Piccirillo JF, et al. Evaluation, classification, and staging. In: Myers EN, Suen JY, eds. *Cancer of the Head and Neck*. Philadelphia, Pa: WB Saunders Co; 1996:33-49.

Pick TP, Howden R, eds. *Gray's Anatomy*. New York, NY: Bounty Books; 1977:77-80, 113-117, 884-886.

Pickford MA, et al. Sebaceous carcinoma of the periorbital and extraorbital regions. *Br J Plast Surg*. 1995;48:93-96.

Pinnell SR, et al. New and improved daily photoprotection: microfine zinc oxide (Z-Cote). *Aesthet Surg J*. 1999;19:260-263.

Pinski JB. Hair transplantation and bald-scalp reduction. *Dermatol Clin*. 1991;9:151-168.

Pinzur MS, et al. Amputation surgery in peripheral vascular disease. *Instructional Course Lectures*. 1999;48:687-691.

Pittman GH. *Liposuction and Aesthetic Surgery*. Saint Louis, Mo: Quality Medical Publishing, Inc; 1993:169.

Place MJ, et al. Basic techniques and principles in plastic surgery. In: Aston SJ, Beasley RW, Thorne CH, eds. *Grabb & Smith's Plastic Surgery*. 5th ed. Philadelphia, Pa: Lippincott-Raven; 1997:13-26.

Pokrovsky AV, et al. Arterialization of the foot venous system in the treatment of the critical lower limb ischaemia and distal arterial bed occlusion. *Ang Vasc Surg*. 1996;4:73-93.

Polley JW, et al. Longitudinal analysis of mandibular asymmetry in hemifacial microsomia. *Plast Reconstr Surg*. 1997;99:328-339.

Polley JW, et al. Management of severe maxillary deficiency in childhood and adolescence through distraction osteogenesis with an external, adjustable, rigid distraction device. *J Craniofac Surg*. 1997;8:181-185.

Polley JW, et al. Rigid external distraction: its application in cleft maxillary deformities. *Plast Reconstr Surg*. 1998;102:1360.

Polley JW. Bone grafts. In: Cohen M, ed. *Mastery of Plastic and Reconstructive Surgery*. Boston, Mass: Little, Brown & Co; 1994;1:102-112.

Popkin GL. Tumors of the skin: a dermatologist's viewpoint. In: McCarthy JG, ed. *Plastic Surgery*. Philadelphia, Pa: WB Saunders Co; 1990;5:3560-3613.

Posner MA. Differential diagnosis of wrist pain: tendinitis, ganglia, and other syndromes. In: Peimer CA, ed. *Surgery of the Hand and Upper Extremity*. New York, NY: McGraw-Hill, Inc; 1996:837-851.

Posnick JC, et al. Normal cutaneous sensibility of the face. *Plast Reconstr Surg*. 1990;86:429-433.

Posnick JC, et al. Pediatric facial fractures: evolving patterns of treatment. *J Oral Maxillofac Surg*. 1993;51:836.

Posnick JC, et al. Surgical correction of temporomandibular joint ankylosis. *Clin Plast Surg*. 1989;16:725-732.

Posnick JC. Management of facial fractures in children and adolescents. *Ann Plast Surg*. 1994;33:442-457.

Posnick JC. Surgical correction of mandibular hypoplasia in hemifacial microsomia: a personal perspective. *J Oral Maxillofac Surg*. 1998;56:639-650.

Posnick JC. The craniofacial dysostosis syndromes. *Clin Plast Surg*. 1994;21:585.

Posnick JC. Treacher Collins syndrome. In: Aston SJ, Beasley RW, Thorne CH, eds. *Grabb & Smith's Plastic Surgery*. 5th ed. Philadelphia, Pa: Lippincott-Raven; 1997:313-319.

Press B. Thermal, electrical, and chemical injuries. In: Aston SJ, Beasley RW, Thorne CH, eds. *Grabb & Smith's Plastic Surgery*. 5th ed. Philadelphia, Pa: Lippincott-Raven; 1997:161-191.

Preston DS, et al. Nonmelanoma cancers of the skin. *N Engl J Med*. 1992;327:1649-1662.

Preuss S, et al. Prominent ears. In: Achauer BM, Eriksson E, Guyuron B, et al, eds. *Plastic Surgery: Indications, Operations, and Outcomes*. Saint Louis, Mo: Mosby - Year Book, Inc; 2000;2:1057-1065.

Pribaz JJ, et al. Prelaminated free flap reconstruction of complex central facial defects. *Plast Reconstr Surg*. 1999;104:357-365.

Price CI, et al. Endoscopic transaxillary subpectoral breast augmentation. *Plast Reconstr Surg*. 1994;94:612-619.

Price VH. Treatment of hair loss. *N Engl J Med*. 1999;341:964-973.

Prockop DJ, et al. The biosynthesis of collagen and its disorders. *N Engl J Med*. 1979;301:13.

Proffit WR. Treatment Planning: the search for wisdom. In: Proffit WR, White RP, eds. *Surgical Orthodontic Treatment*. Saint Louis, Mo: Mosby - Year Book; 1991:158-161.

Proffitt WR, et al. Early fracture of the mandibular condyles: frequentlly and unsuspected cause of growth disturbances. *Am J Orthod*. 1980;78:1-24.

Prosser R. Splinting in the management of proximal interphalangeal joint flexion contracture. *J Hand Ther*. 1996;9:378-386.

Puckett CL. Lymphedema of the upper extremity. In: McCarthy JG, ed. *Plastic Surgery*. Philadelphia, Pa: WB Saunders Co; 1990;7:5023-5031.

Putnam MD, et al. Malignant bony tumors of the upper extremity. *Hand Clin*. 1995;11:265-286.

Putterman AM. *Cosmetic Oculoplastic Surgery: Eyelid, Forehead, and Facial Techniques*. Philadelphia, Pa: WB Saunders Co; 1999;429-256.

Putz R, Pabst R, eds. *Sobatta's Atlas of Human Anatomy*. Baltimore, Md: Williams & Wilkins; 1997;1:43.

Pyo DJ, et al. Craniosynostosis. In: Aston SJ, Beasley RW, Thorne CH, eds. *Grabb & Smith's Plastic Surgery*. 5th ed. Philadelphia, Pa: Lippincott-Raven; 1997:281-293.

Quinn MJ, et al. Subungual melanoma of the hand. *J Hand Surg*. 1998;21A:506-511.

Rae V, et al. Wrinkling due to middermal elastolysis: report of a case and review of the literature. *Arch Dermatol*. 1989;125:950.

Ramasastry SS. Chronic problem wounds. *Clin Plast Surg*. 1998;25:367.

Ramasastry SS. Surgical management of massive perianal hidradenitis suppurativa. *Ann Plast Surg*. 1985;15:218.

Ramirez O. Abdominoplasty and abdominal wall rehabilitation: a comprehensive approach. *Plast Reconstr Surg*. 2000;105:425-435.

Ramirez OM, et al. The sliding gluteus maximus myocutaneous flap: its relevance in ambulatory patients. *Plast Reconstr Surg*. 1984;74:68.

Rao RB, et al. Deaths related to liposuction. *N Engl J Med*. 1999;340:1471-1475.

Rao SB, et al. Traumatic and acquired wrist disorders in children. In: Lichtman DM, Alexander AH, eds. *The Wrist and its Disorders*. Philadelphia, Pa: WB Saunders Co; 1997:540.

Rapaport DP, et al. Influence of steroids on postoperatice swelling after facialplasty: a prospective, randomized study. *Plast Reconstr Surg*. 1995;96:1547-1552.

Raulin C, et al. Q-switched ruby laser treatment of tattos and benign pigmented skin lesions: a critical review. *Ann Plast Surg*. 1998;41:555-565.

Rayan GM. Clinical presentation and types of Dupuytren's disease. Hand Clin. 1999;15:87-96.

Rayan GM. Palmar fascial complex anatomy and pathology in Dupuytren's disease. *Hand Clin*. 1999;15:73-86.

Raymond GV. Craniofacial genetics and dysmorphology. In: Achauer BM, Eriksson E, Guyuron B, et al, eds. *Plastic Surgery: Indications, Operations, and Outcomes*. Saint Louis, Mo: Mosby -Year Book, Inc; 2000;2:614-615.

Rayner CR, et al. What is Gorlin's syndrome? The diagnosis and management of the basal cell naevus syndrome, based on a study of thirty-seven patients. *Br J Plast Surg*. 1977;30:62.

Rees TD, et al. Blepharoplasty and facialplasty. In: McCarthy JG, ed. *Plastic Surgery*. Philadelphia, Pa: WB Saunders Co; 1990;3:2320-2414.

Rees TD, et al. The role of the Schirmer's test and orbital morphology in predicting dry-eye syndrome after blepharoplasty. *Plast Reconstr Surg*. 1988;82:619.

Rees TD. *Aesthetic Plastic Surgery*. Philadelphia, Pa: WB Saunders Co; 1980;2:525-580, 601-606.

Rees TD. Chemabrasion and dermabrasion. In: Rees TD, LaTrenta GS, eds. *Aesthetic Plastic Surgery*. 2nd ed. Philadelphia, Pa: WB Saunders Co;1994:757.

Rees TD. Unique problems associated with the lip-columella-tip complex. In: Rees TD, Baker DC, Tabbal N, eds. *Rhinoplasty: Problems and Controversies*. Saint Louis, Mo: 1998:118-123.

Regnault P. Breast ptosis: definition and treatment. *Clin Plast Surg*. 1976;3:193-203.

Reiger RA. A local flap for repair of the nasal tip. *Plast Reconstr Surg*. 1967;40:147-149.

Reintgen DS, et al. Lymphatic mapping and sentinel lymphadenectomy. In: Balch CM, Houghton AN, Sober AJ, et al, eds. *Cutaneous Melanoma*. 3rd ed. Saint Louis, Mo: Quality Medical Publishing, Inc; 1998:227-244.

Renehan A, et al. An analysis of the treatment of 114 patients with recurrent pleomorphic adenomas of the parotid gland. *Amer J Surg*. 1996;172:7-10.

Restifo RJ, et al. Timing, magnitude, and utility of surgical delay in the TRAM flap: II: clinical studies. *Plast Reconstr Surg*. 1997;99:1217-1223.

Rettig A. Management of acute scaphoid fractures. *Hand Clin*. 2000;16:381-394.

Rettig ME, et al. Fractures of the distal radius. In: Lichtman DM, Alexander AH, eds. *The Wrist and Its Disorders*. Philadelphia, Pa: WB Saunders Co; 1997;347-372.

Reus WF III, et al. Tobacco smoking and complications in elective microsurgery. *Plast Reconstr Surg*. 1992;89:490.

Reus WF, et al. Acute effects of tobacco smoking on blood flow and cutaneous micro circulation. *Br J Plast Surg*. 1994;37:213.

Ricciardelli E, et al. Anatomy/physiolgy/embryology. In: Ruberg RL, Smith DJ, eds. *Plastic Surgery: A Core Curriculum*. Saint Louis, Mo: CV MosbyCo; 1994:251-259.

Rice DH. Diseases of the salivary glands - nonneoplastic. In: Bailey BJ, Calhoun KH, Deskin RW, et al, eds. *Head and Neck Surgery - Otolaryngology*. 2nd ed. Philadelphia, Pa: Lippincott-Raven; 1998;1:561-570.

Richmond JD, et al. The significance of incomplete excision in patients with basal cell carcinoma. *Br J Plast Surg*. 1987;40:63-67.

Ridenour BD. The nasal septum. In: Cummings CW, Fredrickson JM, Harker LA, eds. *Otolaryngology Head & Neck Surgery*. 3rd ed. Saint Louis, Mo: Mosby - Year Book, Inc; 1998;2:921-848.

Riefkohl R, et al. Gynecomastia. In: Georgiade GS, Riefkohl R, Levin LS, eds. *Textbook of Plastic, Maxillofacial and Reconstructive Surgery*. Baltimore, Md: Williams & Wilkins; 1997:820-828.

Ritchie JM, et al. Local anesthetics. In: Goodman G, Gilman AG, eds. *Goodman & Gilman's The Pharmacological Basis of Therapeutics*. 6th ed. New York, NY: Macmillan Publishing Co, Inc; 1980:300-322.

Rizio L, et al. Finger deformities in rheumatoid arthritis. *Hand Clin*. 1996;12:531-539.

Robb GL. Free scapular flap reconstruction of the head and neck. *Clin Plast Surg.* 1994;21:45-58.

Robbins KT. Neck dissection. In: Cummings CW, Fredrickson JM, Harker LA, et al, eds. *Otolaryngology Head Neck Surgery.* 3rd ed. Saint Louis, Mo: Mosby - Year Book, Inc; 1998;3:1787-1810.

Roberts TL, et al. Aesthetic laser surgery. In: Achauer BM, Eriksson E, Guyuron B, et al, eds. *Plastic Surgery: Indications, Operations, and Outcomes.* Saint Louis, Mo: Mosby - Year Book, Inc; 2000;5;2457-2486.

Robertson B, et al. Orthognathic Surgery. In: Evans GR, ed. *Operative Plastic Surgery.* New York, NY: McGraw-Hill, Inc; 2000:585-593.

Robson MC, et al. Cold injuries. In: McCarthy JG, ed. *Plastic Surgery.* Philadelphia, Pa: WB Saunders Co; 1990;1:849-866.

Robson MC, et al. Prevention and treatment of post burn scars and contracture. *World J Surg.* 1992;16:87.

Robson MC, et al. Wound repair: principles and applications. In: Ruberg RL, Smith DL, eds. *Plastic Surgery - A Core Curriculum.* Saint Louis, Mo: Mosby - Year Book, Inc; 1994;1:5-6.

Rockwell WB, et al. Extensor tendon: anatomy, injury, and reconstruction. *Plast Reconstr Surg.* 2000;106:1592.

Rockwell WB, et al. Keloids and hypertrophic scars: a comprehensive review. *Plast Reconstr Surg.* 1989;84:827-837.

Rockwell WB, et al. Nail bed injuries and reconstruction. In: Peimer CA, ed. *Surgery of the Hand and Upper Extremity.* New York, NY: McGraw-Hill, Inc; 1996;2:1101-1111.

Rodeheaver GT, et al. Wound cleansing by high pressure irrigation. *Surg Gynecol Obstet.* 1975;141:357-362.

Roenigk HH Jr. Dermabrasion: state of the art. *J Dermatol Surg Oncol.* 1985;11:306.

Rohrich RJ, et al. A simplified algorithm for the use of Z-plasty. *Plast Reconstr Surg.* 1999;103:1513-1517.

Rohrich RJ, et al. Aesthetic management of the breast following explantation: evaluation and mastopexy options. *Plast Reconstr Surg.* 1998;101:827-837.

Rohrich RJ, et al. An analysis of silicone gel-filled breast implants: diagnosis and failure rates. *Plast Reconstr Surg.* 1998;102:2304-2308.

Rohrich RJ, et al. An update on the role of subcutaneous infiltration in suction-assisted lipoplasty. *Plast Reconstr Surg.* 2003;111:926-927.

Rohrich RJ, et al. Early results of vermilion lip augmentation using acellular allogenic dermis: an adjunct in facial rejuvination. *Plast Reconstr Surg.* 2000;105:409.

Rohrich RJ, et al. Evolving concepts of craniomaxillofacial fracture management. *Clin Plast Surg.* 1992;19:1-10.

Rohrich RJ, et al. Management of frontal sinus fractures: changing concepts. *Clin Plast Surg.* 1992;19:219-232.

Rohrich RJ, et al. Nasal aesthetics. In: Aston SJ, Beasley RW, Thorne CH, eds. *Grabb & Smith's Plastic Surgery.* 5th ed. Philadelphia, Pa: Lippincott-Raven; 1997:513.

Rohrich RJ, et al. Nasal fracture management: minimizing secondary nasal deformities. *Plast Reconstr Surg.* 2000;106:266-273.

Rohrich RJ, et al. Nasal tip blood supply: an anatomic study validating the safety of the transcomellar incision in rhinoplasty. *Plast Reconstr Surg.* 1995;95:795.

Rohrich RJ, et al. Optimizing the management of orbitozygomatic fractures. *Clin Plast Surg.* 1992;19:149-165.

Rohrich RJ, et al. Rationale for submucous resection of hypertrophied inferior turbinates in rhinoplasty: an evolution. *Plast Reconstr Surg.* 2001;108:536-544.

Rohrich RJ, et al. Secondary rhinoplasty. In: Grotting JC, ed. *Reoperative Aesthetic and Reconstructive Surgery.* Saint Louis, Mo: Quality Medical Publishing, Inc; 1995;401-510.

Rohrich RJ, et al. Subungual glomus tumors: an algorithmic approach. *Ann Plast Surg*. 1994;33:300-304.

Rosen GM. When osteotomies should be considered. *Clin Plast Surg*. 1991;18:205-212.

Rosen HM. Chin Surgery. In: Rosen HM, ed. *Aesthetic Perspectives in Jaw Surgery*. New York, NY: Springer-Verlag; 1999:248-249.

Rosenthal JS. The thermally injured ear: a systematic approach to reconstruction. *Clin Plast Surg*. 1992;19:645-661.

Ross JJ, et al. Squamous cell and adnexal carcinomas of the skin. *Clin Plast Surg*. 1997;24:687-703.

Rosse C, Gaddum-Rosse P, eds. *Hollinshead's Textbook of Anatomy*. 5th ed. Philadelphia, Pa: Lippincott-Raven; 1997:359, 767-793.

Roth DA, et al. Immunolocalization of transforming growth factor beta 1, beta 2, and beta 3 and insulin-like growth factor I in premature cranial suture fusion. *Plast Reconstr Surg*. 1997;99:300-309.

Roth DA, et al. Studies in cranial suture biology: part I. Increased immunoreactivity for TGF-beta isoforms (beta 1, beta 2, and beta 3) during rat cranial suture fusion. *J Bone Miner Res*. 1997;12:311.

Rowe NL. Fractures of the jaws in children. *J Oral Surg*. 1969;27:497-507.

Rowland LP. Stroke, spasticity, and botulinum toxin. *N Engl J Med*. 2002;347:382-383.

Rowland SA. Fasciotomy: the treatment of compartment syndrome. In: Green DP, ed. *Operative Hand Surgery*. 3rd ed. New York, NY: Churchill Livingstone, Inc; 1993;2:661-710.

Rowland SA. Fasciotomy: the treatment of compartment syndrome. In: Green DP, Hotchkiss RN, Pederson WC, eds. *Operative Hand Surgery*. 4th ed. New York, NY: Churchill Livingstone, Inc; 1999;1:689-710.

Ruan CM, et al. Magnetic resonance imaging of nonhealing pressure ulcers and myocutaneous flaps. *Arch Phys Med Rehabil*. 1998;79:1080.

Rubenstein R, et al. Atypical keloids after dermabrasion of patients taking isotretinoin. *J Acad Dermatol Surg Oncol*. 1986;15:280.

Ruberg R, et al. *Plastic Surgery: A Core Curriculum*. Saint Louis, Mo: CV Mosby Co; 1994:251.

Rubin MG, ed. *Manual of Chemical Peels: Superficial and Medium Depth*. Philadelphia, Pa: JB Lippincott Co; 1995:3.

Rubin MG. Trichloroacetic acid and other non phenol peels. *Clin Plast Surg*. 1992;19:525-536.

Rudolph R, et al. Skin grafts. In: McCarthy JG, ed. *Plastic Surgery*. Philadelphia, Pa: WB Saunders Co; 1990;1:221-274.

Ruff GL. Progressive hemifacial atrophy: Romberg's disease. In: McCarthy JG, ed. *Plastic Surgery*. Philadelphia, Pa: WB Saunders Co; 1990;5:3135-3143.

Ruggles G. Coincidence of palmaris longus and plantaris muscles. Rushton DH. Management of hair loss in women. *Dermatol Clin*. 1993;11:47.

Sadler TW, ed. *Langman's Medical Embryology*. Baltimore, Md: Williams & Wilkins; 1990:328-337.

Sakar M, et al. Thrombocytopenic coagulopathy (Kasabach-Merrit phenomenon) is associated with Kaposiform hemangioendothelioma and not with common infantile hemangioma. *Plast Reconstr Surg*. 1997;100:1377.

Salisbury RE. Thermal burns. In: McCarthy JG, ed. *Plastic Surgery*. Philadelphia, Pa: WB Saunders Co;1990;2:787-813.

Salmerk L, et al. Studies of antithrombotic effects of Dextran 40 following microarterial trauma. *Br J Plast Surg*. 1991;44:15.

Salmerk L, et al. The effect of Dextran 40 on patency following severe trauma in small arteries and veins. *Br J Plast Surg*. 1995;48:121.

Salmons S. Muscles and fasciae of the head. In: *Gray's Anatomy*. 38th ed. New York, NY: Churchill Livingstone, Inc; 1995;796-802.

Salyer KE. Primary correction of the unilateral cleft lip nose: a 15-year experience. *Plast Reconstr Surg*. 1986;77:558-568.

Samuels TH, et al. Poland's syndrome: a mammagroaphic presentation. *Am J Roentgenol*. 1996;347-348.

Sanders GH, et al. Are keratoacanthomas really squamous cell carcinomas? *Ann Plast Surg*. 1982;9:307-309.

Sandow MJ, et al. Single-cross grasp siz-strand repair for acute flexor tenorrhaphy: modified Savage technique. In: Taras SJ, Schneider LH, eds. *Atlas of the Hand Clinics*. Philadelphia, Pa: WB Saunders Co; 1996:65-77.

Sanz-Gallen P, et al. Hypocalcemia and hypomagnesemia due to hydrofluoric acid. *Occup Med (Lond)*. 2001;51:294-295.

Sasaki GH, et al. Pathogenesis and treatment of infant skin strawberry hemangiomas: clinical and in vitro studies of hormonal effects. *Plast Reconstr Surg*. 1984;73:359.

Sasaki GH, et al. Pathophysiology of skin flaps raised on expanded pigskin. *Plast Reconstr Surg*. 1984;74:59.

Schaffer JV, et al. The clinical spectrum of pigmented lesions. *Clin Plast Surg*. 2000;27:391-408.

Schall SB, et al. Tissue pressures in pyogenic flexor tenosynovitis of the finger. *J Bone Joint Surg*. 1996;78B:793-795.

Schenck RE. Full thickness skin grafts to the hand. In: Blair WF, ed. *Techniques in Hand Surgery*. Baltimore, Md: Williams & Wilkins; 1996:13-18.

Schenck RR. Dynamic traction and early passive movement for fractures of the proximal interphalangeal joint. *J Hand Surg*. 1986;11A:850-858.

Schendel SA. Cephalometrics and orthognathic surgery. In: Bell WH, ed. *Modern Practice in Orthognathic and Reconstructive Surgery*. Philadelphia, Pa: WB Saunders Co; 1992;1:85-99.

Schendel SA. Orthognathic surgery. In: Achauer BM, Eriksson E, Guyuron B, et al, eds. *Plastic Surgery: Indications, Operations, and Outcomes*. Saint Louis, Mo: Mosby - Year Book, Inc; 2000;2:871-895.

Schendel SA. Vertical maxillary deformities. In: Ferraro JW, ed. *Fundamentals in Maxillofacial Surgery*. New York, NY: Springer-Verlag; 1997:284-286.

Schenkler JD, et al. The abdominohypogastric skin flap for hand and forearm coverage. In: Strauch B, Vasconez LO, eds. *Grabb's Encyclopedia of Flaps*. Boston, Mass: Little, Brown & Co; 1990;2:1158-1160.

Schlenz I, et al. The sensitivity of the nipple-areolar complex: an anatomic study. *Plast Reconstr Surg*. 2000;105:905-909.

Schmitz JP, et al. Reconstruction of bone using calcium phosphate bone cements: a critical review. *J Oral Maxillofac Surg*. 1999;57:1122-1126.

Schneider JM, et al. Bilateral forearm compartment syndrome resulting from neuroleptic malignant syndrome. *J Hand Surg*. 1996;21A:287-289.

Schneider LH. Flexor tendons - late reconstruction. In: Green DP, Hotchkiss RN, Pederson WC, eds. *Operative Hand Surgery*. 4th ed. New York, NY: Churchill Livingstone, Inc; 1999;2:1898-1949.

Schneider MS, et al. The tensiometric properties of expanded guinea pig skin. *Plast Reconstr Surg*. 1988;81:398.

Schuller DE, et al. A technique to treat wrestlers' auricular hematoma without interrupting training or competition. *Arch Otolaryngol Head Neck Surg*. 1989;15:202-206.

Schwartz RA. The actinic keratoses: a prospective and update. *Dermatol Surg*. 1997;23:1009.

Schwartz SI, ed. *Principles of Surgery*. New York, NY: McGraw-Hill, Inc;1999.

Sclafani AP, et al. Prevention of earlobe keloid recurrence with postoperative corticosteroid injections versus radiation therapy: a randomized, prospective study and review of the literature. *Dermatol Surg*. 1996;22:569-574.

Scott SM. Pulmonary infections. In: Sabiston DC, ed. *Textbook of Surgery*. Philadelphia, Pa: WB Saunders Co; 1991:1701-1717.

Searles JM Jr, et al. Foot reconstruction in diabetes mellitus and peripheral vascular insufficiency. *Clin Plast Surg*. 1991;18:467-483.

Seckel BR. *Facial Danger Zones: Avoiding Nerve Injury in Facial Plastic Surgery*. Saint Louis, Mo: Quality Medical Publishing, Inc; 1994.

Seibert JW, et al. Blood supply of the Le Fort I maxillary segment: an anatomic study. *Plast Reconstr Surg*. 1997;100:843.

Seitz A, et al. The anatomy of the angular branch of the thoracodorsal artery. *Cells Tissues Organs*. 1999;164:227-236. Seitz WH Jr. Complications and problems in the management of distal radius fractures. *Hand Clin*. 1994;10:117-123.

Semple JL, et al. Breast milk contamination and silicone implants: preliminary results using silicon as a proxy measurement for silicone. *Plast Reconstr Surg*. 1998;102:528-533.

Senturk S, et al. Calciphylaxis: cutaneous necrosis in chronic renal failure. *Ann Plast Surg*. 2002;48:104-105.

Serafin D. Radial forearm flap. In: *Atlas of Microsurgical Composite Tissue Transplantation*. Philadelphia, Pa: WB Saunders Co; 1996:389.

Servelle M. Klippel and Trenaunay's syndrome: 768 operated cases. *Ann Surg*. 1985;201:365.

Seyfer AE, et al. Poland's anomaly: natural history and long-term results of chest wall reconstruction in 33 patients. *Ann Surg*. 1988;208:776-782.

Shack RB, et al. Is aggressive surgical management justified in the treatment of Merkel cell carcinoma? *Plast Reconstr Surg*. 1994;94:970-975.

Shah JP. Cervical lymph nodes. In: Shah JP, ed. *Head and Neck Surgery*. London, England: Mosby-Wolfe; 1996:355-392.

Shankar R, et al. Hematologic, hematopoietic, and acute phase response. In: Herndon DN, ed. *Total Burn Care*. 2nd ed. Philadelphia, Pa: WB Saunders Co; 2002:334-335.

Shapiro PS, et al. Non-neoplastic tumors of the hand and upper extremity. *Hand Clin*. 1995;11:133-160.

Shaw JH, et al. Merkel cell tumour: clinical behaviour and treatment. *Br J Surg*. 1991;78:138-142.

Sheen JH, et al. Applied anatomy and physiology. In: *Aesthetic Rhinoplasty*. Saint Louis, Mo: Quality Medical Publishing; 1998:14.

Sheen JH, et al. Problems in secondary rhinoplasty. In: *Aesthetic Rhinoplasty*. Saint Louis, Mo: Quality Medical Publishing; 1998:1135-1408.

Sheen JH. Closed vs. open rhinoplasty. *Plast Reconstr Surg*. 1997;85:99.

Sheen JH. Spreader graft: a method of reconstructing the roof of the middle nasal vault following rhinoplasty. *Plast Reconstr Surg*. 1984;73:230-239.

Sheen JH. Tip graft: a 20 year retrospective. *Plast Reconstr Surg*. 1993;91:48.

Shenaq SM, et al. Principles of microvascular surgery. In: Aston SJ, Beasley RW, Thorne CH, eds. *Grabb & Smith's Plastic Surgery*. 5th ed. Philadelphia, Pa: Lippincott-Raven; 1997:73.

Shepard DD. Betadine: ophthalmic preparation and intraocular lens surgery. In: *Proceedings of the World Congress on Antiseptics*. Lahn, Germany: Mundipharma Limberg; 1979.

Shepard GH. Nail grafts for reconstruction. *Hand Clin*. 1990;6:79-102.

Sheridan RL, et al. Long-term consequences of toxic epidermal necrolysis in children. *Pediatr.* 2002;109:74-78.

Sheridan RL, et al. The acute burned hand: management and outcome based on 10-year experience with 1047 acute hand burns. *J Trauma.* 1995;38:406-411.

Shermak MA, et al. Butyl-2-cyanoacrylate fixation of mandibular osteotomies. *Plast Reconstr Surg.* 1998;102:319-324.

Sherman R, et al. Lower extremity reconstruction. In: Achauer BM, Eriksson E, Guyuron B, et al, eds. *Plastic Surgery: Indications, Operations, and Outcomes.* Saint Louis, Mo: Mosby - Year Book, Inc; 2000;1:475-496.

Shiffman MA, et al. Fat transfer techniques: the effect of harvest and transfer methods on adipocyte viability and review of the literature. *Dermatol Surg.* 2001;27:819.

Shprintzen RJ. Velocardiofacial syndrome. *Otolaryngol Clin North Am.* 2000;33:1217-1240.

Sidoti EJ Jr, et al. Long-term studies of metopic synostosis: frequency of cognitive impairment and behavioral disturbances. *Plast Reconstr Surg.* 1996;97:276-281.

Siegel RJ, et al. Intradermal implantation of bovine collagen: humoral immune responses associated with clinical reactions. *Arch Dermatol.* 1984;120:183-187.

Siftan DW, ed. *Physician's Desk Reference.* 54th ed. Montvale, NJ: Medical Economics Co; 2000.

Siftan DW, ed. *Physician's Desk Reference.* Montvale, NJ: Medical Economics Co; 2002.

Silkiss RZ, et al. Transconjunctival surgery. *Ophthalmic Surg.* 1992;23:288-291.

Silverstein MJ, et al. Mammographic measurements before and after augmentation mammaplasty. *Plast Reconstr Surg.* 1990;86:1126-1130.

Simmons BP, et al. Juvenile rheumatoid arthritis. *Hand Clin.* 1989;5:157-168.

Simmons KE. Orthodontic role in clefts. In: Booth PW, Schendel SA, Hausamen JE, eds. *Maxillofacial Surgery.* London, England: Churchill Livingstone, Inc; 1999;2:1101-1111.

Simon BE, et al. Classification and surgical correction of gynecomastia. *Plast Reconstr Surg.* 1973;51:48-52.

Simon MS, et al. Cellulitis after axillary lymph node dissection for carcinoma of the breast. *Am J Med.* 1992;93:543-548.

Simon RR, et al. Subungual hematoma: association with occult laceration requiring repair. *Am J Emerg Med.* 1987;5:302-304.

Sims NM. Upper extremity anesthesia. In: McCarthy JG, ed. *Plastic Surgery.* Philadelphia, Pa: WB Saunders Co; 1990;8:4302-4328.

Singleton GT, et al. Frey's syndrome: incidence related to skin flap thickness in parotidectomy. *Laryngoscope.* 1980;90:1636.

Skandalakis JE, et al. The anterior body wall. In: Skandalakis JE, ed. *Embryology for Surgeons.* Baltimore, Md: Williams & Wilkins; 1994:540-593.

Smith B. Superior oblique paresis after blepharoplasty. *Plast Reconstr Surg.* 1980;66:287.

Smith DG. Principles of partial foot amputations in the diabetic. *Instructional Course Lectures.* 1999;48:321-329.

Smith DJ, et al. Microbiology and healing of the occluded skin-graft donor site. *Plast Reconstr Surg.* 1993;91:1094-1097.

Smith MA, et al. Burns of the hand and upper limb - a review. *Burns.* 1998;24:493.

Smith ML, et al. Management of orbital fractures. *Operative Techniques Plast Reconstr Surg.* 1998;5:312-324.

Smith P, et al. Syndactyly. In: Gupta A, Kay SP, Scheker LR, eds. *The Growing Hand.* London: Mosby - Year Books, Inc; 2000:225-230.

Smith RJ. Intrinsic contracture. In: Green DP, Hotchkiss RN, Pederson WC, eds. *Operative Hand Surgery*. 4th ed. New York, NY: Churchill Livingstone, Inc; 1999;1:611.

Smith RJ. Tendon transfers following injuries about the elbow. In: *Tendon Transfers of the Hand and Forearm*. Boston, Mass: Little, Brown & Co; 1987.

Smith RJ. Tendon transfers to restore thumb opposition. In: *Tendon Transfers of the Hand and Forearm*. Boston, Mass: Little, Brown & Co; 1987.

Snell RS, ed. *Clinical Anatomy for Medical Students*. 5th ed. Boston, Mass: Little, Brown & Co; 1995:671-682.

Snyder MC, et al. Early versus late gold weight implantation for rehabilitation of the paralyzed eyelid. *Laryngoscope*. 2001;111:2109-2113.

Sood S, et al. Frey's syndrome and parotid surgery. *Clin Otolaryngol*. 1998;23:291-301.

Sotereanos DG, et al. Hand and digital amputations. In: Peimer CA, ed. *Surgery of the Hand and Upper Extremity*. New York, NY: McGRaw-Hill, Inc; 1996;2:1000-1002.

Souba WW. Evaluation and treatment of benign breast disorders. In: Bland KI, Copeland EM, eds. *The Breast: Comprehensive Management of Benign and Malignant Diseases*. Philadelphia, Pa: WB Saunders Co; 1991:715.

Soucacos PN, et al. Reflex sympathetic dystrophy of the upper extremity. *Hand Clin*. 1997;13:339-354.

Soucacos PN. Indications and selection for digital amputation and replantation. J Hand Surg. 2001;26B:572-581.

Soutar DS, et al. The radial forearm flap in the management of soft tissue injuries of the hand. *Br J Plast Surg*. 1984;37:18.

Soxanas MT. Surgical anatomy of the eyelids and orbit. In: Wright DW, ed. *Color Atlas of Ophthalmic Surgery*. Philadelphia, Pa: JB Lippincott Co; 1992;1-16.

Sparkes BG. Immunological responses to thermal injury. *Burns*. 1997;23:106-113.

Spear SL, et al. Concentric mastopexy revisited. *Plast Reconstr Surg*. 2001;107:1294.

Spear SL, et al. Experience with reduction mammaplasty following breast conservation and radiation therapy. *Plast Reconstr Surg*. 1998;102:1913.

Spear SL, et al. Guidelines in concentric mastopexy. *Plast Reconstr Surg*. 1990;85:961-966.

Spear SL, et al. Reduction mammoplasty and mastopexy. In: Aston SJ, Beasley RW, Thorne CH, eds. *Grabb & Smith's Plastic Surgery*. 5th ed. Philadelphia, Pa: Lippincott-Raven; 1997:742-751.

Spear SL, et al. Staged breast reconstruction with saline-filled implants in the irradiated breast: recent trends and therapeutic implications. *Plast Reconstr Surg*. 2000;105:930.

Spencer JM, et al. Indoor tanning: risks, benefits, and future trends. *J Am Acad Dermatol*. 1995;33:288-298.

Spira M, et al. Injectable soft tissue substitutes. *Clin Plast Surg*. 1993;20:181-188.

Spira M. Otoplasty: what I do now - a 30-year perspective. *Plast Reconstr Surg*. 1999;104:834-840.

Spiro RH, et al. The importance of clinical staging of minor salivary gland carcinoma. *Am J Surg*. 1991;162:330-336.

Spiro RH. Salivary neoplasms: overview of 35-year experience with 2,807 patients. *Head Neck Surg*. 1986;8:177-184.

Sporn MB, et al. Transforming growth factor-beta: biologic function and chemical structure. *Science*. 1986;233:532.

Sriprachya-Anunt S, et al. Infectious complications of pulsed carbon dioxide laser resurfacing for photoaged skin. *Dermatol Surg*. 1997;23:527-536.

Stal GH, et al. Hemangiomas, lymphangiomas, and vascular malformations of the head and neck. *Otolaryngol Clin North Am.* 1986;19:769.

Stal S, et al. Basal and squamous cell carcinoma of the skin. In: Aston SJ, Beasley RW, Thorne CH, eds. *Grabb & Smith's Plastic Surgery.* 5th ed. Philadelphia, Pa: Lippincott-Raven; 1997:107-120.

Stal S, et al. Correction of secondary cleft lip deformities. *Plast Reconstr Surg.* 2002;109:1672-1681.

Stanton RA, et al. Skin resurfacing for the burned patient. *Clin Plast Surg.* 2002;29:29-51.

Stark HH, et al. Operative treatment of intra-articular fractures of the dorsal aspect of the distal phalanx of digits. *J Bone Joint Surg.* 1987;69A:892-896.

Stark WJ, et al. Current concepts in the surgical management of traumatic auricular hematoma. *J Oral Maxillofac Surg.* 1992;50:800-802.

Starkweather KD, et al. Collagenase in the treatment of Dupuytren's disease: an in vitro study. *J Hand Surg.* 1996;21A:490-495.

Steinmann SP, et al. Use of the 1,2 intercompartmental supraretinacular artery as a vascularized pedicle bone graft for difficult scaphoid union. *J Hand Surg.* 2002;27A:391-401.

Stern PJ, et al. Evaluation, staging, and principles of tumor surgery. In: Peimer CA, ed. *Surgery of the Hand and Upper Extremity.* New York, NY: McGraw-Hill, Inc;1996;2:2221-2263.

Stern PJ. Fractures of the metacarpals and phalanges. In: Green DP, Hotchkiss RN, Pederson WC, eds. *Operative Hand Surgery.* 4th ed. New York, NY: Churchill Livingstone, Inc; 1999;1:711-771.

Stevens DL. Invasive streptococcal infections. *J Infect Chemother.* 2001;7:69-80.

Stoelinga P. Orthognathic surgery: maxilla, Le Fort I, II, and III. In: Langdon J, Patel M, eds. *Operative Maxillary Facial Surgery.* New York, NY: Chapman and Hall Medical; 1998:447-461.

Stokes RB, et al. Arterial vascular anatomy of the umbilicus. *Plast Reconstr Surg.* 1998;102:761-764.

Stratoudakis AC. Craniofacial anomalies and principles of their correction. In: Georgiade GS, Riefkohl R, Levin LS, eds. *Textbook of Plastic, Maxillofacial and Reconstructive Surgery.* 3rd ed. Baltimore, Md: Williams & Wilkins; 1992:273-296.

Stratoudakis AC. Principles of bone transplantation. In: Georgiade GS, Riefkohl R, Levin LS, eds. *Textbook of Plastic, Maxillofacial and Reconstructive Surgery.* 3rd ed. Baltimore, Md: Williams & Wilkins; 1992:39-46.

Strauch B, Vasconez LO, Hall-Findlay EJ, eds. *Grabb's Encyclopedia of Flaps.* 2nd ed. Philadelphia, Pa: Lippincott-Raven; 1998.

Strauch B, Yu HL, eds. *Atlas of Microvascular Surgery: Anatomy and Operative Approaches.* New York, NY: Thieme Medical Publishers, Inc; 1993.

Strauch B. User of nerve conduits in peripheral nerve repair. *Hand Clin.* 2000;16:123-130.

Strickland JW, et al. Anatomy and pathogenesis of the digital cords and nodules. *Hand Clin.* 1991;7:645-671.

Strickland JW. Flexor tendons - acute injuries. In: Green DP, Hotchkiss RN, Pederson WC, eds. *Operative Hand Surgery.* 4th ed. New York, NY: Churchill Livingstone, Inc; 1999;2:1851-1897.

Stromberg BV, et al. Anisocoria following reduction of bilateral orbital wall fractures. *Ann Plast Surg.* 1988;2:486-488.

Struewing JP, et al. The risk of cancer associated with specific mutations of BRCA1 and BRCA2 among Ashkenazi Jews. *N Engl J Med.* 1997;336:1401-1408.

Stuzin GM. Anatomy of the frontal branch of the facial nerve: the significance of the temporal fat pad. *Plast Reconstr Surg.* 1989;83:265.

Stuzin JM, et al. Reoperative rhytidectomy. In: Grotting JC, ed. *Reoperative Aesthetic & Reconstructive Surgery*. Saint Louis, Mo: Quality Medical Publishing, Inc; 1995;205-244.

Stuzin JM. Phenol peeling and the history of phenol peeling. *Clin Plast Surg*. 1998;25:1-19.

Su CW, et al. Frostbite of the upper extremity. *Hand Clin*. 2000;16:235-247.

Suen JY, et al. Cancer of the neck. In: Myers EN, Suen JY, eds. *Cancer of the Head and Neck*. Philadelphia, Pa: WB Saunders Co; 1996:462-484.

Sugino H. Surgical correction of Stahl's ear using the cartilage turnover and rotation method. *Plast Reconstr Surg*. 1989;83:160.

Sunderland S. *Nerve and Nerve Injuries*. Baltimore, Md: Williams & Wilkins; 1968:758-762.

Suzuki H. Treatment of traumatic tattoos with the Q-switched neodymium:YAG laser. *Arch Dermatol*. 1996;132:1226-1229.

Swanson AB, et al. Evaluation and treatment of the upper extremity in the stroke patient. *Hand Clin*. 1989;5:75.

Swartz WM, et al. Distally based vastus lateralis muscle flap for coverage of wounds about the knee. *Plast Reconstr Surg*. 1987;80:255.

Swartz WM, et al. The osteocutaneous scapular flap for mandibular and maxillary reconstruction. *Plast Reconstr Surg*. 1986;77:530.

Szabo RM, et al. Acute carpal fractures and dislocations. In: Peimer CA, ed. *Surgery of the Hand and Upper Extremity*. New York, NY: McGraw-Hill, Inc; 1996:711-726.

Szabo RM. Entrapment and compression injuries. In: Green DP, Hotchkiss RN, Pederson WC, eds. *Operative Hand Surgery*. 4th ed. New York, NY: Churchill Livingstone, Inc; 1999;2:1404-1447.

Tang CL, et al. A follow-up study of 105 women with breast cancer following reduction mammaplasty. *Plast Reconstr Surg*. 1999;103:1687-1690.

Tang CL, et al. Breast cancer found at the time of breast reduction. *Plast Reconstr Surg*. 1999:103:1682-1686.

Tang L, et al. Fibrin(ogen) mediates acute inflammatory responses to biomaterials. *J Exp Med*. 1993;178:2147-2156.

Tang L, et al. Natural responses to unnatural materials: a molecular mechanism for foreign body reactions. *Molec Med*. 1999;5:351-358.

Tanzer R. The constricted ear. *Plast Reconstr Surg*. 1975;55:406.

Tanzer RC. Microtia: a long-term follow-up of 44 reconstructed auricles. *Plast Reconstr Surg*. 1978;61:161.

Tardy ME Jr, et al. The over projecting nose: anatomic component analysis and repair. *Facial Plast Surg*. 1993;9:275.

Tardy ME Jr, et al. Transdromal suture refinement of the nasal tip: long-term outcomes. *Facial Plast Surg*. 1993;9:275.

Taylor CR. Laser ignition of traumatically embedded firework debris. *Lasers Surg Med*. 1998;22:157-158.

Taylor RS, et al. Distal venous arterialisation for salvage of critically ischaemic inoperable limb. *Lancet*. 1999;354:1962-1965.

Tebbetts JB. Blepharoplasty: a refined technique emphasizing accuraccy and control. *Clin Plast Surg*. 1992;19:329-349.

Teimourian B, et al. Rejuvination of the upper arm. *Plast Reconstr Surg*. 1998;102:545-553.

Teimourian B. Blindness following fat injections (letter). Plast Reconstr Surg. 1988;82:361.

Tellioglu AT, et al. Temporoparietal fascia: an anatomic and histologic reinvestigation with new potential clinical applications. *Plast Reconstr Surg*. 2000;105:40-45.

Terino EO. Alloplastic facial contouring by zonal principles of skeletal anatomy. *Clin Plast Surg*. 1992;19:487-510.

Tessier P. Anatomical classification of facial, craniofacial and latero-facial clefts. *J Maxillofac Surg*. 1969;4:69.

Thomas JM. Premalignant and malignant epithelial tumors. In: Sams WM Jr, Lynch PJ, eds. *Principles and Practice of Dermatology*. New York, NY: Churchill Livingstone, Inc; 1996:225-239.

Thomas WO, et al. Congenital cutis laxa: a case report and review of loose skin syndromes. *Ann Plast Surg*. 1993;30:252.

Thompson H. Cutaneous hemangiomas and lymphangiomas. *Clin Plast Surg*. 1987;13:341-356.

Thomson HG, et al. Microtia reconstruction: does the cartilage framework grow? *Plast Reconstr Surg*. 1989;84:908.

Thorne CH, et al. Aesthetic Surgery of the aging face. In: Aston SJ, Beasley RW, Thorne CH, eds. *Grabb & Smith's Plastic Surgery*. 5th ed. Philadelphia, Pa: Lippincott-Raven; 1997:633-649.

Thorne CH, et al. Aesthetic Surgery of the face. In: Aston SJ, Beasley RW, Thorne CH, eds. *Grabb & Smith's Plastic Surgery*. 5th ed. Philadelphia, Pa: Lippincott-Raven; 1997:617.

Thorne CH, et al. Reconstructive surgery of the lower extremity. In: McCarthy JG, ed. *Plastic Surgery*. Philadelphia, Pa: WB Saunders Co; 1990;6:4029-4092.

Titus-Ernstoff L. An overview of the epidemiology of cutaneous melanoma. *Clin Plast Surg*. 2000;27:305-316.

Tobin HA, et al. Lip augmentation using an alloderm graft. *J Oral Maxillofac Surg*. 1998;56:722-727.

Tomaino MM, et al. Arthroplasty. In: Herndon JH, ed. *Surgical Reconstruction of the Upper Extremity*. Stamfod, Conn: Appleton & Lange; 1999:963-995.

Tomaino MM. Treatment of Eaton stage I trapeziometacarpal disease: ligament reconstruction or thumb metacarpal extension osteotomy? *Hand Clin*. 2001;17:197-205.

Tortora GJ, Grabowski SR, eds. The special senses. In: Tortora GJ, Grabowski SR, eds. *Principles of Anatomy and Physiology*. 9th ed. New York, NY: John Wiley & Sons, Inc; 2000:512-529.

Tran N, et al. Comparison of immediate and delayed free TRAM flap breast reconstruction in patients receiving postmastectomy radiation therapy. *Plast Reconstr Surg*. 2001;108:78-82.

Trent JT, et al. Diagnosing necrotizing fasciitis. *Adv Skin Wound Care*. 2002;15:135-138.

Troilius AM. Effective treatment of traumatic tattoos with a Q-switched Nd:YAG laser. *Lasers Surg Med*. 1998;22:103-108.

Trott SA, et al. Safety considerations and fluid resuscitation in liposuction: an analysis of 53 consecutive patients. *Plast Reconstr Surg*. 1998;102:2220-2229.

Trumble TE, et al. Repair of peripheral nerve defects in the upper extremity. *Hand Clin*. 2000;16:37-52.

Truppman ES, et al. Major electrocardiographic changes during chemical face peeling. *Plast Reconstr Surg*. 1979;63:44.

Tsuge K. Management of established Volkmann's contracture. In: Green DP, Hotchkiss RN, Pederson WC, eds. *Operative Hand Surgery*. 4th ed. New York, NY: Churchill Livingstone, Inc; 1999;1:591-603.

Tsuge K. Tendon transfers for radial nerve palsy. *Amer NZ J Surg*. 1980;50:767.

Tubiana R, Gilbert A, Masquelet AC, eds. *An Atlas of Surgical Techniques of the Hand and Wrist*. Baltimore, Md: Williams & Wilkins; 1999:38-39.

Tuerk M. Medications that cause gynecomastia. *Plast Reconstr Surg*. 1993;92:1411.

Tung TC. Endoscopic shaver with liposuction for treatment of axillary osmidrosis. *Ann Plast Surg*. 2001;46:400-404.

Turpin IM. Microsurgical replantation of the external ear. *Clin Plast Surg*. 1990;17:397.

Uebel CO. Micrografts and minigrafts: a new approach for baldness surgery. *Ann Plast Surg*. 1991;27:246.

Ueda K, et al. Keloids have continuous high metabolic activity. *Plast Reconstr Surg*. 1999;104:694-698.

Upton J, et al. Congenital anomalies: shoulder region. In: Peimer CA, ed. *Surgery of the Hand and Upper Extremity*. New York, NY: McGraw-Hill, Inc; 1996;3:2001-2048.

Upton J, et al. Vascular malformations of the upper limb: a review of 270 patients. *J Hand Surg*. 1999;24A:1019-1035.

Upton J. Congenital anomalies of the hand and forearm. In: McCarthy JG, ed. *Plastic Surgery*. Philadelphia, Pa: WB Saunders Co; 1990;8:5213-5398.

Upton J. Congenital anomalies of the hand. In: Cohen M, ed. *Mastery of Plastic and Reconstructive Surgery*. Boston, Mass: Little, Brown & Co; 1994;3:1424-1453.

Urban MA, et al. Management of radial dysplasia. *Hand Clin*. 1990;6:589-605.

Urken ML, et al. Lateral thigh. In: Urken ML, Cheney ML, Sullivan MJ, eds. *Atlas of Regional and Free Flaps for Head and Neck Reconstruction*. New York, NY: Raven Press; 1995:169-182.

Vallis CP. Hair replacement surgery. In: McCarthy JG, ed. *Plastic Surgery*. Philadelphia, Pa: WB Saunders Co; 1990;2:1514-1537.

Van Adrichem LN, et al. The effect of cigarette smoking on the survival of free vascularized and pedicled epigastric flaps in the rat. *Plast Reconstr Surg*. 1996;97:86.

van der Velden EM, et al. Tattoo removal: tannic acid method of variot. *Int J Dermatol*. 1993;32:276-180.

Van Hoest AE, et al. Upper extremity surgical treatment of cerebral palsy. *J Hand Surg*. 1999;24:323-330.

Van Hoest AE. Congenital disorders of the hand and upper extremity. *Pediatr Clin North Am*. 1996;43:1123.

Van Uchelen J, et al. Complications of abdominoplasty in 86 patients. *Plast Reconstr Surg*. 2001;107:1869-1873.

VanderKolk CA. Craniofacial surgery. *Clin Plast Surg*. 1994;21:481-631.

Verpaele AM, et al. The superior gluteal artery perforator flap: an additional tool in the treatment of sacral pressure sores. *Br J Plast Surg*. 1999;52:385.

Verwoerd CD. Present day treatment of nasal fractures: closed versus open reduction. *Facial Plast Surg*. 1992;8:220.

Villafane, et al. Endoscopic transaxillary subglandular breast augmentation using silicone gel textured implants. *Aesthetic Plast Surg*. 2000;24:212-215.

Vlachos CC. Orthodontic treatment for the cleft palate patient. *Semin Orthod*. 1996;2:197-204.

Von Heimburg HD, et al. The tuberous breast deformity: classification and treatment. *Br J Plast Surg*. 1996;49:339-345.

Wagner JD, et al. Salivary gland disorders. In: Achauer BM, Eriksson E, Guyuron B, et al, eds. *Plastic Surgery: Indications, Operations, and Outcomes*. Saint Louis, Mo: Mosby - Year Book, Inc; 2000;3:1355-1395.

Wallace JF. Disorders caused by venoms, bites, and stings. In: Isselbacher KJ, Braunwald E, Wilson JD, et al, eds. *Harrison's Principles of Internal Medicine*. 13th ed. New York, NY: McGraw-Hill, Inc; 1994;2:2467-2473.

Walton RL, et al. Pedicled flaps and grafts. In: Achauer BM, Eriksson E, Guyuron B, et al, eds. *Plastic Surgery: Indications, Operations, and Outcomes*. Saint Louis, Mo: Mosby - Year Book, Inc; 2000;4:1793-1817.

Wang KC, et al. Irreducible volar rotary dislocation of the proximal interphalangeal joint. *Orthop Rev*. 1994;23:886-888.

Warpeha RL. Resurfacing of the burned face. *Clin Plast Surg*. 1981;8:255.

Warso M, et al. Melanoma of the hand. *J Hand Surg*. 1997;22A:354-360.

Warwick R, Williams P, eds. *Gray's Anatomy*. Philadelphia, Pa: WB Saunders Co; 1993:1050.

Watson HK, et al. Pathologic anatomy. *Hand Clin*. 1991;7:661-668.

Watson JD. Hidradenitis suppurativa: a clinical review. *Br J Plast Surg*. 1985;38:567.

Watson KH, et al. Intercarpal arthrodesis. In: Green DP, Hotchkiss RN, Pederson WC, eds. *Operative Hand Surgery*. 4th ed. New York, NY: Churchill Livingstone, Inc; 1999;1:122-216.

Watson KH, et al. Stiff joints. In: Green DP, Hotchkiss RN, Pederson WC, eds. *Operative Hand Surgery*. 4th ed. New York, NY: Churchill Livingstone, Inc; 1999;1:552-561.

Watson S. The principles of management of congenital anomalies of the upper limb. *Arch Dis Child*. 2000;83:10-17.

Watson WL, et al. Blood vessel and lymph vessel tumors: a report of 1056 cases. *Surg Gynecol Obstet*. 1940;71:569.

Weber ER, et al. Chronic wrist instability. In: Peimer CA, ed. *Surgery of the Hand and Upper Extremity*. New York, NY: McGraw-Hill, Inc; 1996:727-758.

Weber RA, et al. A randomized prospective study of polyglycolic acid conduits for digital nerve reconstructions in humans. *Plast Reconstr Surg*. 2000;106:1036-1045.

Weber RS, et al. Clinical assessment and staging. In: Weber RS, Miller MJ, Goepfert H, eds. *Basal and Squamous Cell Skin Cancers of the Head and Neck*. Baltimore, Md: Williams & Wilkins; 1996:65-77.

Weber RS, et al. Surgical principles. In: Weber RS, Miller MJ, Goepfert H, eds. *Basal and Squamous Cell Skin Cancers of the Head and Neck*. Baltimore, Md: Williams & Wilkins; 1996:115-132.

Weedon D. The granulomatous reaction pattern. In: Weedon D, ed. *Skin Pathology*. 2nd ed. London, England: Churchill Livingstone; 2002:193-209.

Wei W, et al. Free split and segmental latissimus dorsi transfer in one stage for facial reanimation. *Plast Reconstr Surg*. 1999;103:473-482.

Weiland AJ, et al. Vascularized bone transfers. In: Yaremchuk MJ, Burgess AR, Brumback RJ, eds. *Lower Extremity Salvage and Reconstruction: Orthopedic and Plastic Surgical Management*. Stamfod, Conn: Appleton & Lange; 1989.

Weinstein C, et al. Aesthetic skin resurfacing with the high-energy ultrapulsed CO_2 laser. *Clin Plast Surg*. 1997;24:379-405.

Weinstein C, et al. Simultaneously combined Er:YAG and carbon dioxide laser (derma K) for skin resurfacing. *Clin Plast Surg*. 2000;27:273-285.

Weinstein C. Erbium laser resurfacing: current concepts. *Plast Reconstr Surg*. 1999;103:602.

Weisberg NK, et al. Repair of nasal ala defects with conchal bowl composite grafts. *Dermatol Surg*. 2000;26:1047-1051.

Weiss JS, et al. Topical tretinoin improves photoaged skin: a double-blind vehicle-controlled study. *JAMA*. 1988;259:527.

Wellisz T. Reconstruction of the burned external ear using a Medpor porous polyethylene pivoting helix framework. *Plast Reconstr Surg*. 1993;91:811.

Wells MD, et al. Surgical management of facial palsy. *Clin Plast Surg*. 1990;17:645.

Wesley RE, et al. Superior oblique paresis after blepharoplasty. *Plast Reconstr Surg*. 1980;66:283.

West BR, et al. Ultrasound debridement of trabeculated bome: effective and atraumatic. *Plast Reconstr Surg*. 1994;93:561-566.

Westesson P. Magnetic resonance imaging of the temporomandibular joint. *Oral Maxillofac Surg Clin North Am*. 1992;4:183-206.

Westfall CT, et al. Operative complications of the transconjunctival inferior fornix approach. *Ophthalmology*. 1991;98:1525-1528.

Wexler A, et al. Conservative treatment of cutis aplasia. *Plast Reconstr Surg.* 1990;86:1066.

Wexler A. Anatomy of the head and neck. In: Ferraro JW, ed. *Fundamentals in Maxillofacial Surgey.* New York, NY: Springer-Verlag; 1997:53-113.

Wheatley MJ, et al. The use of intra-arterial urokinase in the management of hand ischaemia secondary to palmar and digital arterial occlusion. *Ann Plast Surg.* 1996;37:356.

Wheeler DR. Reconstruction for radial nerve palsy. In: Peimer CA, ed. *Surgery of the Hand and Upper Extremity.* New York, NY: McGraw-Hill, Inc; 1996:1363-1379.

White B, et al. The use of carbon dioxide laser in head and neck injuries. *Laser Surg Med.* 1986;6:293.

White CW, et al. Treatment of childhood angiomatous diseases with recombinant interferon alfa-2a. *J Pediatr.* 1991;118:59-66.

Wider TM, et al. Simultaneous osseous genioplasty and meloplasty. *Plast Reconstr Surg.* 1997;99:1273-1287.

Wiedrich TA. Congenital constriction band syndrome. *Hand Clin.* 1998;14:29-37.

Wieland U, et al. Erythoplasia of Queyrat: coinfection with cutaneous carcinogenic human papillomavirus type 8 and genital papillomaviruses in a carcinoma in situ. *J Invest Dermatol.* 2000;115:396-401.

Wilgis EF. Evaluation and treatment of chronic digital ischemia. *Ann Surg.* 1981;193:693-696.

Wilhelmi BJ, et al. Upper blepharoplasty with bony anatomical landmarks to avoid injury to trochlea and superior oblique muscle tendon with fat resection. *Plast Reconstr Surg.* 2001;108:2137-2140.

Williams CN Jr, et al. Fingernail and fingertip injuries. In: Cohen M, ed. *Mastery of Plastic and Reconstructive Surgery.* Boston, Mass: Little, Brown & Co; 1994;3:1493-1507.

Williams CW. Silicone gel granuloma following compressive mammography. *Aesthet Plast Surg.* 1991;15:49.

Williams HB. Vascular neoplasms. *Clin Plast Surg.* 1980-;7:397-411.

Williams JK, et al. Nonsyndromic craniosynostosis. In: Achauer BM, Eriksson E, Guyuron B, et al, eds. *Plastic Surgery: Indications, Operations, and Outcomes.* Saint Louis, Mo: Mosby Year - Book, Inc. 2000;2:683-706.

Williams PL, Warwick R, Dyson M, et al, eds. *Gray's Anatomy.* 37th ed. Edinburgh, Scotland: Churchill Livinstone, Inc; 1989:337-367, 570-575,1098-1107, 1564.

Williams WG, et al. Pathophysiology of the burn wound. In: Herndon DN, ed. *Total Burn Care.* Philadelphia, Pa: WB Saunders Co; 1996:63-67.

Wilson BC, et al. Comparison of complications following frontal sinus fractures managed with exploration with or without obliteration over 10 years. *Laryngoscope.* 1988;98:516.

Wilson M, et al. Complications of upper blepharoplasty. In: Putterman A, ed. *Cosmetic Oculoplastic Surgery.* Philadelphia, Pa: WB Saunders Co; 1993:342.

Wilson MR, et al. Poland's syndrome: variable expression and associated anomalies. *J Hand Surg.* 1988;13A:880-882.

Wind GG, et al. *Anatomic Exposures in Vascular Surgery.* Baltimore, Md: Williams & Wilkins; 1991.

Wisnicki JL. Hemangiomas and vascular malformations. *Ann Plast Surg.* 1984;12:41.

Witt PD. Velopharyngeal insufficiency. In: Achauer BM, Eriksson E, Guyuron B, et al, eds. *Plastic Surgery: Indications, Operations, and Outcomes.* Saint Louis, Mo: Mosby Year - Book, Inc. 2000;2:819-933.

Wolfe SA, et al. Avoidance of lower-lid contraction in surgical approaches to the inferior orbit. *Operative Techniques Plast Reconstr Surg.* 1998;5:201-212.

Wolfe SA, et al. *Facial Fractures.* New York, NY: Thieme Medical Publishers, Inc; 1993;41-61.

Wolfe SA, et al. Frontal sinus injuries: primary care and management of late complications. *Plast Reconstr Surg*. 1988;82:781-791.

Wolfe SA, et al. Surgery of the jaws. In: Aston SJ, Beasley RW, Thorne CH, eds. *Grabb & Smith's Plastic Surgery*. 5th ed. Philadelphia, Pa: Lippincott-Raven; 1997:321-333.

Wolfe SW, et al. Metacarpal and carpometacarpal trauma. In: Peimer CA, ed. *Surgery of the Hand and Upper Extremity*. New York NY: McGraw-Hill, Inc; 1996;1:883.

Wolfe SW. Tenosynovitis. In: Green DP, Hotchkiss RN, Pederson WC, eds. *Operative Hand Surgery*. 4th ed. New York, NY: Churchill Livingstone, Inc; 1999;2:2022-2044.

Wolford LM, et al. Surgical Planning. In: Booth PW, Schendel SA, Hausamen JE, eds. *Maxillofacial Surgery*. London, England: Churchill Livingstone, Inc; 1999;2:1205-1257.

Wolfort FG, et al. Pearls and pitfalls: how to avoid and manage complications. In: Wolfort FG, Kanter WR, eds. *Aesthetic Blepharoplasty*. Boston, Mass: Little, Brown & Co; 1995;189-218.

Wolfort FG, et al. Retrobulbar hematoma and blepharoplasty. *Plast Reconstr Surg*. 1999;104:2154.

Wolfort FG, et al. Suction-assisted lipectomy for lipodystrophy syndromes attributed to HIV-protease inhibitor use. *Plast Reconstr Surg*. 1999;104:1814-1820.

Wong RJ, et al. Cancer of the nasal cavity in the paranasal sinuses. In: Shah JP, ed. *Cancer of the Head and Neck*. Hamilton, Ontario: BC Decker Inc; 2001.

Wray CR. Fractures and joint injuries of the hand. In: McCarthy JG, ed. *Plastic Surgery*. Philadelphia, Pa: WB Saunders Co; 1990;7:4617-4627.

Wray RD, et al. A comparison of conjunctival and subciliary incisions for orbital fractures. *Br J Plast Surg*. 1977;30:142-145.

Wright SW, et al. Clinical presentation and outcome of brown recluse spider bite. *Ann Emerg Med*. 1997;30:28-32.

Wright T. Anatomy and development of the ear and hearing. In: Ludman H, Wright T, eds. *Diseases of the Ear*. 6th ed. London, England: Arnold; 1998:8-13.

Wrobel JS, et al. Making the diagnosis of osteomyelitis: the role of prevalence. *J Am Podiatr Med Assoc*. 1998;88:337-343.

Wuring E. Refinement of central pedicle reconstruction by application of the ligamentous suspension. *Plast Reconstr Surg*. 1999;103:1400-1409.

Wyrick JD, et al. Secondary nerve reconstruction. *Hand Clin*. 1992;8:587-598.

Yaghoubian R, et al. Diagnosis and management of acute fracture-dislocations of the carpus. *Ortho Clin North Am*. 2001;32:295-305.

Yajima H, et al. Osteocutaneous radial forearm flap for hand reconstruction. *J Hand Surg*. 1999;24A:594.

Yamaguchi Y, et al. Effect of burn injury on glucose and nitrogen metabolism in the liver: preliminary studies in a perfused liver system. *Surgery*. 1997;121:295.

Yaremchuk MJ, et al. Soft tissue alterations associated with acute extended open reduction and internal fixation of orbital fractures. *J Craniofac Surg*. 1992;3:134-140.

Yaremchul MJ. Fractures of the maxilla. In: Cohen M, ed. *Mastery of Plastic and Reconstructive Surgery*. Boston, Mass: Little, Brown & Co; 1994:1156-1165.

Yin HQ, et al. Comparative evaluation of antimicrobial activity of Acticoat antimicrobial barrier dressing. *J Burn Care Rehab*. 1999;20:195-200.

Yotsuyanagi T, et al. Nonsurgical treatment of various auricular deformities. *Clin Plast Surg*. 2002;29:327-332.

Young AE. Venous and arterial malformations. In: Mulliken JB, Young AE, eds. *Vascular birthmarks: Hemangiomas and malformations*. Philadelphia, Pa: WB Saunders Co; 1988;196-214.

Yu GY, et al. Carcinoma of the salivary gland: a clinicopathologic study of 405 cases. *Semin Surg Oncol*. 1987;3:240-244.

Zaias N, ed. *The Nail in Health and Disease*. 2nd ed. Stamford, Conn: Appleton & Lange; 1990:67-85.

Zampino G, et al. Opitz C trigonocephaly syndrome and midline brain anomalies. *Amer J Med Genet*. 1997;73:484-488.

Zancolli E, ed. *Structural and Dynamic Bases of Hand Surgery*. 2nd ed. Philadelphia, Pa: JB Lippincott Co; 1979;19-20.

Zancolli E. Surgery for the quadriplegic hand with active, strong wrist extension preserved: a study of 97 cases. *Clin Orthop*. 1975;112:101-113.

Zarem HA, et al. Benign growths and generalized skin disorders. In: Aston SJ, Beasley RW, Thorne CH, eds. *Grabb & Smith's Plastic Surgery*. 5th ed. Philadelphia, Pa: Lippincott-Raven; 1997:141-159.

Zawacki BE. The natural history of reverible burn injury. *Surg Gynecol Obstet*. 1974;139:867.

Zempsky WT, et al. EMLA versus TAC for topical anesthesia of extremity wounds in children. *Ann Emerg Med*. 1997;30:163-166.

Zhang B, et al. Dextran's antithrombotic properties in small arteries are not altered by low-molecular-weight heparin or the fibrinolytic inhibitor tranexamic acid: an experimental study. *Microsurg*. 1993;14:289

Zide B, et al. Cephalometric analysis for upper and lower midface surgery: part II. *Plast Reconstr Surg*. 1981;68:961.

Zide B, et al. Cephalometric analysis: part I. *Plast Reconstr Surg*. 1981;68:816.

Zide BM, et al. Chin surgery I: augmentation--the allures and the alerts. *Plast Reconstr Surg*. 1999;104:1843-1862.

Zide BM, et al. Chin surgery II: submental ostectomy and soft-tissue excision. *Plast Reconstr Surg*. 1999;104:1854-1860.

Zide BM, et al. Chin surgery III: revelations. *Plast Reconstr Surg*. 2003;111:1542-1550.

Zide BM, et al. How to block and tackle the face. *Plast Reconstr Surg*. 1998;101:840-851

Zide BM, et al. *Surgical Anatomy of the Orbit*. New York, NY: Raven Press; 1985.

Zide BM. Nasal anatomy: the muscles and tip sensation. *Aesthetic Plast Surg*. 1985;9:193.

Zide BM. The temporomandibular joint. In: McCarthy JG, ed. *Plastic Surgery*. Philadelphia, Pa: WB Saunders Co; 1990;2:1475-1513.

Zide MF, et al. Indications for open reduction of mandibular condyle fractures. *J Oral Maxillofac Surg*. 1983;41:89-98.

Zook EG, et al. A study of nail bed injuries: causes, treatment, and prognosis. *J Hand Surg*. 1984;9A:247-252.

Zook EG, et al. Anatomy and physiology of the perionychium: a review of the literature and anatomic study. *J Hand Surg*. 1980;5:528-536.

Zook EG, et al. The perionychium. In: Green DP, Hotchkiss RN, Pederson WC, eds. *Operative Hand Surgery*. 4th ed. New York, NY: Churchill Livingstone, Inc; 1999;1:1353-1380.

Zook EG. Anatomy and physiology of the perionychium. *Hand Clin*. 2002;18:553-559.

Zook EG. Surgically treatable problems of the perionychium. In: McCarthy JG, ed. *Plastic Surgery*. Philadelphia, Pa: WB Saunders, Co; 1990;8:4499-4515.